Sixth Edition

T0195350

Ross-Kerr and Wood's
CANADIAN NURSING
ISSUES & PERSPECTIVES

Lynn McCleary, RN, BScN, MSc, PhD
Professor
Graduate Program Director, Master of Applied Gerontology Program
Department of Nursing
Faculty of Applied Health Sciences
Brock University
St. Catharines, ON

Tammie R. McParland, RN, BScN, MN, PhD
Assistant Professor
School of Nursing
Faculty of Education and Professional Studies
Nipissing University
North Bay, ON

ELSEVIER

ROSS-KERR AND WOOD'S CANADIAN NURSING:
ISSUES & PERSPECTIVES, SIXTH EDITION

ISBN: 978-0-323-68336-4

Notice

Practitioners and researchers must always rely on their own experience and knowledge in evaluating and using any information, methods, compounds, or experiments described herein. Because of rapid advances in the medical sciences in particular, independent verification of diagnoses and drug dosages should be made. To the fullest extent of the law, no responsibility is assumed by Elsevier, authors, editors, or contributors for any injury and/or damage to persons or property as a matter of products liability, negligence, or otherwise, or from any use or operation of any methods, products, instructions, or ideas contained in the material herein.

Library of Congress Control Number: 2020941976

VP Education Content: Kevonne Holloway
Content Strategist, Canada Acquisitions: Roberta A. Spinosa-Millman
Director, Content Development: Laurie Gower
Content Development Specialist: Sandy Matos
Publishing Services Manager: Deepthi Unni
Project Manager: Manchu Mohan
Copy Editor: Micheila Storr
Design Direction: Ryan Cook

Last digit is the print number: 9 8 7 6 5 4 3 2 1

Working together
to grow libraries in
developing countries

www.elsevier.com • www.bookaid.org

We dedicate this book to our mothers,
Rosemary McCleary, a nurse, and Rita May Hall,
a social worker, two women who inspire us every day
to embody nursing, service to the public,
and lifelong learning. We also dedicate this book to
nurses everywhere. We have been and continue to
be inspired by our teachers, our colleagues, and our
students—the future generation of nurses—who will
continue to transform the nursing profession.

ACKNOWLEDGEMENTS

It is an honour to be entrusted with creating the new edition of this iconic account of issues in, and for, the nursing profession in Canada. Following in the footsteps of the amazing editors of and contributors to previous editions of the book was daunting and we want to thank the previous editors, contributors, and Elsevier for this opportunity.

We thank Roberta Spinosa-Millman and Laurie Gower at Elsevier for their faith in us and their support. We especially thank Sandy Matos, Content Developmental Specialist, who worked tirelessly to support us and the contributors to this book, keeping us on track, guiding us, and encouraging us. Sandy, we would be lost without you. Thank you also to our copy editor, Micheila Storr, for your work on this edition. We also acknowledge and thank those who reviewed the previous edition of the book, providing recommendations and ideas for the new edition, and those who reviewed this new edition, providing helpful criticism and suggestions for improvements. To say we learned so much through the process of creating this book would be an understatement.

We gratefully acknowledge the contributors of the various chapters in this book for their dedication to maintaining the high calibre of the content in each chapter they contributed. They are located across the country and represent all nursing domains: nursing research, clinical practice, nursing administration, and nursing education and practice areas. They took a lot of time and effort to honour the previous edition and its contributors, thoroughly update and revise their chapters, and meet the publication deadlines, some of them contributing more than one chapter. We sincerely appreciate the opportunities that editing this book provided us, as we had the good fortune to work with experts across Canada and meet several new colleagues.

Finally, we thank our family and friends for their unwavering support throughout the writing process and their understanding of the time we spent on this project.

Dr. McCleary is a Professor in the Department of Nursing and Graduate Program Director of the Master of Applied Gerontology Program in the Faculty of Applied Health Sciences at Brock University. She is a mental health and gerontological nurse who works with research teams and service providers on health and social care for older people and their families. Her research and practice emphasize improving dementia care services as well as improving gerontology and geriatrics education in the health professions. She is a past president of the Canadian Gerontological Nursing Association. She is coauthor of *Ebersole and Hess' Gerontological Nursing and Healthy Aging* (First and Second Canadian Editions) and co-editor of *Evidence-Informed Approaches for Managing Dementia Transitions: Riding the Waves.*

Dr. McParland is an Assistant Professor in the School of Nursing at Nipissing University. She has extensive nursing experience spanning several practices—rural, remote, medical-surgical, telepractice, labour and delivery, intensive and critical care, and education. She is a founding member of the Ontario Simulation Alliance and CANSim, which focuses on the use of all forms of simulation pedagogy in nursing education. She has served on the board of directors for the Registered Nurses' Association of Ontario as the education member-at-large. She has taught Issues and Trends in undergraduate nursing education for the past several years.

CONTRIBUTORS

Barbara Astle, RN, PhD
Associate Professor and Director
MSN Program
School of Nursing
Director
Centre for Equity & Global
    Engagement
Trinity Western University
Langley, BC

Cynthia Baker, RN, BA, MN, MPhil, PhD
Executive Director
Management
Canadian Association of Schools of
    Nursing
Ottawa, ON
Professor Emerita
Nursing
Queen's University
Kingston, ON

R. Lisa Bourque Bearskin, RN, BScN, MN, PhD
Associate Professor
School of Nursing
Thompson Rivers University
Kamloops, BC

Susan M. Duncan, BScN, MSN, PhD
Professor and Director
School of Nursing
University of Victoria
Victoria, BC

Joyce K. Engel, RN, BEd, MEd, PhD
Adjunct Professor
Department of Nursing
Brock University
St. Catharines, ON

Dr. John H.V. Gilbert, C.M., PhD, LLD, FCAHS
Professor Emeritus
Audiology & Speech Sciences
The University of British Columbia
Vancouver, BC
Senior Scholar
WHO Collaborating Centre on Health
    Workforce Planning & Research
Dalhousie University
Halifax, NS
Dr. TMA Pai Endowment Chair in
    Interprofessional Education &
    Practice
Manipal University
Manipal, Karnataka
India

Sharon M. Goodwin, RN, BScN, MN, DHA
Senior Vice President
Home & Community Care Quality and
    Operations
VON Canada
Ottawa, ON

Lyle G. Grant, RN, BComm, BSN, MSN, JD, PhD
Director, Acute Care Services
Saskatchewan Health Authority
Lloydminster, SK

Linda Haslam-Stroud, RN
Past President
Ontario Nurses' Association
Utterson, ON

Sonya L. Jakubec, RN, BHScN, MN, PhD
Professor
School of Nursing
Faculty of Health & Community Studies
Mount Royal University
Calgary, AB

Margaret Ann Kennedy, BScN, MN, PhD
President
Kennedy Health Informatics Inc.
Halifax, NS
Chief Nursing Informatics Officer
Centres of Excellence
Gevity Consulting Inc.
Halifax, NS

Dr. Kelly A. Lackie, BScN, MN, PhD, RN, CCSNE
Assistant Professor
School of Nursing
Faculty of Health Junior Scholar
WHO/PAHO Collaborating Centre
    on Health Workforce Planning &
    Research Centre for Transformative
    Nursing and Health Research
    (CTNHR)
Dalhousie University
Halifax, NS
Adjunct Professor
School of Education
Acadia University
Wolfville, NS

Amanda E. McEwen, RN, BSc, BScN, MSCN
Ancillary Academic Staff II -
    Experiential Learning Specialist
Faculty of Nursing
University of Windsor
Windsor, ON

Robert J. Meadus, BN, BVocEd, MSc(N), PhD, CPMHN(C)
Associate Professor
Faculty of Nursing
Memorial University
St. John's, NL

Noeman A. Mirza, BScN, PhD
Associate Professor
School of Nursing
Thompson Rivers University
Kamloops, BC

Ndolo Njie-Mokonya, BScN, MScN, PhD (C)
Nurse Educator
General Internal Medicine
The Ottawa Hospital
Ottawa, ON

Linda J. Patrick, RN, BScN, MA, MScN, PhD
Dean
Faculty of Nursing
University of Windsor
Windsor, ON

Pauline Paul, PhD, RN
Professor
Faculty of Nursing
University of Alberta
Edmonton, AB

Pammla Lusenga Petrucka, RN, PhD
Professor
College of Nursing
University of Saskatchewan
Regina, SK

Lynn Anne Rempel, BScN, MASc, PhD
Associate Professor
Department of Nursing
Brock University
St. Catharines, ON

Lori Schindel Martin, PhD, RN, GNC(C)
Professor
Daphne Cockwell School of Nursing
Ryerson University
Toronto, ON

Victoria Smye, RN, BA, MHSc, PhD
Associate Professor and Director
Arthur Labatt Family School of Nursing
Western University
London, ON

The authors would like to thank these additional experts for their contributions in the following chapters:

Chapter 10
Leanne M. Currie, RN, PhD
Associate Professor
School of Nursing
The University of British Columbia
Core Faculty, UBC Designing for
People (DFP) Initiative
Co-Director Research, Canadian
Nursing Informatics Association
Steering Committee, Centre for
Artificial Intelligence Decision-
Making and Action
Vancouver, BC

Tania Gayle Dick, RN, BScN, MN-NP
Elected Councillor
First Nations Health Council
Kwakwaka'wakw Region, BC

Kelly S. Davison, MN, MSc, RN, CPMHN(C), G.Cert-HTS, CTSS
Doctoral Student
School of Health Information Science
University of Victoria
Victoria, BC

Jacquelyn MacDonald, RN, BN, MN, CCHN(C)
Regional eHealth Nurse
eHealth Program
Health Assessment and Surveillance
Directorate
First Nations and Inuit Health Branch
Atlantic Region
Indigenous Services Canada
Halifax, NS

Chapter 19
Amber Alecxe, BAHons, MA, PhD(C)
Director of Government Relations
Saskatchewan Union of Nurses
Regina, SK

Dan Anderson, BComm
Director, Labour Relations/Chief
Negotiator (retired)
Ontario Nurses' Association
Toronto, ON

Doug Anderson
Assistant to the President
Ontario Nurses' Association
Toronto, ON

Melanie Benard, BCL/LLB
National Director of Policy and
Advocacy
Canadian Health Coalition
Ottawa, ON

Vanessa Bevilacqua
Conseillère syndicale, secteur
Sociopolitique
Fédération interprofessionnelle de la
santé du Québec
Papineau, QC

David Cournoyer, BA
Communications Advisor
United Nurses of Alberta
Edmonton, AB

Paul Curry, BA, MA, PhD
Researcher/Educator/Government
Relations Advisor/Health and Safety
Advisor
Nova Scotia Nurses' Union
Halifax, NS

Debbie Forward, RN, BN, MEd
President
Registered Nurses' Union
Newfoundland and Labrador
St. John's, NL

Janet Hazelton
President
Nova Scotia Nurses' Union
Halifax, NS

Cathryn Hoy, RN
First Vice President
Political Action & Professional Issues
Ontario Nurses' Association
Toronto, ON

Manitoba Nurses Union
Winnipeg, MB

Vicki McKenna, RN
President
Ontario Nurses' Association
Toronto, ON

Linda Silas, RN, BScN
President
Canadian Federation of Nurses Unions
Ottawa, ON

Heather Smith
President
United Nurses of Alberta
Edmonton, AB

Christine Sorensen, BScN, ICD.D
President
British Columbia Nurses' Union
Burnaby, BC

Jane Sustrik, RN
First Vice President
United Nurses of Alberta
Edmonton, AB

Pauline Worsfold, RN
Chair
Canadian Health Coalition
Secretary Treasurer
Canadian Federation of Nurses Unions
Ottawa, ON

Tracy M. Zambory, RN
President
Saskatchewan Union of Nurses
Regina, SK

REVIEWERS

June Anonson, RN, MEd,
Postsecondary Certificate, PhD
Professor (previous Assistant
    Dean)
College of Nursing
University of Saskatchewan
Saskatoon, SK

Catherine Aquino-Russell, RN,
MN, PhD
Professor
Faculty of Nursing
University of New Brunswick
Moncton, NB

Monique Bacher, RN, BScN,
MSN/Ed
Professor
Practical Nursing Program
Sally Horsfall Eaton School of
    Nursing
George Brown College
Toronto, ON

Lois Berry, RN, BN, MCEd, PhD
Professor
College of Nursing
University of Saskatchewan
Saskatoon, SK

Sandra MacDonald, RN, MN, PhD
Professor
School of Nursing
Memorial University of
    Newfoundland
St. John's, NL

Elaine Schow, RN, BScN, MN
Associate Professor
Bridge to Canadian Nursing
    Program
Mount Royal College
Calgary, AB

Lisa Seto Nielsen, RN, BScN,
MN, PhD
Associate Professor
School of Nursing
Faculty of Health
York University
Toronto, ON

Barb Shellian, RN, MN
Director Rural Health
Alberta Health Services Calgary
    Zone
Adjunct Professor
Faculty of Nursing
University of Calgary
Calgary, AB

At the time of the first edition of *Canadian Nursing: Issues & Perspectives*, there was no comprehensive written information that students could read to learn about a range of Canadian nursing issues. Since it is an impossible task for any instructor to present, by word of mouth, all the background on issues of concern to Canadian nurses, the idea emerged for developing a text to serve as a resource on a wide variety of issues. Janet Ross-Kerr and Jannetta MacPhail, co-authors of the first three editions, and Janet Ross-Kerr and Marilynn Wood, co-editors of the fourth and fifth editions, identified and evaluated developments in the profession and monitored progress over the first 22 years following publication of the first edition. Lynn McCleary and Tammie R. McParland, editors of the sixth edition, are carrying on this tradition, now 32 years on. Thirty-two years may seem like a long time, but it is short relative to the development of a profession. Twelve years ago, when the fifth edition was published, the editors noted that there had been steady and measurable progress, with continued challenges for nurses and the nursing profession. It is evident that progress continues. For some issues, it is a case of two steps forward, one step back, repeated.

This book attends to historical perspectives of issues in nursing, a valuable approach given the back-and-forth nature of progress in this profession. Having a long-term perspective and considering the history and broad context of issues makes it easier to see progress and recognize the lack of it. Some issues that had preoccupied nursing for years prior to the last edition seem to have been resolved. For example, baccalaureate education is the norm for entry into nursing practice in all provinces except Quebec. Other issues that seemed to be resolving at the time of the last edition have faced setbacks. Conversely, when the fifth edition was published, nursing research funding was plentiful. Currently, diminished funding for health research in Canada is having as much of an impact on nursing as it is on other health professions. Some issues that have emerged since the last edition were not anticipated when the previous edition was published, such as the move to licensing via an American-based exam. Some longstanding issues were suppressed and are only now beginning to be addressed, such as diversity within the nursing profession and the devastating repercussions of colonization.

Nurses continue to be held in high esteem by the public and remain at the forefront of innovating new ways to deliver the high-quality care Canadians deserve and expect. Health care is being shaped by policy and legislative changes, new directions, and new realities such as climate change. Nurses are at the forefront of change management and will continue to play a key role in navigating the new paths we will travel. The new directions and how to navigate them are discussed in this edition.

FEATURES OF THE SIXTH EDITION

Content in all chapters has been reworked and updated to reflect current developments in nursing and health care.

New student-friendly pedagogy has been introduced, including the following features:

- Updated and expanded art program with graphs, charts, and photos throughout;
- Learning objectives at the beginning of each chapter to help students identify key content;
- New Personal Perspectives boxes in each chapter that present relevant topics and real-world situations to introduce the chapter;
- Bolded key terms identifying important terms in each chapter and a new glossary at the end of the book;
- Updated Research Focus boxes that highlight current and relevant research in content areas specific to each chapter;
- New Case Study boxes that introduce new theories and clinical practice;
- New Gender Considerations and Cultural Considerations boxes as they relate to the LGBTQ2 community, race and ethnicity, and Indigenous peoples are threaded throughout all applicable chapters;
- Every chapter includes Applying Content Knowledge boxes that provide focused opportunities for reflection and discussion about the chapter's content;
- Balanced national coverage from coast to coast, including updated Canadian Nurses Association's *Code of Ethics* and updated Canadian Association of Schools of Nursing Standards; and
- Critical Thinking Questions at the end of each chapter to help students apply learning to practice. Answers are available on the Evolve website.

CHAPTER UPDATES

Chapter 1: The Canadian Health Care System

Update on current trends and challenges for the Canadian health care system, such as rapid health system reforms, increasing expenditures, population diversification, evolving health care workforce, and situating Canada's health leadership within the global context. Recognizes and highlights inclusiveness and participation, embedding the Truth and Reconciliation Commission of Canada's Calls to Action and the United Nations Sustainable Development Goals.

Chapter 2: Nursing in Canada, 1600s to the Present: A Brief Account

Chapter structure maintained, with updated content reflecting new historical developments. New content was added concerning Indigenous women healers and nurses in southern Alberta between 1880 and 1930, the Canadian Indigenous Nurses Association, and recent history about nurses in the Canadian Armed Forces.

Chapter 3: Professionalization in Canadian Nursing

Updated with a new focus on contemporary legislation for the regulation of registered nurses in each province and territory. Discussion of the evolution of the profession and its current status includes reference to the role of Indigenous nurses in Canada, differentiation of concepts such as vocation and profession, and the role of program approval and accreditation in Canada.

Chapter 4: The Professional Image: Impact and Strategies for Change

Substantially revised to reflect contemporary contexts that impact upon image as understood by nurses, nursing students, and the public. The chapter explores relevant concepts such as health and policy advocacy, role diversity, nursing entrepreneurship, as well as professional image branding and self-marketing across interprofessional and global networks.

Chapter 5: Gender in Nursing

New chapter expands upon and updates content in previous editions. Thorough update of issues of gender diversity in the nursing workforce and among patient populations. A strong emphasis on men in nursing and on nursing responses to health and health care barriers experienced by members of the LGBTQ2 community. Framed within an understanding of feminism and the relationship between feminism and nursing.

Chapter 6: Theoretical Issues in Nursing in the Twenty-First Century: Nursing Theorizing as Everyday Practice

Substantially revised and updated with a central focus on theorizing in everyday practice in the context of nursing's epistemology and ontology as well as the current Canadian health care context, including the use of big data and information technologies, regulation, competency-based education, the market economy, evidence-informed practice, and decolonization.

Chapter 7: Thinking Philosophically in Nursing

Revision focused on helping readers understand the requirement to think philosophically in nursing practice in addition to the need for evidence-informed decision making. More in-depth examination of the impact of moving away from wondering and thinking deeper about what nursing is about.

Chapter 8: Nursing Research in Canada

Substantially revised and updated, including historic trends in funding nursing research, the emergence of patient engagement strategies in nursing, the impact of the Canada Research Chairs programs on nursing research, the impact of strategic funding policies within federal research funding agencies, the emergence of bibliometrics and altmetrics, and research using standardized data that demonstrates the value of nursing.

Chapter 9: Knowledge Translation and Evidence-Informed Practice

Maintains focus on the significance of evidence-informed practice for nursing. Substantially updated content organized according to the CIHR knowledge-to-action process model of knowledge translation and Rogers' diffusion of innovations model. Includes strategies to decrease barriers to evidence-informed practice and increase sustained adoption of new evidence in nursing practice. Includes discussion of the emerging role of knowledge brokers.

Chapter 10: Nursing Informatics and Digital Health

Substantially updated to include a focus on digital health and the progression of technological innovations influencing nursing and health care; standardized languages and terminology; standardized nursing data; and nursing data science, with highlights on progress made by key industry organizations in terms of digital health maturity.

Chapter 11: Primary Health Care: Challenges and Opportunities for the Nursing Profession

Substantially revised and updated, including a stronger focus on primary health care as the responsibility of all nurses; updated history of primary health care; increased coverage of health equity and social determinants of health, especially for Indigenous peoples; enhanced examples of Canadian nurses providing primary health care; and an expanded focus on primary health care research and evaluation.

Chapter 12: Quality of Care: From Quality Assurance and Improvement to Cultures of Patient Safety

Updated with a focus on new research and scholarly work on nursing-sensitive outcomes, nursing best practice guidelines, patient safety, and information about how "lean" ideas fit into the continuous quality improvement methods that are becoming increasingly common in health care settings.

Chapter 13: The Practising Nurse and the Law

Updated considerations of electronic health and medical records, including discussion about associated privacy and confidentiality issues. Further in-depth discussion of the complexities of informed consent, including considerations for medical assistance in dying. Modifications to the discussion of negligence.

Chapter 14: Decolonizing and Anti-Oppressive Nursing Practice: Awareness, Allyship, and Action

Substantially revised to examine nursing leadership practices of awareness, allyship, anti-oppression, and decolonization in consideration of contemporary environments of oppression related to age, ability, gender, sexuality, language, race, and culture.

Chapter 15: Ethical Issues and Dilemmas in Nursing Practice

Extensively updated and revised to include relational, virtue, deontological, and utilitarian ethics as well as bioethics. Discussion of contemporary issues and concerns includes medical assistance in dying and euthanasia; use of assistive reproductive technology; equity and equality for historically disadvantaged persons such as Indigenous peoples and members of the LGBTQ2 community; therapeutic lying with persons with dementia; fitness to practice; and conscientious objection.

Chapter 16: Collaboration in Nursing Practice

New chapter that introduces readers to the concept of interprofessional education for collaborative patient/client/family-centred and community-centered practice. Competencies necessary for interprofessional collaborative practice are highlighted from various frameworks. Macro-, meso-, and micro-level factors that impact both education and practice are introduced.

Chapter 17: Shortage or Oversupply? The Registered Nursing Workforce Pendulum

Revised to present the current and future state of health human resources in the context of the nursing profession.

Updated statistics about the nursing workforce in Canada. Discussion of the changes to the profession that impact health human resources.

Chapter 18: Political Influence in Nursing

Substantially revised to recognize the imperative of nursing's political influence for global health, with an emphasis on critical perspectives on power. Reference to contemporary examples of how nurses act politically as individuals and as collectives to influence decisions on contemporary health issues.

Chapter 19: Nursing Unions as a Social Force in Canada: Advocating for Nurses, Patients, and Health Care

Substantially revised and updated. Addition of new material related to contemporary issues including PTSD, occupational health and safety, violence, staff–patient ratios, professional responsibility, and Canadian and provincial–territorial advocacy campaigns.

Chapter 20: The Origins and Development of Nursing Education in Canada

Chapter structure maintained, with content updated to reflect new historical developments. Content added on the following topics: men in nursing, Indigenous nurses, responding to the Truth and Reconciliation Commission of Canada's Calls to Action, and preparing nurses to serve francophone official language minority populations.

Chapter 21: Licensure, Credentialling, and Entry to Practice in Nursing

Two chapters were integrated to highlight the linkage of licensure, credentialling, and entry to practice and the changes that have occurred, including the implementation of the American-written NCLEX-RN exam. Changes to the scope of practice of registered nurses and other regulated nurses are also discussed.

Chapter 22: The Growth of Graduate Education in Nursing in Canada

Substantially updated and revised to include sections on the expansion of graduate programs across Canada and the growth of opportunities for nurse practitioner and doctoral studies. The development of research as a requirement for graduate program growth is discussed.

Chapter 23: Career Development in Nursing

Substantially revised to provide information on developing one's career in nursing. The role of research and advanced graduate studies is explored. Developing a career plan as well as selecting graduate education is discussed.

Chapter 24: Monitoring Standards in Nursing Education

Substantially revised to update accreditation, approval, and institutional evaluations in Canada. Provides a more in-depth historical context to the quality assurance of nursing education in Canada. The chapter also situates assessment and monitoring of nursing education in the literature about quality assurance in postsecondary education.

Chapter 25: Global Nursing: Emerging Issues and Events Locally and Beyond

Substantially revised with fully updated sections on the re-emergence of global diseases such as Ebola and COVID-19, and global issues such as planetary health and climate change. The chapter also addresses localized emerging health issues such as antimicrobial resistance, vaping, legalization of cannabis, and opioid misuse. Includes the United Nations Sustainable Development Goals and the critical role of nurses in achieving them. Discussion of the Nursing Now 2020 initiative launched by the International Council of Nurses and the World Health Organization.

Chapter 26: Internationalization in Canadian Nursing

Substantially revised and updated to reflect practice and educational experiences of internationally educated nurses as they integrate into the Canadian health care system. Research and future research directions regarding their integration is discussed, as well as the socioeconomic and ethical implications of the globalization of nursing.

STUDENT RESOURCES ON EVOLVE

An accompanying Evolve website offers additional student learning resources, including answers to the Critical Thinking Questions, case studies, review questions for each chapter, chapter web links, and printable key points for each chapter.

NEXT GENERATION NCLEX™

The National Council of State Boards of Nursing (NCSBN) is a not-for-profit organization whose members include nursing regulatory bodies. In empowering and supporting nursing regulators in their mandate to protect the public, the NCSBN is involved in the development of nursing licensure exams such as the NCLEX-RN®. In Canada, the NCLEX-RN® was introduced in 2015 and is, as of the writing of this text, the recognized licensure exam required for practising registered nurses in Canada.

As of 2023, the NCLEX-RN® will be changing to ensure that the exam's item types adequately measure clinical judgement, critical thinking, and problem-solving skills on a consistent basis. The NCSBN will also be incorporating into the exam what they refer to as the Clinical Judgement Measurement Model, a framework created by the NCSBN to measure a novice nurse's ability to apply clinical judgement in practice.

These changes to the exam arose in response to findings indicating that novice nurses are making a higher than desirable number of errors with patients (i.e., errors causing patient harm). Upon investigating these errors, the NCSBN discovered that the majority were caused by failures of clinical judgement.

Clinical judgement has been a foundation underlying modern nursing education and is based on the work of several nursing theorists. The theory of clinical judgement that most closely aligns with the NCSBN's Clinical Judgement Measurement Model is the work of Christine A. Tanner.

The new version of the NCLEX-RN® is identified loosely as the Next Generation NCLEX, or NGN, and will feature the following:

- Six key skills in the Clinical Judgement Measurement Model: recognizing cues, analyzing cues, prioritizing hypotheses, generating solutions, taking actions, and evaluating outcomes.
- Approved item types as of June 2020: multiple response, extended drag and drop, cloze (drop-down), enhanced hot-spot (highlighting), and matrix/grid. More question types may be added.
- All new item types are accompanied by mini case studies with comprehensive patient information—some of it relevant to the question, and some of it not.
- Case information may present a single, unchanging moment in time (a "single episode" case study) or multiple moments in time as a patient's condition changes (an "unfolding" case study).
- Single-episode case studies may be accompanied by one to six questions; unfolding case studies are accompanied by six questions.

For more information regarding the NCLEX-RN® and upcoming changes to the exam, visit the NCSBN's website at https://www.ncsbn.org/11447.htm and https://ncsbn.org/Building_a_Method_for_Writing_Clinical_Judgment_It.pdf.

For further NCLEX-RN® exam preparation resources, see *Silvestri's Canadian Comprehensive Review for the NCLEX-RN Examination* (2nd ed.), ISBN 9780323709385.

Before preparing for any nursing licensure exam, please refer to your provincial or territorial nursing regulatory body to determine which licensure exam you are required to take in order to practise in your chosen jurisdiction.

CONTENTS

Part III: Nursing Care Delivery

Part V: Canadian and International Nursing

The Profession in Canada

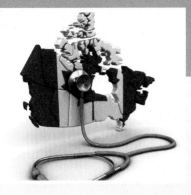

The Canadian Health Care System

Pammla Lusenga Petrucka

ⓔ http://evolve.elsevier.com/Canada/Ross-Kerr/nursing

LEARNING OBJECTIVES

After reading this chapter, you will be able to:
- Explain the Canadian health care system—past, present, and future—as it relates to Medicare and universal health care.
- Discuss the various legislative, regulatory, and rights-based elements constituting Canada's existing, reforming, and emerging health care system.
- Explain the philosophical and fiscal elements of Canadian health care.
- Reflect on the capacities and challenges of meeting the needs of all Canadians, including an understanding of Indigenous peoples' health within current Truth and Reconciliation efforts.
- Compare the Canadian health care system across current local, regional, and global contexts.

OUTLINE

KEY TERMS

accessibility
comprehensiveness
decentralized
devolved
equality
equity
gross domestic product
portability

privatization
public administration
refugee
registered nurses
social safety net
sustainability
universal health care
universality

As the wave of health care reform across Canada became a tsunami, many communities lost hospitals, entire programs disappeared, and individuals experienced uncertainty and vulnerability. Health care reform may have been written into policy by senior government officials, but it was nurses who took on a key leadership role in translating the policy into action. For example, one community introduced a clinic led by a nurse practitioner and a pharmacist who reviewed medications for individuals with chronic disease. The clinic reduced travel and properly prioritized patients for physician visits and referrals. In another setting, nurse navigators began to coordinate the care and information needs of cancer patients while liaising with the health care team, thereby improving patient and family satisfaction and reducing wait times for services. Across the country, we saw innovative nurse-led activities ranging from grassroots activities (such as becoming local first responders) to national advocacy activities (such as establishing best practice guidelines). Nurses quickly expanded their leadership roles in more interdisciplinary teams: nurse–paramedic mobile teams reached out to street youth and homeless people, and seniors' rapid response teams (made up of nurse practitioners, nurses, paramedics, occupational therapists or physiotherapists, pharmacist, physicians) worked to avert senior admissions to nursing homes or hospitals through a home-based response. We continue to see nurses leading health care transformation using innovative patient-centred approaches that span primary, secondary, and tertiary care. These innovations focus on new ways of communicating and cooperating, such as telehealth, text-message appointment reminders, and health call-lines. Care teams that include **registered nurses** and nurse practitioners can now be found all over the country—in schools, sports complexes, malls, vans, and even online!

INTRODUCTION

As a relatively young settler-colonial state, Canada has a 150-year history of nationhood and more than a 50-year history of striving for a **universal health care** system. Despite the many challenges facing the health care system, Canadians have remained steadfast in their commitment to providing health care based on need and not on ability to pay; unfortunately, over half the world's population still lacks coverage for essential health needs. The world is now tasked with responding to the United Nations Sustainable Development Goal of providing universal health coverage. This chapter takes the reader through the history, policy and legislative enablers, and the challenges in the quest to build a robust health care system in Canada. It recognizes our achievements and our failures on this arduous path to health **equity**. While much work remains to achieve equity, we are journeying on this path together with a wealth of knowledge and experience as well as ongoing resolve to remain a health care leader that inspires other jurisdictions around the world.

Canada's strong reputation as a global leader in universal health coverage has not wavered, but the need to intensify innovation and risk taking in the health sector over the next 50 years is apparent. We cannot rest on our laurels; rather, we must be cognizant of the present and look to the future to build a solid, equitable, and sustainable health care system in Canada. Now is the time to bravely commit to creating a new social contract that will serve all Canadians regardless of socioeconomic, cultural, ethnic, geographic, or demographic status.

THE CANADIAN HEALTH CARE SYSTEM: PAST, PRESENT, AND FUTURE

Tracing the evolution of Canada's health care system and oft-cited role as a global exemplar for universal health coverage leads one to discover that it has been a difficult journey punctuated by complex political, social, cultural, and contextual "moving" targets. Canadians' national identity is strongly rooted in universal health care (Martin, 2017) despite our diverse populations, histories, and geographies, with nearly 90% of Canadians identifying it as a source of collective national pride (The Canadian Press, 2012). We are, however, at a critical juncture, as the system itself is in need of care, sustenance, and innovation. To understand what is perhaps Canada's greatest "trademark," one must consider the health care system's past and present to determine its optimal future path.

Health care services were originally designed to meet pressing or emergent needs, and thus began the legacy of the Canadian health care system. When Indigenous peoples encountered the first European settlers, it was the burden of infectious diseases (tuberculosis and smallpox) rather than the potential for trade and other opportunities that left an indelible mark on the Indigenous population. As European populations and settlements grew, a series of short-term approaches to solving sanitation problems, epidemics, and medical needs were attempted and often failed. By 1867, when the *British North America Act* led to the creation of Canada as a nation, the provincial and federal governments divided responsibilities for maintaining the health of Canadians; the provinces and territories would oversee public health (including hospitals), while the federal government would manage public policy aspects of health (such as pharmaceutical safety, data collection, and health research) as well as health services for Indigenous peoples (Storch, 2006). The provinces and territories enacted a critical measure during the early 1900s by introducing local health boards, which focused primarily on sanitation, care of the poor, and the levy of taxes to cover related costs. However, the continued lack of funding for health services led to significant hardships for individuals and an absence of sustainable solutions for communities, resulting in the increased involvement of volunteer and religious entities in **social safety net** programs (Taylor, 1978). Health care was rapidly becoming inaccessible to the majority of Canadians. As Taylor (1978) wrote,

> *Our heritage of the Elizabethan Poor Law had placed responsibility for the sick poor on local government, (leading to) near or actual bankruptcy from the combination of declining revenues and expanding relief payment for food, clothing and shelter. Medical care, except in the direct emergency conditions, was a luxury that only few individuals or municipalities could afford.* (p. 4)

These challenges did not go unrecognized, as the Liberals made the first references to a national health care system in their 1919 election platform (Taylor, 1978). Although universal health care was still years away, the emergence of prepayment plans for hospital care marked the beginning of an insurance scheme to reduce hardships on patients, providers, and communities. Two world wars sandwiching the Great Depression gave the issue of health insurance further traction as part of postwar political rhetoric (Taylor, 1978). Postwar, few people could afford to pay their health care bills (Agnew, 1974); in turn, many health care providers also remained unpaid (*Report of the Saskatchewan Department of Public Health* (1933), as cited in Taylor, 1978). This situation would be partially addressed by the *Employment and Social Insurance Act, 1935*. Though the Act was later rescinded as unconstitutional, it set in motion efforts to launch an insurance framework. In the interim, commercial insurance plans arose that were either local (e.g., Edmonton Group Hospitalization plan) or provincial (e.g., Manitoba Blue Cross plan) premium-based voluntary plans focused on covering hospitalization costs only (Vayda, Evans, & Mindell, 1979).

However, because different authorities were responsible for developing and maintaining the plans offered in different provinces, there was considerable variation in benefits from plan to plan. A substantial segment of the Canadian population was not covered by any form of prepaid insurance owing to ineligibility for plans limited to specific groups of people or inability to pay the required premium. These issues were addressed head on at a 1945 federal–provincial conference with the proposal of a cost-sharing universal health insurance plan (Vayda, Evans, & Mindell, 1979). The legislation once again failed to gain royal assent, but the effort catalyzed a new wave of provincially driven efforts that would soon change the face of Canada's health care environment forever.

In 1947, Premier of Saskatchewan Tommy Douglas introduced the first mandatory universal hospital insurance plan in North America, with general revenues (and later a provincial sales tax) as the funding source; the rest of Canada would receive universal health coverage two decades later. This chapter reflects on Canada's next steps locally, regionally, and globally as champions and innovators for universal health coverage.

APPLYING CONTENT KNOWLEDGE

Based on your understanding of universal health care, do you think Canada currently has a universal health care system? Why or why not?

LEGISLATIVE, REGULATORY, AND RIGHTS-BASED GUIDELINES

Framing the Canadian Health Care System

The Canadian health care system has its origins in constitutional processes first laid out in the *British North America Act, 1867*. The legislation clearly delineated the roles and responsibilities for health and health care at the provincial/territorial and federal levels of government. These were later reaffirmed in the *Constitution Act, 1982* (s. 92) (Government of Canada, 2019). The roles of different levels of government are summarized in Table 1.1.

TABLE 1.1 Canadian Federal and Provincial/Territorial Jurisdictional Differences	
Federal Jurisdiction	**Provincial/Territorial Jurisdiction**
Financing through transfer payment arrangements	Financing and managing health services as specified in the *Canada Health Act*
Enforcing relevant Acts and legislative documents, especially the *Canada Health Act*	Arranging for payments or co-payments for services as specified in the *Canada Health Act* or relevant legislation
Co-delivery or delivery of health services to target groups	Developing and implementing the health care insurance plan for their jurisdiction
Establishing and enacting national agendas in core areas such as consumer health and safety, pharmaceuticals, public health, and health research	

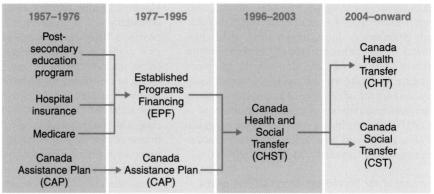

Figure 1.1 Historical timeline of Canada's funding for postsecondary education, social transfers, and health care. (Reproduced with the permission of the Department of Finance, 2020, https://www.fin.gc.ca/fedprov/his-eng.asp)

This **devolved** approach to health care is significantly different from the approach used by the United States and most European countries, all of which have a centralized (federalist) controlled health care mandate. Wallace (1980) reflected on how social evolution shifted the health care context beyond the expectations and anticipations of the Fathers of Confederation, stating that they

> clearly thought they were assigning the provinces the less important and inexpensive functions of government, among which education, hospitals, charities and municipal institutions were then reasonably numbered. They could scarcely have foreseen the way in which time would reverse their expectations, so that the costliness of the responsibilities laid upon the provinces subsequently increased to the point where it was financially impossible to defray them. (p. 27)

Figure 1.1 traces the progression of Canada's funding programs since 1957. The *Canada Health Act* (1984), as mentioned, articulates the requirements for selected publicly financed health services. The *Canada Health Act* is rooted in five guiding principles: **portability, universality, accessibility, comprehensiveness,** and **public administration** (as described in Table 1.2). These principles are supported through transfer payment mechanisms that prohibit user fees or copayments from insured individuals for covered services. Certain individuals or groups are exempt from the coverage offered under the *Canada Health Act*, which means their health care services are provided or paid for by the federal government. Exempt from coverage under the *Canada Health Act* are members of the Royal Canadian Mounted Police and Canadian Armed Forces (both active and eligible veterans), members of Parliament, eligible

TABLE 1.2　Overview of the Principles of the *Canada Health Act, 1984*

Principle	Description
Portability	Mobility between provinces or territories (as well as outside of Canada in the short term) is not to be a deterrent to receiving insured health service benefits (some conditions apply)
Universality	All insured residents (regardless of age, gender, ethnicity, income) receive the same health service benefits
Accessibility	Reasonable access to insured health services by all insured residents
Comprehensiveness	No out-of-pocket charges (i.e., copayment or deductible) for all insured benefits (medically necessary) provided in hospital and through physician services, health services, and dental services in hospital
Public Administration	Administration on a nonprofit basis by a public authority (such as a regional health authority)

Sources: Adapted from Health Canada. (2016a). *Canada's health care system.* Retrieved from https://www.canada.ca/en/health-canada/services/canada-health-care-system.html; Martin, D., Miller, A. P., Quesnel-Vallée, A., et al. (2018). Canada's universal health-care system: Achieving its potential. *Lancet, 391*(10131), 1718–1735. https://doi.org/10.1016/S0140-6736(18)30181-8.

TABLE 1.3 Examples of Relevant Canadian Health Legislation	
Legislation	**Focus**
Canadian Environmental Protection Act, 1999 (amended 2018) http://www.ec.gc.ca/lcpe-cepa	Addresses, regulates, and enforces pollution prevention and environmental protection in partnership with Environment Canada for sustainable development
Canadian Institutes of Health Research Act, 2000 http://www.cihr-irsc.gc.ca/e/9466.html	Strategically plans research agendas and manages funding of health-related research through 13 virtual institutes
Cannabis Act, 2018 https://laws.justice.gc.ca/eng/acts/C-24.5/	Monitors and protects public health and safety through product safety and quality controls
Controlled Drugs and Substances Act, 1996 http://laws-lois.justice.gc.ca/eng/acts/C-38.8/	Controls certain drugs, precursors, and related substances
Emergency Management Act, 2007 http://laws-lois.justice.gc.ca/eng/acts/E-4.56	Develops and implements civil emergency plans; facilitates and coordinates across government levels and institutions, foreign governments, and international organizations
Food and Drugs Act, 1985 (amended 2018) http://laws-lois.justice.gc.ca/eng/acts/F-27/	Regulates food, food additives, drugs, blood products, cosmetics, and therapeutic devices
Tobacco and Vaping Products Act, 1997 (amended 2018) http://laws.justice.gc.ca/eng/acts/T-11.5/	Regulates the manufacture, sale, labelling, and promotion of tobacco and vaping products with a focus on protection of young persons and nonusers

Source: Government of Canada. (2019). *Lists of acts and regulations*. Retrieved from https://www.canada.ca/en/health-canada/corporate/about-health-canada/legislation-guidelines/acts-regulations/list-acts-regulations.html.

Indigenous groups, and all federal inmates (Health Canada, 2016a). Health coverage for newcomers (**immigrants** and **refugees**) to Canada is managed outside the *Canada Health Act* until individuals have obtained residency status. For immigrants to Canada, there is significant variability in coverage depending on the type of residency/permit (i.e., permanent resident; student visa), waiting periods, and provincial rules that need to be considered on a situational basis. For refugees, refugee claimants, and resettled individuals, the Interim Federal Health Program provides limited short-term health care coverage if individuals are not covered under provincial or territorial programs (Government of Canada, 2017a). Visitors to Canada are not covered and require personal travel insurance.

Under the *Canada Health Act*, the federal government is obligated to "to protect, promote and restore the physical and mental well-being of residents of Canada and to facilitate reasonable access to health services without financial or other barriers" (Health Canada, 2011). However, Canada continues to face challenges to delivering on this commitment owing to decentralization, regional variability (fragmentation), multiple points of entry, and **sustainability** issues. The *Canada Health Act* is not specific on the range of covered health services other than provider payment and hospital care, an ambiguity that has led to the variability in coverage across the country. Health Canada oversees the administration,

implementation, and ongoing consultations for a number of laws and regulations, which are listed in Table 1.3.

A well-articulated legislative agenda in Canada serves to keep stakeholders and the public informed about efforts to protect, regulate, control, and report on the health care system and health-related issues, threats, and opportunities. However, the elephant in the room is the issue of the "right to health care," which was never made explicit in the *Canadian Charter of Rights and Freedoms, 1982*, or the *Canada Health Act*, though most Canadians believe it is a legally protected right. Many legislative and policy vehicles create the illusion of this right, but only Quebec has embedded health as a right in its provincial legislative framework. According to Martin, Miller, Quesnel-Vallée et al. (2018, p. 1718), the Canadian health care system is based on an "implicit social contract between governments, health-care providers, and the public."

Reframing the Canadian Health Care System

In this legislative context, the federal and provincial governments have implemented continuous improvements and restructuring in pursuit of creating a quality, responsive, and equitable health care system that delivers safe, integrated, and progressive health care to Canadians. The reality of funding limitations will be further explored later in this chapter, but suffice to say that funding is one of several elements that drive health care efficiency and quality.

As the federal government became a lesser contributor, an apparent shift took place in who controlled the mandate and vision of the national health insurance program (Brown, 1980). This shift led to discussions about the potential restructuring and reorganization of the health care system. Within the 1964 *Royal Commission on Health Services* report, early conversations and recommendations about health reform had begun emerging (Royal Commission on Health Services, 1965). These hints at reform were met with resistance on a number of fronts; most notably, the provinces and territories demonstrated an unwillingness to revisit the constitutional parameters of their roles and responsibilities. The introduction of the *Canada Health Act* was also met with resistance by the same provincial and territorial voices as well as by physicians unwilling to lose control as gatekeepers to entry into the health care system. As new models (e.g., nurse practitioner–led clinics) and technologies (e.g., digital imaging; telepsychiatry) emerged, the need to reconsider the future elements of the Canadian health care system became apparent.

Political and fiscal pressures, along with growing social expectations for public engagement in the future of health care, prompted a series of public commissions in the early 2000s. Several national and provincial reports were published almost in tandem in 2002: the national reports included the *Kirby Report* (Kirby, 2002) and a report by the Commission on the Future of Health Care in Canada (Romanow, 2002), while the provincial reports included Alberta's *Mazankowski*

Report (Premier's Advisory Council on Health, 2002). Both national reports contained recommendations to increase funding to stabilize and sustain the system, as well to increase the accountability of the federal government to honour the Act while preserving Medicare. Conversely, the authors of the Alberta report were highly critical of the status quo, suggesting that a private–public model (two-tiered) was essential to meeting the needs of all Canadians. Although contradictory in approach, the synergy in the messages was clear: the health care system needed to be reimagined and restructured if it was to meet the needs of Canadians.

In response to these reports and a litany of other commissions, forums, and reviews (see Table 1.4), the provinces and territories undertook a range of activities to restructure and regionalize the planning and delivery of health services. These activities were purportedly designed to streamline services and meet local needs, but their cost-saving intent soon became apparent (McIntosh, Ducie, Burka-Charles et al., 2010). Even the language to describe the reforms varied, with some provinces referring to these new administrative and delivery areas as districts and others as regions—often defined according to geographic boundaries—that would be responsible for the delivery and administration of publicly funded health care services. For instance, Saskatchewan originally had 32 health districts and British Columbia 20 regions. Regionalization efforts swirled and faltered as the locus of control shifted from a central authority to regions and districts; moreover, decentralization provided inadequate resources to facilitate this new model of planning and delivery (Collier, 2010). Shortly thereafter, recentralization efforts

TABLE 1.4 **Major Commissions and Reports on the Canadian Health System**	
Review Name, Year	**Key Recommendations**
Royal Commission on Health Services (Hall Commission), 1964	Comprehensive health coverage for all Canadians
	Strengthened national policy on health care and health financing
Health Services Review, 1980	Reviewed post-1964 commission changes
	Determine status of extra-billing and user fee compliance
Royal Commission on Aboriginal Peoples, 1996	Representative training of health care providers
Standing Senate Committee on Social Affairs, Science, and Technology Study on the State of the Health Care System in Canada (Kirby Committee), 2002	Increased federal government oversight of all dimensions of health care
	Advanced need for equity in human resources and health service across geographies
Commission on the Future of Health Care in Canada (Romanow Commission), 2002	Renewal of commitment to philosophical values of equity and a single-payer health care system
Truth and Reconciliation Commission of Canada, 2015	Establish a comprehensive response to abuses experienced by Indigenous peoples throughout the era of residential schools (see additional discussion later in this chapter)
Advisory Panel on Healthcare Innovation, 2015	Imperative for a health care system that uses modern technologies and leads on innovations to improve patient outcomes

began to dominate Canadian health care. Prince Edward Island was the first jurisdiction to revert to a single entity (Health PEI) in 2005 (Institute of Public Administration in Canada, 2013). Alberta followed suit in 2008 with the dissolution of its nine regional health authorities and the creation of Alberta Health Services. Within the span of a decade, Canadians had endured the decentralization and recentralization of their health care system, with proponents of each of the models claiming that theirs was superior and would streamline services, address fiscal constraints, improve governance, and meet the care needs of Canadians. Although these efforts have been disjointed and minimally successful, health reforms have advanced opportunities for community and home-based care as well as health prevention/promotion services.

APPLYING CONTENT KNOWLEDGE

Looking at the principles of the *Canada Health Act*, do you believe that they are sufficient and reflective of today's realities? Should sustainability be an additional pillar? What would sustainability add to the future Canadian health care system? What are the risks of adding sustainability to the principles?

PHILOSOPHICAL AND FISCAL ELEMENTS OF CANADA'S HEALTH CARE SYSTEM

As mentioned earlier, the *Canada Health Act* of 1984 defined the principles under which the health care system would operate across provincial and territorial boundaries, between federal–provincial–territorial jurisdictions, within subsets of the population, and across time. However, the *Canada Health Act* was also the vehicle for managing funding in a manner that would inhibit the formation of a two-tiered health care system—one for the haves and another for the have-nots. As part of these funding deliberations, the federal government took a hardline stance to disallow extra-billing and user fees; otherwise, the provinces and territories risked incurring a financial penalty. This meant that insured health services and programs would be provided free of charge across the country, with each jurisdiction individually deciding how these constraints would be managed. Hence, some provinces (i.e., New Brunswick, Nova Scotia, Prince Edward Island, and Saskatchewan) allowed physicians to extra-bill and still claim for services within the plan; others, such as Quebec, allowed physicians to opt in or out of the plan (Collier, 2015). While the Canadian Medical Association opposed the legislation,

the Canadian Nurses Association (CNA) lauded the Act's entrenching of access to health care regardless of ability to pay and lobbied for the end to extra-billing and user fees (CNA, 1983). A direct fallout from the Act was that specialized services delivered by nurses were for the first time reimbursable under provincial health insurance plans. The CNA continued to call for action through extensive lobbying. They campaigned for health insurance to be extended beyond the traditional hospital-based delivery to include home, community, and other settings (such as schools and clinics) and for full recognition of health care practitioners other than physicians, as reflected in the words of CNA President Dr. Helen Glass:

> It's our responsibility to make nursing's voice heard—and soon. Even if you have already contacted your Minister of Health, we strongly urge you to keep up your lobbying efforts. Health department officials, leaders of opposition parties, opposition health critics and members of standing committees on health will be key targets. (Glass, 1983, p. 1)

The pride and commitment of Canadians to their universal health care system reflects both a national achievement and national misconceptions. Regardless of how the health system functions, it is the philosophical and fiscal foundations that have thus far enabled Medicare to deliver health care services. Ongoing efforts are critical to ensure that Medicare will survive and thrive.

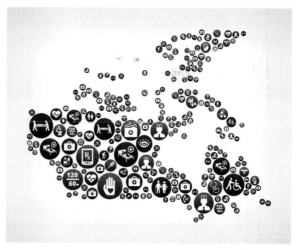

Medicare: A context of diversity (istock.com/bubaone)

Two key features are foundational to the Canadian Medicare approach and differentiate it from the national health insurance programs of other countries. For one,

Canada's health care system is highly **decentralized;** each province and territory retains significant latitude in the provision and allocation of selected services but ascribes to a common set of financing principles. This decentralization has, in part, enabled physicians to act as independent contractors who remain somewhat at arm's length from the system (Allin & Rudoler, 2017). Second, Canadians are inherently resistant to **privatization,** which is frequently mentioned in times of recession or shortfalls (such as wait-lists for surgeries). Private clinics exist and are growing for the provision of some services, especially fertility, surgical, and diagnostic services. The argument around private clinics has many dimensions, including whether these private clinics save time, money, or both; whether they create a two-tiered system; whether competition actually leads to quality and efficiency; and whether there is a risk of prioritizing profit over people (Government of British Columbia, 2007). Recently, there has also been much discussion regarding the cost of universal health coverage and its long-term sustainability (Kondro, 2010).

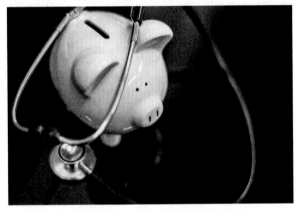

Is health care really free? (istock.com/FatCamera)

The perception that health care is free is a misnomer on both sides of the equation, as health care expenditures involve costs for both the funder (i.e., through taxes) and the user (e.g., prescription drugs or dental care). In Canada, these combined expenditures have long neared or exceeded double-digit percentages of Canada's **gross domestic product** (GDP; the total value of goods and services produced in a country in a year). Canada's health care expenditures were estimated to be 11.6% of the GDP in 2019, up from 10.4% in 2018, with over $264 billion being invested by governments and citizens directly (through personal payments and private insurance) (Canadian Institute for Health Information [CIHI], 2019). This GDP percentage

is fairly consistent among some developed countries (e.g., Australia, 9.4%; France, 11.5%), but is markedly higher in the United States (17.1%) and dramatically lower in low- and middle-income countries (Democratic Republic of Congo, 4.3%; Ghana, 5.9%; Thailand, 3.8%) (World Bank, 2017).

The split in funding between the Canadian government (70.9%) and other sources (personal, 13.6%; private insurance, 15.5%) is approximately 70:30, respectively (Organisation for Economic Co-operation and Development [OECD], 2019a; CIHI, 2016). In other jurisdictions, the public–private split ranges widely: it is 49%–51% in the United States, 80%–20% in New Zealand and the United Kingdom, and 84%–16% in Germany and Sweden. We see further variance in actual health expenditures per capita across geographic and economic regions. For example, in Canada, the total expenditure per person per year in US dollars is $4,974; this is nearly half of the US expenditure of $10,586 but closely mirrors that of France ($4,965) and Australia ($5,005). Where we start to see significant deviation is in Africa ($34 in Tanzania; $66 in Sierra Leone), South America ($381 in Paraguay), and Central America ($282 in El Salvador) (OECD, 2019a; CIHI, 2016; World Bank Group, 2019).

As we come to understand the variability in health care expenditures by both public and private sources, we need to look at many implicit and explicit considerations. In the Canadian health care system, these considerations are reflected in a three-tiered pattern (Martin, Miller, Quesnel-Vallée et al., 2018; CIHI, 2019). The first layer contains the Medicare "bundle," which includes publicly financed hospital care and physician services. Although this layer is available to most Canadians, some individuals fall outside the legal mandate (see previous discussion); other individuals who cannot access these services are subgroups of refugees and temporary residents with expired permits. The second layer contains a range of packages of health services, such as ambulance services, extended care, and pharmacare; these services are often co-paid or cost shared through public and private funding (CIHI, 2019). In 2017, the amount Canadians spent on pharmaceuticals alone was $860 US dollars per capita at the household level (OECD, 2019b). Finally, the third layer consists of services that are predominantly or entirely privately funded, such as physiotherapy, chiropody, private duty nursing, and vision care (Marchildon, 2013).

This three-tiered model is highly reliant on individuals having access to sufficient financial resources or adequate private insurance to offset the real costs in layers two and three. Yet, nearly one-third of Canadians lack a private insurance plan (similar to the proportion of Americans without health insurance), leaving them vulnerable beyond the essential services package offered under Medicare. This has led to calls to extend the services included under Medicare (Law, Kratzer, & Dhalla, 2014; American Institute of Medical Sciences and Education, 2018).

The federal funding approach evolved through several stages in the post–World War II era. Initially, federal legislation took a two-pronged approach, focusing on ensuring capital construction of hospitals and providing hospital care insurance (Vayda, Evans, & Mindell, 1979). As early as 1948, the National Health Grants Programs disseminated the message that a publicly funded hospital insurance program was forthcoming. By 1957, the *Hospital Insurance and Diagnostic Services Act* offered an option for provinces to co-share universal services such as hospital care, with the federal government paying "an amount equal to 25% of its own per capita cost (less authorized charges) plus 25% of the national per capita cost multiplied by the number of insured persons" (Brown, 1980, p. 523). By 1961, with all provinces having signed onto the *Hospital Insurance and Diagnostic Services Act* (Vayda, Evans, & Mindell, 1979), the environment seemed conducive to establishing a federal plan that would reimburse physician services using the same cost-sharing formula. However, nearly a decade passed before all provinces and a highly resistant physician group agreed (not until after an unprecedented strike action by the group in 1962) to the federal *Medical Care Act, 1966*.

As hospitalization rates and health care costs escalated, so did costs associated with a physician-driven health care system (physicians were the only health care providers cited within the legislation respecting remuneration). Soon it became obvious that the cost-sharing method was not sustainable. The federal government established the *Fiscal Arrangements and Established Programs Financing Act* of 1977, which dramatically reduced their contribution from 50% to 25% of the costs in the co-shared services. Thus arrived an era of block transfer payments and a complicated funding formula for the wider array of health services provided, which included extended care and home care services. As a result, there was a lowering of federal taxes accompanied by the provinces' increased powers to tax Canadians in order to offset the funding deficits incurred under this new model. This opened the flood gates to extra-billing or premiums by hospitals and providers from the latter part of the 1970s into the 1990s, which catalyzed a significant trend in health reform discussed later in this chapter (CIHI, 2000).

The next major reconfiguration of funding occurred in 2004 through the federal government's 10-Year Plan to Strengthen Health Care. It was introduced purportedly to plan and build a more sustainable and equitable Canadian health care system (Health Canada, 2006).

Despite the rhetoric, little changed. By 2017, a new iteration of the Canada Health Transfer was implemented. This plan shifted over $37 billion to the provinces and territories, based on population served, known as per capita (or per person) funding. These transfers continued to meet the requirements of the *Canada Health Act* (Government of Canada, 2017a), which sets out the responsibilities of the federal and provincial/territorial governments with respect to funding and provision of services. Through separate commitments outside of the *Canada Health Act*, the federal government committed to out-of-hospital health benefits, such as home care and mental health services ($6 billion and $5 billion, respectively, over 10 years); pharmaceutical system investments ($140.3 million); data management and evidence-informed decision making ($53 million); and technology innovations ($300 million) (Government of Canada, 2017a).

The *Canada Health Act* continues to address the requirements associated with federal transfer payments, which are currently about 20% of the provincial/territorial health care budgets, while provinces and territories are committing about 38% of their budgets (on average) to health care spending (Martin, Miller, Quesnel-Vallée et al., 2018; Health Canada, 2017; Sibbald, 2017).

> ### 🔒 APPLYING CONTENT KNOWLEDGE
>
> Do you think Canada should strive to be a leader in the area of universal health care? What are the implications of taking on such a role? How will this role impact universal health care in Canada?

REPRESENTING THE NEEDS OF ALL CANADIANS WITHIN THE CANADIAN HEALTH CARE SYSTEM

To say that Canada is diverse hardly captures the complexity and potential of this country. It is an immense undertaking to build a responsive and equitable health system in a country with a sprawling land mass of nearly 10 million km² and a mere 37 million people. Consider Canada's closest neighbour, the United States, a country with a nearly identical land mass yet 10 times the population. In Canada, the number of people under 15 years of age (16%) mirrors the number over 65 years of age (17%). Life expectancy is 82.14 years (fourteenth in the world), which is comparable to that of most OECD countries. Canada's human development index of 0.920 gives it a global ranking very similar to Australia's index of 0.939 (second place), where the geographic and cultural challenges are often comparable.

🌐 CULTURAL CONSIDERATIONS

Equity Explored

For nurses, the term "equity" translates into a personal epiphany on accepting difference and understanding cultural humility. More than just thinking outside the box, it means not seeing the box to begin with. Far from the pristine linens of hospital wards, nurses are handing out blankets and clean needles to the homeless, climbing into boxcars to talk about STIs and Narcan kits with street-engaged youth, and even walking the nights with local sex workers to provide free testing and condoms. Far from the idyllic mother–baby hospital units, nurses and nurse practitioners are counseling drug-addicted pregnant mothers, advocating for decent housing conditions for adolescent mothers, and working in community gardens to increase food security for immigrant and newcomer families. Far from the security of the nursing station, nurses and nurse practitioners are petitioning city hall for school-based nutrition programs, advocating for barrier-free access to menstrual hygiene products, and being heard on issues of climate change, anti-poverty campaigns, and human rights. Nurses working with an equity lens are building a Canadian health care system that aims for far more than the lowest common denominator in health and health services—the system must aim to achieve optimal health outcomes for all.

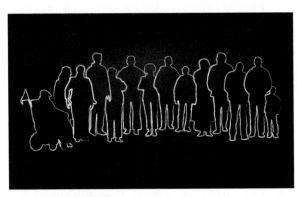

(istock.com/A-Digit)

However, the challenges reflected by selected health care indicators document the failure of the health care system to achieve equity. For example, 63% of Canadians reported difficulty accessing after-hours care compared with 51% of Americans and 44% of Australians. Sixteen percent of Canadians report cost-related barriers to accessing care; this is a proportion similar to that in France (17%),

markedly higher than that in the United Kingdom (7%), and significantly lower than that in the United States (33%). Yet another disturbing indicator is the above-average use of emergency rooms due to many Canadians' lack of a regular family physician, with 17% of Canadians visiting emergency rooms as opposed to a mere 7% of their British and French counterparts (OECD, 2019a; United Nations Development Programme [UNDP], 2019; World Bank, 2017, 2018).

▣ RESEARCH FOCUS

A study by Chan and colleagues focused on timely access to health care for individuals with one or more chronic health conditions, as chronic illnesses are the leading cause of death globally. The study considered a range of influences (i.e., age, gender, living circumstances, costs, and availability) on patients' perceptions of the appropriateness of and accessibility to care. The research showed that younger females living alone were more likely to perceive their access to care negatively than were other participants. The study was informed by the evidence that health care expenditures are disproportionately distributed to people with multiple chronic care conditions, with a significant shift coinciding with aging. With a rapidly aging population, we see more chronic disease diagnoses. It is important that we find ways to manage this.

Source: Chan, C. W. T., Gogovor, A., Valois, M. F., & Ahmed, S. (2018). Age, gender, and current living status were associated with perceived access to treatment among Canadians using a cross sectional survey. *BMC Health Services Research, 18,* 471. https://doi.org/10.1186/s12913-018-3215-6.

As a relatively young settler-colonial nation, Canada has a population consisting of a mosaic of Indigenous peoples, newcomers, and the descendants of recent immigrants. Each of these groups has unique needs, challenges, and opportunities that merit consideration. Given that Canada has often been lauded as promoting and spearheading health and human equity globally, so too must we be held to task to ensure that equity is achieved domestically (Nixon, Lee, Bhutta et al., 2018).

First Nations, Inuit, and Métis (hereinafter referred to as Indigenous peoples) represent about 5% (1.7 million) of the population in Canada; this population continues to grow at more than four times the rate of the non-Indigenous population (The Canadian Press, 2017; Statistics Canada, 2017a). Indigenous peoples are also significantly younger, with a national average age of 32.1 years compared with an average of 40.9 years for the non-Indigenous population (Statistics Canada, 2017a). Between

2006 and 2016, the over-65 age grouping for Indigenous peoples has also seen an upswing from 4.8% to 7.3% of the population (Statistics Canada, 2017b).

Treaties, which predate Confederation, and recent comprehensive land claims (Government of Canada, 2018) embed the government's commitment to Indigenous peoples for the provision of services, including health care, as well as long-term land rights. In the *Indian Act* of 1985, the federal government assumed responsibility for health services. However, what was once seen as "the great promise" has become "the great shame" (Trudeau, 2018). There are persistent inequities in the health and living standards of Indigenous peoples in Canada. Nearly one-quarter live below the poverty line. Health outcomes for Indigenous peoples are similar to those for people living in developing countries (Martin, Miller, Quesnel-Vallée et al., 2018). Nationally, these unfavourable health outcomes are reflected in higher rates of infant mortality; higher rates of intentional injury; higher rates of respiratory, digestive, mental and behavioural, endocrine, genitourinary, and musculoskeletal diseases; and numerous other suboptimal health outcomes (Guèvremont, Carrière, Bougie, & Kohen, 2017; Sheppard, Shapiro, Bushnok et al., 2017). According to Statistics Canada (2017b), the life expectancy of Indigenous peoples in Canada is significantly lower than that of the non-Indigenous population (e.g., statistics for males: First Nations, 74 years; Inuit, 64 years; non-Indigenous, 80 years). These egregious trends are similar to the experiences of Indigenous peoples in the settler-colonial societies of Australia and New Zealand (Pulver, Haswell, Ring et al., 2010)

Negative trends in unemployment, substandard housing, lack of clean drinking water on reserve, incarceration, suicide, homicide, noncommunicable diseases, and so on quickly make apparent the complexity and far-reaching impacts of a colonial past on Indigenous peoples (Garner, Varriere, & Sanmartin, 2010). For instance, the tuberculosis rate is over 50 times higher among First Nations living on reserve than among non-Indigenous people born in Canada. The legacy of residential schools, cultural genocide, the epidemic of Missing and Murdered Indigenous Women and Girls, the loss of traditional lands and practices, racism, social exclusion, as well as the loss of self-determination over the span of hundreds of years have perpetuated large inequities in Indigenous peoples' socioeconomic, political, historical, and environmental contexts (Allan & Smylie, 2015; Reading, 2015).

Further adding to this complexity is the disjointed delivery of health services to Indigenous peoples, with on-reserve services to First Nations primarily rendered by federal programs, whereas off-reserve services fall under provincial Medicare or federal government supplemental insurance (Health Canada, 2016a). In the 2016 through 2018 budgets, nearly $12 billion was allocated to address the social determinants of health for Indigenous peoples (Philpott, 2018). Health care services are presently delivered through collaborative intergovernmental efforts (federal, provincial and territorial, and Indigenous) that all recognize these realities and inequities.

Many recent efforts have been informed by the multivolume Truth and Reconciliation Commission of Canada report, which issued 94 Calls to Action, of which seven were health oriented. These seven Calls to Action emphasized the need to establish sustainable funding, embed cultural healing practices, provide cultural safety and competency training for care providers, and build a representative cadre of health professions inclusive of Indigenous peoples (Truth and Reconciliation Commission of Canada [TRCC], 2015). The TRCC is being used as vector for "establishing and maintaining a mutually respectful relationship between Aboriginal and non-Aboriginal peoples in this country. For that to happen, there has to be awareness of the past, acknowledgement of the harm that has been inflicted, atonement for the causes, and action to change behaviour" (TRCC, 2015, p. 3). The current imperative is for all leaders and all Canadians to seek genuine reconciliation, thereby catalyzing a new and shared vision for a Canadian health care system that brings equity, dignity, and hope.

Another group that faces significant health challenges and inequities in Canada is newcomers. Canada has long welcomed migrants (though at various times government policies have limited immigration from specific source countries). Like many G7 countries, Canada relies heavily on immigration for population and economic growth. According to Statistics Canada (2016), the foreign-born population in Canada was 21.9% (more than 1 in 5 people) in 2016 versus 13.6% (~1 in 7 people) in the United States, and 29.6% (~1 in 3 people) in Australia (OECD, 2018). In 2016, Canada's population increased by 1% owing to immigration alone (Statistics Canada, 2016). By 2036, 30% of Canadians are expected to be immigrants (The Canadian Press, 2017).

As we look at the health status of newcomers and immigrants, a range of profiles emerge. Canada is home to economic migrants, refugees, and immigrants, some of whom have been here for decades; hence, there is an imperative to recognize this diversity (Vang, Sigouin, Flenon, & Gagnon, 2017). The health characteristics and burden borne by these individuals, especially in the period immediately following migration, are strongly linked to country of origin, recent living situation (e.g., refugee camp, internment), reason for migration, and preexisting conditions (Citizenship and Immigration Canada, 2013). Compared with the Canadian population, subgroups of immigrants often exhibit a higher prevalence of specific disease-related morbidities and mortality such as HIV, hepatitis C, tuberculosis, sexually transmitted infections, and mental health conditions (Aldridge, Yates, Zenner et al., 2014; Redditt, Janakiram, Graziano, & Rashid, 2015). The prevalence of tuberculosis in the foreign-born population of Canada is 20 times that in the non-Indigenous, general population. And although immigrants and refugees from HIV-endemic countries constitute about 2% of the Canadian population, they disproportionately represent 1 in 7 HIV cases (International Coalition on AIDS and Development, 2016).

Another major issue for recent immigrant subgroups is initiation into the health care system as well as access to care. The challenges often begin with strict rules regarding eligibility for and commencement of health insurance coverage in Canada (Government of Canada, 2017c). Although the health profile of immigrants begins to match the overall Canadian profile over time, particularly with respect to having a regular family physician, recent immigrants experience more difficulties in access to care and are less likely to seek care (McKreary & Newbold, 2010; Setia, Quesnel-Vallée, Abrahamowicz et al., 2011). Most newcomers report that language and cultural differences in care are significant deterrents to access and can contribute to a distrust of both health care providers and the health care system (Joshi, Russel, Cheng et al., 2013; McKreary & Newbold, 2010; Wayland, 2006). These issues are likely best addressed in the short term through the use of navigators and health interpreters; however, the health care system, through its agents, must be reformed to address cultural safety, competency, and humility to meet the needs of these and other populations (Joshi, Russel, Cheng et al., 2013; Setia, Quesnel-Vallée, Abrahamowicz et al., 2011).

This dialogue on cultural safety, competence, and humility within the Canadian health care system is in its formative stages, and while we speak liberally of these desired attributes, they are exceedingly difficult to understand and deliver. Greenwood, de Leeuw, and Lindsay (2018) discuss transformative interdisciplinary and intersectoral practices, policies, and systems that are reflective and respectful of the populations served. But we are not there yet and can only reach these goals through true collaboration, recognizing the imperative for self-reflection and humility to effect the changes needed (Schuessler, Wilder, & Byrd, 2012). See Chapter 14 for more discussion.

👤 APPLYING CONTENT KNOWLEDGE

Consider three unique Canadian subpopulations. Where do you see these groups experiencing inequities in health care services? Are you aware of any programs and services that address the inequities in any or all of these groups?

RE-ENVISIONING THE CANADIAN HEALTH CARE SYSTEM

The First 50 Years

In the relatively short span of 50 years, the Canadian health care system has continually encountered demographic shifts, competing agendas (e.g., public–private split), and unanticipated innovation (especially technologies). These pressures and challenges have driven the health care system to evolve as we maintain the vision of a national program that is comparable to or supersedes regional and global models.

The Canadian health care system faces local, regional, and global challenges. For example, when we consider aging, the populations of many developed countries skew much older than those of developing countries. In Canada, some subpopulations have high birth rates (and therefore younger population statistics), while the majority of the population is part of a rapidly aging demographic. Hence, one quickly realizes that solutions for health and health care are complex and may vary considerably across the globe, within regions, and even within nations. As another example, consider access issues. In North America and Europe, access is often addressed through advanced paramedical services, but these solutions are not available in most African contexts. A lack of access to adequately trained health care providers is a ubiquitous challenge that leads to excessive wait times, delayed access to care, and even morbidity and mortality in all health care systems around the world.

By 2030: The Global Imperatives

As we embark on the next set of challenges facing the Canadian health care system, all relevant sectors must engage in dialogues that will change the health of people within our borders and beyond. We must also look to the United Nations Development Programme's 17 Sustainable Development Goals (SDGs) (see Figure 1.2), which are "a universal call to action to end poverty, protect the planet and ensure that all people enjoy peace and prosperity" (UNDP, 2019). The call for universal health coverage has been a recent focus of the SDGs. Universal health coverage will address the lack of quality and affordable essential services to over half the world's population, with nearly 100 million people being pushed into extreme poverty by the need to access essential health care services (Martin, Miller, Quesnel-Vallée et al., 2018). Universal health coverage means "that all people and communities can use the promotive, preventive, curative, rehabilitative and palliative health services they need, of sufficient quality to be effective, while also ensuring that the use of these services does

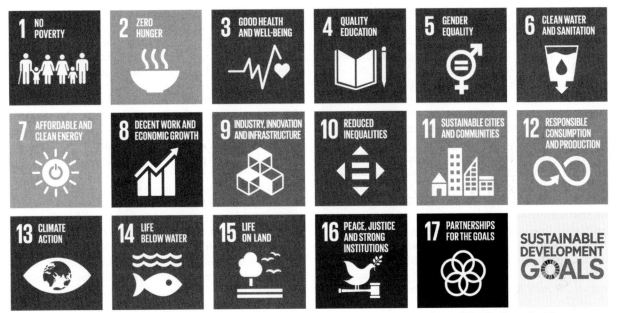

Figure 1.2 Global Sustainable Development Goals. (From United Nations. [2015]. *Sustainable Development Goals kick off with start of new year*. Retrieved from https://www.un.org/sustainabledevelopment/)

not expose the user to financial hardship" (World Health Organization, n.d.).

Consider how important it is to look at integrated and intersectoral approaches to issues such as urbanization, where major geographic and demographic shifts are significantly altering global land use, environment, and health (Haase, Güneralp, Dahiya et al., 2018). Urbanization aligns with multiple SDGs; these include SDG 3, Good Health and Well-Being; SDG 7, Affordable and Clean Energy; SDG 11, Sustainable Cities and Communities; SDG 12, Responsible Consumption and Production; and SDG 13, Climate Action (see Figure 1.2). There is an expectation that, between now and 2050, the urban population will grow from 55% to 68% of all people but, perhaps more significantly, 90% of the increase in urban dwellers will be in African and Asian centres (United Nations Department of Economic and Social Affairs, 2018).

Canada features diverse geography and demographic characteristics. Although the country is becoming increasingly urbanized, about 18.9% of the population remains in rural and remote communities (Sibley & Weiner, 2011). A significant problem facing these communities has been the lack of health care providers; solutions must address local transportation issues and alternative means of connecting people to their health care providers (i.e., telemedicine, remote monitoring) (Nagle, Sermeus, & Junger, 2017). The issue of having enough trained health care providers closely aligns with SDG 3, Good Health and Well-Being (see Figure 1.2). However, urbanization is bringing increased attention to other important issues across Canada; food deserts, transportation, poverty, climate extremes management, homelessness, and substandard housing are beginning to dominate these health care system dialogues (Allen & Farber, 2019; Gough & Rozanov, 2002; Harcourt & Seymour, 2017; Slater, Epp-Koop, Jakilazek, & Green, 2017). These broader urban issues align with SDG 1, No Poverty; SDG 3, Good Health and Well-Being; SDG 11, Sustainable Cities and Communities; and SDG 13, Climate Action (see Figure 1.2).

Globally, the population aged 65 and over continues growing faster than all other age groups; the proportion aged 65 and over is expected to increase from the current 9% (1 in 11 people) to 16% (1 in 6 people) by 2050 (United Nations, 2019). This trend is mirrored in Canada's demographics, where the aging baby boomer population (also the fastest-growing age group in Canada) is anticipated to increase use of the health care system because of the increasing prevalence of chronic and age-related diseases. According to the Conference Board of Canada (2017), the demand for nursing in continuing care for seniors will increase annually by 3.4%. To meet the growing pressures, the health care system will need to remain nimble and responsive through design alternatives that shift its typical focus away from acute care.

The demographics are also shifting for regulated nurses, who make up 48% of all Canadian health care providers (CIHI, 2018). According to the Canadian Institute for Health Information (2018), "Declining numbers of new nursing graduates, growing numbers leaving the profession late in their careers and an increase in part-time and casual positions are the trends we see impacting the nursing landscape in Canada today." According to the CNA (2009), we will see a deficit of 60,000 registered nurses by 2022 if major steps are not taken to bridge the shortfall. The shortages projected in the health care workforce between 2017 and 2026 are significant—these include nurses (registered nurses (RNs), registered practical nurses (RPNs), licensed practical nurses (LPNs)), general and family practitioners, optometrists, physical therapists, and occupational therapists (Government of Canada, 2017b; see Chapter 17). Such shortages will be even more problematic in rural and remote locations, necessitating a concerted effort for future health human resources planning (Health Canada, 2016b). Globally, there are 20.7 million nurses and midwives, with an anticipated shortage of 7.6 million by 2030, primarily in Africa and eastern Mediterranean regions (World Health Organization, 2016).

A significant challenge in Canada, and indeed globally, is that universal health coverage has persistently failed to achieve equity, affordability, accessibility, and sustainability (Tuohy, 2012). Many countries, including the United States, continue to struggle with the implementation of Medicare and Medicaid-like programs. The first indications of an interest in a federal health insurance scheme in the United States is credited to President Roosevelt as part of the *Social Security Act* of 1935, but it was never formally launched (LBJ Presidential Library, n.d.). Following this initial effort, President Truman blocked a bill for health insurance for seniors in 1949. However, in 1965, President Johnson signed the first official Medicare law in the United States despite outcries that it was socialized medicine and therefore un-American (LBJ Presidential Library, n.d.). However, much resistance remains in the United States against "socialized medicine," with its full implementation and even clear directions elusive in the current political context.

In the United Kingdom, the National Health Service has existed since 1948, and it is likely one of the most comprehensive health care systems. It recently shifted to a two-tiered system of health care financing, thereby enabling both public and private systems to coexist.

In Canada, the tenacious commitment to a single-payer health care system has led some to suggest the need for more investment and a more action-oriented approach (Clark & Horton, 2018) that will allow the system to survive and thrive.

Given all we have learned so far about the Canadian health care system, what is the best way forward? Martin, Miller, Quesnel-Vallée, et al. (2018) proposed that governments, providers, and the public work together through a three-party social contract to redesign the next iteration of Canada's health care system. This redesign will require building a health care system that reflects Canadian values, maintains a single-payer (government) Medicare system, and demonstrates a financially and operationally sound approach that is sustainable. According to these authors, this decentralized model would delineate the roles and interrelationships between governments at provincial, territorial, federal, and Indigenous levels. In working through the redesign, the three parties (i.e., governments, providers, and the public) would need to recognize, anticipate, and facilitate the roles of interprofessional health teams in addressing disparities, improving the continuum of care, and building accountabilities (and co-stewardship) into the delivery of quality evidence-informed care (Nohr, 2016). One example of this three-party effort could be the passing of legislation that enables and catalyzes these interprofessional efforts.

The third stakeholder group is the public, which is often forgotten yet imperative to getting this next phase right. There is no precedent on how to fully engage the public in these dialogues and build a shared understanding, but there have been some indications of potential ways forward through targeted public-engaged health research (Canadian Institutes of Health Research, 2017).

Canada's health care system has long been admired in other jurisdictions. To maintain our position as a global leader now and in the future, we must show leadership from within as well. Our health care system has become static and, like any system, it must be maintained and rebuilt to remain current, responsive, and accountable. The next chapter of Canada's health care system has yet to be written, but the last word belongs to the Father of Medicare in Canada, the Honourable Tommy Douglas:

Let's not forget that the ultimate goal of Medicare must be to keep people well rather than just patching them up when they get sick… It means expanding and improving Medicare by providing pharmacare and denticare programs. It means promoting physical fitness through sports and other activities… It seems to me that this is the task that lies before us, and I suggest to you that programs of this kind can be organized under Medicare.

We can't stand still. We can either go back or we can go forward. The choice we make today will decide the future of Medicare in Canada!

Courage my friends, 'tis not too late to build a better world. (Douglas, 1982)

👤 APPLYING CONTENT KNOWLEDGE

You have the opportunity to question the candidates in your upcoming provincial or territorial election on their position on the future of nursing. What two questions might you pose to these candidates?

SUMMARY OF LEARNING OBJECTIVES

- The core value of the Canadian health care system is that access be based on need and not on ability to pay. Although this value is laudable, it is challenging to meet this goal equitably, efficiently, and in a fiscally responsible manner.
- The Canadian Medicare "system" is actually a cluster of 13 provincial and territorial health insurance plans that address hospital and medical services for selected members of the Canadian population through a single-payer model.
- Through legislation and policy, Canada's federal–provincial–territorial government triad has managed to adhere to the principles of the *Canada Health Act* through a social contract and numerous reformations, which has ensured co-funding, co-administration, and role delineation.

- The next phase of Medicare must involve the inclusion of all Canadians, particularly reconciliation with Indigenous peoples. The status quo is not acceptable in an environment in which certain populations are experiencing poorer health outcomes, inequities, and lack of affordable and accessible services.
- The Canadian health care system is challenged by local, regional, and global shifts, constraints, and agendas. These complex challenges create a dynamic and high-risk environment that requires a range of high-impact strategies and innovations to ensure an equitable and sustainable health care system.
- The Canadian health care system requires a clearly articulated action plan that is inclusive of all stakeholders (i.e., governments, providers, and the public) to meet the challenges of health care for generations to come.

CRITICAL THINKING QUESTIONS

1. Discuss the five principles outlined in the *Canada Health Act*, giving an applied example of each.
2. Explore reconciliation as an imperative in the Canadian health care system. What does reconciliation mean in terms of health and health care for Indigenous peoples? Governments? Non-Indigenous people?

3. Reflecting on the contents of this chapter as a new practitioner, identify three actions or key roles you might undertake to influence or contribute to the evolution of universal health care locally or globally.

REFERENCES

Agnew, G. H. (1974). *Canadian hospitals, 1920 to 1970: A dramatic half century.* Toronto, ON: University of Toronto Press.

Aldridge, R. W., Yates, T. A., Zenner, D., et al. (2014). Pre-entry screening programmes for tuberculosis in migrants to low-incidence countries: A systematic review and meta-analysis. *The Lancet Infectious Diseases, 14*(12), 1240–1249. https://doi.org/10.1016/S1473-3099(14)70966-1.

Allan, B., & Smylie, J. (2015). *First Peoples, second class treatment: The role of racism in the health and well-being of Indigenous peoples in Canada.* Toronto, ON: Wellesley Institute.

Allen, J., & Farber, M. (2019). Sizing up transport poverty: A national scale accounting of low-income households suffering from inaccessibility in Canada, and what to do about it. *Transport Policy, 74*, 214–223. https://doi.org/10.1016/j.tranpol.2018.11.018.

Allin, S., & Rudoler, D. (2017). *The Canadian health care system. International Health Care Systems Profiles.* Toronto,

ON: University of Toronto and Centre for Addiction and Mental Health. Retrieved from http://international.commonwealthfund.org/countries/canada/.

American Institute of Medical Sciences and Education. (2018, March 29). *US vs Canadian healthcare: What are the differences?* Retrieved from https://www.aimseducation.edu/blog/us-vs-canadian-healthcare-differences/.

Brown, M. C. (1980). The implications of established program finance for national health insurance. *Canadian Public Policy, 3*, 521–532.

Canadian Institute for Health Information. (2000). *Health care in Canada 2000: A first annual report.* Retrieved from https://secure.cihi.ca/free_products/eng-brochure.pdf.

Canadian Institute for Health Information. (2016). *National health expenditure trends, 1975 to 2016.* Retrieved from https://secure.cihi.ca/free_products/NHEX-Trends-Narrative-Report_2016_EN.pdf.

Canadian Institute for Health Information. (2018, June 14). *Canada's nursing workforce experiences slowest growth in a decade.* Retrieved from https://www.cihi.ca/en/canadas-nursing-workforce-experiences-slowest-growth-in-a-decade.

Canadian Institute for Health Information. (2019). *National health expenditure trends, 1975 to 2019.* Retrieved from https://www.cihi.ca/en/national-health-expenditure-trends-1975-to-2019.

Canadian Institutes of Health Research. (2017). *Strategy for patient-oriented research.* Retrieved from http://www.cihr-irsc.gc.ca/e/41204.html.

Canadian Nurses Association. (1983). *An information package on CNA's recommendations for the proposed Canada Health Act.* Ottawa, ON: Author.

Canadian Nurses Association. (2009). *Tested solutions for eliminating Canada's registered nursing shortage.* Ottawa, ON: Author. Retrieved from https://www.cna-aiic.ca/-/media/cna/page-content/pdf-en/rn_highlights_e.pdf?.

The Canadian Press. (2012, November 25). Poll: Canadians are most proud of universal medicare. *CTV News.* Retrieved from http://www.ctvnews.ca/canada/poll-canadians-are-most-proud-of-universal-medicare-1.1052929#.

The Canadian Press. (2017, January 25). Immigrants could make up one-third of Canada's population by 2036: StatsCan. *Toronto Star.* Retrieved from https://www.thestar.com/news/canada/2017/01/25/immigrants-could-make-up-one-third-of-canadas-population-by-2036-statscan.html.

Citizenship and Immigration Canada (2013). *Panel members' handbook.* Ottawa, ON: Author. Retrieved from https://www.canada.ca/en/immigration-refugees-citizenship/corporate/publications-manuals/panel-members-handbook-2013.html.

Clark, J., & Horton, R. (2018). Canada's time to act. *The Lancet, 391,* 1643–1645. https://doi.org/10.1016/S0140-6736(18)30176-4.

Collier, R. (2010). Is regionalization working? *Canadian Medical Association Journal, 182,* 331–332. https://doi.org/10.1503/cmaj.109-3167.

Collier, R. (2015). Doctors v. government: The first major fight over pay. *Canadian Medical Association Journal, 187,* E146–E147. https://doi.org/10.1503/cmaj.109-4990.

Conference Board of Canada. (2017). *Demand for nursing services challenging to meet as Canada's population ages.* Retrieved from https://www.conferenceboard.ca/press/newsrelease/17-03-14/Demand_for_Nursing_Services_Challenging_to_Meet_as_Canada_s_Population_Ages.aspx?.

Douglas, T. C. (1982, January 1). *The future of Medicare — 1982. Speeches of Tommy Douglas.* Retrieved from http://tommydouglas.blogspot.com/1982/.

Garner, R., Varriere, G., & Sanmartin, C. (2010). *The health of First Nations living off-reserve, Inuit, and Métis adults in Canada: The impact of socio-economic status on inequalities in health.* Ottawa, ON: Statistics Canada. Retrieved from https://www150.statcan.gc.ca/n1/pub/82-622-x/82-622-x2010004-eng.pdf.

Glass, H. P. (1983). *Letter to Dr. Janet Kerr. Provincial health insurance plans: Extra-billing/user charges by hospitals.* Ottawa, ON: Health and Welfare Canada.

Gough, W. A., & Rozanov, Y. (2002, May). *Impact of urbanization on the climate of Toronto, Ontario, Canada.* Toronto, ON: Paper presented at Cool Toronto—Urban Heat Island Summit.

Government of British Columbia. (2007). *Part II: Summary of Input on the Conversation on Health. Public private debate.* Retrieved from https://www.health.gov.bc.ca/library/publications/year/2007/conversation_on_health/PartII/PartII_PublicPrivateDebate.pdf.

Government of Canada. (2017a). *Budget 2017. Chapter 3—A strong Canada at home and in the world.* Retrieved from https://www.budget.gc.ca/2017/docs/plan/chap-03-en.html.

Government of Canada. (2017b). *Canadian Occupational Projection System: Data for figures in imbalances between labour demand and supply (2017–2026).* Retrieved from http://occupations.esdc.gc.ca/sppc-cops/content.jsp?cid=53&lang=en.

Government of Canada. (2017c). *Health Care in Canada.* Retrieved from https://www.canada.ca/en/immigration-refugees-citizenship/services/new-immigrants/new-life-canada/health-care-card.html.

Government of Canada. (2018). *Treaties and agreements.* Retrieved from https://www.rcaanc-cirnac.gc.ca/eng/1100100028574/1529354437231.

Government of Canada. (2019). *Lists of acts and regulations.* Retrieved from https://www.canada.ca/en/health-canada/corporate/about-health-canada/legislation-guidelines/acts-regulations/list-acts-regulations.html.

Greenwood, M., de Leeuw, S., & Lindsay, L. (2018). Challenges in health equity for Indigenous peoples in Canada. *Lancet, 391*(10131), 1645–1648. http://dx.doi.org/10.1016/S0140-6736(18)30177-6.

Guèvremont, A., Carrière, G., Bougie, E., & Kohen, D. (2017). Acute care hospitalization of Aboriginal children and youth. *Health Reports, 28*(7), 11–17. Statistics Canada, Catalogue No. 82-003-X.

Haase, D., Güneralp, B., Dahiya, B., et al. (2018). Global urbanization. In T. Elmqvist, X. Bai, N. Frantzeskaki et al.,

(Eds.), *Urban planet: Knowledge towards sustainable cities* (pp. 19–44). Cambridge, UK: Cambridge University Press.

Harcourt, M., & Seymour, N. K. (2017, March 4). Opinion: Canadian cities face complex problems in the urban century. *Vancouver Sun*. Retrieved from https://vancouversun.com/opinion/opinion-canadian-cities-in-the-urban-century/.

Health Canada. (2006). *Health care system—A 10-year plan to strengthen health care*. Retrieved from https://www.canada.ca/en/health-canada/services/health-care-system/health-care-system-delivery/federal-provincial-territorial-collaboration/first-ministers-meeting-year-plan-2004/10-year-plan-strengthen-health-care-backgrounders.html.

Health Canada. (2011). *Canada Health Act—Frequently asked questions*. Retrieved from https://www.canada.ca/en/health-canada/services/health-care-system/canada-health-care-system-medicare/canada-health-act-frequently-asked-questions.html.

Health Canada. (2016a). *Canada's health care system*. Retrieved from https://www.canada.ca/en/health-canada/services/canada-health-care-system.html.

Health Canada. (2016b). *Health care system—Committee on Health Workforce*. Retrieved from https://www.canada.ca/en/health-human-resources/committee-health-workforce.html.

Health Canada. (2017). *Canada Health Act Annual Report 2015–2016*. Retrieved from https://www.canada.ca/en/health-canada/services/publications/health-system-services/canada-health-act-annual-report-2015-2016.html.

International Coalition on AIDS and Development. (2016). *International literature review of newcomer, migrant and refugee health*. Retrieved from http://www.icad-cisd.com/pdf/NMRH/NMRH-International-Lit-Review-FINAL.pdf.

Institute of Public Administration of Canada. (2013). *Healthcare governance models in Canada: A provincial perspective*. Retrieved from https://neltoolkit.rnao.ca/sites/default/files/Healthcare%20Governance%20Models%20in%20Canada_A%20Provincial%20Perspective_Pre-Summit%20Disscussion%20Paper%20March%202013.pdf.

Joshi, C., Russell, G., Cheng, I., et al. (2013). A narrative synthesis of the impact of primary health care delivery models for refugees in resettlement countries on access, quality and coordination. *International Journal of Equity in Health, 12*, 88. https://doi.org/10.1186/1475-9276-12-88.

Kirby, M. J. L. (2002). *The health of Canadians—The federal role. Volume six: Recommendations for reform*. Ottawa, ON: Standing Senate Committee on Social Affairs, Science and Technology. Retrieved from https://sencanada.ca/content/sen/committee/372/soci/rep/repoct02vol6-e.htm.

Kondro, W. (2010). Nation's physicians urge re-opening of Canada Health Act. *Canadian Medical Association Journal, 182*(13), 1408. https://doi.org/10.1503/cmaj.109-3352.

Law, M. R., Kratzer, J., & Dhalla, I. A. (2014). The increasing inefficiency of private health insurance in Canada. *Canadian Medial Association Journal, 186*, E470–E474. https://doi.org/10.1503/cmaj.130913.

LBJ Presidential Library. (n.d.). *Medicare and Medicaid*. Retrieved from http://www.lbjlibrary.org/press/media-kit/medicare-and-medicaid.

Marchildon, G. P. (2013). Canada: Health system review. *Health Systems in Transition, 15*, 1–179.

Martin, D. (2017). Better now: Six ideas to transform Canadian health care. Retrieved from http://www.6bigideas.ca/assets/uploads/sbi/Better-Now-Toolkit.pdf.

Martin, D., Miller, A. P., Quesnel-Vallée, A., et al. (2018). Canada's universal health-care system: Achieving its potential. *Lancet, 391*(10131), 1718–1735. https://doi.org/10.1016/S0140-6736(18)30181-8.

McIntosh, T., Ducie, M., Burka-Charles, M., et al. (2010). Population health and health system reform: Needs-based funding for health services in five provinces. *Canadian Political Science Review, 4*, 42–61.

McKeary, M., & Newbold, B. (2010). Barriers to care: The challenges for Canadian refugees and their health care providers. *Journal of Refugee Studies, 23*, 23–45. https://doi.org/10.1093/jrs/feq038.

Nagle, L., Sermeus, W., & Junger, A. (2017). Evolving role of the nursing informatics specialist. In J. Murphy, W. Goossen, & P. Weber. (Eds.), *Forecasting informatics competencies for nurses in the future of connected health* (pp. 212-221). https://doi.org/10.3233/978-1-61499-738-2-212.

Nixon, S. A., Lee, K., Bhutta, Z. A., et al. (2018). Canada's global health role: Supporting equity and global citizenship as a middle power. *Lancet, 391*(10131), 1736–1748. https://doi.org/10.1016/S0140-6736(18)30322-2.

Nohr, C. W. (2016). *Stewardship in an integrated health care system*. Retrieved from https://www.albertadoctors.org/services/media-publications/newsletters-magazines/digest/digest-archive/integrated-health-care-system-stewardship.

Organisation for Economic Co-operation and Development. (2018). *Foreign-born population*. Retrieved from https://data.oecd.org/migration/foreign-born-population.htm.

Organisation for Economic Co-operation and Development. (2019a). *Health expenditure and financing*. Retrieved from https://stats.oecd.org/Index.aspx?DataSetCode=SHAcd.

Organisation for Economic Co-operation and Development. (2019b). *Pharmaceutical spending (indicator)*. https://doi.org/10.1787/998febf6-en.

Philpott, J. (2018). *Speech of Minister Jane Philpott on The Lancet Series: Canada's global leadership on health*. Retrieved from https://www.canada.ca/en/indigenous-services-canada/news/2018/04/the-lancet-series-canadas-global-leadership-on-health.html.

Premier's Advisory Council on Health. (2002). *A framework for reform: Report of the Premier's Advisory Council on Health (Mazankowski report)*. Edmonton, AB: Government of Alberta. Retrieved from https://open.alberta.ca/publications/0778515478#detailed.

Pulver, L. J., Haswell, M. R., Ring, I., et al. (2010). *Indigenous Health—Australia, Canada, Aotearoa New Zealand and the United States—Laying claim to a future that embraces health for us all*. World Health Report, Background Paper 33. Geneva, Switzerland: World Health Organization. Retrieved from http://www.who.int/healthsystems/topics/financing/healthreport/IHNo33.pdf.

Reading, C. (2015). Structural determinants of Aboriginal peoples' health. In M. Greenwood, S. de Leeuw, N. N. Lindsay,

& C. Reading (Eds.), *Determinants of Indigenous peoples' health in Canada: Beyond the social* (pp. 3–13). Toronto, ON: Canadian Scholars' Press.

Redditt, V. J., Janakiram, P., Graziano, D., & Rashid, M. (2015). Health status of newly arrived refugees in Toronto, Ont. Part 1: Infectious diseases. *Canadian Family Physician, 61*, e303–e309.

Romanow, R. J. (2002). *Building on values: The future of health care in Canada—Final report.* Ottawa, ON: Commission on the Future of Health Care in Canada.

Royal Commission on Health Services. (1965). *Hall Commission Report (Vol. 2).* Ottawa, ON: Author.

Schuessler, J. B., Wilder, B., & Byrd, L. W. (2012). Reflective journaling and development of cultural humility in students. *Nursing Education Perspectives, 33*(2), 96–99. https://doi.org/10.5480/1536-5026-33.2.96.

Setia, M. S., Quesnel-Vallée, A., Abrahamowicz, M., et al. (2011). Access to health care in Canadian immigrants: A longitudinal study of the National Population Health Survey. *Health and Social Care in the Community, 19*(1), 70–79. https://doi.org/10.1111/j.1365-2524.2010.00950.x.

Sheppard, A. J., Shapiro, G. D., Bushnok, T., et al. (2017). *Birth outcomes among First Nations*, Inuit and Métis populations. Health Reports, *28*(11), 11–16. Statistics Canada, Catalogue No. 82-003-X.

Sibbald, B. (2017). Impasse over federal health transfers. *Canadian Medical Association Journal, 189*, E127–E128. https://doi.org/10.1503/cmaj.109-5376.

Sibley, L. M., & Weiner, J. P. (2011). An evaluation of access to health care services along the rural–urban continuum in Canada. *BMC Health Services Research, 11*, 20.

Slater, J., Epp-Koop, S., Jakilazek, M., & Green, C. (2017). Food deserts in Winnipeg, Canada: A novel method for measuring a complex and contested construct. *Health Promotion for Chronic Disease Prevention in Canada, 37*(10), 350–356. https://doi.org/10.24095/hpcdp.37.10.05.

Statistics Canada. (2016). Immigration and ethnocultural diversity in Canada. Ottawa, ON: Author. Retrieved from http://www12.statcan.gc.ca/nhs-enm/2011/as-sa/99-010-x/99-010-x2011001-eng.cfm.

Statistics Canada. (2017a). *Aboriginal peoples in Canada: Key results from the 2016 Census.* Retrieved from https://www150.statcan.gc.ca/n1/daily-quotidien/171025/dq171025a-eng.htm.

Statistics Canada. (2017b). *Life expectancy.* Retrieved from https://www150.statcan.gc.ca/n1/pub/89-645-x/2010001/life-expectancy-esperance-vie-eng.htm.

Storch, J. (2006). Canadian health care system. In M. McIntyre, E. Thomlinson, & C. McDonald (Eds.), *Realities of Canadian nursing: Professional, practice, and power issues* (pp. 29–53). Philadelphia, PA: Lippincott Williams & Wilkins.

Taylor, M. G. (1978). *Health insurance and Canadian public policy: The seven decisions that created the Canadian health insurance system and their outcomes.* Montreal, QC: McGill–Queen's University Press.

Trudeau, J. (2018). Canada's vision for global health and gender equality. *Lancet, 391*, 1651–1653. https://doi.org/10.1016/S0140-6736(18)30180-6.

Truth and Reconciliation Commission of Canada. (2015). *Honouring the truth, reconciling for the future: Summary of the final report.* Retrieved from http://www.trc.ca/assets/pdf/Honouring_the_Truth_Reconciling_for_the_Future_July_23_2015.pdf.

Tuohy, C. H. (2012). Reform and the politics of hybridization in mature health care states. *Journal of Health Politics, Policy, and Law, 37*, 611–632. https://doi.org/10.1215/03616878-1597448.

United Nations. (2019). *Ageing.* Retrieved from https://www.un.org/en/sections/issues-depth/ageing/.

United Nations Department of Economic and Social Affairs. (2018). *World urbanization prospects: The 2018 revision.* Retrieved from https://www.un.org/development/desa/en/news/population/2018-revision-of-world-urbanization-prospects.html.

United Nations Development Programme. (2019). *Sustainable Development Goals.* Retrieved from https://www.undp.org/content/undp/en/home/sustainable-development-goals.html.

Vang, Z. M., Sigouin, J., Flenon, A., & Gagnon, A. (2017). Are immigrants healthier than native-born Canadians? A systematic review of the healthy immigrant effect in Canada. *Ethnicity and Health, 22*, 209–241. https://doi.org/10.1080/13557858.2016.

Vayda, E., Evans, R., & Mindell, W. R. (1979). Universal health insurance in Canada: History, problems, trends. *Journal of Community Health, 4*(3), 217–231.

Wallace, E. (1980). The origin of the social welfare state in Canada, 1867–1900. In C. A. Meilicke & J. L. Storch (Eds.), *Perspectives on Canadian health and social services policy: History and emerging trends* (pp. 25–37). Ann Arbor, MI: Health Administration Press.

Wayland, S. V. (2006). *Unsettled: Legal and policy barriers for newcomers to Canada.* Retrieved from https://dalspace.library.dal.ca/bitstream/handle/10222/10465/Wayland%20Research%20Immigrant%20Settlement%20EN.pdf.

World Bank. (2017). Current health expenditures (% of GDP). Retrieved from https://data.worldbank.org/indicator/SH.XPD.CHEX.GD.ZS.

World Bank. (2018). *World Development Indicators.* Retrieved from https://databank.worldbank.org/source/world-development-indicators.

World Bank Group. (2019). *Current health expenditures per capita (current US$).* Retrieved from https://data.worldbank.org/indicator/SH.XPD.CHEX.PC.CD.

World Health Organization. (n.d.). *Health financing.* Retrieved from https://www.who.int/health_financing/universal_coverage_definition/en/.

World Health Organization. (2016). *Global strategy on human resources for health: Workforce 2030.* Geneva, Switzerland: Author. Retrieved from https://www.who.int/hrh/resources/globstrathrh-2030/en/.

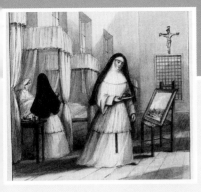

Nursing in Canada, 1600s to the Present: A Brief Account

Pauline Paul

http://evolve.elsevier.com/Canada/Ross-Kerr/nursing

LEARNING OBJECTIVES

After reading this chapter, you will be able to:
- Explain the influence of historical factors on contemporary nursing trends and issues.
- Describe the unique contribution of nurses from New France to the development of nursing in Canada in the seventeenth century.
- Describe the survival and gradual expansion of nursing between 1763 and 1874.
- Describe the link between the advent of modern nursing in Canada in the late 1800s and Florence Nightingale's reforms.

- Explain why nurses saw the need to create professional nursing organizations in the early 1900s.
- Describe the roles Canadian nurses have played during major armed conflicts.
- Describe the roles of Canadian nurses in community and hospital settings throughout history.

OUTLINE

KEY TERMS

apothecary
cloistered (noncloistered) order of nuns
Crusades
New France

nuns
Nursing Sisters
nursing order

PERSONAL PERSPECTIVES

For many years, nurses wore a nursing pin attached to their uniforms. Some nurses still do. Nursing pins are one of the oldest traditions of nursing. According to Rode (1989), these pins are descendants of the Maltese Cross that adorned the habits of the Hospitallers of Saint John of Jerusalem. The Hospitallers were knights who provided care to those who traveled during the **Crusades**. Graduates of the Nightingale Saint Thomas' Hospital in London were given a badge with a Maltese Cross on it. Eventually, badges became pins, with each school of nursing designing its own pin. The pin depicted here is from the Winnipeg General Hospital Training School of Nursing. The school opened its doors in 1887 and was the second in Canada. It would have been worn by a Canadian Nursing Sister during World War I. Like many school pins in the country, a red cross was a prominent feature. When in clinical settings, the reader should check to see whether some nurses wear their school pins.

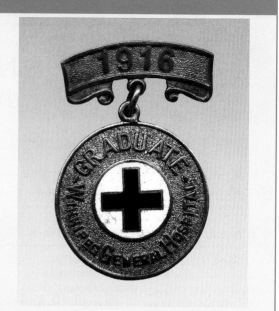

(Canadian War Museum. With permission from National Library of Medicine.)

INTRODUCTION

Studying the history of nursing reveals the contextual factors that continue to shape contemporary nursing issues. Many of the factors influencing nursing today, albeit in a slightly different form, have been with the profession for decades, if not longer. As stated by the American Association for the History of Nursing (2001, p. 1), "The social pressures that have shaped nursing in the past persist today in new forms. Today's challenges are not easily understood or addressed in the absence of such insight." The ample attention given to history in this text is essential to understanding nursing in the twenty-first century.

This chapter provides a cursory review of the evolution of nursing as a profession in Canada; a review of the development of nursing education is presented in Chapter 20. Additional insights into the historical background of nursing and nursing education have been integrated into detailed analyses of the major issues facing the profession in Canada; these analyses are dispersed throughout this text. The observant reader may be surprised to discover that many older references are used in this chapter. However, these older references are seminal and remain the best sources available.

NURSING IN NEW FRANCE: 1600 TO 1759

As a result of Jacques Cartier's numerous voyages across the Atlantic, including his 1535 landing in Newfoundland, France laid claim to the vast area along the St. Lawrence River that would one day be known as Canada. This land would be explored and settled over the next century. Samuel de Champlain established the first French settlement in what is now called Nova Scotia. He later founded a settlement in 1608 that would become the city of Québec; this beautiful sheltered spot would serve as an ideal trading centre for the growing fur trade.

The story of the early colonization of **New France** parallels the development of nursing, because the establishment of hospitals and a health care system preceded the general settlement of the colony. The development of health care in the new colony was of prime importance, as the French had a long tradition of providing care to the ill. At the outset, and for many years thereafter, human services—including health care, education, and social welfare—were primarily provided to the many First Nations living in the region. Spurred by religious fervour, **nuns** and priests made great efforts to befriend and subsequently convert Indigenous peoples to Christianity. However, historians have also shed light on how settlers who arrived from France were in turn influenced by Indigenous peoples. For example, French settlers were introduced to new means of transportation, new food, and new ways of thinking (Mouhot, 2002). The role of nurses in colonization and the impact of colonization on the health of Indigenous peoples is examined in greater depth in Chapter 14.

The First Nurses in New France

The first nurses in New France demonstrated exceptional courage, altruism, and skill and thus left behind an important legacy. Long before the first Europeans arrived, however, the thousands of Indigenous peoples living in the region were already following their own health practices; these practices were holistic and included the use of medicinal plants (Wytenbroek & Vanderberg, 2017). The first Europeans to tend the sick, in the region that would become Canada, were male attendants at a "sick bay" established in 1629 at the French garrison in Port Royal in Acadia (Gibbon & Mathewson, 1947). At that time, the Jesuit priests, who were missionary immigrants to New France, found themselves caring for the sick in the course of performing their primary duties as Christian missionaries. They "singly or in pairs travelled in the depth of winter from village to village, ministering to the sick and seeking to commend their religious teachings by their efforts to relieve bodily distress" (Parkman, 1897, p. 176).

Marie Rolet

The first European laywoman who cared for the sick in her home in the community was Marie Rolet, who was married to **apothecary** Louis Hébert. The Hébert family emigrated to Quebec in 1617, and Marie Rolet became the first woman to emigrate from France (Bennett, 1966/1979, n.p.). In Quebec, Louis Hébert's "apothecary skill and his small store of grain were a godsend to the sick and starving winterers. In spite of the company's demands on his and his servant's time, he succeeded in clearing and planting some land" (Bennett, 1966/1979, n.p.), and "Marie Rolet aided her husband in caring for the sick" (Bennett, 1966/2018, n.p). Rolet's involvement was quite natural, as it was common for French wives in the early seventeenth century to collaborate with their husbands in their work.

She also expressed genuine concern for the First Nations people. Her and her husband's efforts to care for First Nations people and to share their health knowledge appear to have been welcomed (Thwaites, 1959). European settlers also benefited from the knowledge of Indigenous peoples. For example, records show that the First Nations of the St. Lawrence River valley knew of the healing properties of conifers, particularly for treating conditions like scurvy. By boiling pine needles and parts of the bark, vitamin C was released; this decoction saved Jacques Cartier and his critically ill crew during the winter of 1536 (Durzan, 2009).

A Call for Nurses

The people of France learned about the new colony through the *Jesuit Relations*, informative reports written regularly by the Jesuit missionary priests to spread word about colonial life and stimulate much-needed financial support. These reports were written over a 72-year period and provide a marvellous account of life in early Canada: "It was clear to the fathers that their ministrations were valued solely because their religion was supposed by many to be a 'medicine' or charm, efficacious against disease and death" (Parkman, 1897, p. 179). The priests sent urgent requests for nurses to join the colony to assist with their work. In 1634, Father LeJeune wrote in his *Jesuit Relations*:

> If we had a hospital here, all the sick people of the country, and all the old people, would be there. As to the men, we will take care of them according to our means; but, in regard to the women, it is not becoming for us to receive them into our houses. (Kenton, 1925, p. 49)

Questions of propriety, an important aspect of the culture at the time, made it difficult for the Jesuit priests to treat Indigenous women who were ill on missionary premises. This issue presented another pressing reason for female members of a **nursing order** to bring their skills to Canada to assist with this work. Consider how curious it is that "Quebec, as we have seen, had a seminary, a hospital, and a convent, before it had a population" (Parkman, 1897, p. 259).

Hospitalières de la Miséricorde de Jésus

The Duchesse d'Aiguillon, a niece of Cardinal Richelieu—who, besides being a cardinal, was a powerful minister in the French government of King Louis XIII—read and was moved by the *Jesuit Relations* and developed a plan to build the Hôtel-Dieu at Québec. She used her influence to obtain a grant of land and arranged for the careful selection of three Augustinian nuns of the Hospitalières de la Miséricorde de Jésus, also known as Les Augustines, to go to Canada to establish the hospital. The three nuns, who all came from good families, were Marie Guenet de St. Ignace (later Mère de St. Ignace), Anne Lecointre de St. Bernard, and Marie Forestier de St. Bonaventure de Jésus. Aboard the ship at Dieppe, the "hospital nuns" encountered three Ursuline nuns, whose mission was to teach Indigenous people, and Madame de la Peltrie, who intended to help establish a convent school for Indigenous children. The voyage was perilous, lasting from May to August 1639 (Juchereau & Duplessis, 1939/1984). Upon their arrival, the women began work immediately:

> The Hospital Nuns arrived at Kebec on the first day of August of last year. Scarcely had they disembarked

*before they found themselves overwhelmed with pa-
tients. The hall of the hospital being too small, it was
necessary to erect some cabins, fashioned like those of
the [Aboriginal people], in their garden. Not having
furniture for so many people, they had to cut in two
or three pieces part of the blankets and sheets they had
brought for these poor sick people . . . The sick came
from all directions in such numbers, their stench was
so insupportable, the heat so great, the fresh food so
scarce and so poor, in a country so new and strange.*
(Kenton, 1925, p. 157)

The smallpox epidemic, which was raging upon the
sisters' arrival and for a considerable time thereafter, also
required the labour of the Ursuline nuns, whose school convent became a hospital and who "found themselves nursing instead of teaching" (Millman, 1965, p. 424). Jamieson
commented that the Ursulines used Indigenous women for
assistance in their hospitals and that "their teacher training was instrumental in providing the earliest instruction
and supervision of nurses in America" (Jamieson, Sewall, &
Gjertson, 1959, p. 196).

New recruits from Dieppe were sought, and the first two
arrived the following summer. The nuns also moved their
base of operations to Sillery, a settlement outside Québec,
in a more convenient location for the Indigenous people.
The structure in which the nuns had spent their first winter had proved inadequate for withstanding the winter elements, and a new building was constructed in Sillery. Soon
the hospital was inundated with Indigenous patients, and
many had to be cared for in adjacent cabins. With considerable regret, the nuns had to abandon their white habits for
a more serviceable brown. They also applied themselves to
learning the language of the Hurons and Algonquins, the
First Nations people for whom they provided care (Gibbon
& Mathewson, 1947). These statements about the early
days of the Augustines in Quebec by classic authors such
as Gibbon and Mathewson (1947), Jamieson, Sewall, and
Gjertson (1959), and Millman (1965) can be confirmed by
reading *Les Annales de l'Hôtel-Dieu de Québec 1636–1716*.
The *Annales* were a daily account written in old French by
sisters Juchereau and Duplessis. First published in 1939,
they were reprinted in 1984.

In 1644, Governor de Montmagny implored the sisters
to return to the safety of Québec, because the Iroquois were
reported to be threatening an attack, and the sisters would
be in danger if they remained in Sillery. They returned
and were lodged in temporary quarters while a new hospital was constructed, with the latter being completed only
2 years later. During the smallpox epidemic of 1650, the
number of patients received was so great that they could
not all be accommodated in the hospital. The sisters also

considered it their duty to assist new settling families in the
province of Quebec as much as they could. The archives of
the Hôtel-Dieu de Québec contain a letter from Vincent de
Paul, written in April 1652, in which he states "I consider
this enterprise as one of the greatest accomplished within
fifteen hundred years" (Gibbon & Mathewson, 1947, p. 15).
By 1671, the nuns were obtaining sufficient local recruits to
the order that they no longer depended on assistance from
France.

In 1690, hostilities broke out once more between the
British and the French, and the sisters of the Hôtel-Dieu de
Québec found themselves in the middle of the conflict. It
is reported that 26 cannonballs hit the hospital on a single
day of heavy fighting. The siege was over in 4 days, and the
British withdrew. Epidemics recurred from time to time;
the worst appears to have been a smallpox epidemic in
1703, when more than a quarter of the nuns died:

*Our sisters fell ill in such numbers from the very first
that there were not enough of those who were well to
look after the infected cases in our rooms and wards.
We accepted the offer of service from several good
widows.* (Gibbon & Mathewson, 1947, p. 35)

Jeanne Mance

Born in 1606 to wealthy parents of 12 children in Langres,
France, Jeanne Mance attended a girls' school and decided
at an early age that she was going to devote her life to God.
Following the death of her parents, she looked after her
younger brothers and sisters. When Langres was hit by
an epidemic of the plague, Jeanne Mance assisted other
women in the community in caring for the sick. She also
gained experience nursing casualties of the Thirty Years'
War. A cousin who was a Jesuit priest made plans to go
to New France, and this interested Mance, who began to
investigate how she could be of service in the New World
(Daveluy, 1966/2017).

La Société de Notre Dame de Jésus was composed of a
group of philanthropists who wanted to establish a colony
of a religious character to work with First Nations on the
Island of Montreal. This was no easy matter because they
had to secure the charter for the land and raise sufficient
funds to send a carefully selected group of people to create the society they had in mind. They thought, however,
that the hospital might be begun at once. Mance had been
reading the *Jesuit Relations* regularly and believed she was
being called to serve in the New World. Through the wealth
of Madame de Bullion, Mance was asked to take charge of
building a hospital in the settlement that was to be established at Montreal. Thus, she sailed from La Rochelle in
1641, along with three women and 40 men, under the
leadership of Paul de Chomédey, sieur de Maisonneuve

(Canadian Nurses Association [CNA], 1968). Their two ships arrived in Quebec, but their reception was not a welcoming one:

> They arrived too late in the season to ascend to Montreal before winter. They encountered distrust, jealousy, and opposition. The agents of the company of the Hundred Associates looked on them askance; and the Governor of Quebec, Montmagny, saw a rival governor in Maisonneuve. Every means was used to persuade the adventurers to abandon their project, and settle at Quebec. (Parkman, 1897, p. 296)

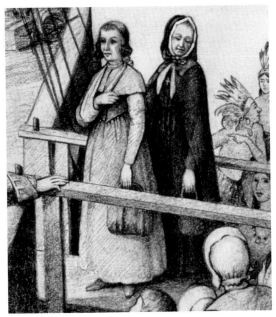

Marguerite Bourgeoys and Jeanne Mance, her broken arm in a sling, are depicted boarding a ship to France in 1657 to solicit funds for the struggling colony of Montreal. (Marguerite Bourgeoys and Jeanne Mance, Rose-Alma Dufresne, CND, Marguerite Bourgeoys Museum, Montreal)

Steadfast in his resolve to accomplish the mission to establish a settlement at Montreal, Maisonneuve "expressed his surprise that they should assume to direct his affairs. 'I have not come here,' he said, 'to deliberate, but to act. It is my duty and my honour to found a colony at Montreal; and I would go, if every tree were an Iroquois!'" (Parkman, 1897, pp. 296–297). The group had difficulty finding housing for the winter, but through the generosity of one colonist, they were housed at St. Michel. Jeanne Mance found that her neighbours were the hospital nuns who lived in their mission at Sillery, not far from Québec. Here she spent a good deal of her time assisting in the work of the hospital, and this undoubtedly served her well as she ventured to Montreal as the only person with health care knowledge.

When, on May 17, 1642, Maisonneuve and his followers landed at Ville-Marie (Montreal), the Associates of Montreal took possession of the land that "Champlain, thirty-one years before, had chosen as the fit site of a settlement" (Parkman, 1897, p. 302). They gave thanks and then proceeded to establish their settlement. The hospital was one of the first buildings constructed in the colony, although there were apparently some misgivings:

> It is true that the hospital was not wanted, as no one was sick at Villemarie, and one or two chambers would have sufficed for every prospective necessity; but it will be remembered that the colony had been established in order that a hospital might be built... Instead then of tilling the land to supply their own pressing needs, all labourers of the settlement were set at this pious though superfluous task. (Parkman, 1897, p. 362)

The hospital was 46 m by 18.5 m and contained a kitchen, living quarters for Jeanne Mance and for the servants, and two large areas for the patients. "It was amply provided with furniture, linen, medicine and all necessaries and had two oxen, three cows and 20 sheep. A small oratory of stone was built adjoining it" (Parkman, 1897, pp. 362–363). A palisade was constructed around it because of the considerable danger of Iroquois attacks. "Here Mademoiselle Mance took up her abode and waited the day when wounds or disease should bring patients to her empty wards" (Parkman, 1897, p. 363). All the new settlers were committed to the objective of converting the First Nations people to Christianity and sought to gain their favour in whatever way they could: "If they could persuade them to be nursed, they were consigned to the tender care of Mademoiselle Mance" (Parkman, 1897, p. 364). A year after its founding, Montreal became the target of the Iroquois, and Mance had

> her hands full attending to men wounded by their arrows. She dressed wounds of all kinds. Chilblains and frostbite frequently required her attention. According to the Clerk of the Court, she had mortar, scales, a syringe with ivory tube, razors and lances. She had sufficient skill to compound her own medicines, and also had experience in blood letting. (Gibbon & Mathewson, 1947, pp. 25–26)

Mance was soon in need of more help than the one young girl who had come with her, so she enlisted the assistance of two others to cope with the patient load. Mance made three voyages back to France: one 4 years after her arrival, one in 1657, and one in 1663. Her mission was to meet with members of the Associates of Notre Dame of Montreal and other benefactors to generate financial resources for her hospital. Just like today, funding was necessary to operate a hospital. Jeanne Mance was also worried about succession. She arranged for assistance from a nursing order in France in 1659; three nuns of St. Joseph de la Flèche arrived thereafter to assist in nursing the sick in her hospital, of which she remained the administrator. By 1663, the Associates were bankrupt and could no longer continue their assistance to the colony and the hospital. They transferred their interests to the Gentlemen of Saint Sulpice, and Mance witnessed the transfer of ownership to this group. When she died in 1673, she was "universally respected and beloved by the Colony which she had helped to found" (Gibbon & Mathewson, 1947, p. 30).

Jeanne Mance is one of the most celebrated nurses in Canadian nursing history. Co-founder of the city of Montreal, she was held in high regard for the hospital she founded and the work she did ministering to First Nations people and settlers alike. She was Maisonneuve's confidante, advisor, and accountant. Without her, the colony would not have become as strong. Today, the highest award of the Canadian Nurses Association for contribution to the profession is named the Jeanne Mance Award.

The Grey Nuns of Montreal

Marie-Marguerite Dufrost de Lajemmerais was born in Varennes, Quebec. Niece of the famed explorer La Vérendrye, she became Marguerite d'Youville after marrying a fur trader who was also notorious as a bootlegger and gambler and who died in less than a decade, leaving his family in debt. After his death, Marguerite d'Youville drew on her religious faith and gathered a group of like-minded women to assist her. The Sisters of Charity of Montreal, or les Soeurs Grises (the Grey Nuns), the nursing order of nuns she founded in 1736, are considered the first visiting nurses in Canada. The Grey Nuns order was the first **non-cloistered order** to be established in Canada, patterned after the model initiated by St. Vincent de Paul. Madame d'Youville organized this group of women with charitable intentions, and they "agreed to combine their possessions in a house of refuge chiefly for the poor" (Gibbon & Mathewson, 1947, p. 45).

Life was by no means easy for them because they had to raise funds to subsist and carry on their work with the sick and the poor. For the purpose of raising money, wealthy paying guests were taken in, and the sisters did handiwork that they sold. Because it was not a **cloistered order**, and because it took up the nursing of patients in their homes (something not previously done in Canada),

there was originally some mistrust of its work and intentions. "Though they usually did their visiting in pairs for self-protection, the Grey Nuns were innovators and subject to misunderstanding" (Gibbon & Mathewson, 1947, p. 46). The other orders of nuns working in Canada, the Augustinians in Québec and the St. Joseph's Hospitallers of Montreal, were cloistered and thus not permitted to venture into the community except in an emergency by special permission of the bishop.

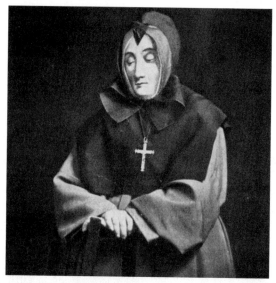

Canonized in 1990, Marguerite d'Youville, founder of the Grey Nuns, pioneered home visits and was renowned for her excellent care regardless of a patient's race, status, or religion. (Albert Ferland. Vénérable Mère d'Youville, 1900. Musée de la civilisation, dépôt du Séminaire de Québec, 1993.21409)

A fire in 1745 destroyed their house, and the Grey Nuns were forced to move from one place to another for the next 2 years to carry on their work. Then, the Gentlemen of Saint Sulpice gave permission for d'Youville and the Grey Nuns to take over the General Hospital under a charter as the Soeurs de la Charité de l'Hôpital Général de Montréal. The Grey Nuns' debts were so great that they had to resort to all sorts of new fundraising activities, including making military garments and tents, establishing a brewery and a tobacco plant, and operating a freight and cartage business. Patients who regained health as a result of the nuns' charitable efforts were put to work to aid in the fundraising effort (Gibbon & Mathewson, 1947, p. 47).

When war broke out between the British and the French in 1756, a section of the hospital called the Ward of the

English was opened to care for wounded English soldiers. The sisters were sufficiently generous of spirit to provide refuge to escaped English soldiers. "One of these English showed his gratitude, in 1760, by saving the hospital from the artillery fire of the army of invasion" (Gibbon & Mathewson, 1947, p. 48). In 1760, the transfer of authority over Montreal to the British brought with it statements testifying to the high regard in which the sisters were held. General Amherst spoke

"of the goodwill I have to a Society so worthy of respect as that of the Monastery of St. Joseph de l'Hôtel-Dieu de Montréal, which can count so far as the British Nation is concerned on the same protection that it has enjoyed under French rule" (Gibbon & Mathewson, 1947, p. 48).

The Status of Nursing in Canada in the Seventeenth and Eighteenth Centuries

There was a marked contrast between Canada and Britain in the status of nursing and the quality of care provided in the seventeenth and eighteenth centuries. Nursing in Britain had fallen into disrepute after Henry VIII's renunciation of the Catholic Church. The nursing orders of nuns, which had previously provided the nursing service in the large London hospitals, were expelled, leading to a challenging period when nursing deteriorated.

This decline in nursing was barely evident in early Canada because the first settlement at Québec had developed as a colony of France. In France, nursing was spared the regressive period that had occurred in England. Young women of good character from reputable families continued to be recruited to nursing in France—primarily under the auspices of the Catholic Church—throughout this time.

If the settlements along the St. Lawrence River had been colonized in the seventeenth century by the English instead of the French, the history of nursing in Canada might have been very different. Circumstances, however, decided in favour of the French, a fortunate outcome for the White pioneers. In the wake of the arrival of the fur traders and coureurs de bois came several orders of French nuns—the Augustinian Hospitallers or nursing sisters of Dieppe to Québec, and the St. Joseph Hospitallers of La Flèche to Montreal—on their missions of healing and mercy; these missions had no counterpart in the colonizing efforts of the Protestant English in North America (Gibbon & Mathewson, 1947, p. 1). Consequently, the Huron and Algonquin also suffered fewer deaths due to influenza, measles, and smallpox (which had been unwittingly introduced by the French settlers) thanks to the care of the French nuns.

Health care in New France also developed unique characteristics. From its inception, the Hôtels-Dieu of New France were devoted to patient care and were more than refuges for the poor. In contrast with the Hôtels-Dieu of France, those in the colony provided care to patients of all social classes (Violette, 2005). The birth of the truly Canadian Grey Nuns was also an important milestone, since, as will be seen, they played a central role in the development of health care in Western Canada.

The health care system that had developed in the colony was firmly established when the English defeated the French in 1759 in the battle of the Plains of Abraham. Undoubtedly, the geographic separation from England and the political climate in North America ensured the continuation of the French tradition of good nursing in Canada.

SURVIVAL AND GRADUAL EXPANSION OF NURSING: 1763 TO 1874

After the war of 1756 to 1763, the transition to British rule was difficult for Quebec nursing orders. The nuns received little or no financial support because their wealthy benefactors had returned to France, and donations dwindled. Without a regular income, the nuns were impoverished at the outset of the new regime. However, in correspondence with the Duchesse d'Aiguillon, William Pitt, prime minister of Great Britain, stated that the commanding general of the British troops had "the satisfaction to be able to state that our officers, who are very strong in their praises of the charitable care of our sick and wounded by these nuns, have paid them every attention required by piety and misfortune" (Gibbon & Mathewson, 1947, p. 52). In addition, there is a record of some financial assistance from the British for the sisters. "By instruction of Pitt, General Murray relieved the Hôtel-Dieu of a debt of taxes to the extent of 3,389 livres, which had reverted to the British at the change of the regime, and also paid £808 for rent of lodgings to the troops, and £3,085 for the use of furniture, laundry and utensils of the hospital" (Gibbon & Mathewson, 1947, pp. 52–53). Nevertheless, all the hospital systems remained in place at the transfer of power.

The subsequent decades were tumultuous for the British colonies, as Americans were seeking independence. From 1775 to 1776, during the American War of Independence, the American attack on the Canadian border brought patients from each side of the battle to the Hôtel-Dieu de Québec, where all were cared for with warmth and humanity. An American lieutenant recorded the following in his diary on March 10, 1776:

Was removed to the Hotel Dieu, sick of the scarlet fever, and placed under the care of the Mother Abbess, where I had fresh provisions and good attendance. For several nights the nuns sat up with me, four at a time, every two hours. Here I feigned myself sick after I had recovered, for fear of being sent back to the Seminary to join my fellow officers, and was not discharged until I acknowledged that I was well. When I think of my captivity, I shall never forget the time spent among the nuns who treated me with so much humanity. (Gibbon & Mathewson, 1947, p. 55)

Among other hospitals that also cared for the sick and wounded was the Hôtel-Dieu de Trois-Rivières, which had been established in 1697. The tradition of caring for all regardless of race, nationality, or creed was paramount, and preservation of human life and nourishment of the spirit through religious beliefs and practices remained central characteristics of the nuns' work.

Effects of Immigration on Nursing

After the defeat of the French forces at the Plains of Abraham, the Treaty of Paris of 1763 established certain rules for the government of the colony of Quebec. Its thrust was Anglicization to attract English-speaking settlers to help rebuild the shattered economy after the war. Although the British had imagined a flood of settlement would soon help anglicize Quebec, "in fact, few people came" (Morton, 1983, p. 23). Soon the people of Quebec were recognized as Canadians, and the *Quebec Act* of 1774 restored many of their former freedoms and rights. The Act was also designed to win the support of these new Canadians in the upcoming conflict with the Americans. With some difficulty, the British were able to hold Quebec in that conflict.

After the American War of Independence, United Empire Loyalists, who wanted to remain loyal to Britain, immigrated to Canadian territory. Their numbers eventually totalled 50,000. These settlers were joined by large numbers of immigrants from Britain and Ireland. "Late Loyalists" followed during the early nineteenth century. There was also a sizeable increase in the French Canadian population, from 60,000 in 1760, to 110,000 by 1784, to 330,000 by 1860. The *Constitutional Act* of 1791 divided Quebec into Upper Canada and Lower Canada, each with its own system of government, and confirmed the rights of French Canadians as laid down earlier in the *Quebec Act*.

The devastating effects of the Napoleonic Wars (1803–1815) on trade in England led many in the British Isles to emigrate to overcome poverty. "Factory folk, miners, and farmers became equally distressed, and the British Government could do little more than divert the resulting emigration to countries where the British flag still flew" (Gibbon & Mathewson, 1947, p. 71). A majority of these immigrants were poorly nourished and travelled in "vessels which were overcrowded and unsanitary," so disease found easy prey among the new settlers.

The United Empire Loyalists, who travelled by land, avoided the unsanitary conditions of disease-infested ships and thus escaped the devastation that followed the voyages of the Europeans. Nevertheless, diseases brought by new arrivals spread rapidly among residents of the new colony. Dramatic increases in the population gave epidemic diseases more scope, and immigrants brought with them cholera, typhus, smallpox, and trachoma. In 1832, an epidemic of cholera wiped out one-seventh of the population of Montreal, or 4,000 people (Gibbon & Mathewson, 1947). To protect the Canadian population, the British imposed health examinations for immigrants, and a quarantine station and hospital were established at Grosse-Île in the St. Lawrence River. This hospital was staffed by lay nurses, including Irish and French Canadian nurses and even a Norwegian nurse (Young & Rousseau, 2005).

The rapid increase in the population of English-speaking Canada in the late eighteenth and early nineteenth centuries led to a shortage of the health care facilities made necessary by persistent waves of epidemics. The dismal state of nursing in Britain was paralleled in new areas of the colony opened up by the English and not yet served by the French nursing orders, such that "nursing in English-speaking Canada remained primitive for many years" (CNA, 1968, p. 30). Laywomen attempted nursing in the hospitals that were established, but they were largely without the proper training and skills to do what was needed. The established French-speaking sisterhoods expanded their work across the country, and new English-speaking orders were formed.

Because so many of the arriving settlers were destitute and ill, they needed a great deal of assistance. The Female Benevolent Society was organized in Montreal in 1816 and was responsible for the establishment of what would become Montreal General Hospital. In Kingston, the Kingston Compassionate Society secured a grant of land from the government and constructed the first version of Kingston General Hospital. Likewise, in York, Toronto General Hospital was founded by a philanthropic group with funds designated to buy medals for the War of 1812 (Gibbon & Mathewson, 1947). The introduction of lay nurses in areas previously served by nursing sisterhoods met with some opposition at first, but the needs of the sick and the poor had to be met,

The Grey Nuns and the Opening Up of the West

On April 24, 1844, four Grey Nuns set out in long canoes bound for St. Boniface, Manitoba. The measure of courage required for the strenuous journey is difficult to appreciate in an age when we commonly travel on superhighways. For example, on May 2, Sister Lagrave wrote,

> What shall I tell you? I can hardly collect a few thoughts. I believe the high wind has scattered them over Lake Huron, I sit on a rock: my head is spinning, my heart is fluttering . . . I have not slept since our departure . . . The bad weather is lasting and when the rain stops, contrary winds delay our progress. (Drouin, 1988, pp. 170–171)

The nuns were greeted by a series of epidemics upon their arrival in 1846, and thus from the outset they found themselves stretched far beyond their capacity. These epidemics were devastating, and the death toll was high. Sister Laurent described how they coped with the patient load:

> Each of us was appointed to do that which she was best fitted for. Some of us went into the houses where sick people were. They used to have measles and dysentery and inflammatory rheumatism, and smallpox sometimes. We had medicines from Montreal, but we also learned the uses of herbs that grew in this country, and how to help the sick people so as to ease their pain and aid them to get better. (Gibbon & Mathewson, 1947, p. 89)

In Saskatchewan and Alberta, the Grey Nuns were again the pioneers who trekked west to establish health care facilities and systems for the populace. In 1859, after a long journey first from Montreal to St. Boniface, and then by ox cart to Lac Ste. Anne (in modern-day Alberta), three Grey Nuns established their mission and began to minister to the First Nations people through nursing. Four years later, the nuns moved to St. Albert. Upon their arrival, they took the sick into their convent if they required constant care. In 1870, they added a hospital wing to their convent, and in 1881, they built a separate building. In 1860, three nuns of this order from St. Boniface arrived at Île à La Crosse, Saskatchewan, a fur trade settlement 200 miles north of Prince Albert.

Arriving before most of the settlers, the sisters established systems of quality health care. The Grey Nuns performed a great deal of visiting nursing, regularly attending to the sick in their homes, working tirelessly as one epidemic after another devastated the local population. For example, in St. Albert, Alberta, Sister Emery wrote that during the last 6 months of 1870, the sisters made 692 home visits, provided wound care to 22 patients, and vaccinated 218 children and 133 adults against smallpox (Emery, 1871).

THE ADVENT OF MODERN NURSING IN CANADA IN THE LATE 1800s

Florence Nightingale is often credited as the mother of modern nursing worldwide. Her influence on the development of modern nursing in Canada was critically important, and the principles she espoused were consistent with those of the French-Canadian **nursing sisters**.

One of Nightingale's most important contributions was the creation of the first nursing school for laywomen at St. Thomas Hospitals in London, England. Nursing schools began to open in North America soon after, and hospitals began to rely on nursing students for the provision of care (McPherson, 2005). The first Canadian school of nursing in Canada was created at St. Catharines, Ontario in 1874. Chapter 20 provides details about the development of nursing schools in Canada.

During this period, English Canada embraced nursing, and nurses who were nuns were joined by lay nurses in shaping the future of the profession in Canada. However, nursing orders remained strong and were often the first to offer services to those who ventured west. The settling of Western Canada, particularly Alberta and British Columbia, saw the arrival of other **religious orders** that would play significant roles in health services. Most of these were of French Canadian or British origin. A notable exception was the Sisters Servants of Mary Immaculate, who came from Ukraine in 1902 to provide nursing care to Ukrainian settlers in Alberta (Paul, 2005). The rise of the modern hospital, scientific developments, industrialization, and immigration were all forces that changed the nature of nursing. As the network of religious and secular hospitals gradually expanded, nursing schools flourished, and graduates began to seek recognition. In order to become recognized, nurses began creating organizations that would speak on their behalf.

🌐 CULTURAL CONSIDERATIONS
Immigrants and Health Care

In this chapter, we mention the arrival of the Sisters Servants of Mary Immaculate, who came from Ukraine in 1902. Many Ukrainian families settled in Alberta in the 1890s. They were one of the largest group of settlers who did not speak French or English when they arrived in Canada. From a patient point of view, it would have been very reassuring to be able to receive health care services in Ukrainian. Receiving services in one's mother tongue continues to be valued by patients. Today, we would describe the provision of services in the patient's preferred language, when possible, as part of cultural competence.

🌐 CULTURAL CONSIDERATIONS

Indigenous Women Healers and Nurses in Southern Alberta

> Historian Kristin Burnett (2006) has explored the role of women in providing health services between 1880 and 1930 in Southern Alberta. Her doctoral dissertation documents that settlers to this region relied on Indigenous women during childbirth. Women from the Blackfoot, Blood, Peigan, Stoney, and Sarcee First Nations were capable midwives and knowledgeable about medicinal plants; they had used this essential knowledge for centuries. As the Grey Nuns and other nurses came to the region, the First Nations people began to use their services as well. What is clear from Burnett's work is that the role of women in the provision of health services is often neglected. For example, anthropologists who came to study the Indigenous populations tended to focus on the activities of men, thus making invisible the contribution of Indigenous women. Similarly, the history of health care has focused on male physicians and thus ignored the fact that settler populations often relied on the services of nurses.

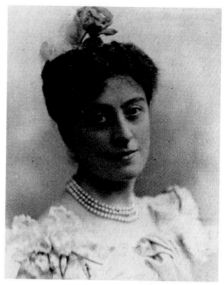

Ethel Bedford-Fenwick, 1899–1904, British nurse and lobbyist who conceived the idea of professional nursing organizations and helped form the International Council of Nurses. (Courtesy Stephen Callander-Grant, consultant editor for www.internurse.com)

ESTABLISHMENT OF NATIONAL PROFESSIONAL NURSING ORGANIZATIONS AND THEIR EVOLUTION

A leading figure in British nursing was Ethel Bedford-Fenwick. Bedford-Fenwick was influential in the formation of the first nursing organizations and was editor of the forerunner of the *British Journal of Nursing*. Attending the 1893 Congress of Charities, Corrections, and Philanthropy in Chicago, Bedford-Fenwick met the leaders in American nursing: Isabel Hampton, Adelaide Nutting, and Lavinia Dock. Interestingly, of these three nurses, two were Canadians living and working in the United States—Isabel Hampton and Adelaide Nutting. They discussed the need for a drive to secure legislation for the registration of nurses to raise the standard of professional nursing and to ensure those practising were qualified and able.

Bedford-Fenwick had been struggling to achieve comparable legislation in Britain at the time. She became convinced that to succeed, nurses had to band together and form professional organizations. The three American leaders were so impressed with the case for establishing nursing organizations that they immediately organized the American Society of Superintendents of Training Schools for Nurses of the United States and Canada, of which Isabel Hampton Robb became the first president. The major thrust of the organization never strayed from its original goal "to work for higher standards of nurse preparation." It was the forerunner of the National League for Nursing that formed in 1912 (CNA, 1968, p. 35).

Soon after, alumnae associations were established at schools of nursing in the United States. In 1896, under the leadership of its first president, Isabel Hampton Robb, the Nurses' Associated Alumnae of the United States and Canada took root. Criteria for membership included graduation from a 2-year program at minimum and association with a hospital with at least 100 beds. The organization, the forerunner of the American Nurses Association, first directed its efforts at improving the quality of educational programs and then advocating for legislation to ensure the registration of nurses. The *American Journal of Nursing* began to publish in 1900 and served as a way of communicating with nurses who could assist with developing the organization (CNA, 1968).

One of Bedford-Fenwick's major goals was the formation of an international organization of nurses. She had initiated discussions about this endeavour with American nursing leaders in Chicago, and together they decided that formation of national groups was the first priority. Although the North American organization had initially included both Canada and the United States, it was deemed necessary to separate the organizations. Since the responsibility for health care was vested at provincial and state levels, the campaign for registration of nurses would have to be decentralized. Therefore, to pursue the goal of registering nurses, separate national organizations needed to be established to assist in the development of provincial and state organizations. The International Council of Nurses (ICN) was formed in 1899, with Britain, the United States, and Germany as charter members. Canada was represented at this meeting by five nurses; Mary Agnes Snively, superintendent of nurses at Toronto General Hospital, became the first honorary treasurer of the fledgling organization.

In Canada, the Canadian Society of Superintendents of Training Schools for Nurses was the first completely Canadian national organization of nurses. It was formed in 1907 with Mary Agnes Snively as its president. The next year, the society invited representatives from all nursing organizations in Canada to meet and establish a national association of nurses. The meeting resulted in the inception of the Provisional Society of the Canadian National Association of Trained Nurses (CNATN), and Mary Agnes Snively was inducted as the founding president. Initially, members were enrolled through membership societies composed primarily of graduate nurse and alumnae associations. The first alumnae association in Canada was founded in 1894 at Toronto General Hospital (Gibbon & Mathewson, 1947). Nearly every school formed such an organization shortly thereafter, and many of these were amalgamated with other groups, at first by region and eventually by province and territory.

The CNATN applied for membership in the ICN in 1908, and formal admission took place the next year at the international meeting in London. Because the CNATN had been organized somewhat hastily for the purpose of joining the ICN, a structure that would be suitable for the national organization and would recognize the historical division of powers between the provincial–territorial and federal governments had yet to be considered.

A full-time executive secretary, Jean Wilson, was appointed to the CNATN in 1923. The first national office was opened in Winnipeg, moving later to Montreal and then to Ottawa. In the meantime, the *Canadian Nurse* had begun publication in 1905. Membership of affiliated organizations in the CNATN went from 28 in 1911 to 52 in 1924, when the association changed its name to the Canadian Nurses Association (CNA). In 1930, CNA became "a federation of the nine provincial associations, a move that has the effect of eliminating duplicate membership and making possible the first calculation of CNA individual membership" (CNA, 2013, p. 213). In 2018, the CNA announced changes to its membership criteria:

> Since its beginnings in 1908, CNA has been the national professional voice of registered nurses, which includes nurse practitioners. However, on June 18, 2018, voting delegates at CNA's annual meeting of members voted overwhelmingly in favour of expanding CNA's membership to include licensed practical nurses (known as registered practical nurses in Ontario) and registered psychiatric nurses (regulated in the four western provinces and Yukon). (CNA, 2018, n.p.)

This motion has the potential to bring these other regulated nurses into the CNA in the near future, a change that is likely the result of similar provincial trends.

Through its journal, the *Canadian Nurse*, which was first published in 1905, the CNA has a vehicle to reach nurses. At first, most articles were written by physicians, but the publication grew into a peer-reviewed journal containing research articles, general articles, columns, and professional information. The CNA also created the Canadian Nurse Portal in 2007, NurseONE, which is now known as MyCNA. This membership site provides access to the Canadian Nurse website, a learning centre, information about CNA certification, search engines, and other documents.

The Provisional Council of the Canadian Association of University Schools and Departments of Nursing held its first meeting in 1942, when representatives from eight nursing schools and departments met to respond to a proposed program of federal financial assistance. The organization was small for a considerable period of time after its founding, with the work being carried out by volunteers. In 1970, a part-time executive secretary was hired, and the name changed to the Canadian Association of University Schools of Nursing (CAUSN). It was not until 1984 that the position of executive secretary became full time. The organization changed its name to the Canadian Association of Schools of Nursing (CASN) in 2002 to reflect the expansion of its membership to include nursing schools at universities, university college partnerships, and colleges. Membership increased from 31 university schools in 1994 to 93 schools of all types in 2019. Responsibility for accreditation was incorporated into its mandate in 1973, and the first standards were published in 1987. In 2006 and 2007, a new accreditation program was initiated to reflect the various types of baccalaureate programs in nursing. A major review and revision of the accreditation program occurred in 2013 (Canadian Association of Schools of Nursing, 2019).

APPLYING CONTENT KNOWLEDGE

Nurses have developed many organizations over the years. Can you think of some common purposes behind the creation of all these organizations?

In 1962, the Canadian Nurses Foundation (CNF) was incorporated as an organization separate from the CNA to provide scholarships, bursaries, and fellowships for graduate study in nursing. Because the CNF was a charitable organization, donations could be accepted on a tax-exempt basis, thus facilitating the collection of funds for scholarships. A grant of $150,000 from the W.K. Kellogg Foundation in 1962 helped to build the fund at its inception. Membership fees, collected on a voluntary basis, provided the financial base. However, in response to continuing financial difficulties, the CNF would later develop sophisticated corporate fundraising campaigns.

Initially, the CNA and CNF operated autonomously, but developed closer links when it became clear that the financial structure of the CNF was weak. The executive director of the CNA is the secretary–treasurer of the CNF, housed in CNA House in Ottawa. During CNA biennial convention years, annual meetings of the CNF are held in association with the CNA meeting. Over time, the CNF broadened its activities to work closely with the CNA on matters of importance to both organizations.

Although it is reported that a provision was made by the CNF in 1966 to include assistance for study at the baccalaureate level (CNA, 1968, p. 11), in practice, fellowships were awarded almost exclusively for master's and doctoral study. A resolution, passed at the 1982 annual meeting in St. John's, Newfoundland, provided a mandate to award one scholarship for baccalaureate study in each province and territory each year. Today, the CNF provides awards for study at the baccalaureate, master's, and doctoral levels and some research awards (Canadian Nurses Foundation [CNF], 2019).

Created in 1975, the Canadian Indigenous Nurses Association (CINA) was the brainchild of a dedicated group of Indigenous nurses. At the time, there were no statistics on the number of Indigenous nurses in the country, so word of mouth had to be used to find a potential membership base. At its onset, the association had 41 members and was named Registered Nurses of Canadian Indian Ancestry. Its first president was Jean Goodwill, a Cree nurse from Saskatchewan. In 2010, the association updated its goals to include working on Indigenous health nursing issues, engaging in research on Indigenous Health Nursing, and promoting awareness of the health needs of Indigenous people (Canadian Indigenous Nurses Association [CINA], 2019). Data from the 2016 census confirmed that there were "13,010 health professionals identifying as Aboriginal; of which 9,695 are nurses" (University of Saskatchewan College of Nursing and CINA, 2018, n.p.) These nurses represent 74.5% of Indigenous health professionals.

NURSING IN TIMES OF CONFLICT

Nurses have played pivotal roles during military conflicts throughout Canadian history. The nursing sisters of the Hôtel-Dieu hospitals in Québec and Montreal are legendary: they remained bipartisan despite intense French–English hostilities that damaged the hospitals and injured fellow nurses. During the Northwest Rebellion of 1885, a military request for nursing services showed the influence of Florence Nightingale (see Box 2.1) and the experience gained during the American Civil War: "No volunteer nurses. If you can send an organized body under a trained head, they will be welcome" (CNA, 1968, p. 63). Two groups of nurses responded, one headed by Mother Hannah Grier from the Anglican order of St. John the Divine in Toronto, the other by Miss Miller, a head nurse at the Winnipeg General Hospital (CNA, 1968). In 1898, nurses with the Victorian Order of Nurses (VON) attached to the Yukon Military Force were praised for their efforts (Gibbon & Mathewson, 1947).

In 1899, the Canadian government made an offer to Joseph Chamberlain, England's colonial secretary, to send a Canadian contingent of nurses to assist during the Boer War. The first group of four nurses was sent to assist in South Africa under the leadership of Georgina Fane Pope, a Bellevue Hospital–educated nurse from Prince Edward Island. She recounted the conditions under which nursing took place:

We nursed in huts and found the work at times very heavy . . . We received our first convoy of wounded a few days after the Battle of Maggersfontein and Modder River when the beds were filled with men of the Highland Brigade . . . No. 3 General Hospital of 600 beds was pitched under canvas at Rondesbosch, a few miles away . . . having at times very active service; sometimes covered with sand during a "Cape South-Easter"; at others delayed with a fore-runner of the coming rainy season, and at all times in terror of scorpions and snakes as bedfellows. (Gibbon & Mathewson, 1947, pp. 290–291)

The South African nursing experience was sufficient to persuade the Canadian Army Medical Corps that an army nursing service ought to be an integral part of the permanent corps. Georgina Pope and Margaret Macdonald were appointed to the staff on a permanent basis in 1906. When World War I broke out, the Army Nursing Corps consisted of five nurses. However, within 3 weeks of the declaration of war, thousands of nurses had volunteered for service overseas. Margaret Macdonald, who was appointed matron-in-chief of the Army Nursing Corps, described the first group of volunteers:

The selection, from coast to coast, of over one hundred nurses from thousands of applicants, the vast majority of whom were entirely unacquainted with Army Life

BOX 2.1 The Influence of Florence Nightingale on Nursing in Canada

In 1854, Florence Nightingale set off with her small band of 38 carefully selected nurses to tend to the British soldiers in Crimea. Until that time, British military hospitals had been staffed by male attendants only. It had not been easy for the Nightingale to secure permission to nurse the sick and wounded military personnel during the Crimean War. However, Nightingale came from a prominent and wealthy family and had connections with many powerful people. She had been well educated at home and had travelled widely before setting out to learn how to nurse the sick. She first went to Germany, where she stayed for some time at Pastor Fliedner's Lutheran hospital, and later went to work with the nursing nuns at the Hôtel-Dieu in Paris. Upon her return to England, she obtained a position in charge of a private Harley Street hospital. When the Crimean War broke out, Nightingale managed to not only obtain permission to go to Crimea but also to raise the British consciousness about the need for good nursing for the sick. "Her onslaught on the appalling lack of sanitation in the wards of the General and Barrack hospitals at Scutari contributed greatly to the reduction in the deaths of cases treated from 315 per thousand to 22 per thousand" (Gibbon & Mathewson, 1947, pp. 109–110). Recent scholarship further confirms that Nightingale had a profound impact on the well-being of troops (Gill & Gill, 2005).

The outpouring of public support for Nightingale's cause was overwhelming, and a fund was established, even before she returned from Crimea, to allow her to organize a training school for nurses (Nutting & Dock, 1937). At last, nursing was to become a suitable occupation for women in Great Britain:

> Mark what by breaking through customs and prejudices Miss Nightingale has effected for her sex. She has opened to them a new profession, a new sphere of usefulness . . . a claim for more extended freedom of action, based on proved public usefulness in the highest sense of the word. (Gibbon & Mathewson, 1947, p. 110)

Florence Nightingale's reputation had worldwide influence. Her work reached Canada by way of both Britain and

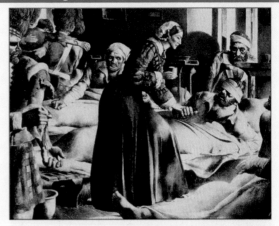

Florence Nightingale revolutionized nursing practice and training through her work with the British Army during the Crimean War, when many were "surviving the battles and being killed by the hospitals." (The U.S. National Library of Medicine)

the United States when, during the American Civil War, there was an attempt to establish Nightingale's standard of nursing to minimize suffering. In 1873, training schools based on the Nightingale model were opened in three American hospitals: Bellevue in New York, Massachusetts General, and New Haven (Gibbon & Mathewson, 1947). Canadian hospitals, particularly the secular hospitals in English-speaking settlements, considered that educating nurses to raise the standards of care was a direct result of Nightingale's influence. She had a profound influence on the initiation of an organized system of nursing education for lay nurses throughout the world. Chapter 20 discusses the establishment of nursing schools.

A number of scholars (e.g., McDonald, 2001; Nelson & Gordon, 2004; Gill & Gill, 2005; McPherson, 2005; Kudzma, 2006) have re-examined Nightingale's legacy. As is the case for most historical figures of her stature, there are debates about the place she is given in history. Nonetheless, she is likely the most recognized name in nursing worldwide.

and regulations, constituted somewhat of a problem. However, when all the formalities incident to the appointment of these Nursing Sisters were concluded, it was astonishing how quickly and naturally in becom-

ing military minded they fell into place. Their example and esprit de corps became the pattern for the many hundreds that followed. (Gibbon & Mathewson, 1947, p. 296)

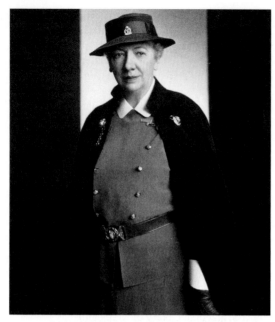

Elizabeth Smellie, Victorian Order of Nurses, became matron-in-chief of the Army Medical Corps during World War II and was the first Canadian woman to reach the rank of colonel. (Courtesy Victorian Order of Nurses for Canada)

There are many accounts of the services rendered by Canadian nurses during the war, all of which remark upon the flexibility and devotion to duty that was required. Matron Macdonald described the introduction of the first group of **Nursing Sisters** to field nursing:

Their first introduction to Field Nursing began at Salisbury Plain in 1914; patients, many seriously ill, poured into huts that were ill-equipped to receive them. Cold, damp weather with continuous rain prevailed, adding much to the general discomfort. The sisters literally ploughed their way through mud and water from hut to hut; their living quarters left much to be desired. (Gibbon & Mathewson, 1947, p. 297)

Major Margaret Macdonald was succeeded by Edith Rayside as matron-in-chief of the nursing service. In all, approximately 3100 nurses saw service during World War I, 47 losing their lives as a result of the conflict (Toman, 2015; Veterans Affairs Canada, 2019a). Fourteen nurses perished in the sinking of the Canadian hospital ship *Llandovery Castle* (CNA, 1968). The significance of nurses' service during World War I led to the establishment of a permanent corps of Nursing Sisters by the Royal Canadian Army Medical Corps (RCAMC).

Elizabeth Smellie served as matron-in-chief of the nursing service of the Army Medical Corps during World War II, from 1940 to 1944. In civilian life, Smellie had been chief superintendent of the VON. She became the first Canadian woman to achieve the rank of colonel. A somewhat larger number of nurses, 4473, served during World War II than in World War I (Toman, 2015; Veterans Affairs Canada, 2019a). However, the number of nurses who volunteered far exceeded the number of positions available (Toman, 2005). Twenty-four Canadian general hospitals were established to care for the wounded during World War II, compared with 16 during World War I. In addition, there was a convalescent hospital in France, a neurologic and plastic surgery hospital in England, and casualty clearing stations, totalling 34 overseas hospitals. Sixty hospitals and two hospital ships were maintained in Canada, all staffed with nurses (Gibbon & Mathewson, 1947). In response to a request from South Africa, nurses under the leadership of Matron-in-Chief Gladys Sharpe were sent to care for wounded British soldiers.

For most of the war, Canadian nurses staffed the military hospitals in England and Canada and did not serve under battle conditions in Europe until 1943, when they were sent to assist following the invasion of Italy:

Canadian nurses were the first to reach Sicily after the invasion . . . The unit was recruited largely from Winnipeg, and other Western cities, but the first girl ashore was Lieutenant Elizabeth Lawson of St. John, New Brunswick . . . Lieutenant Trennie Hunter, of Winnipeg, was a close second. The Matron of this hospital is Miss Agnes J. MacLeod, of Edmonton. They were described as a "group of grimy, tin-hatted girls, perspiring in the terrific heat and burdened with cumbersome equipment." (Gibbon & Mathewson, 1947, p. 465)

Gladys Sharpe described conditions in South Africa and the response to the nurses' arrival:

Our beds filled rapidly, the first convoy via hospital train brought casualties from Burma, Madagascar, the Middle East and Singapore, at the rate of 257 admitted in just two hours—the highlight was the official opening ceremony at which Field Marshall Smuts took the opportunity of publicly thanking "Canada" for sending nurses. (Gibbon & Mathewson, 1947, p. 462)

Up to this point, nurses in military service held the relative rank of officers but did not actually have the official status or authority of officers. During the war, the Privy Council granted nurses commissions equivalent to those of other commissioned officers. In contrast, British and American nurses did not achieve this until the end of the war (CNA, 1968, p. 65).

Sixty Nursing Sisters served in the Korean War (1950–1953) (Toman, 2015). Today, Nursing Sisters are referred to as Nursing Officers. Since the Korean War, they have served in other conflicts, including the Gulf War, Bosnia and Herzegovina, Rwanda, Somalia, and Afghanistan. (Veterans Affairs Canada, 2019a). During a video interview in 2008, veteran First Lieutenant Joanna Streppa recounted her experiences at the Kandahar field hospital in Afghanistan:

The injuries that we saw were gunshot wounds definitely. We saw mine blasts so a lot of times traumatic amputations. We would see stabbings. You would see rollovers. A lot of vehicles rolled over. You would see blast injuries, lots of burns, burns, burns, burns . . . . You do six months in Afghanistan, it's like doing ten years in a trauma centre. You can never ever imagine the amount of trauma we see. (Veterans Affairs Canada, 2019b)

RESEARCH FOCUS

In her book, nursing professor Sonia Grypma explores the life of Canadian nursing missionaries who worked in China and were interned in Japanese war camps during World War II. The book focuses on the extensive diary of Betty Gale. Gale's story is captivating, as she had decided to stay in occupied China during the war and was in an internment camp for 4 years. Grypma had access to other documents provided by Gale's daughter and other written records found at various archives. Through her work, Grypma informs the reader about this little-known chapter of Canadian nursing and Protestant missionary history.

Source: Grypma, S. (2012). *China interrupted. Japanese internment and the reshaping of a Canadian missionary community.* Waterloo, ON: Wilfrid Laurier University Press.

PUBLIC HEALTH NURSING

Public health nursing developed as both an area of specialization in nursing and an integral part of nursing in all settings largely during the twentieth century. The idea of preventing illness and the spread of disease by educating people about beneficial health practices and lifestyle modifications had not been recognized until that time. And although good nutritional practices were important for all, they were especially essential to the health of young children and pregnant women. Some of the first public health nursing took place in the home, when nurses cared for patients with tuberculosis and taught preventive measures.

The first school nurses were appointed in Hamilton, Ontario, in 1909 and Toronto in 1910. Lina Rogers, a graduate of The Hospital for Sick Children, achieved international fame for her work correlating the absence of children from school with lack of medical care. Her appointment to the School Nursing Service of the Toronto Board of Education led to the recruitment of a staff of nurses and dentists whose mandate was to teach children and their families hygienic practices to prevent disease. The Nursing Service was transferred to the health department several years later, providing a model for a system of public health nursing in each province and territory (Gibbon & Mathewson, 1947).

The development of public health nursing has been a gradual process. The entrenchment of a hospital-based system of health care, encouraged by Canadian federal health legislation since 1948, undoubtedly limited recognition of the need for preventive services, home-based services, and consumer involvement in health care. The Lalonde Report (Lalonde, 1975) provided the first evidence of the federal government's concern about disease prevention and health maintenance. However, the skyrocketing costs of care in hospitals focused attention on the need to care for people in different ways. Day surgery, ambulatory care, outpatient services, and home care are now used extensively, with heavy reliance on nurses in each of these. Even though many of these services can be described as "illness care," the need to teach health practices for disease prevention and health maintenance is an important facet of nursing care. The continued emphasis of the Epp Report (Epp, 1986) on prevention, poverty reduction, and enhancing people's ability to cope with their lives was further evidence of federal support for health promotion.

The Declaration of Alma-Ata, adopted in 1978 at the International Conference on Primary Health Care and jointly sponsored by the World Health Organization and UNICEF, established the goal of "health for all" by the year 2000. This stimulated a strong commitment to promoting health and preventing disease in Canada. Although the initial target year has passed, work continues on many of the initiatives. In 1994, the National Forum on Health was established under the direction of Prime Minister Jean Chrétien with a mandate to consult with Canadians and advise government on innovative ways to improve the health of Canadians. The forum concluded its work in 1997 and published two reports: *Canada Health Action Building on the Legacy, Volume I: Final Report* and *Canada Health Action Building on the Legacy Volume II: Synthesis Reports and Issue Papers.* These are available on the Health Canada website. In view of the continuing debate about the future of Medicare and pressure by some provinces to move to privately funded health care, the Commission on the Future of Health Care in Canada, chaired by Roy Romanow, was appointed in 2001 by Prime Minister Chrétien. The *Romanow Report* recommended policies and measures to ensure the long-term sustainability of a universally accessible, publicly funded health care system (Romanow, 2002).

The initial impetus for the development of public health nursing took place at a time when there were no antibiotics and few immunizations to combat disease. Thus, good health practices to prevent the spread of infectious diseases were essential. As antibiotics and immunization against a number of diseases became available, the incidence and prevalence of communicable diseases subsided. This decrease may have led to complacency on the part of governments and citizens. However, with the increasing incidence of AIDS, tuberculosis, and hepatitis C since the late 1980s and the emergence of SARS in the early 2000s, it became clear that the battle against communicable diseases was far from over. It was further troubling that despite the official discourse on health promotion and the repeated suggestions for more community nursing, during the 2000s only 14.1% of registered nurses worked in the community (Canadian Institute for Health Information [CIHI], 2008). In 2017, only 15.7% of nurses were working in the community (CNA, 2018). See Chapter 11 for more details about public health nursing, prevention, and the principles of primary health care.

NURSING IN HOSPITALS

Prior to the 1950s, hospitals were primarily staffed by nursing students. During those years, nurses who had completed their studies tended to work in what was called "private duty nursing." Private duty nurses provided services in patients' homes. In the 1960s, hospitals became the primary place of employment of registered nurses. In 2007, 63% of registered nurses in Canada worked in the hospital sector (CIHI, 2008), while in 2017, 63.6% of nurses worked in hospitals (CNA, 2018). In the 1990s, hospital restructuring led to the layoff of thousands of nurses. The number of nurses employed in hospitals decreased by over 20%, while the number employed in the community increased by 2%.

Many of the nurses and new graduates laid off during the 1990s found work abroad. It has been argued that this migration contributed to the shortage of nurses in Canada in the 2000s (Heitlinger, 2003). One way governments used to address workforce issues was to increase the number of licensed practical nurses (LPNs; known as registered practical nurses in Ontario). In 2003, LPNs represented 21% of regulated nurses (CIHI, 2007), while by 2019, they represented 28.9% of regulated nurses (CIHI, 2020). See Chapter 21 for a detailed discussion of these trends.

APPLYING CONTENT KNOWLEDGE

Why were hospitals predominantly staffed by nursing students prior to the 1950s?

The last two decades have also been characterized by increased patient acuity and changes in technology, as well as an aging registered nurse workforce. Although hospitals remain dependent on the availability of registered nurses, they also increasingly depend on other regulated nurses. The challenge for the profession is to ensure that the high standards of nursing and nursing education are not compromised.

The history of nursing in Canada is long and distinguished. Nurses have been caring for people from the time of the earliest French settlements on the shores of the St. Lawrence. Likewise, nurses have been at the heart of new developments in high-technology acute care and strong advocates for health promotion. Altruism has characterized nursing and nurses from the outset, and commitment to the public good has been a firmly entrenched principle guiding professional activities. As the Canadian health care system evolves, nurses will continue to successfully meet the new and difficult challenges facing them.

SUMMARY OF LEARNING OBJECTIVES

- Before the arrival of European settlers, Indigenous peoples were knowledgeable about the use of medicinal plants and considered health from a holistic point of view.
- The provision of health care and the establishment of hospitals came early in New France.
- French Canadian nursing sisters played a prominent role in spreading nursing across Canada.
- British colonies did not have the organized nursing that French colonies had. Without French Canadian nursing sisters, nursing would not have developed as rapidly.

- Florence Nightingale was influential in reforming nursing in her country and in other parts of the world, including Canada. After the reforms of Nightingale, women of English origin began to see nursing as a possible occupation.
- Modern nursing was brought to Canada by the creation of the first nursing school in St. Catharines, Ontario. This school was primarily patterned on the Nightingale model. However, it differed in one important respect: it did not have an independent budget from the hospital.
- The desire for professionalization and better standards of care brought about the development of national

nursing organizations. These organizations have evolved to serve various sectors of nursing and groups of nurses.
- Nurses played and continue to play a significant role during armed conflicts. Nurses have served during all modern conflicts, providing health services to soldiers.
- Nurses have played key roles in both public health and hospital care. Nurses were particularly involved in pub-

lic health in the early 1900s. During that time, most nurses provided their services in patients' homes. In the 1950s, as hospitals gradually abandoned their reliance on nursing students to provide care, more nurses became employed by hospitals. Today, the majority of nurses work in hospitals.

CRITICAL THINKING QUESTIONS

1. Organized nursing in this country was established under a French regime. What influence did this have on Canadian nursing?
2. It is said that nursing began with Florence Nightingale. What argument is used to support this statement? How would you explain that this is not the case? Give examples supporting your views.
3. Consider the nursing leaders described in this chapter. What characteristics were common to most, if not all, of

them? What lessons can today's nurses take from these characteristics?
4. Consider the history of how public health nursing emerged, and reflect on your knowledge of the health care system in your province. Can you think of a few factors that explain why so few nurses are working in public health to this day?

REFERENCES

American Association for the History of Nursing. (2001). *Position paper—Nursing history in the curriculum: Preparing nurses for the 21st century.* Retrieved from https://www.aahn.org/position-paper-on-history-in-curriculum1.

Bennett, E. M. G. (1966/1979). "Hébert, Louis" in *Dictionary of Canadian Biography,* vol. 1, University of Toronto/Université Laval. Retrieved from http://www.biographi.ca/en/bio/rollet_marie_1E.html.

Bennett, E. M. G. (1966/2018). "Rolet (Rollet), Marie (Dufeu; Hébert; Hubou)," in *Dictionary of Canadian Biography,* vol. 1, University of Toronto/Université Laval. Retrieved from http://www.biographi.ca/en/bio/rollet_marie_1E.html.

Burnett, K. (2006). *The healing work and nursing care of Aboriginal women, medical missionaries, nursing sisters, public health nurses, and female attendants in Southern Alberta first nations communities, 1880–1930* [Doctoral dissertation]. York University, Toronto, ON.

Canadian Association of Schools of Nursing. (2019). *CASN accreditation.* Retrieved from https://www.casn.ca/accreditation/casn-and-accreditation/.

Canadian Indigenous Nurses Association. (2019). *About us.* Retrieved from http://indigenousnurses.ca/about.

Canadian Institute for Health Information. (2008). *Regulated nurses: Trends, 2003 to 2007.* Retrieved from https://secure.cihi.ca/free_products/nursing_report_2003_to_2007_e.pdf.

Canadian Institute for Health Information. (2007). *Canada's health care providers.* Ottawa, ON: CIHI. Retrieved from https://secure.cihi.ca/free_products/HCProviders_07_EN_final.pdf.

Canadian Nurses Association. (1968). *The leaf and the lamp.* Ottawa, ON: Author.

Canadian Institute for Health Information. (2020). *Nursing in Canada, 2019—Chartbook.* Ottawa, ON: CIHI. Retrieved from https://www.cihi.ca/en/nursing-in-canada-2019.

Canadian Nurses Association. (2013). *Canadian Nurses Association: One hundred years of service, 1908–2008.* Ottawa, ON: Author.

Canadian Nurses Association. (2018). *LPNs/RPNs & RPNs.* Ottawa, ON: Author. Retrieved from https://www.cna-aiic.ca/en/membership/lpnrpn.

Canadian Nurses Foundation. (2019). *Our history.* Retrieved from http://cnf-fiic.ca/who-we-are/our-stories/our-history/.

Daveluy, M. C. (1966/2017). "Mance, Jeanne" in *Dictionary of Canadian Biography,* vol. 1, University of Toronto/Université Laval. Retrieved from http://www.biographi.ca/en/bio/mance_jeanne_1E.html.

Drouin, C. (1988). *Love spans the centuries* (pp. 1821–1853). (Vol. 2). Montreal, QC: Meridian Press.

Durzan, D. J. (2009). Argine, scurvy and Cartier's "tree of life". *Journal of Ethnobiology and Ethnomedicine, 5,* 1–25. https://doi.org/10.1186/1746-4269-5-5.

Emery, Sister. (1871). Letter from Saint-Albert to Mother Slocombe at Montréal, 6 January 1871. In *Lettres de Saint-Albert, 1858–1877* (pp. 247–253). Montreal, QC: Archives des Soeurs Grises de Montréal.

Epp, J. (1986). *Achieving health for all: A framework for health promotion.* Ottawa, ON: Health and Welfare Canada.

Gibbon, J. M., & Mathewson, M. S. (1947). *Three centuries of Canadian nursing.* Toronto, ON: Macmillan.

Gill, C. J., & Gill, G. C. (2005). Nightingale in Scutari: Her legacy re-examined. *Clinical Infectious Diseases, 40,* 1799–1805. https://doi.org/10.1086/430380.

Heitlinger, A. (2003). The paradoxical impact of health care restructuring in Canada on nursing as a profession. *International Journal of Health Services, 23*(1), 37–54. https://doi.org/10.2190/RMAY-NJA9-KFW7-1UEW.

Jamieson, E., Sewall, M., & Gjertson, L. (1959). *Trends in nursing history.* Philadelphia, PA: W.B. Saunders.

Juchereau, J.-F., & Duplessis, M.-A. (1939/1984). *Les annales de l'Hôtel-Dieu de Québec: 1636–1716.* Québec, QC: L'Hôtel-Dieu de Québec.

Kenton, E. (1925). *The Jesuit Relations and allied documents.* New York, NY: Vanguard Press.

Kudzma, E. C. (2006). Florence Nightingale and healthcare reform. *Nursing Science Quarterly, 19*(1), 61–64. https://doi.org/10.1177/0894318405283556.

Lalonde, M. (1975). *A new perspective on the health of Canadians.* Ottawa, ON: Health and Welfare Canada. Retrieved from http://www.phac-aspc.gc.ca/ph-sp/pdf/perspect-eng.pdf.

McDonald, L. (Ed.). (2001). *Florence Nightingale: An introduction to her life and family.* Waterloo, ON: Wilfrid Laurier University Press.

McPherson, K. (2005). The Nightingale influence and the rise of the modern hospital. In C. Bates, D. Dodd, & N. Rousseau (Eds.), *On all frontiers: Four centuries of Canadian nursing* (pp. 73–88). Ottawa, ON: University of Ottawa Press.

Millman, M. B. (1965). Nursing in Canada. In G. Griffin & J. Griffin (Eds.), *Jensen's history and trends of professional nursing* (pp. 423–439). St. Louis, MO: C.V. Mosby.

Morton, D. (1983). *A short history of Canada.* Edmonton, AB: Hurtig.

Mouhot, J.-F. (2002). L'influence amérindienne sur la société en Nouvelle-France. *Une exploration de l'historiographie de Francoi-Xavier Garneau à Allan Greer (1845-1997). Revue internationale d'études québécoises, 5*(1), 123–157. https://doi.org/10.7202/1000668ar.

Nelson, S., & Gordon, S. (2004). The rhetoric of rupture: Nursing as a practice with a history. *Nursing Outlook, 52,* 255–261. https://doi.org/10.1016/j.outlook.2004.08.001.

Nutting, M. A., & Dock, L. (1937). *A history of nursing* (Volumes 1–4). New York, NY: Putnam.

Parkman, F. (1897). *The Jesuits in North America in the seventeenth century.* Boston, MA: Little, Brown.

Paul, P. (2005). Religious nursing orders of Canada: A presence on all western frontiers. In C. Bates, D. Dodd, & N. Rousseau (Eds.), *On all frontiers: Four centuries of Canadian nursing* (pp. 125–138). Ottawa, ON: University of Ottawa Press.

Rode, M. W. (1989). The nursing pin: Symbol of 1,000 years of service. *Nursing Forum, 24*(1), 15–17. https://doi.org/10.1111/j.1744-6198.1989.tb00813.x.

Romanow, R. J. (2002). *Building on values. The future of health care in Canada.* Ottawa, ON: Queen's Printer. Retrieved from http://publications.gc.ca/site/eng/237274/publication.html.

Thwaites, R. G. (1959). *The Jesuit Relations and allied documents: Travels and explorations of the Jesuit missionaries in New France* (Volumes I–XII). New York, NY: Pageant. Retrieved from Library and Archives Canada. http://epe.lac-bac.gc.ca/100/206/301/lac-bac/jesuit_relations-ef/jesuit-relations/h19-151-e.html.

Toman, C. (2005). "Ready, Aye Ready": Canadian military nurses as an expandable and expendable workforce (1920–2000). In C. Bates, D. Dodd, & N. Rousseau (Eds.), *On all frontiers: Four centuries of Canadian nursing* (pp. 169–181). Ottawa, ON: University of Ottawa Press.

Toman, C. (2015). Nursing sisters, in *Canadian Encyclopedia.* Toronto, ON: Historica Canada. Retrieved from https://www.thecanadianencyclopedia.ca/en/article/nursing-sisters.

University of Saskatchewan College of Nursing and CINA (2018). *2018 University of Saskatchewan & CINA's fact sheet: "Aboriginal Nursing in Canada."* Retrieved from http://indigenousnurses.ca/sites/default/files/inline-files/Nursing_AborigNursing_sheet_2018_3.pdf.

Veterans Affairs Canada. (2019a). *The nursing sisters of Canada.* Retrieved from https://www.veterans.gc.ca/eng/remembrance/those-who-served/women-and-war/nursing-sisters.

Veterans Affairs Canada. (2019b). 2008 recording of 1st Lieutenant Joanna Streppa: Injuries and Traumas, in the series *Heroes to Remember.* Retrieved from https://www.veterans.gc.ca/eng/video-gallery/video/6097.

Violette, B. (2005). Healing the body and saving the soul: Nursing sisters and the first Catholic hospitals in Quebec (1639–1880). In C. Bates, D. Dodd, & N. Rousseau (Eds.), *On all frontiers: Four centuries of Canadian nursing* (pp. 57–71). Ottawa, ON: University of Ottawa Press.

Wytenbroek, L., & Vanderberg, H. (2017). Reconsidering nursing's history during Canada 150. *The Canadian Nurse, 113*(4), 16–18.

Young, J., & Rousseau, N. (2005). Lay nursing from the New France era to the end of the nineteenth century (1600-1891). In C. Bates, D. Dodd, & N. Rousseau (Eds.), *On all frontiers: Four centuries of Canadian nursing* (pp. 11–25). Ottawa, ON: University of Ottawa Press.

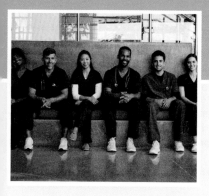

Professionalization in Canadian Nursing

Joyce K. Engel

http://evolve.elsevier.com/Canada/Ross-Kerr/nursing

LEARNING OBJECTIVES

After reading this chapter, you will be able to:

- Analyze nursing with respect to the characteristics of a profession.
- Explain changes in nursing education that have led to a more highly prepared workforce.
- Describe how the nursing profession has endeavoured to extend its knowledge base over the past century.
- Analyze the challenges the nursing profession has faced in its quest to raise its standards of education.
- Describe the legislation governing nursing practice in each province and territory.

OUTLINE

KEY TERMS

accreditation
associations
code of ethics
discipline
program approval
mandatory registration

occupation
profession
regulatory colleges
unions
vocation

PERSONAL PERSPECTIVES

Melanie is excited to begin her nursing education and future career. She has dreamed of becoming a nurse since her accident at 14 years of age, when she spent several weeks in hospital. Yesterday, she received an acceptance from the nursing program to which she had applied. And today, she is sharing her enthusiasm about the acceptance with her best friend. Her friend responds, "Melanie, you are so smart. Why don't you go into medicine instead? Everyone thinks doctors are so smart and it is a real profession." Melanie wonders whether she has made the right decision. Will she find the same challenges and satisfaction in nursing that she would find in medicine?

INTRODUCTION

The evolution of nursing as a **profession** in Canada is a story of courage, conviction, and altruism. In 1639, three Augustinian nuns arrived from France to provide nursing care to the small population at Québec. From this humble beginning, nursing evolved as an essential service in the New World at a time when knowledge of disease was primitive, technology was virtually nonexistent, and a few herbal remedies were the only drug therapies available.

Over the centuries, as the practice of nursing was refined, it began to be perceived as important to the health and well-being of communities. In the twentieth century, a concerted effort was made to develop educational standards and programs to prepare nurses for practice. Efforts were also made to gain control over the practice of nursing through the registration of nurses and development of professional standards. At the beginning of the twenty-first century, the expansion of educational requirements and opportunities, nursing practice, and nursing knowledge is leading to greater specialization in nursing. In turn, this is creating opportunities to broaden nursing's influence on health systems and delivery as well as the interprofessional teams of which nurses are a part.

There is much diversity of opinion about what constitutes a profession and no real agreement on the definition of professionalism (Akhtar-Danesh, Baumann, Kolotylo et al., 2013). The process of professionalization in nursing can be clearly seen and identified. The first two decades of the twentieth century signalled the beginning of the struggle to define the nature, scope, and object of nursing and the subsequent campaign for professional recognition and regulation. The latter movement has spread worldwide, although its status varies from one country to another (Duncan, Thorne, & Rodney, 2015).

Within Canada, there is relative uniformity of opinion, because nursing has been recognized as a self-governing profession that is a legislated right in each province and territory. In the twenty-first century, this right has been legislatively amended to more fully acknowledge the roles of nurses and their place in health care, especially in relation to advanced practice and nurses' influence on improving health care accessibility and sustainability. Legislation also continues to strengthen and clarify the role of regulatory bodies in nursing.

DEVELOPMENT OF PROFESSIONS

Within the context of present-day nursing, it may seem odd that the status of nursing as a profession has been questioned. Yet historically, much debate has surrounded whether nursing is a profession, a semi-profession, or an **occupation**—or even whether, as a reflection of its nineteenth-century roots, it remains a **vocation**. This debate is both practically and ethically important (White, 2002), because it is pivotal to understanding the roots of nursing as well as its current iterations. Although not directly synonymous, the concepts of occupation, vocation, and profession are interrelated. An occupation refers to habitual employment (White, 2002), or what one does for a living or work; it encompasses the future goal of many who enter the profession of nursing. A vocation requires a strong dedication to certain types of work (e.g., caring for others who are ill) and reflects the belief that such a career or occupation is a calling.

The view of nursing as a vocation has been especially enduring and includes identification with strong norms such as the importance of caring about patients and how their experience of illness matters to them (White, 2002). The characteristics of nursing as a vocation, such as ideals of service to others and requirements for deference to authority, search for perfection, and self-sacrifice, were particularly dominant into the 1960s and were reinforced by the nurse apprenticeship model of education in hospital-based nursing programs (Bradshaw, 2010).

However, the view of nursing as a vocation is seen by some as problematic. Historically, nursing as a vocation has been associated with traditional feminine roles, such as mothers, whose physical and emotional work also involves the concepts of altruism and caring (Yam, 2004) but not the extensive theoretical knowledge base and formal education required of those in a profession. In addition, the concept of vocation has been associated with charitable work, low pay, and long hours, a perspective that may seem incongruent with how some contemporary nurses view their work (Carter, 2014). Nonetheless, the legacy of caring inherent in

BOX 3.1 Flexner's Characteristics of a Profession

1. It is basically intellectual, carrying with it high responsibility.
2. It is learned in nature, because it is based on a body of knowledge.
3. It is practical rather than theoretical.
4. Its technique can be taught through educational discipline.
5. It is well organized internally.
6. It is motivated by altruism.

Source: Flexner, A. (1915). Is social work a profession? *Proceedings of the National Conference of Charities and Corrections* (pp. 578–581). Chicago, IL: Heldermann.

the vocational perspective remains an integral component of the profession today.

The ongoing debate about the definition of nursing underscores the reality that professionalization is a gradual process involving movement along a defined continuum, from a vocation or occupation at one end to a profession at the other. The measurement of progress along this continuum focuses on the extent to which an occupational group meets the criteria deemed to characterize a profession.

The debate about nursing as a profession began shortly after the beginning of the twentieth century, when Abraham Flexner (Box 3.1) identified six characteristics of a profession based on his observations of law, medicine, and theology. Flexner (1915) observed that nursing did not appear to be a profession because "the responsibility of the trained nurse is neither original nor final" (p. 581). However, his assessment of how nursing met the stated criteria was made before the passage of laws regulating the practice of nursing in most provinces and before nursing education first appeared in a university prospectus in Canada. His determination also occurred at a time when women had yet to be considered "persons" under the original provisions of the 1867 *British North America Act*, in which only male nouns and pronouns were used; thus, while women were considered persons in personal circumstances such as pain, they were not persons in relation to public responsibilities such as voting or holding office (Munroe, 2019).

In a classic study by Bixler and Bixler (1945) on the status of nursing as a profession, the authors examined the extent to which nursing met the standard criteria for designation as a profession. They reached the conclusion that although nursing was well into professionalization, it had further to go before it could be described as a profession. Edward Bernays, a public relations expert—hired by the *American Journal of Nursing* in 1945 to raise the profile

of nurses in the United States and an influential catalyst in the development of a **code of ethics** by the American Nurses Association (ANA)—contended that nurses could not achieve professional status without prestige. Bernays suggested that the route to increased prestige, and thus to professional status, included a clear definition of the profession, articulation of educational requirements, and specification of the experience required. Importantly, as a fourth step in increasing the status and visibility of nursing, he underscored the need for a code of ethics to solidify the place of nursing as a trusted profession (Philbin & Keepnews, 2014).

Wilensky (1964) was the first to refer to the "natural history of professionalism" as a description of the milestones in the development of professions. Some of these milestones include the date the profession first became a full-time occupation, the date of the first educational program to prepare practitioners, and the date the first university school for the profession was established. Also included as significant events are the date the first national professional association was formed, the date of the enactment of the first provincial registration act, and the date of the development and adoption of a formal code of ethics.

Flexner (1915) saw the development of a formal base of knowledge, the first criterion, as the most central for professions. An articulated knowledge base is common to most categorizations of professions. Since the knowledge needed to practise a profession is complex and cannot be mastered by an ordinary person, practitioners require a lengthy period of preparation and supervised practice before they can function competently on an independent basis. The educational process is considered important and complex enough that programs are offered within universities, and the first professional degree often follows a four-year university arts or science degree. The knowledge base of a profession is continually upgraded through research performed by members to expand and update knowledge for practice. To ensure that new practitioners have the knowledge necessary to engage in their profession, members also maintain control over educational standards for the admission of new practitioners into the profession and must use their knowledge to serve and benefit the public.

Because professions are inherently important to the public, some form of licensing or registration of those qualified to practise is necessary. Control of this process, while vested in legislation, is normally left to the profession. Professions are organized for the purpose of regulating practice, which includes retaining the authority to remove from practice those who are incompetent. Professional commitment to the public is demonstrated by the development of a code of ethics, or statement of moral or ethical duty. Although codes of ethics are important for the health professions, there are limitations in that they are expressed as general principles and may not be helpful in specific issues and situations. Nevertheless, Fowler (2010) suggests that a code of ethics is the central and necessary mark of a profession because it lays out the social contract between the profession and the public that it serves and signifies its accountabilities and responsibilities to its members and the public. This is important in gaining the trust of the public, as indicated by a recent Gallup poll in which nursing was ranked the highest of 22 occupations, for the sixteenth consecutive year, on honesty and ethics (Gallup, 2017).

EVOLUTION OF NURSING AS A PROFESSION

In Canada, the nursing profession has held a prominent place in society since the first nurses were encouraged to immigrate to the shores of New France. The history of nursing in Canada points to the importance of the French Catholic and British nursing apprenticeship traditions in the evolution of nursing in this country. The history of nursing also points to a failure to acknowledge the vital role that Indigenous healers and midwives occupied in their own communities and in those of settlers. The eradication of Indigenous cultures following Confederation further diminished the importance of this contribution and often prevented Indigenous women from entering nursing programs until the 1930s (Wytenbroek & Vandeberg, 2017).

In the nineteenth century, members of the Order of the Sisters of Charity of Montreal (the Grey Nuns) bravely set out, without the benefit of reliable transportation, to provide needed health care to remote parts of the country where small settlements were opening. These women placed mission before profit and were creative leaders who sometimes pushed against the hierarchies in the church at a time when women had limited status. By 1947, nursing sisters had well over 100 hospitals across Canada and wielded considerable power as managers, accountants, and owners of nurse-run hospitals (Wytenbroek & Vandenberg, 2017).

Around the turn of the twentieth century, a movement began in support of securing legislation to regulate nursing practice as a means to differentiate qualified from unqualified practitioners. The first provincial statute governing the practice of nursing was passed in Nova Scotia in 1910. By 1922, with the passage of legislation in Ontario, statutes governing nursing had been established in all provinces. The development of stronger legislation, which would differentiate the actual practice of nursing with the title of Registered Nurse (RN), occurred later, with the initial passage of legislation in Newfoundland in 1953. All provinces have now moved to mandatory forms of legislation governing nursing (Table 3.1), either through inclusion in umbrella legislation that covers regulation of various health professions or through nursing-specific legislation. Achieving the legislated privilege to practise, embodied in law, was an important step in professionalizing nursing.

TABLE 3.1	Legislation Regulating Nursing Practice by Province and Territory	
Province or Territory	Legislation Governing Registered Nurses	Legislative Authority
Alberta	*Health Professions Act, 2000*	Umbrella legislation that includes the regulation of registered nurses, licensed practical nurses, and registered psychiatric nurses (Alberta Queen's Printer, 2019).
British Columbia	*Health Professions Act, 1996*	Umbrella legislation that includes the regulation of registered nurses, licensed practical nurses, and registered psychiatric nurses. The British Columbia College of Nursing Professionals was established in 2018 as the regulatory college for all nurses (British Columbia College of Nursing Professionals, 2019; College of Registered Nurses of British Columbia, 2018).
Manitoba	*Regulated Health Professions Act, 2009*	Umbrella legislation that governs registered nurses, effective May 31, 2018. Prior to 2018, registered nurses were regulated under the *Registered Nurses Act* (College of Registered Nurses of Manitoba, n.d.).

TABLE 3.1 Legislation Regulating Nursing Practice by Province and Territory (*Cont.*)

Province or Territory	Legislation Governing Registered Nurses	Legislative Authority
New Brunswick	*Nurses Act, 2002*	Regulates registered nurses (Nurses Association of New Brunswick, 2008).
Newfoundland	*Nurses Act, 2008*	Regulates registered nurses and nurse practitioners. Amendments to the Act in 2019 will change the name of the regulatory body for registered nurses to that of a college and will remove the requirement to have a legislated standards committee approve nurse practitioner scope of practice (Government of Newfoundland, 2019).
Northwest Territories and Nunavut	*Nursing Profession Act, S.N.W.T. 2003*; *Nunavut Nursing Act, S.N.W.T. 1998*	Regulates registered nurses (Registered Nurses Association of the Northwest Territories and Nunavut, 2015).
Nova Scotia	*Nursing Act, 2019*	Act created a single college for registered nurses, nurse practitioners, and licensed practical nurses (Nova Scotia Legislature, 2019).
Ontario	*Regulated Health Professions Act, 1991*; *Nursing Act, 1991*	Together with the *Regulated Health Professions Act*, an umbrella legislation for self-regulating professions in Ontario, the *Nursing Act* regulates registered nurses and registered practical nurses (College of Nurses of Ontario, 2018).
Prince Edward Island	*Regulated Health Professions Act, 2018*	Act regulates registered nurses and transitioned the regulatory body for nurses from an association to a college (Legislative Counsel Office, 2019).
Quebec	*Nurses Act, 2003*	Act regulates nurses (Ordre des infirmières et infirmiers du Québec, 2010).
Saskatchewan	*Registered Nurses Act, 1988*	Act regulates registered nurses (Saskatchewan Registered Nurses Association, 2019).
Yukon	*Registered Nurses Profession Act, R.S.Y. 2002* (O.I.C. 2012/197) and pursuant regulations	Regulates registered nurses (Yukon Registered Nurses Association, 2019).

Sources: Alberta Queen's Printer. (2019). *Revised statutes of Alberta 2000: Chapter H-7. Office consolidation (current as of April 1, 2019).* Edmonton, AB: Queen's Park Printer.

College of Registered Nurses of Manitoba. (n.d.). *Policy and legislation.* Retrieved from https://www.crnm.mb.ca/about/policies-and-legislation

College of Nurses of Ontario. (2018). *Legislation and regulation: an introduction to the Nursing Act, 1991.* Retrieved from http://www.cno.org/globalassets/docs/prac/41064_fsnursingact.pdf

Government of Newfoundland. (2019). *Amendments proposed to strengthen the Nurses' Act.* Retrieved from https://www.releases.gov.nl.ca/releases/2014/health/1202n09.aspx

Legislative Counsel Office. (2019). *Regulated Health Professions Act.* Retrieved from https://www.princeedwardisland.ca/sites/default/files/legislation/r-10-1-regulated_health_professions_act.pdf

Nova Scotia Legislature (2019). Bill No. 121 (*Nursing Act*). Retrieved from https://nslegislature.ca/legc/bills/63rd_2nd/3rd_read/b121.htm

Ordre des infirmières et infirmiers du Québec. (2010). *Preparation guide for professional examination of the Ordre de infirmières et infirmiers du Québec.* Retrieved from https://www.oiiq.org/sites/default/files/uploads/pdf/publications/publicationsoiiq/Supplement-anglais.pdf

Registered Nurses Association of the Northwest Territories and Nunavut. (2015). *Acts and legislation.* Retrieved from http://www.rnantnu.ca/documents/acts-legislation

Saskatchewan Registered Nurses Association. (2019). *Act and bylaws.* Retrieved from https://www.srna.org/about-us/how-we-govern/act-bylaws/

Yukon Registered Nurses Association. (2019). *Regulatory authority.* Retrieved from https://yukonnurses.ca/index.php?option=com_content&view=article&id=304&Itemid=276

Nursing education in Canada began in 1874 in St. Catharines, Ontario, after worldwide recognition of Florence Nightingale's efforts to establish formal education for nurses. Nightingale believed that nurses needed to be educated to care for patients properly. Her point was demonstrated in Crimea in 1856, when she and a small group of trained nurses provided care for wounded soldiers, dramatically lowering the soldiers' mortality and morbidity rates. Nursing education moved into Canadian universities in 1918, when courses in public health nursing were run at the University of Alberta. The first Canadian degree program in nursing was offered at The University of British Columbia, under the direction of Ethel Johns. Today, a number of baccalaureate degree program options are available to nursing students across Canada.

The impetus for baccalaureate preparation in nursing was supported by early initiatives such as the 1932 *Weir Report*, in which the admission and education standards for nurses were deemed insufficient. Recommendations from the report included bringing nursing programs into the general education system (Canadian Association of Schools of Nursing [CASN], 2016) and requiring university preparation, as in other professions. What brought about these changes decades later was the adoption and active promotion by the Canadian Nurses Association (CNA) and other professional associations of the baccalaureate degree as an entry-to-practice requirement. Currently, all provinces and territories except Quebec require nurses entering the profession to have a baccalaureate degree. Quebec offers diploma programs, however, and supports the development of baccalaureate programs between its Collèges d'enseignement général et professionnel (CEGEP) and universities (Canadian Nurses Association [CNA], 2019a).

In 1959, a master's degree program in nursing was initiated at the University of Western Ontario, and nursing research development began in earnest. Master's programs have flourished since then, with a growing number of programs and specializations available and accessible to students across Canada. Specializations at the master's level include gerontology, clinical nurse specialist, Indigenous health, mental health, and nurse practitioner. The first doctoral program, at the University of Alberta, admitted students on January 1, 1991, and others followed suit such that doctoral preparation became available in all regions of the country. Graduation from master's programs in nursing increased from 617 graduates in 2013 to just over 700 graduates in 2017. Graduation from doctoral programs remained relatively stable during the same period, with 64 students graduating in 2017 (CASN, 2018).

Provincial and territorial colleges and **associations** are responsible for approving entry-level nursing programs, and the Canadian Association of Schools of Nursing (CASN) provides a national accreditation program for undergraduate and nurse practitioner programs. **Program approval** and program accreditation are distinct processes. In addition to ensuring that graduates of a program can meet the entry-to-practice competencies set out by provinces and territories and thus ensure public safety, program approval is required for graduates of a program to write licensing examinations. **Accreditation** promotes excellence in nursing programs and assists programs with identifying strengths and weaknesses (CASN, n.d.).

Both program approval and accreditation are guided by the entry-to-practice competencies established by provincial and territorial regulatory bodies and the National Nursing Education Framework, a consensus-based national framework that outlines the core expectations for Canadian baccalaureate, master's, and doctoral programs in nursing. This framework clearly establishes baccalaureate education as generalist preparation for nursing and sets out the progression from baccalaureate to graduate education (CASN, 2015). Core expectations for each level of nursing education in the national framework are consistent with those in non-nursing degree programs, as outlined in the Canadian Degree Qualifications Framework, which attests to the maturation of nursing as a **discipline** as well as a profession. The evolution of the unique knowledge base considered necessary for a discipline has been fostered through the development of nursing education and nursing research and provides the foundation for the profession, the focus of which is service (Parse, 1998).

The development of a code of ethics normally occurs relatively late in the process of professionalization: "Toward the end, legal protection appears; at the end, a formal code of ethics is adopted" (Wilensky, 1964, pp. 143–144). A historical review indicates that this was the case for the nursing profession in Canada. The first North American code of ethics for nursing was published by the American Nurses Association in 1950; in 1953, the International Council of Nurses (ICN) approved a code of ethics. Finally, in 1980, the first CNA code of ethics was developed. The CNA regularly reviews the code of ethics, with the most recent code approved in 2017 (CNA, 2017). (See Chapter 15 for further discussion of the code).

> **APPLYING CONTENT KNOWLEDGE**
>
> How well do you think nursing meets the criteria for professional status compared with other health care professions?

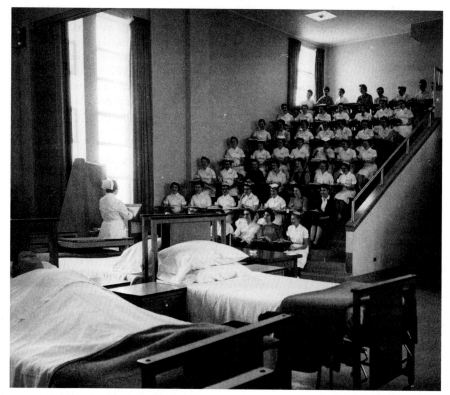

A University of Saskatchewan nursing classroom in the 1950s. (University of Saskatchewan, University Archives and Special Collections, Photograph Collection. A-1603.)

EMERGENCE OF A SCIENTIFIC KNOWLEDGE BASE FOR NURSING

Research to build and extend the knowledge base in nursing, and thus to advance nursing as a discipline, has been enhanced by the establishment of master's and doctoral programs in nursing across the country. Many of these programs have a strong research thrust, and their graduates are engaged in advancing the scientific basis of nursing.

The importance of studying nursing questions has been emphasized by leaders in the profession, who have stressed the need for scientific testing of traditional nursing practices. With the development and expansion of graduate programs, research in schools and faculties of nursing has increased exponentially. This growth in research has been accompanied by a movement to ensure that nursing practice is evidence informed, as the public expects practitioners to provide high-quality nursing care that is based on the best available evidence.

RESEARCH FOCUS

Using interpretive narrative methodology guided by Polkinghorne's theory of narrative identity, journal entries and face-to-face interviews with six millennial nursing students were analyzed. Three main themes were identified (Real Nursing: Making a Difference; The Good Nurse: Defined by Practice; and Creating Career–Life Balance). The study highlighted the importance of providing new graduates with formal and informal supports and professional development to assisting with professional socialization. These supports would enable students to remain close to their professional ideal of making a difference in the lives of others.

Sources: Price, D., McGillis Hall, L., Murphy, G., & Pierce, B. (2018). Evolving career choice narratives of new graduate nurses. *Nurse Education in Practice, 28*, 86–91. https://doi.org/10.1016/j.nepr.2017.10.007.

The movement to develop the science of nursing using an evidence-informed approach has been a critical step forward in the professionalization of nursing in the twenty-first century, and Canada's progress in this area is notable. Developing strong underpinnings for nursing practice through links with theory and research is essential for the continued growth of nursing as an evidence-based profession.

PROFESSIONAL EDUCATION FOR NURSING

Issues of Status and Control

Nursing education has been the subject of considerable controversy. While requiring a baccalaureate degree for entry to practice is now widely accepted, the initial proposal for this requirement, made in Alberta in 1975, was met by heated debate. Eventually, the position was ratified by the CNA and provincial and territorial associations because of the

- Increasing complexity of nursing and health care;
- Expanding knowledge bases in nursing and health care;
- Rapidly expanding technologies in knowledge translation and utilization;
- Need for lifelong learning to adapt to rapid changes in health care, technology, and knowledge;
- Accountability to the public for safe, effective, ethical, and compassionate care;
- Need to understand and practice within the pluralistic cultural, social, and political contexts of Canadian society; and
- Cultural, geographic, and demographic diversity of Canada (Adapted from CNA, 2015, p. 12. © Canadian Nurses Association. Reprinted with permission. Further reproduction prohibited.).

A frequent argument against the requirement of a baccalaureate degree for entry to practice was that it would result in higher health care costs. However, following cost-benefit analyses, the CNA suggested that it was unwise to assume that entry-level baccalaureate education would result in higher health care costs; instead, various studies have linked this education with lower mortality rates, fewer complications of care such as decubitus ulcers, and shorter hospital stays (CNA, 2015), all of which have positive economic and financial implications.

The Vancouver General Hospital and the University of British Columbia were the first to implement the baccalaureate degree as an entry-to-practice standard when they initiated a collaborative degree program in 1989. This was followed by a collaborative program between the University of Alberta and Red Deer College in 1990. Expansion of these early collaborations has led to 41 college–university partnered programs in Canada, with baccalaureate programs offered in every province and territory, except the Yukon, which does not have registered nurse education programs (CASN, 2018). Implementation of the baccalaureate degree as an entry-to-practice requirement prompted growth in graduate programs and enrollments and eventually was instrumental in the introduction of doctoral programs (CASN, 2016).

Provinces and territories have their own program approval processes, as set out by their associations or **regulatory colleges**. An important element of program approval is consideration of how well graduates are prepared in entry-to-practice competencies. Approval processes may include utilization or integration of the results of CASN accreditation to determine approval of programs (CASN, 2016).

Both education and licensure are impacted by national and regional trends, as well as by history, health priorities, and emerging social and health issues (see Gender Considerations box). The aging population, for example, has put increased emphasis on organizational models that facilitate access to primary care. This in turn has raised the profile of nurse practitioner programs and resulted in expanded scopes of practice for nurse practitioners. Transnational workforce migration and projected nursing shortages may increase pressure on regulatory bodies to consider additional measures that decrease delays in registration for internationally prepared nurses (Stievano, Caruso, Pittella et al., 2018). Workforce trends have prompted and will likely continue to prompt innovations in the structure of nursing programs such as year-round programming for second-degree graduates and bridging programs for practical nurse graduates. Nurses increasingly work within and lead interprofessional teams and

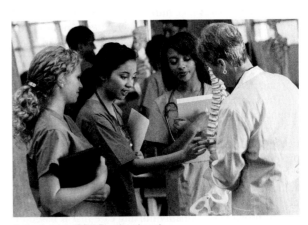

(istock.com/SDI Productions)

must be prepared with the skills to effectively function within this context.

Certifications are fast becoming a necessary component of continuing education and lifelong learning because of the increasing specialization of nursing practice. These different areas of specialization include the age of the client, health problems (e.g., pain management), diagnostic group (e.g., mental health), practice setting (e.g., operating room), and type of care (e.g., critical care). CNA certifications are nationally recognized specialty credentials that are awarded for a 5-year duration after completion of rigorous testing. Currently, the CNA offers 22 specialty certifications for registered nurses and one for licensed practical nurses in a variety of areas such as pediatrics, oncology, gerontology, emergency, and mental health or psychiatric nursing (CNA, 2019b).

CONTROL OF PROFESSIONAL NURSING PRACTICE

The first phase of nurses' efforts to gain control of professional nursing practice began with the enactment of the first provincial legislation regulating nursing, in Nova Scotia in 1910, and ran until Ontario introduced its legislation in 1922, the final province in Canada to do so. By that point, all nine provinces had some form of registration act.

The second phase involved the development of acts requiring mandatory registration. These acts regulate nursing in each province, with each act containing a definition of nursing and a description of the scope of nursing practice. This legislation ensured that nursing practice and practitioners would be more strictly regulated. The first mandatory nursing registration legislation in Canada was enacted in 1953 in Newfoundland. Other provinces did not follow suit until Prince Edward Island passed such legislation in 1972.

Today, all provinces and territories have enacted legislation on **mandatory registration**, and legislation and regulations pertaining to nursing practice continue to evolve (see Table 3.1). Recent changes in legislation and regulations enable registered nurses to prescribe medications, a move prompted by evidence suggesting that allowing nurses to administer medication improves accessibility to care. Such changes are accompanied by the development of new standards and guidelines, as well as by requirements for continuing education.

Complementing the nursing legislation and regulations governing the nursing profession is the realm of nursing **unions,** associations, and regulatory colleges, each of which serves relatively distinct functions (see Case Study). Unions negotiate working conditions such as pay and hours of work, and advocate for appropriate staffing and other factors that impact on the workplace and work life. Professional associations advance the interests of the profession and its members through advocacy and professional development (Duncan, Thorne, & Rodney, 2015). Regulatory colleges protect and serve the public according to their statutory obligations (Government of

GENDER CONSIDERATIONS

Fowler (2017) suggests that the links between nursing and women's rights and status, as well as hard-fought battles to overcome patriarchy, sexism, and oppressive social structures, have created a sense of shelter in sisterhood community; such connections may or may not make it difficult for nurses to be empathetic to the cause of trans persons or even to fully address the issue of men in the profession and women's "privileged rise in the profession" (Fowler, 2017, p. 4). Nonetheless, Fowler (2017) suggests that, within the profession itself, we need to consider the extent to which we welcome trans persons or cis males (those who were assigned male at birth and are comfortable with this designation) and how our views affect recruitment, retention, and curriculum. These questions are timely, particularly in relation to curriculum design and the education of nurses, given that the House of Commons Standing Committee on Health (House of Commons, 2019) recently presented a report pointing to disparities in the health of LGBTQ2 communities. In response to the issues identified, the committee made several recommendations aimed at the following: improving the health of trans people; overcoming bias and stereotypes; increasing trans people's access to health care; and improving the collection of information about trans people and their health needs. Importantly, the report recommended training health care providers, including nurses, to ensure that they understand gender diversity and sexual orientation, as well as how to interact with trans people, but also to foster changes in the attitudes of providers. Inclusion of knowledge and skills related to the health of trans persons in nursing programs is consistent with how nursing education continues to evolve in response to health priorities and social and health issues.

Sources: Fowler, M. (2017). "Unladylike commotion': Early feminism and nursing's role in gender/trans dialogue. *Nursing Inquiry, 24*(1), 1–6. https://doi.org/10.1111/nin.12179; House of Commons. (2019, June 17). *Report 28: The Health of LGBTQIA2 Communities in Canada. Report of the Standing Committee on Health.* Retrieved from https://www.ourcommons.ca/DocumentViewer/en/42-1/HESA/report-28/.

CASE STUDY

John, a recently graduated registered nurse, has been hired by an acute medical care unit. He is delighted to have a full-time nursing position and eager to prove his competency alongside his quick-thinking colleagues, as well as be accepted by his new peers. There are often too few staff to assist effectively with patient care on the unit. Even when tired from his regularly scheduled shifts, John accepts overtime hours to help alleviate the short staffing, gain favour from his colleagues, and increase his income with student loan repayments looming. His colleagues, however, start to notice that John is often tired and sometimes curt with patients and peers. Recently, he has been taking shortcuts in his patient care, such as failing to adequately check the identity of patients before administering medication. On one particularly short-staffed and hectic day, John administers potassium to one of his patients without checking the patient's identification. The patient's partner questions John about the medication, but John is dismissive about the partner's concern. When the patient, who is in renal failure and whose potassium levels are already elevated, begins to experience chest pain and dyspnea, the patient's worried partner calls another nurse. The patient's medication orders are quickly reviewed and John is asked what he gave to the patient. The physician is immediately contacted for further orders. Later, John and the unit manager review the incident for reporting purposes, as well as to debrief the factors that led to the error—staffing, caregiver fatigue, and breach of practice guidelines—and to discuss strategies to mitigate these issues. How might a union become involved in preventing errors like these? If John continues to make errors, how might his regulatory college become involved? What is John's responsibility as a professional nurse? What is the role of his professional association in promoting quality care and preventing these errors?

Alberta, 2019), which include the maintenance of a registry, establishment of continuing education and practice recency requirements, management of misconduct by members, and approval of nursing programs (Stievano, Caruso, Pittella et al., 2019).

Historically, professional nursing associations encompassed the functions of associations, unions, and regulatory colleges. In some provinces and territories, where not prohibited, the regulatory body and the professional association are still represented by one organization (e.g., the Saskatchewan Registered Nurses Association). Changes in provincial legislation, particularly in the last decade, have emphasized the regulatory rather professional functions of nurse-led organizations, with provinces such as Prince Edward Island transitioning their professional nursing association to a regulatory college (Legislative Counsel Office, 2019). Such legislation has also increasingly separated the functions of regulatory colleges and professional associations. This move has led some experts to express concern that the diminished role of professional associations and their dwindling capacity to influence the health care system and education might also impact the competence of individual nurses and the quality of patient care (Duncan, Thorne, & Rodney, 2015).

 APPLYING CONTENT KNOWLEDGE

Reflect on how, in the last century, nursing has progressively improved its standards of education and practice.

THE FUTURE OF THE NURSING PROFESSION IN CANADA

Changes in nursing practice will likely continue to unfold as the profession responds to the challenges of chronic disease and an aging population, increasing diversity, advanced technology, changes in health care delivery, the evolution of nursing education, changes in legislation that affect nursing practice, the need for increased specialization in practice, and the advancement of nursing knowledge. These changes are already evident in the broadening role of registered nurses in medication administration and that of nurse practitioners in various settings. What is clear is that nursing has evolved far beyond its early days as the vocation of lay and Indigenous healers and religious orders. Nursing is now a self-regulating profession in which entry-level knowledge and skills are learned through baccalaureate education; knowledge and skills are advanced and informed by research and theory; scope of practice is a legislated privilege; and a code of ethics articulates nursing's moral obligation to and contract with society. The growth of nursing as a profession has been aided by education and research and has, in turn, demanded the evolution of nursing-specific education and research. In so doing, nursing has been positioned for roles in a wide variety of settings and as a valuable resource for health care in Canada while retaining its original focus on caring, compassion, and service to others.

SUMMARY OF LEARNING OBJECTIVES

- There is no clear consensus on the definition of profession. The characteristics of a profession put forward by Flexner and others include a formal body of knowledge that is both intellectual and applied, self-regulation, service to others, development of a code of ethics, and acquisition of the knowledge through university education.

- Nursing education has progressed from hospital-based apprenticeship programs to university programs. At the university level, these programs include significant collaborations with college partners to provide access to the baccalaureate education now required for entry to practice in most Canadian jurisdictions. This has been followed by the introduction of graduate programs, the creation of a national framework for nursing educa-

tion, and formal approval and accreditation processes that assure the public of a well-prepared and competent nursing workforce. The development of graduate programs has fostered the growth of nursing research and evidence-informed practice to ensure quality patient care.

- Initial proposals for a baccalaureate degree as an entry-to-practice requirement were resisted because of fears that such a change would result in increased health care costs.

- Each province and territory has legislation that provides nursing with the privilege of self-regulation, which includes mandatory registration for practice, maintenance of a registry of members, management of misconduct, and monitoring of curricula and approval of programs.

CRITICAL THINKING QUESTIONS

1. How would you distinguish a profession from a vocation?
2. Why is a code of ethics important for a profession like nursing?

3. Explain why nursing faced so many challenges in implementing university-level education for members of the profession.

REFERENCES

Akhtar-Danesh, N., Baumann, A., Kolotylo, C., et al. (2013). Perceptions of professionalism among faculty and nursing students. *Western Journal of Nursing Research, 35*, 248–271. https://doi.org/10.1177/0193945911408623.

Bixler, G. K., & Bixler, R. W. (1945). The professional status of nursing. *American Journal of Nursing, 45*(9), 730–735. https://doi.org/10.2307/3416626.

Bradshaw, A. (2010). An historical perspective on the treatment of vocation in the Briggs Report (1972). *Journal of Clinical Nursing, 19*, 3459–3467. https://doi.org/10.1111/j.1365-2702.2010.03359x.

British Columbia College of Nursing Professionals. (2019). *Regulation of nurses*. Retrieved from https://www.bccnp.ca.

Canadian Association of Schools of Nursing. (n.d.). *Accreditation*. Retrieved from https://www.casn.ca/accreditation.

Canadian Association of Schools of Nursing. (2015). *National Nursing Education Framework*. Retrieved from https://www.casn.ca/wp-content/uploads/2014/12/Framwork-FINAL-SB-Nov-30-20151.pdf.

Canadian Association of Schools of Nursing. (2016). *Ties that bind: The evolution of education for professional nursing in the 17th to the 21st century*. Retrieved from https://www.casn.ca/wp-content/uploads/2016/12/History.pdf.

Canadian Association of Schools of Nursing. (2018). *Registered nurses education in Canada statistics*. Retrieved from https://www.casn.ca/wp-content/uploads/2018/12/2016-2017-EN-SFS-FINAL-REPORT-supressed-for-circulation.pdf.

Canadian Nurses Association. (2015). *Framework for the practice of registered nurses in Canada* (vol. 2) (p. 12). Retrieved from https://www.cna-aiic.ca/~/media/cna/page-content/pdf-en/framework-for-the-pracice-of-registered-nurses-in-canada.pdf.

Canadian Nurses Association. (2017). *Code of ethics for registered nurses*. Retrieved from https://www.cna-aiic.ca/~/media/cna/page-content/pdf-en/code-of-ethics-2017-edition-secure-interactive.

Canadian Nurses Association. (2019a). *RN and baccalaureate education*. Retrieved from https://www.cna-aiic.ca/en/nursing-practice/the-practice-of-nursing/education/rn-baccalaureate-education.

Canadian Nurses Association. (2019b). *CNA certification program*. Retrieved from https://www.cna-aiic.ca/en/certification.

Carter, M. (2014). Vocation and altruism in nursing: the habits of practice. *Nursing Ethics, 21*, 695–706. https://doi.org/10.1177/0969733013516159.

College of Nurses of Ontario. (2018). *Legislation and regulation: an introduction to the Nursing Act, 1991*. Retrieved from http://www.cno.org/globalassets/docs/prac/41064_fsnursingact.pdf.

College of Registered Nurses of British Columbia. (2018). *Legislation relevant to nurses' practice*. College of Registered Nurses of British Columbia: Vancouver, BC.

College of Registered Nurses of Manitoba. (n.d.). *Policy and legislation*. Retrieved from https://www.crnm.mb.ca/about/policies-and-legislation.

Duncan, S., Thorne, S., & Rodney, P. (2015). Evolving trends in nurse regulation: what are the policy impacts for nursing's social impact? *Nursing Inquiry, 22*(1), 27–38. https://doi.org/10.1111/nin.12087.

Flexner, A. (1915). Is social work a profession? *Proceedings of the National Conference of Charities and Corrections* (pp. 578–581). Chicago, IL: Heldermann.

Fowler, M. (2010). *Guide to the code of ethics for nurses: Interpretation and application.* Silver Spring, MD: American Nurses Association.

Gallup. (2017). *Nurses keep healthy lead as most honest, ethical profession.* Retrieved from https://news.gallup.com/poll/224639/nurses-keep-healthy-lead-honest-ethical-profession.aspx?g_source=CATEGORY_SOCIAL_POLICY_ISSUES&g_medium=topic&g_campaign=tiles.

Government of Alberta. (2019). *Regulated health professions and colleges.* Retrieved from https://www.alberta.ca/regulated-health-professions.aspx.

Government of Newfoundland. (2019). *Amendments proposed to strengthen the Nurses' Act.* Retrieved from www.releases.gov.nl.ca.

Legislative Counsel Office. (2019). *Regulated Health Professions Act.* Retrieved from https://www.princeedwardisland.ca/sites/default/files/legislation/r-10-1-regulated_health_professions_act.pdf.

House of Commons. (2019, June 17). *Report 28: The Health of LGBTQIA2 Communities in Canada. Report of the Standing Committee on Health.* Retrieved from https://www.ourcommons.ca/DocumentViewer/en/42-1/HESA/report-28/.

Munroe, S. (2019). *The persons case: a milestone in the history of Canadian women.* Retrieved from https://www.thoughtco.com/the-persons-case-508713.

Nurses Association of New Brunswick. (2008). *Nurses Act.* Retrieved from http://www.nanb.nb.ca/media/resource/NANB-NursesAct-2008-Bilang.pdf.

Ordre des infirmières et infirmiers du Québec. (2010). *Preparation guide for the Ordre de infirmières et infirmiers du Québec.*

Retrieved from https://www.oiiq.org/sites/default/files/uploads/pdf/publications/publicationsoiiq/Supplement-anglais.pdf.

Parse, R. (1998). Nursing: The discipline and the profession. *Nursing Science Quarterly, 12,* 275–276. https://doi.org/10.1177/089431849901200401.

Philbin, G., & Keepnews, D. (2014). Edward L. Bernays and nursing's code of ethics: An unexplained history. *Nursing History Review, 22,* 144–158. https://doi.org/10.1891/1062-8061.22.144.

Registered Nurses Association of the Northwest Territories and Nunavut. (2015). *Acts and legislation.* Retrieved from http://www.rnantnu.ca/documents/acts-legislation.

Saskatchewan Registered Nurses Association. (2019). *Acts and by-laws.* Retrieved from https://www.srna.org/about-us/how-we-govern/act-bylaws/.

Stievano, A., Caruso, R., Pittella, F., et al. (2019). Shaping nursing professional regulation through history: a systematic review. *International Nursing Review, 66*(1), 17–29. https://doi.org/10.1111/inr12449.

White, K. (2002). Nursing as vocation. *Nursing Ethics, 9,* 279–290. https://doi.org/10.1191/0969733002ne510oa.

Wilensky, H. L. (1964). The professionalization of everyone? *American Journal of Sociology, 70*(2), 137–187. https://doi.org/10.1086/223790.

Wytenbroek, L., & Vandenberg, H. (2017). Reconsidering nursing's history during Canada 150. *Canadian Nurse, 113*(4), 16–18.

Yam, B. (2004). From vocation to profession: the quest for professionalization of nursing. *British Journal of Nursing, 9,* 978–982. https://doi.org/10.12968/bjon.2004.13.16.15974.

Yukon Registered Nurses Association. (2019). *Regulatory authority.* Retrieved from https://yukonnurses.ca/index.php?option=com_content&view=article&id=304&Itemid=276.

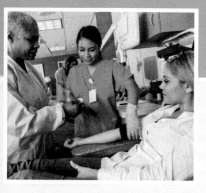

4

The Professional Image: Impact and Strategies for Change

Lori Schindel Martin

ⓔ http://evolve.elsevier.com/Canada/Ross-Kerr/nursing

LEARNING OBJECTIVES

After reading this chapter, you will be able to:

- Examine the impact of the image of nursing on the profession.
- Describe historical factors that have influenced the image of nursing.
- Appreciate the influence of mass and social media in shaping the public image of nursing.
- Recognize the impact of image on educational experience, recruitment, and emergent professional self-identity.
- Discuss how the self-image of nursing affects the ongoing development of the nursing profession.
- Apply strategies to strengthen a positive professional image of nursing.

OUTLINE

KEY TERMS

professional image
professional self-identity
positive professional image
public image of nursing

professional image enactment
professional brand image
professional image marketing

PERSONAL PERSPECTIVES

Leroy graduated with a nursing degree in 1983. His mother, Constance, was a surgical nurse who received a hospital-based diploma in 1948. When he was still a young boy, Constance gave Leroy a book titled *Nurses Who Led the Way: Real Life Stories of Courageous Women in an Exciting Profession* (De Leeuw & De Leeuw, 1961). Leroy and his mother shared many conversations about the contributions to professional image by nurse influencers such as Florence Nightingale. Constance believed that the great strength of nursing is its roots in diversity. She returned to full-time nursing in 1969 as a nursing supervisor, taking courses about postoperative nursing to help direct-care nurses implement acute change of condition protocols. Constance encouraged Leroy to consider a baccalaureate nursing degree as the gateway to a career that would satisfy his intellectual curiosity and desire to experience professional caregiving across many specialties. Leroy completed a baccalaureate nursing program and began his career on an in-patient chronic disease management unit. He stayed there for 3 years after becoming a team leader. He then transferred to a diabetic education role while studying for a Master of Nursing, graduating in 1990. He became a clinical nurse specialist in cardiac care in a teaching hospital, then joined an elder care research team evaluating chronic congestive heart failure protocols in nursing homes. Preparing for retirement, Leroy came across the book Constance had given him all those years ago. He realized that the strong images of nursing contributed to his positive professional self-identity. From an early age, Leroy recognized that nursing was an influential profession from its historical beginnings; nursing practice had always involved data collection, informed decision making, theory, policy analysis, advocacy, equitable distribution of resources, and public education. After transitioning into full retirement, he began writing a new book, in collaboration with his mother, to educate children about professional nurses, their backgrounds, and the important roles they played.

INTRODUCTION

The **professional image** of nursing has evolved since the discipline's inception in the 1850s. There is agreement that, by definition, a professional health care discipline must incorporate specialized knowledge and skills, legislated accountabilities for public safety, standards of practice established by bona fide regulatory and organizational bodies, and a formalized process of licensure for protected titles such as "Registered Nurse" (Ayala, Vanderstracten, & Bracke, 2014) (see Chapter 3). Professional image reflects a philosophical "way of being" shared by members within a professional discipline. Nursing scholars and professional bodies believe that a strongly **positive professional image** in nursing is associated with high-quality evidence-informed education that equips nurses with the knowledge and courage to risk public advocacy. This advocacy mobilizes resources for the development of policy to support excellent patient outcomes (Gordon, 2010; Marafion & Pera, 2015).

Professional image involves two sets of perceptions: those from outside the discipline, who witness group member behaviour, and those within the discipline, who enact the professional role. Professional image is never static; it is in a continual process of development, shifting from moment to moment throughout nurses' lives and across time according to context (Neishabouri, Ahmadi, & Kazemnejad, 2017; Marafion & Pera, 2015). In nursing, political, social, economic, environmental, and interpersonal factors shape the context and meanings of professional image (Emeghebo, 2012; Price & McGillis Hall, 2014; Tuckett, 2015). Professional image and **professional self-identity** are interrelated. Professional image emerges from real, tangible actions in the clinical field represented by symbols, metaphors, stories, and clinical examples. It is significant that self-image is shaped by nurses' perceptions of the public image of nursing (Browne, Wall, Batt, & Bennett, 2018). Therefore, strategies to strengthen the professional image of nursing must address the perceptions of both nurses and those of the public.

Across jurisdictions in Canada, there are inconsistencies with respect to the characteristics that constitute professional "image." There is no single accepted definition of professional image in nursing; common elements reflect both direct and indirect performance indicators. Direct indicators include conduct, competence, evidence-informed care delivery, physical appearance and interprofessional collaboration (Akhtar-Danesh, Baumann, Kolotylo et al., 2013; Daigle, 2018). Professional image is also a set of indirect indicators that guide practice such as values, beliefs, knowledge, intellect, critical thinking, and inquiry (Rezaei-Adaryani, Salsali, & Mohammadi, 2012).

The varying images of nursing as a profession have captured the attention of the nursing literature and professional associations because of how inconsistencies in the image affect educational experience, recruitment, retention, turnover, career development, career success, professional self-esteem, and professional self-identity

CASE STUDY
Nursing is Multifaceted and Complex

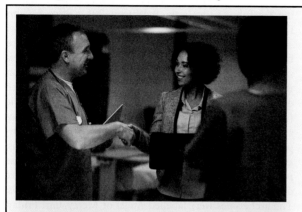
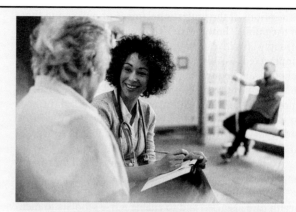
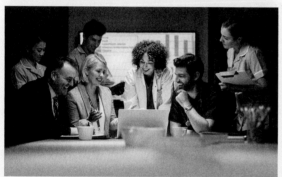
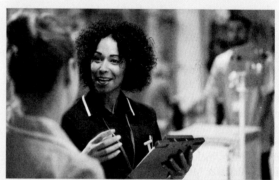

(istock.com/sturti)

While Yoo-Hee and Juan were preparing a presenta-tion about professional image in nursing, Juan stated, "Remember when Student Council proposed a new pro-fessional design for school uniforms? I didn't understand what that meant!" Yoo-Hee replied, "Yes, I didn't yet have an informed opinion, but now I think professional image is something that all nurses are accountable for and it goes beyond appearance and how we 'care.' Think about the way our preceptor quoted research-based assessment and non-pharmacological strategies for delirium dur-ing the team meeting. Jennifer looked polished and her words had power." Juan and Yoo-Hee agreed that Jennifer projected a positive professional image by being knowl-edgeable, competent, and convincing and by facilitating team implementation of delirium protocols, mentoring students, and serving on the board of a nursing organi-zation. Yoo-Hee and Juan interviewed Jennifer to identify

strategies for novice nurses to build their own profession-al self-image. Jennifer explained, "About six months into my first job, my manager asked me to co-lead our unit's fall prevention working group. I was nervous, but I chan-neled that energy to get the group talking, researching protocols, and putting their ideas together into a practical plan. Our team reduced fall rates and won a practice in-novation award. Collaborative leadership has been part of my professional self-identity ever since." As part of their presentation, Juan and Yoo-Hee reported on nursing roles for implementing a delirium protocol. They asked their peers to develop short messages about principles for as-sessment of delirium that would support the use of the protocol during team huddles.

List the characteristics and actions that contributed to Jennifer's professional image and self-identity. How might this experience influence Yoo-Hee and Juan?

(Liu & Liu, 2016; Masters & Liu 2016; Toren, Kerzman, & Kagan, 2011). Historically, tension has existed between "what actually is" and "what could be" with respect to perceptions of the professional image of nurses and those of the public (Emeghebo, 2012; Nelson & Gordon, 2006). Strongly positive images are crystallizing toward an empowered worldview of professional nursing. Nurse scholars and educators around the world are working toward a positive professional image. Most G20 nations and several neighbouring states have recognized the need to develop strategies that invoke and sustain a positive individual and collective identity and public image of nursing.

A strongly positive professional image of nursing is important to attract strong students to the profession, to provide nurse administrators with educated staff for health care agencies, and to enable nurse scholars to mentor the next generation of researchers. Continuous efforts to refine and polish the professional image of nursing are the responsibility of all nurses, regardless of career stage. Projecting a shared positive professional image will provide all nurses with confidence, pride, and influence when identifying themselves as nurses during interactions across social, health care, and community situations. Currently, Canada's health care system is changing to one in which innovation and creativity are required of all workers, the use of technology is ever increasing, and the roles of health care providers, including nurses, are shifting for economic reasons (Price & McGillis Hall, 2014; Canadian Institute for Health Information, 2019). More than ever before, the nursing profession needs bright, articulate leaders and mentors who can pave the way to success by aligning practices to shifting needs and by taking on professional roles that new technologies and global health requirements bring into play.

HISTORICAL IMAGES OF NURSES AND NURSING

In addressing the image of nursing, nurses ought to reflect on the historical factors that influence these images. Such a perspective will contribute to ongoing efforts to enhance the image of nursing using a cache of impactful strategies that support strongly positive images of professional nurses. Images of any profession or work group are influenced by the values and orientations learned from family and friends and by individuals' experiences with particular members of a profession, including nurse managers (Milisen, De Busser, Kayaert et al., 2010; Morris-Thompson, Shepherd, Plata, & Marks-Maran, 2011; Varaei, Vaismoradi, Jasper, & Faghihzadeh, 2012). Images are also influenced

by mass and social media messages, both past and current. These include television programs, films, books, newspapers, radio reports, and social media platforms, including YouTube (Kelly, Fealy, & Watson, 2012; Price & Gillis Hall, 2014).

A seminal study on the image of nursing, conducted by Kalisch and Kalisch (1982, p. 5), involved a historical survey of mass media products pertaining to nursing that were published between the nineteenth and mid-twentieth centuries. These media sources included "the print media (200 novels, 143 magazine short stories, poems and articles and 20,000 newspaper clippings), as well as the newer nonprint media (204 motion pictures, 122 radio programs, and 320 television episodes)." Through an analysis of these products, the researchers classified the image into five dominant types characterizing five successive time periods. The archetypes were labelled Angel of Mercy, Girl Friday, Heroine, Mother, and Sex Object (Table 4.1).

APPLYING CONTENT KNOWLEDGE

The emergence of the careerist nurse (Kalisch & Kalisch, 1982) has shifted the professional image of nursing toward realizing its full potential for practice change. How does the nurse in this photo portray a professional image that mirrors that of the contemporary careerist? Consider the sociopolitical contexts of Canada's current health care system that have contributed to the evolution of the contemporary careerist nurse. Reflect upon the professional image you wish to portray. What positive attributes of professional image do you believe you already portray? What do you consciously wish to change? Why?

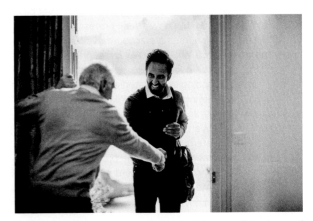

Professional nurse greets client at home. (istock.com/ Dean Mitchell)

TABLE 4.1   Nursing Typologies from 1854 to the Present

Typology	Time Period	Characteristics	Context
Angel of Mercy	1854–1919	Noble, moral, religious, virginal, ritualistic, self-sacrificing	• Crimean War • World War I
Girl Friday	1920–1929	Subservient, cooperative, methodical, dedicated, modest, loyal	• Industrial growth and urbanization • Development of hospital systems
Heroine	1930–1945	Brave, rational, dedicated, decisive, humanistic, autonomous	• Great Depression • World War II
Mother	1946–1965	Maternal, nurturing, sympathetic, passive, expressive, domestic	• Decommissioned soldiers return to an economic boom across North America • Working women and married nurses are expected to return to domestic work
Sex Object	1966–1981	Sensual, romantic, hedonistic, frivolous, irresponsible, promiscuous	• Sexual revolution • Feminist movement • First baccalaureate programs in Canada
Careerist	1982–1999	Intelligent, logical, progressive, sophisticated, empathic, and assertive woman or man who is committed to attaining higher and higher standards of health care	• Emergence of nursing theorists, career nurse scientists, graduate degrees, first doctoral programs in nursing science and nursing research • Emergence of best practice guidelines, professional practice standards of nursing, and evidence-informed nursing • Emergence of specialized certification under the auspices of the Canadian Nurses Association
Contemporary careerist	2000– present	Well educated, sophisticated, interprofessional collaborator, international and global health advocate, media savvy, and contributor to policy and change advocacy	• Expansion of advanced practice nursing roles • Emergence of nurse-led clinics and health services • Expansion of nurses appointed as leaders of national and international committees

Sources: Adapted from Kalisch, B., & Kalisch, P. (1982). Anatomy of the image of the nurse: Dissonant and ideal models. In C. Williams (Ed.), *Image-making in nursing* (pp. 3–23). Kansas City, MO: American Academy of Nursing; Price, S. L., & McGillis Hall, L. (2014). The history of nurse imagery and the implications for recruitment: A discussion paper. *Journal of Advanced Nursing, 70*(7), 1502–1509. https://doi.org/10.1111/jan.12289.

Without a doubt, various contextual factors have influenced these changing images. Socioeconomic and political influencers have informed the direction of the nursing self-identity and professional image. For instance, during the Victorian period, when nurses were practising in the Crimean battlefield, nurses came to be perceived as Angels of Mercy. Since that time, the image of nursing has aligned with various social and political movements representing significant change or upheaval. These include, for example, World War I and World War II, economic booms and busts, urbanization, hospitalization, feminism, technological innovation, evidence-based knowledge, credentialling, and globalization. Nursing will continue to shift and change according to the world within which individuals and the entire discipline practises and builds new knowledge.

CHANGING IMAGES OF NURSES AND NURSING

It could be said that nursing has come full circle since the era of Florence Nightingale. Nightingale consciously chose nursing as a career, despite the objections of her family, and contributed to developing the vision for what it means to be a professional nurse. Nightingale has been referred to as the first nurse researcher. Her contributions and achievements were astounding. She saved the lives of many wounded soldiers during the Crimean War, restoring order from chaos by assuming responsibility for the soldiers' environment as well as nursing care, despite strong resistance from the physicians in charge. Nightingale brought innovation and advancement to the fields of nursing, health, and hospital planning. She was well educated, used knowledge and scientific thinking to develop and test new methods for health care, and wrote essays, policy briefs, and reports. Nightingale wrote the seminal work *Notes on Nursing: What It Is and What It Is Not* (Nightingale, 1969), first published in 1859. She met regularly with politicians to advocate for funding and better health conditions. She set the path for future nurses to engage in the practice of evidence-informed care delivery (McDonald, 2014).

Two recent studies of easily accessible texts and images have identified how messaging might influence the public's perception of nurses and nursing and reflect the earlier work of Kalisch and Kalisch (Carroll & Rosa, 2016; Koo & Lin, 2016). Carroll and Rosa (2016) conducted a qualitative media analysis to explore the roles and images of nursing found in 30 children's books published for audiences from prekindergarten through Grade 2. Seven themes about nurses emerged from the media analysis: unlikely, minimal, caring, subordinate, skillful, diverse, and obvious. The images of nursing across the storybooks were simple yet inaccurate portrayals; the depiction of nursing behaviour was positive for the most part. The researchers discussed the potential for inaccurate portrayals of nurses in children's literature to continue influencing individual viewpoints of nursing over a lifetime. They recommended that the image of nursing in children's storybooks be modified to reflect an accurate portrayal of both the art and science of nursing by emphasizing the knowledge, skills, diversity, and complexity of nursing care.

Similarly, Koo and Lin (2016) analyzed the first 100 images obtained through a search for the term "nurse" using Google Images and Shutterstock. A total of 171 portrayals of nursing behaviour were found within the 100 images. The images were predominantly of women, the majority of them smiling, often with a stethoscope and holding documents, clip boards, or tablet computers. A small number of images depicted the application of medical or technological devices. While the researchers concluded that the majority of images were professional looking, role performance was limited to acts of comfort or recording data. A paucity of images depicted nurses engaging in scientific activities such as research. The authors recommended that nurses advocate for more accurate and comprehensive representation of the nursing profession on the Internet. These studies identified a gap that current nurses can fill with respect to promoting strongly positive messages about the nature of nurses' work. Shifting messages in this direction will have a positive impact on how the profession is regarded by the public and will attract potential recruits who are seeking a careerist path.

RESEARCH FOCUS

The purpose of this study was to build knowledge about the factors influencing turnover and retention of new graduate nurses. The hypothesis was that the combined effects of nurses' pre-entry expectations, perceived intensity of work practices, and professional self-image would influence nurses' decisions to leave or remain in first-career nursing jobs. The prospective, longitudinal study recruited 160 nurses affiliated with the Quebec Nurses' Association and followed them for over 3 years. Researchers collected baseline survey data regarding pre-entry work expectations and professional image at the time of nursing program graduation (Time 1). At 6 months postwork entry, participants were asked to complete a survey capturing their perceptions of high-involvement work practices, professional self-image, and intention to leave the organization (Time 2). Finally, 3 years after Time 2, participants were surveyed about organizational and professional turnover. Data analysis consisted of structural equation modelling to examine relationships among and between the main constructs. The study's main finding is that perceived high-involvement work practices were positively related to professional self-image, although professional self-image held by participants did not seem to affect turnover. The researchers concluded that early and meaningful engagement of novice nurses in high-involvement work practices contributes to the development of a positive professional self-image. They recommended that nurse administrators, educational leaders, and advanced clinical practice nurses could strengthen professional self-image and identity by providing novice nurses with opportunities to contribute to membership on committees, project evaluations, development of best practice guidelines, and facilitating workplace educational presentations for peers.

Source: Chênevert, L., Jourdain, G., & Vandenberghe, C. (2016). The role of high-involvement work practices and professional self-image in nursing recruits' turnover: A three-year prospective study. *International Journal of Nursing Studies*, 53, 73–84. https://doi.org/10.1016/j.ijnurstu.2015.09.005.

PUBLIC PERCEPTION OF NURSES AND NURSING

Nurses have become increasingly aware that they are accountable and responsible for the public's inaccurate and outdated perceptions of nursing. The **public image of**

nursing is paradoxical: nurses are respected for their caring role, but not the complex interplay of their scientific knowledge, skills, and competencies (Gordon, 2010; Ben Natan, 2016; Kelly, Fealy, & Watson, 2012). Public perception influences recruitment into nursing programs and the retention of nurses in the workforce (Ben Natan, 2016). Research suggests that a barrier to the recruitment of talented individuals is the prevalence of an over-simplified image of nursing that omits the complexity, scholarship, and robust science of nursing practice (Girvin, Jackson, & Hutchison, 2016; Morris-Thompson, Shepherd, Plata, & Marks-Maran, 2011; Price & McGillis Hall, 2014; Price, McGillis Hall, Angus, & Peter, 2013). Professional discourse that trivializes nursing knowledge, standards, and competencies minimizes nursing influence in the policy arena (Gordon, 2010). Continuous mobilization of strongly positive and accurate portrayals of the complexity of nursing work will provide the social platform upon which nurses can better advocate for themselves and for better health care system outcomes.

Popular culture often depicts nurses as undervalued heroes rather than the careerists envisioned by Kalisch and Kalisch (1982). Television shows like *Grey's Anatomy* and *Kim's Convenience* and the film *Meet the Parents* all portray both female and male nurses as capable, but with serious flaws, including uncertainty and clumsiness. For the most part, nursing characters are shown in situations involving unskilled bodywork (e.g., taking a patient's pulse or temperature, holding a patient's hand, and sharing a joke or a smile) rather than those involving skillful leadership, the application of research-informed knowledge, or the teaching of clients and families.

Nursing is far more complex than its image lets on. Developing the knowledge, skills, attitudes, and values needed to practice nursing is a complicated undertaking. The knowledge and skills needed to be a competent nurse are considerable. Nurses often situate caring as the central component of relational practice, requiring authentic communication and interpersonal connection (Gottlieb, 2013; Tuckett, 2015). The public image of nursing reflects the caring aspect of the nursing role. It is now the collective responsibility of nurses to expand the public's understanding of nursing to include recognition that scientific knowledge and empirical evidence forms the basis of interpersonal caring acts in the same way that evidence underpins clinical knowledge, skills, and competencies (Girvin, Jackson, & Hutchinson, 2016). While caring requires authentic altruism, its **professional image enactment** requires strong interpersonal skills and clinical knowledge.

The public image of nursing does not typically reflect power or authority. In contrast, a positive professional image is a form of power that brings respect and enables nurses to create changes to improve conditions for their patients (ten Hoeve, Jansen & Roodbol, 2014; Tuckett, 2015; Tuckett & Turner, 2016). Purposeful action on the part of nurse administrators, educators, and researchers can create and support a positive image of nursing. Emergent communication platforms offer genuine opportunities for nurses to immerse themselves deeply and meaningfully in networking, advocacy, and practice change initiatives to build and maintain their professional self-identity and experience self-mastery with respect to influencing care. The marketing and branding of the discipline of nursing as a profession with a powerful collective voice could be an excellent vehicle through which to effect change in the public's image of nursing.

SELF-IMAGE OF NURSING

Nurses' professional identity may be understood as inextricably linked to self-image or internal image. Self-image is vitally important, because people's perceptions of nurses and nursing are influenced by their interactions and experiences with nurses. Discussion papers, literature reviews, and research studies indicate that professional image is related to recruitment, work engagement, job satisfaction, retention, turnover, and professional advancement (Chauke, Van Der Wal, & Botha, 2015; Emeghebo, 2012; Rezaei-Adaryani, Salsali, & Mohammadi, 2012; Tuckett, Kim, & Huh, 2017). The studies cited indicate that these factors were considerably more influential in shaping nurses' self-image than were inaccurate messages distributed through the media. Thus, nurse educators, clinicians, and administrative leaders, in collaboration with nursing students and novice nurses, must develop and evaluate their own strategies to strengthen self-image and share this broadly throughout the public sphere (Chauke, Van Der Wal, & Botha, 2105; Tuckett, Kim, & Huh, 2017).

Canadian researchers have conducted studies examining how nurses perceive their own self-image (Price & McGillis Hall, 2014; Price, McGillis Hall, Angus, & Peter, 2013). Their findings suggest that the stereotypical view that places virtuous caring at the centre of nursing represents a one-dimensional, dissatisfying understanding of nursing. The authors recommend that marketing of a more complete image of nursing should emphasize messaging about opportunities for career diversification, specialization, graduate education, as well as mentorship and teaching.

A recent study introduced three measurement scales to study brand image in nursing (Godsey, Hayes, Schertzer et al., 2018). The research team consisted of nursing and business scholars interested in measuring factors that might contribute to the development of a consistent **professional brand image**. The researchers hypothesized that a clear professional image will ultimately lead to cohesive and transformative leadership within nursing. The aim of this study was to complete a factor analysis across three scales: nurse brand image scale (42 items describing the profession); nursing's current brand position scale (10 items), and nursing's desired brand position scale (10 items). A sample of 286 nursing alumni and faculty representing 28 states from Florida to Alaska completed the scales through an electronic survey. The study's findings provide strong preliminary evidence for the factor structure and internal consistency reliability of the three scales.

Although this work is at an early stage, the research team established that nurse participants were most likely to describe their professional brand image with terms reflecting the interpersonal aspects of practice, such as communication, caring, and compassion. Participants were least likely to relate professional brand image with factors associated with influential leadership. The study points to the need to educate nursing students such that their emergent professional brand image is more strongly associated with influence, decision making, and authority.

Nurses have often reported struggling to build and maintain a positive professional self-image, particularly one that extends beyond their role as a caregiver; these relational aspects of nursing seem to be the easiest to market to the public and to potential recruits. The centrality of the nurse–patient relationship as the focus of nursing competence may be reflected in appearance, approach to patients, relationships with other health care providers, and behaviour in the community. Many factors contribute to the development of self-image, including the values and attitudes one brings to a profession. These values and attitudes are influenced by life experiences before entering the educational system to prepare for the profession (Carroll & Rosa, 2016). The educational system then influences the learner's concept of nursing practice, the role of the nurse, relationships with other health care providers, and professional responsibilities as a member of the profession and the community.

Nurse educators can help to cultivate a positive self-image of nursing through teaching and role modelling. They may also contribute unknowingly to some negative aspects of image development. The importance that they attach to the individual nurse and to the work of nursing can have a major effect on how the students view themselves for many years. Nurse educators can assist students with developing their own professional brand image through assignments about nursing advocacy (writing policy briefing notes) and entrepreneurship (developing business plans, brochures, and business cards). Students are also strongly influenced by the nurses—practitioners, administrators, researchers—with whom they interact in clinical practice settings and by the relationships they observe between nurses and other health care providers (Schuler, 2016). There is some evidence that seasoned nurses feel hopeful that younger generations of nurses, who have been educated in evidence-based nursing and practice at the baccalaureate level, will assume leadership roles that engage the public in shifting the image of nursing (Ben Natan, 2016; Girvin, Jackson, & Hutchison, 2016; Marcinowicz, Owlasiuk, & Perkowska, 2016). Seasoned nurses are well positioned to act as mentors and role models for younger nurses, collaborating to build a strongly positive collective vision for nursing identity.

Nurses have the opportunity to effect changes now and assume responsibility for the future of nursing. Individuals can affect the image of nursing through their daily performance in nursing practice and their reactions to various members of the public—patients, family members, friends, students, potential recruits, other professionals, legislators, policy makers, or colleagues. As indicated by the studies cited, these interactions contribute to other people's views of nursing. Moreover, one's personal experiences as a nurse and one's own perception of nursing have a great impact on daily encounters with the public.

The self-image of nursing affects whether nurses encourage others to enter the discipline, including their own children. A strong self-image of nursing influences how nurses think students should be educated. A positive professional image inspires nurses to conduct research, translate new knowledge into practice, and engage in **professional image marketing** to ensure nursing services are applied effectively for desired outcomes. A professional image motivates nurses to improve how nursing services are organized and encourages nurses to advocate for policy change for better health outcomes. A professional image awakens nurses to the importance of helping people take responsibility for their own health and strengthens nurses' commitment to ensuring people can influence decisions about their own care. Although nurses will not always agree on the specifics of recommended policy changes to improve nursing services, they should collaborate together with stakeholders to reach consensus, identify common goals, and have sound rationale to support their positions. A shared professional image embraced by all members of the discipline has the potential to build the power of nurses for influence in both the professional and political arenas.

CULTURAL CONSIDERATIONS
Diversity, Inclusion, and Professional Image

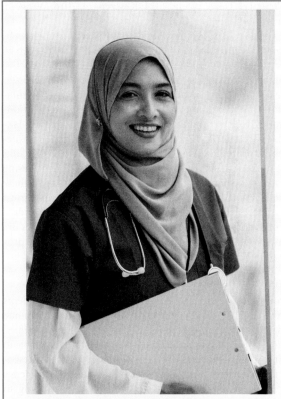

(istock.com/SDI Productions)

Amira's Professional Self-Image Journey

When Amira graduated from her nursing program, she was delighted to accept a position in a small community hospital in rural Saskatchewan. Amira, a Muslim, was not certain how she could gain entrée into the community. She was living away from her family for the first time, at the staff residence across from the hospital. She worried about how members of the small town would see her, and she wondered what strategies she could use to convey a professional image while she simultaneously developed her self-identity as a novice nurse.

After the end of the in-class orientation, a preceptor was assigned to guide Amira through her first set of practice shifts. During Amira's first shift, one client asked questions about her qualifications, saying to the preceptor, "Do they learn enough about nursing where she comes from?" What would Amira's best professional response be to this microaggression? What sort of professional response should Amira expect from her preceptor? What factors might contribute to the client's reaction?

At the end of the shift, Amira noticed a group of staff gathering at the nursing station, preparing to leave together. She suddenly recognized this as an opportunity to promote herself as a professional colleague. What actions would you advise Amira to take? What should she say? What words, phrases, and terms should Amira include in her "1-minute professional nurse branding message"? Why?

STRATEGIES FOR CHANGING THE IMAGE OF NURSES AND NURSING

While some residual negative images of nurses and nursing persist, strategies that will continue enhancing the image of nurses and nursing need to be identified, such as actions that could be undertaken by individuals and the profession through professional associations. These strategies include paying attention to appearance and communication style, enrolling in continuing educational programs, seeking a mentor, volunteering for committees, staying current with professional literature, engaging in political advocacy, and seeking career development programs. Nurses can actively follow the social media presence of professional nurse leaders. Retweeting positive messages about nursing knowledge advancements and advocacy initiatives to family, friends, and network partners will influence public understanding. This action will ensure the broad dissemination of strong professional images that reflect the complex nature of the discipline of nursing.

Leaders for Professional Image

Evidence suggests that both nurse administrators and nurse educators have a strong role to play in strengthening the professional image of nursing students (Milisen, De Busser, Kayaert et al., 2010). Nursing scholars, career mentors, and preceptors all contribute to reinforcing the image of nurses as competent and evidence informed as well as engaged in conducting and disseminating nursing research. Positive growth and expansion in influential nursing roles across Canada in the past decade has led to new graduates who take pride in their nursing work, recommend nursing to others, and quickly engage in ongoing professional development to maintain their currency and expand their knowledge, practice, and skill base.

Experiences That Grow Professional Image

Nurses can seek new opportunities to collaborate with nurses and other professionals who hold different viewpoints or can share new skills or knowledge. Deep immersion in professional development activities such as participating in research projects, developing skills in student mentoring, and enacting these as a formal preceptor will serve to strengthen nurses' self-image and position them to realize their full potential as leaders and changemakers (Girvin, Jackson, & Hutchison, 2016; Kagan, Biran, Telem et al., 2015; Price & McGillis Hall, 2014). These activities will all contribute to a professional identity that leads to greater job satisfaction, higher retention, and an emergent professional self-image that can be shared and modeled within public forums.

Social Media for Professional Image

Tuckett and Turner (2016) conducted a survey of new nursing and midwifery graduates' uptake of social media. Their findings suggest that social media platforms could allow novice nurses to strengthen their self-image by sharing examples of their work as well-educated, scholarly, evidence-informed practitioners. The authors recommended that nurse educators facilitate this use of social media to assist with the development of professional self-identity. Since becoming an effective leader requires developing a positive self-image (Godsey, Hayes, Schertzer et al., 2018; Marcinowicz, Owlasiuk, & Perkowska, 2016), it makes sense that this should be the focus of strategies to improve nursing's image.

Recruitment and Professional Image

In an effort to cultivate the image of nurses as intelligent, capable, and equal partners in health care delivery, a number of universities and professional organizations have produced videos to recruit students into the profession. The videos depict nurses as articulate, compassionate, and innovative professionals who work as key members of a health care team. Links to videos produced by the Registered Nurses' Association of Ontario, the Registered Practical Nurses' Association of Ontario, the Canadian Nurses Association (CNA), and the Canadian Nursing Students' Association (CNSA) could be added to nursing school websites to promote a strongly positive professional image to students interested in nursing as a career.

Regardless of the format or the group to which recruitment strategies are targeted, the materials used to attract people into undergraduate nursing programs and nurses into positions in health care agencies must be scrutinized for the image of nursing presented (Price & McGillis Hall, 2014; Kagan, Biran, Telem et al., 2015). The materials should be relevant to all genders as well as to individuals from diverse backgrounds (Ben Natan, 2016). Care should

be given to the messaging such that recruitment materials address the unique needs of male nurses whose professional self-image is impacted by a specific set of variables (Chan, Lo, Tse, & Wong, 2014; Kluczynska, 2016; Wang, Li, Hu et al., 2011) (see Chapter 5).

Most institutions now make extensive use of their websites for student recruitment. Recruitment strategies can be very effective in presenting a positive image to prospective students. Nursing schools must ensure that their websites are picked up by major search engines to hit as representative a public group as possible. Professional organizations should dedicate financial resources to ensure that the language on their websites is optimized such that the websites appear prominently in Internet searches (Price & McGillis Hall, 2014). A search for the term "nursing Canada" using Google.ca brings up thousands of websites. Many of these sites are prospective employers, and they include most of the Canadian nursing schools, all of which provide a description of nursing as a profession. These websites are an excellent opportunity to present a strongly positive professional image of nursing to the public.

Promoting a Professional Public Image

Professional websites that target nurses and nursing students provide an excellent opportunity to present a professional image of nursing to the public. The sites, if demonstrated during public presentations made by nurses, could serve to reinforce positive professional images. During these presentations, nurses should describe their practice as evidence informed, competency based, and delivered according to expected standards. The focus of practice should be on the promotion and maintenance of health, not only illness care, with the goal of helping people attain, maintain, and regain their optimal levels of health and function. Nurses should be portrayed as being in interdependent practice, where they enact a leadership role in collaborative decision making and in making independent decisions related to nursing care.

During public forums, nurses should explain that they play an active role in creating policies pertaining to health care and its financing and are not merely reacting to circumstances and events (Kagan, Biran, Telem et al., 2015). During public presentations, nurses should explain that they base their practice upon evidence-informed standards and competencies. Professional organizations can educate the public about expected performance and practice guidelines, for example, the Standards of Nursing Practice and Competencies published by the CNA's Certification Program Advisory Group and the Best Practice Guidelines published by the Registered Nurses' Association of Ontario. Broad dissemination to the public about professional standards will also reinforce the public's understanding of the important advocacy role of nurses (see Table 4.2).

TABLE 4.2   Strategies to Influence the Professional Self-Image of Nurses

Strategy	Description
Nurse managers promote professional image	Nurse manager and administrative leader competencies should include promoting, reinforcing, and commending student and staff evidence of professional image (Masters & Liu, 2016; Varaei, Vaismoradi, Jasper, & Faghihzadeh, 2012)
Nurse educators support students' professional image	Nurse educators are responsible and accountable for assisting nursing students in building a strongly positive professional image (Milisen, De Busser, Kayaert et al., 2010)
Nurses contribute to an image that reflects diversity within the profession	All members of the discipline of nursing are responsible and accountable for contributing to the development of a strongly positive professional image that includes equally strong representation of all genders, culturally diverse backgrounds, rural and urban contexts, and so on (Wang, Li, Hu et al., 2011)
Nurses promote a contemporary image of nursing to elementary and high school students	Nurses across all jurisdictions should project and reinforce an updated professional image that reflects the "contemporary careerist" using social media, recruitment posters, and presentations that specifically target students in elementary and high school (Koo & Lin, 2016; Tuckett, Kim, & Hugh, 2017)
Nurses promote a contemporary image through children's stories	Nurses should write children's stories about nursing to contribute to the continued evolution of nurses' image as contemporary careerists (Carroll & Rosa, 2016)
Nurses increase their marketing skills	Nurses should take courses on marketing and brand messaging, and use these skills to drive image building in the discipline (Coke, 2019)
Nurses use reliable and valid measures of self-image	Nurse educators and professional practitioners should teach nurses to use reliable and valid self-image rating measures through their student years and throughout their developing careers (Coke, 2019; Godsey, Hayes, Schertzer et al., 2018)
Support nurses' engagement in social media	Professional organizations should involve their members in annual social media and professional image writing campaigns (Price & McGillis Hall, 2014)
Engage nursing students and novice nurses in leadership	Professional organizations across all general and specialty jurisdictions are responsible and accountable for creating meaningful board and committee opportunities for nursing students and new nursing graduates (Price & McGillis Hall, 2014)

Sources: Carroll, S. M., & Rosa, K. C. (2016). Role and image of nursing in children's literature: A qualitative media analysis. *Journal of Pediatric Nursing, 31*, 141–151. https://doi.org/10.1016/j.pedn.2015.09.009; Coke, L. A. (2019). Integrating entrepreneurial skills into clinical nurse specialist education: The need for improved marketing, negotiation and conflict resolution skills. *Clinical Nurse Specialist, May/June*, 146–148 https://doi.org/10.1097/nur.0000000000000440; Godsey, J. A., Hayes, T., Schertzer, C., et al. (2018). Development and testing of three unique scales measuring the brand image of nursing. *Issues in Healthcare and Pharmacology for Vulnerable Populations, 12*(1), 2–14. https://doi.org/10.1108/IJPHM-09-2016-0052; Koo, M., & Lin, S.-C. (2016). The image of nursing: A glimpse of the Internet. *Japan Journal of Nursing Science, 13*, 496–501. https://doi.org/10.1111/jjns.12125; Masters, J. L., & Liu, Y. (2016). Perceived organizational support and intention to remain: The mediating roles of career success and self-esteem. *International Journal of Nursing Practice, 22*, 205–214. https://doi.org/10.1111/ijn.12416; Milisen, K., De Busser, T., Kayaert, A., et al. (2010). The evolving professional nursing self-image of students in baccalaureate programs: A cross-sectional survey. *International Journal of Nursing Studies, 47*, 688–698. https://doi.org/10.1016/j.ijnurstu.2009.11.008; Price, S. L., & McGillis Hall, L. (2014). The history of nurse imagery and the implications for recruitment: A discussion paper. *Journal of Advanced Nursing, 70*(7), 1502–1509. https://doi.org/10.1111/jan.12289; Tuckett, A., Kim, H., & Huh, J. (2017). Image and message: Recruiting the right nurses for the profession. A qualitative study. *Nurse Education Today, 55*, 77–81. https://doi.org/10.1016/j.nedt.2017.05.007; Varaei, S., Vaismoradi, M., Jasper, M., & Faghihzadeh, S. (2012). Iranian nurses self-perception—factors influencing nursing image. *Journal of Nursing Management, 20*, 551–560. https://doi.org/10.1111/j.1365-2834.2012.01397.x; Wang, H., Li, X., Hu, X., et al. (2011). Perceptions of nursing profession and learning experiences of male students in baccalaureate nursing program in Changsha, China. *Nurse Education Today, 31*, 36–42. https://doi.org/10.1016/j.nedt.2010.03.011

ORGANIZATIONS PROMOTING PROFESSIONAL NURSING IMAGE

Several national professional organizations support the building of nursing's professional image; resources are available on their websites. The Canadian Nurses Foundation (CNF), established in 1962, has awarded over $10 million in scholarships, bursaries, and research grants to more than 1,500 Canadian nurses and nursing students. Not only have these awards transformed the lives of nurses, they have also created far better experiences and outcomes for the millions of patients who have benefited from the CNF's professional investments in Canadian nurses. Most importantly, the CNF provides opportunities for nurses and nursing students to share positive stories of their influence with peers, patients, educators, and communities. Through such professional organizations, nursing students and nurses can network, find mentors, and seek advice regarding career development.

The CNA is another national organization that provides vital support to the growth of a strong professional image. The organization provides resources, including library resources, toolkits, and career development resources; represents the voice of Canadian nurses for policy and advocacy initiatives; circulates media releases about key issues in nursing practice; and provides the infrastructure through which nurses can achieve certification in the 22 nursing specialties associated with the Canadian Network of Nursing Specialties. The CNA also facilitates the annual Dorothy Wylie Health Leaders Institute. The CNA's website is a source of policy briefs, white papers, and reports submitted to governmental agencies as well as various educational webinars cached on the CNA's YouTube channel. The CNA also provides nurses with access to "nurse ambassadors," who provide support and advice for nurses preparing to write a certification exam for specialization. The CNA markets the nursing role as contributing to "… health system transformation" through direct influence on federal leaders and parties (CNA, 2018).

The Canadian Association of Schools of Nursing is another professional organization in Canada that provides evidence-based scholarly resources for undergraduate nursing education and serves as the accreditor for Canadian nursing education programs (see Chapter 21). The organization's website is an excellent resource that includes information on ongoing educational programs to expand teaching–learning skills, mentorship approaches, graduate student facilitation, and entry-to-practice competency documents to guide nursing education. The website has a cache of open-access publications and webinars on various topics such as recovery narratives in mental health nursing, digital health, and simulation.

The CNSA, consisting of almost 30,000 members, is an important organization run by students, for students. It is governed by a board that includes a president, vice-president, governance chair, and regional directors representing jurisdictions across Canada. The board also includes a director of communications, director of Indigenous advocacy, director of membership development, and directors of bilingualism and translation. Committees of the board include the Diversity Committee, National Conference Committee, Research and Education Committee, Global Health Committee, Practical Nurse Committee, and Community and Public Health Committee. There is also an Indigenous health advocacy ally, an administrative officer, and a technology officer. The board consults with a stakeholder representative of the CNA, as the CNSA is an affiliate member of the CNA. The CNSA is actively dedicated to the positive promotion of nurses and the nursing profession as a whole, in addition to promoting the legal, ethical, professional, and educational principles integral to professional nursing.

Nurses are influential, both as individuals and as a collective, when explaining the image of nurses and nursing to the public and to their fellow health care providers. The perception of nursing plays a vital role in nurses' self-image, as does nurses' skill at communicating their professional image to others. As nursing students and novice nurses embrace the concept of the professional contemporary "careerist," as originally proposed by Kalisch and Kalisch (1982), nursing will succeed in changing the image and developing a cadre of intelligent, sophisticated, assertive, competent, empathic, and supportive nurses who are leaders in improving health and the health care system.

BUILDING A PERSONAL NURSING BRAND

Professional nurses are responsible and accountable for engaging in continuous self-reflection as they develop and refine their professional image and self-identity. Each encounter between a nurse and another person or group has the potential to add value and leverage influence. Every nurse should engage in purposeful steps to develop a unique professional self-image that builds upon personal strengths, values, and beliefs.

The strategies identified in Table 4.2 are useful for building one's professional brand; however, it is recommended that nurses first engage in a personal branding exercise (Trepanier & Gooch, 2014) so that workplace and social behaviours align with the image the nurse wishes to project at all times.

Nurses who are successful in building a consistently positive professional image invest in developing their strengths throughout their careers, surround themselves with strong

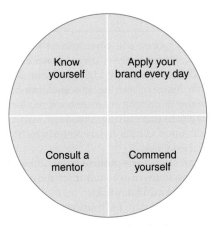

Fig. 4.1 The essential steps to developing your personal brand. (Adapted from Trepanier, S., & Gooch, P. (2014). Personal branding and nurse leader professional image. *Nurse Leader*, *12*(3), 51–57. https://doi.org/10.1016/j.mnl.2014.03.005)

role models, seek opportunities to learn from others, share their knowledge generously, and believe in the importance of leaving a legacy, regardless of which stage they are at in their careers (Trepanier & Gooch, 2014).

Developing a personal brand as a professional nurse can begin with the following concurrent activities (see Figure 4.1):

1. Know yourself—Identify personal strengths, values, and beliefs about what it means to be a professional nurse. Observe role models, just like Yoo-Hee and Juan studied Jennifer's professional performance (see Case Study). Make a list of the qualities that role models enact, and identify those that personally resonate. These traits should align with one's own attributes and values. Draw a picture, sketch a symbol, or find a photographic image that captures what is most important and will serve as a metaphor for a personal brand.
2. Apply your brand every day—Seek opportunities to apply your brand during every interaction in both professional and social settings. Reflect upon whether the brand was realized during each interaction. Refine and polish your brand through continued education and professional development. Make every interaction count.
3. Consult a mentor—Frequently seek feedback from a trusted mentor. Provide the mentor with examples of encounters that matched your professional brand and those that fell short. Discuss strategies that make the brand consistently achievable.
4. Commend yourself—Identify the moments during which the projection of your professional image was strong, knowing that you made a difference, no matter

how small. Congratulate yourself for these positive moments, and recognize that you may well have served as a role model for others.

Over time, if these steps are enacted regularly and mindfully, a personal brand will emerge, take shape, strengthen, and flourish. Personal branding of this kind will assist nurses in gaining trust and credibility, achieving career success, and making strongly positive impressions on colleagues and the public.

CONCLUSION

In spite of significant and rapid advances in technology and health care over the past 30 years, changes in the way nurses are perceived, both within and outside the profession, have been steady but slow. Although images of nurses and nursing might be changing to overcome the collective historical narrative of nurses as Angel of Mercy, Girl Friday, Heroine, Mother, or Sex Object, these images continue lurking within mass and social media messaging. What is called for now is a national plan that engages students, new nurses, and the public. Promoting a professional image of nursing within the discipline itself and in the public sphere will change both the internal and external images of nursing. Only nurses can lead efforts to change their image through sustained action by committed individuals and the profession as a whole.

Provincial and national professional organizations must provide funding to develop and implement robust marketing programs for use by constituent nurses at the local, regional, and national levels. The priority given to enhancing the image of nurses and nursing by professional associations needs to be continued. Such initiatives should target both nurses and the public so that the messages are frequent and consistently powerful, provocative, and engaging.

Individual nurses also need to actively participate in the promotion of the ideal professional image. Nurses can help to attract to the profession those who will advance knowledge, improve practice, and be known as people committed to knowing and doing. By taking every opportunity to promote professional nursing as well as the diversity of opportunities available to nurses, nurses can ensure that the potential positive impact of social media is maximized (Kelly, Fealy, & Watson, 2012; Tuckett & Turner, 2016). Meanwhile, nursing leaders must ensure that students and new graduates are socialized into a professional role within nursing and in interdisciplinary practice (Chênevert, Jourdain, & Vandenberghe, 2016). Working together to develop and communicate a powerful branding message that cultivates a strongly positive professional image will keep nursing on track.

SUMMARY OF LEARNING OBJECTIVES

- Professional image is a complex entity built upon the interplay of the different perceptions of nursing held by members of the discipline, other health care professionals, and the public.
- Professional image is a perception upon which the public builds opinions, beliefs, and attitudes about what nurses are and what they do.
- Self-image, professional self-identity, and positive professional image are inextricably linked, emerging as a set of beliefs and values that inform the direction of professional image enactment.
- Self-image of nursing, held by individuals and groups within the discipline, affects the ongoing development of the nursing profession.
- Professional image mirrors the socioeconomic and political climate within which members of the discipline practice.
- Historically, the image of nurses as agents of change emerged from within the context of limited and poorly developed health care systems, both on the Crimean battlefield and in civilian hospitals.
- Professional image in nursing has been grouped into five types that characterize five successive periods, from 1854 to the early 1980s. These archetypes were labelled Angel of Mercy, Girl Friday, Heroine, Mother, and Sex Object. The primary messaging around these archetypes excluded the importance of nursing science as the basis of practice.
- From the 1980s to the present, the image of nursing shifted to reflect a growing expectation held by both the public and health professionals that practice be based upon evidence. This expectation provided the context for the modern nurse to be perceived as a "contemporary careerist."
- Attributes of the contemporary careerist include education, sophistication, interprofessional collaboration, international and global advocacy, policy and change advocacy, and media fluency.
- The current professional public image of nursing has not yet shifted to align with the reality of the contemporary careerist. This inaccurate public image is sustained by the discipline's pervasive messaging that the core competency of nurses is relational practice. Consequently, public understanding of the role of nursing is dominated by the image of nurses performing acts of physical and emotional comfort.
- Modern professional nursing images do not yet consistently reflect the reality that practice standards and competencies are grounded in empirical scientific research unique to the discipline. This has impacted nursing's capacity to take up advocacy, policy, and governmental leadership roles, wherein health care system changes are realized.
- Mass and social media are highly influential in shaping the public image of nursing. In some cases, media representations of nursing are inaccurate, reinforcing public perceptions that nursing consists primarily of caring acts built upon commonplace knowledge rather than empirical evidence.
- Nurses can strengthen positive public images of nursing by consciously marketing their competencies and evidence-informed knowledge.
- Nurses can also sustain the transformation of their public image by rewriting the narrative of nursing such that it reflects the complexity, autonomy, knowledge, power, and influence of nurses.
- A strongly positive professional image of nursing will contribute to the recruitment of nursing students who have capacity across the multiple competencies required to shape public health policy.
- Educational experiences that facilitate the early emergence of professional self-identity can contribute to new graduates who develop, brand, and market themselves as contemporary careerists.
- A shared positive self-image can generate many powerful outcomes: influential professional organizations with lobbying power; a growing body of evidence-informed practice standards, competencies, and guidelines; availability of strong mentors, researchers, and governmental leaders; and leadership within interprofessional networks.
- Nurse educators, nurse managers, and administrative leaders are responsible and accountable for assisting nurses at all career stages with building a strongly positive professional image and marketing this as a brand, both individually and for the discipline as a whole.
- National professional organizations such as the Canadian Nurses Association, Canadian Nurses Foundation, Canadian Association of Schools of Nursing, and Canadian Nursing Students' Association are excellent sources of promotional materials and professional self-identity tools that can be used by nurses to develop their skills in brand marketing. Provincial professional nursing organizations, which represent nurses' workplace needs, also advocate for a professional image of nursing by disseminating ad campaigns and promotional materials to their members and the public.
- Nurses who are successful in building a consistently positive professional image continuously invest in developing their strengths throughout their careers, surround themselves with strong role models, seek opportunities

to learn from others, share their knowledge generously, and believe in the importance of leaving a legacy.

- All nurses, regardless of which career stage they are at, are responsible and accountable for developing a professional self-identity that contributes to the overall brand image of nursing as positive, effective, empirically based, research informed, and a main driver of public health policy.

CRITICAL THINKING QUESTIONS

1. What strategies could nurses engage in to strengthen their own professional self-image? Which of these strategies resonates the most with you? Why?

2. What impact can the actions of individual nurses have on the public image of nursing?

REFERENCES

Akhtar-Danesh, N., Baumann, A., Kolotylo, C., et al. (2013). Perceptions of professionalism among nursing faculty and nursing students. *Western Journal of Nursing Research*, 35, 248–271. https://doi.org/10.1177/019394591.

Ayala, R. A., Vanderstracten, R., & Bracke, P. (2014). Prompting professional prerogatives: New insights to reopen an old debate about nursing. *Nursing & Health Sciences*, 16, 506–513. https://doi.org/10.1111/nhs.12129.

Ben Natan, M. (2016). Interest in nursing among academic degree holders in Israel: A cross-sectional quantitative study. *Nurse Education Today*, 38, 150–153. https://doi.org/10.1016/j.nedt.2015.11.15.

Browne, C., Wall, P., Batt, S., & Bennett, R. (2018). Understanding perceptions of nursing professional identity in students entering an Australian undergraduate nursing degree. *Nurse Education in Practice*, 32, 90–96. https://doi.org/10.1016/j.nepr.2018.07.006.

Canadian Institute for Health Information. (2019). *Nursing in Canada, 2018: A Lens on Supply and Workforce*. Ottawa ON: Author. Retrieved from https://www.cna-aiic.ca/en/news-room/news-releases/2019/cihi-report-reveals-optimistic-signposts-for-future-of-the-nursing-profession.

Canadian Nurses Association (CNA). (2018). *2018 Year in review*. Ottawa, ON: CNA. Retrieved from https://www.cna-aiic.ca/-/media/cna/page-content/pdf-en/2019-meeting-of-members/2018-annual-report.pdf.

Carroll, S. M., & Rosa, K. C. (2016). Role and image of nursing in children's literature: A qualitative media analysis *Journal of Pediatric Nursing*, 31, 141–151. https://doi.org/10.1016/j.pedn.2016.09.009.

Chan, Z. C. Y., Lo, K. K. L., Tse, K. C. Y., & Wong, W. W. (2014). Self-image of male nursing students in Hong Kong: Multi-qualitative approaches. *American Journal of Men's Health*, 8(1), 26–34. https://doi.org/10.1177/1557988313488929.

Chênevert, L., Jourdain, G., & Vandenberghe, C. (2016). The role of high-involvement work practices and professional self-image in nursing recruits' turnover: A three-year prospective study. *International Journal of Nursing Studies*, 53, 73–84. https://doi.org/10.1016/jjnurstu.2015.09.005.

Chauke, M. E., Van Der Wal, D., & Botha, A. (2015). Using appreciative inquiry to transform student nurses' image of nursing. *Curationis*, 38(1), E1–E8. https://doi.org/10.4102/curationis.v38i1.1460.

Daigle, A. (2018). Professional image and the nursing uniform. *The Journal of Continuing Education in Nursing*, 49(12), 555–557. https://doi.org/10.3928/00220124-20181116-06.

De Leeuw, A., & De Leeuw, C. (1961). *Nurses who led the way: Real life stories of courageous women in an exciting profession*. Racine, WI: Whitman Publishing Company.

Emeghebo, L. (2012). The image of nursing as perceived by nurses. *Nurse Education Today*, 32, e49–e53. https://doi.org/10.1016/j.nedt.2011.10.015.

Girvin, J., Jackson, D., & Hutchinson, M. (2016). Contemporary public perceptions of nursing: A systematic review and narrative synthesis of the international research evidence. *Journal of Nursing Management*, 24, 994–1006. https://doi.org/10.1111/jonm.12413.

Godsey, J. A., Hayes, T., Schertzer, C., et al. (2018). Development and testing of three unique scales measuring the brand image of nursing. *Issues in Healthcare and Pharmacology for Vulnerable Populations*, 12(1), 2–14. https://doi.org/10.1108/IJPHM-09-2016-0052.

Gordon, S. (2010). Nursing needs a new image. *International Nursing Review*, 57(4), 403–404. https://doi.org/10.1111/j.1466-7657.2010.00862.x.

Gottlieb, L. N. (2013). *Strengths-based nursing care: Health and healing for person and family*. New York, NY: Springer.

Kagan, I., Biran, E., Telem, L., et al. (2015). Promotion or marketing of the nursing profession by nurses. *International Nursing Review*, 62, 368–376. https://doi.org/10.1111/inr.12178.

Kalisch, B., & Kalisch, P. (1982). Anatomy of the image of the nurse: Dissonant and ideal models. In C. Williams (Ed.), *Image-making in Nursing* (pp. 3–23). Kansas City, MO: American Academy of Nursing.

Kelly, J., Fealy, G. M., & Watson, R. (2012). The image of you: Constructing nursing identities in YouTube. *Journal of Advanced Nursing*, 68(8), 1804–1813. https://doi.org/10.1111/j.1365-2648.2011.05872.x.

Kluczynska, U. (2016). Motives for choosing and resigning from nursing by men and the definition of masculinity: A qualitative study. *Journal of Advanced Nursing*, 73(6), 1366–1376. https://doi.org/10.1111/jan.13240.

Koo, M., & Lin, S. -C. (2016). The image of nursing: A glimpse of the Internet. *Japan Journal of Nursing Science*, 13, 496–501. https://doi.org/10.1111/jjns.12125.

Liu, J., & Liu, Y. (2016). Perceived organizational support and intention to remain: The mediating roles of career success and self-esteem. *International Journal of Nursing Practice, 22,* 205–214. https://doi.org/10.1111/ijn.12416.

Marafion, A. A., & Pera, P. I. (2015). Theory and practice in the construction of professional identity in nursing students: A qualitative study. *Nurse Education Today, 35,* 859–863. https://doi.org/10.1016/j.nedt.2015.03.014.

Marcinowicz, L., Owlasiuk, A., & Pekowska, E. (2016). Exploring the ways experienced nurses in Poland view their profession: A focus group study. *International Nursing Review, 63,* 336–343. https://doi.org/10.1111/inr.12294.

Masters, J. L., & Liu, Y. (2016). Perceived organizational support and intention to remain: The mediating roles of career success and self-esteem. *International Journal of Nursing Practice, 22,* 205–214.

McDonald, L. (2014). Florence Nightingale and Mary Seacole on nursing and health care. *Journal of Advanced Nursing, 70*(6), 1436–1445. https://doi.org/10.1111/jan.12291.

Milisen, K., De Busser, T., Kayaert, A., et al. (2010). The evolving professional nursing self-image of students in baccalaureate programs: A cross-sectional survey. *International Journal of Nursing Studies, 47,* 688–698. https://doi.org/10.1016/j.ijnurstu.2009.11.008.

Morris-Thompson, T., Shepherd, J., Plata, R., & Marks-Maran, D. (2011). Diversity, fulfilment and privilege: The image of nursing. *Journal of Nursing Management, 19,* 683–692. https://doi.org/10.1111/j.1365-2834.2011.01268.x.

Neishabouri, M., Ahmadi, F., & Kazemnejad, A. (2017). Iranian nursing students' perspectives on transition to professional identity: A qualitative study. *International Nursing Review, 64,* 428–436. https://doi.org/10.1111/inr.12334.

Nelson, S., & Gordon, S. (2006). *The complexities of care.* New York, NY: Cornell University Press.

Nightingale, F. (1969). *Notes on Nursing: What it is, and what it is not* (unabridged republication of first American edition, as published by D. Appleton and Company in 1860). New York, NY: Dover Publications, Inc.

Price, S. L., & McGillis Hall, L. (2014). The history of nurse imagery and the implications for recruitment: A discussion paper. *Journal of Advanced Nursing, 70*(7), 1502–1509. https://doi.org/10.1111/jan.1289.

Price, S. L., McGillis Hall, L., Angus, J. E., & Peter, E. (2013). Choosing nursing as a career: A narrative analysis of millennial nurses' career choice of virtue. *Nursing Inquiry, 20*(4), 305–316. https://doi.org/10.1111/nin.12027.

Rezaei-Adaryani, M., Salsali, M., & Mohammadi, E. (2012). Nursing image: An evolutionary concept analysis. *Contemporary Nurse, 41*(1), 81–89. https://doi.org/10.5172/conu.2012.43.1.81.

Schuler, M. S. (2016). Shadowing in early baccalaureate nursing education and its influence on professional role perspectives. *Nurse Educator, 41*(6), 304–308. https://doi.org/10.1097/NNE.0000000000000276.

ten Hoeve, Y., Jansen, G., & Roodbol, P. (2014). The nursing profession: Public image, self-concept and professional identity. A discussion paper. *Journal of Advanced Nursing, 70*(2), 295–309. https://doi.org/10.1111/jan.12177.

Toren, O., Kerzman, H., & Kagan, I. (2011). The difference between professional image and job satisfaction of nurses who studied in a post-basic education program and nurses with generic education: A questionnaire survey. *Journal of Professional Nursing, 27*(1), 28–34. https://doi.org/10.1016/j.profnurs.2010.09.003.

Trepanier, S., & Gooch, P. (2014). Personal branding and nurse leader professional image. *Nurse Leader,* 51–57. https://doi.org/10.1016/j.mnl.2014.03.005.

Tuckett, A. (2015). Speaking with one voice: A study of the values of new nursing graduates and the implications for educators. *Nurse Education in Practice, 15,* 258–264. https://doi.org/10.1016/j.nepr.2015.02.004.

Tuckett, A., & Turner, C. (2016). Do you use social media? A study into new nursing and midwifery graduates' uptake of social media. *International Journal of Nursing Practice, 22,* 197–204. https://doi.org/10.1111/ijn.12411.

Tuckett, A., Kim, H., & Huh, J. (2017). Image and message: Recruiting the right nurses for the profession. *A qualitative study. Nurse Education Today, 55,* 77–81. https://doi.org/10.1016/j.nwsr.2017.05/007.

Varaei, S., Vaismoradi, M., Jasper, M., & Faghihzadeh, S. (2012). Iranian nurses self-perception – factors influencing nursing image. *Journal of Nursing Management, 20,* 551–560. https://doi.org/10.1111/j.1365-2834.2012.01397.x.

Wang, H., Li, X., Hu, X., et al. (2011). Perceptions of nursing profession and learning experiences of male students in baccalaureate nursing program in Changsha. *China. Nurse Education Today, 31,* 36–42. https://doi.org/10.1016/j.nedt.2010.03.011.

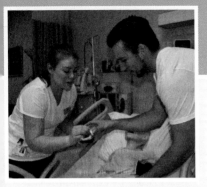

Gender in Nursing

Robert J. Meadus

ⓔ http://evolve.elsevier.com/Canada/Ross-Kerr/nursing

LEARNING OBJECTIVES

After reading this chapter, you will be able to:

- Recognize the contribution of feminism and feminist thinking to nursing.
- Describe the various philosophical views of feminism.
- Understand the relationship between feminism and nursing.
- Understand the impact of feminism on nursing research.
- Describe workforce statistics on the representation of men and women in nursing.
- Understand the barriers to men entering the nursing profession and ways of overcoming these.
- Understand research findings about men in nursing.
- Understand the issues for LGBTQ2 populations accessing health care services as well as nursing strategies to address issues and reduce barriers.

OUTLINE

KEY TERMS

cisgender
cisnormativity
epistemological
gender bias
heteronormativity
homophobia

LGBTQ2
marginalization
nonbinary
social construction
trans (transgender)

PERSONAL PERSPECTIVES

This chapter addresses gender and nursing, a topic that may seem more important to some than others. New students to the profession may lack awareness of how gender has shaped the early development of nursing and how its impact is still relevant today. Students who enter the profession need to be knowledgeable about how societal constructions of gender have shaped all aspects of nursing, from education to practice. Florence Nightingale, the founder of modern nursing, influenced how images of the white female nurse have endured, further limiting the role of men and members of ethnic groups in the profession. Nightingale's efforts enabled nursing to become a gendered profession, and these perceptions continue to hinder the development of a gender-diverse and inclusive workforce.

I recall that when I entered a 3-year nursing diploma program over 40 years ago, I was not thinking about gender. I was in a class of 110 students, four of whom were male, a number that at that time I thought was appropriate. However, I considered myself lucky when, in one of my clinical experiences, our clinical group had a male instructor. When I graduated and went to work in medical-surgical nursing, I was the only male registered nurse. However, being a minority within the profession, I wasn't expecting things to change. It would have been great to have had male mentors along the way.

Today, men entering the profession may have more opportunity to meet male preceptors and mentors, depending upon their clinical practice areas. This gives male nurses the chance to observe and work alongside each other, which can aid their development as registered nurses. As a man and a registered nurse for the past 40 years, I have observed very little change with respect to nursing's lack of gender diversity. Men remain underrepresented, and negligible inroads have been made to dispel the negative stereotypes about men who choose nursing as a career. Nursing needs to remember that health care is not exclusive to one gender. The profession needs to make concerted efforts to value diversity and take action to address stereotypes. This will lead to a balanced nursing workforce that represents all genders and is ready to meet the health care needs of the population it serves. Such endeavours will benefit the profession and the health care system as a whole.

INTRODUCTION

From the beginning, issues of gender have contributed to the formulation of nursing as a women's profession. These gender issues have been prominent since the first formal arrangements were made to care for the sick. In ancient times, religious orders of priests, monks, and nuns worked as caregivers. Although men have served as nurses throughout recorded history, our knowledge of nursing usually begins with Florence Nightingale. In reality, there is a history of men playing important roles in nursing long before that time (Christensen, 2017). The first nursing school on record began in India in about 250 BC, when only men were permitted as students (O'Lynn, 2013). In 330 AD, during the Byzantine Empire, men played a prominent role in organized nursing in hospitals. In Rome, the first known male nurses from the Christian era were from an all-male organization known as the Paraboloni brotherhood (Brothers in Christ). This order of men cared for the sick and dying and also served as health visitors. During the Crusades in the eleventh century, male nursing orders of military knights tended to the sick and injured.

In Canada, the first males to provide nursing care were the Jesuit missionaries and male attendants at the French garrison in Port Royal, Acadia, in 1629. However, in response to the impropriety of male priests' caring for sick women, three nuns who were nurses emigrated from France in 1639 to establish the first hospital at Québec. A pattern thus developed that continued for four centuries, whereby female religious orders built and operated hospitals to care for the sick, prevent illness, and promote health. Later, nuns took on the added responsibility of training nurses to staff the hospitals. After the middle of the twentieth century, religious orders began to withdraw from nursing education and management of hospitals, and secular health agencies prevailed as hospital operations became more expensive and moved into the public sector.

Wars influenced who attended to the sick and injured and who was recruited into nursing. The influence of societal attitudes and norms on military policy meant that only men were permitted to go to war, as it was considered appropriate for men to kill others and die in defence of their country. This belief was apparent in seventeenth-century battles between Europeans and Indigenous peoples and in wars and conflicts until recent years. During World War I, only men in the Medical Corps were permitted to serve on the front lines of battle; while female nurses were also members of the Medical Corps, they staffed Canadian-base hospitals caring for the wounded. In both the First and Second World Wars, women were recruited in great numbers to staff civilian hospitals, because many nurses had left to join the nurse corps of the three armed services divisions, and many men volunteered for, or were conscripted into, the armed services. This increased the number of women entering nursing but decreased the number of men, as men were needed for battle instead.

The practice of having only male attendants care for the sick and injured prevailed until Florence Nightingale, with her small band of nurses, went to Crimea, where she worked to improve the care of wounded soldiers. During her work in the battlefield hospitals, she saved many lives and improved the environmental conditions during recovery through her strong determination, expert knowledge, and nursing skill. She overcame barriers to women's involvement in nursing the sick and wounded during war, and later challenged and finally overcame Victorian barriers to women working outside the home. Nightingale saw nursing as a respectable profession for women. Later, when the first nursing school was established at St. Thomas's Hospital in London in 1860, only women were accepted as applicants. The school was organized separately from the hospital, thus creating an opportunity for employment outside the home and promoting a separate environment for women to work. In the process of overcoming societal pressures for women to conform to Victorian beliefs and customs, Nightingale also excluded men from nursing, resulting in the feminization of the profession. As a result of these various social changes, nursing labour became segregated by gender.

Nursing continues to be a predominantly white and female profession that is lacking in diversity and gender inclusivity. Societal values and expectations about the capabilities of men to assume a nurturing role in the family and outside the home have changed over the past several decades, and it has become more acceptable for men to enter nursing. However, the nursing workforce still lags behind the changing composition of the Canadian population and thus has yet to bridge the gap in gender inclusion and racial and ethnic diversity. To better understand the gender-based issues facing the nursing profession, it is necessary to have some knowledge about feminism and issues related to men. Consequently, a review of feminism and its relationship with nursing will be followed by a review of issues relating to men and men in nursing, concluding with a discussion of gender diversity (**LGBTQ2**) issues that require an immediate call to action in the nursing profession.

INTRODUCTION TO FEMINISM

Feminism is an outgrowth of reactions against forms of social organization in which women are not valued as highly as men. The norms of such a system condone systematic bias toward women. Although feminism is commonly thought of as a movement that grew out of the 1960s, writing by women in the seventeenth century was already reflecting feminist ideas. In the late eighteenth and early nineteenth centuries,

the women's rights movement and the women's suffrage movement had a powerful impact on society, resulting in important changes to how women were treated. Despite strong resistance to this movement, mostly white, middle-class women (i.e., suffragists) campaigned for the right of women to vote at all levels of government (Strong-Boag, 2016).

Nurses were profoundly influenced by the thinking of suffragists and were in an important position to demonstrate women's capabilities. Nursing had recently gained respect as a profession and was one of few careers open to women. Politically active nursing leaders were able to accomplish critical professional goals that would enable remarkable development in the profession throughout the twentieth century. The entrenchment of nursing registration in legislation in Canada and other countries during this period was a victory and an important step forward for the status of women.

The ideology of feminism is threatening to some and may be seen as opposing both men and the traditional structure of the family. Feminist discourse challenges systems and institutions that favour one sex over the other, as the fundamental ideas of feminism espouse valuing both women and men equally. Feminists also model behaviour that may not be thought of as feminine, which is undoubtedly unsettling to some. In this respect, modern feminists share some attributes with early suffragists, particularly in the way that they strived to address equity and justice.

THE RELATIONSHIP BETWEEN FEMINISM AND NURSING

The relationship between feminism and nursing has been somewhat tenuous and uneasy, as nurses did not fully align with its tenets early on. Although Florence Nightingale believed in the right and duty of service that nursing provided, she did not actively support the women's rights movement or the ideology of feminism. The Nightingale-era nurse engendered stereotypical views of women as subservient and obedient. Moreover, the male medical establishment defined nurses' work and influenced nursing education well into the late 1950s.

The second wave of feminism arrived in the early 1960s, a movement symbolized by the burning of bras as women cast off male dominance and oppression. At this time, nurses started to question the feminine ideal of the duty to serve in favor of equal rights and equal pay. Nursing education moved from hospital-run diploma programs to universities and community colleges. These developments enabled nurses to have greater control over their practice and education, leading to more autonomy and independence. Nurses started to emphasize empowerment and equality with other professions. Many became involved in unions and professional associations, advocating for the rights of nurses and patients. These endeavours succeeded in helping the profession gain a voice within the power relations in health care and greater recognition in the public sphere. With the third wave of feminism in the early 1990s, nurses were motivated to advocate for full equality for all people regardless of gender, and the tenets of feminism were emphasized in feminist nursing research (Dixon Vuic, 2009; Im, 2010).

As a predominantly female profession, nursing has been undervalued when measured by the contributions made by its members to society and has sometimes been invisible in the social and professional policy-making arena. In their attempt to obtain equality, nurses have aligned themselves with the tenets of feminism. However, this relationship with feminism and the feminist movement was tenuous in the beginning, as both groups were originally diametrically opposed in their ideals. Feminist discourse devalued nursing as a legitimate professional domain for highly educated women. According to feminist ideology, young women should not have to choose nursing as a career but should feel free to pursue other male-dominated careers like medicine (Gross, 2014; Malka, 2007).

Research and Feminism

Feminism seeks to confront the "social inequities resulting mainly from gender discrimination, oppression, and **marginalization**" (Sundean & Polifroni, 2016, p. 397). Although feminism is informed by different philosophical perspectives, a common view is that patriarchal norms and power imbalances within society contribute to these inequities. The relevance and value of a feminist stance is not limited to research with or about women. Feminist research as a method of social inquiry provides nurses with an opportunity to expose multiple forms of discrimination and health care paternalism as well as advocate for social justice and health equity. Individuals who already feel socially or culturally marginalized because of their race, ethnicity, gender, class, disability, or illness may feel further disempowered when accessing the health care system. These negative experiences undermine the goal of providing respectful care and reinforce health inequities.

Today, feminist research is an integral part of nursing as reflected in the increasing number of studies published in nursing journals. Feminist research in nursing offers numerous perspectives and incorporates a variety of methodologies and methods while reflecting nursing's concern with the experiences of people disempowered by the health care system. Scholars have questioned whether the best approach to feminist research is qualitative or quantitative, with many frequently characterizing it as the former. Contemporary feminists suggest that feminist

methodologies could employ any research method that describes the meaning of the patient's health experience within the sociopolitical context of their daily lives. The use of such approaches, including qualitative, quantitative, or a combination of both, will contribute to better nursing knowledge and elimination of social injustices (Im, 2010).

While it is clear that both qualitative and quantitative approaches are likely to be useful, multiple methods (i.e., triangulation) are being used more frequently in feminist research. To enhance practice knowledge, nurse researchers are using different **epistemological** perspectives to explore nursing phenomena related to underserved and marginalized populations (Im, 2013; MacDonnell, 2014). Nursing research has much to offer in the area of power and oppression, and a feminist perspective can be useful to nursing researchers who wish to go beyond the traditional biomedical model of health. A feminist perspective may foster nurses' capacity to change the institutional and societal conditions that create health inequities. Nurses have just begun to recognize how challenging it is to commit to carrying out impactful work that addresses social justice and inequities in health care systems around the world.

 APPLYING CONTENT KNOWLEDGE

From a feminist perspective, what questions might a nurse ask about health outcomes for people who are living in impoverished conditions?

MEN IN NURSING

Although an increasing number of men have entered nursing in recent decades, men still make up an insignificant proportion of the registered nurse population in Canada and globally, leading to a persistent gender imbalance in the profession. This inequity is remarkable at a time when the proportion of women in traditionally male-dominated professions has increased at a phenomenal rate. Disciplines now open to women include business, dentistry, law, medicine, engineering, and pharmacy. These careers are available to women because of pressure from women's groups, whose allegations of sexism have led to changes in recruitment policies and affirmative action. Thus, as many as half of the admission placements in these disciplines are available to women. In Canada, nursing has not made a similarly concerted effort to recruit men or advocate for specific admission policies for male applicants to undergraduate programs. Meanwhile, other traditionally female-dominated professions, such as teaching and library science, have seen notable increases in the number of male students.

The lack of men in nursing raises important questions: Why has the proportion of men in nursing increased so

TABLE 5.1 Comparison of Female and Male Registered Nurses (RNs) in Canada, 1968–2019

Year	Total No. of RNs	Female		Male	
		No.	%	No.	%
1968	120,000*	119,628	99.7	372	0.3
1974	128,675†	126,745	98.5	1930	1.5
1985	229,345	223,896	97.6	5,449	2.4
1990	256,145	248,153	96.9	7,992	3.1
1995	262,400	252,365	96.2	10,035	3.8
2005	268,376	254,369	94.4	14,007	5.6
2010	284,788	266,247	93.8	17,841	6.2
2015	292,355	270,178	92.4	22,177	7.6
2019	300,669	274,602	91.4	25,728	8.6

*Approximate number employed in nursing.
†Total number employed in nursing; remainder employed elsewhere.
Sources: Cahoon, M. C. (1978). The male/female dichotomy in the nursing profession in a time of social change: More male nurses, but increasing numbers of female patients—An international perspective. *Journal of Advanced Nursing, 3,* 65–72; Canadian Institute of Health Information. (2020). *Nursing in Canada, 2019—Data tables.* Retrieved from https://www.cihi.ca/en/access-data-and-reports; Canadian Nurses Association. (2006). *2005 Workforce profile of registered nurses in Canada.* Ottawa, ON: Author. Retrieved from https://cna-aiic.ca/~/media/cna/page-content/pdf-en/workforce-profile-2005-e.pdf; Mussallem, H. K. (1968). No lack of nurses—but a shortage of nursing. *International Nursing Review, 15*(1), 35–49; Trudeau, R. (1996). Male registered nurses, 1995. *Health Reports, 8*(2), 21–27. Retrieved from https://www150.statcan.gc.ca/n1/en/pub/82-003-x/1996002/article/2828-eng.pdf.

slowly, and why are men not choosing nursing as a career? What factors have influenced the entry of men into nursing, and will these factors continue to exert the same influence? What are the advantages of having more men in nursing? What has the nursing profession done (or not done) to change the proportion of men entering its ranks? What would nursing look like today if it had remained a male-dominated profession? Finally, what implications does the Charter of Rights and Freedoms have for the continued predominance of women or men in any profession?

Proportion of Men and Women in Nursing

The proportion of men in nursing in Canada has increased slowly since the 1960s, as shown in Table 5.1. Currently, men make up only 8% of the Canadian nursing workforce (Canadian Nurses Association, 2018). Even though the number of male registered nurses employed in Canada has increased incrementally, men continue to be underrepresented in the nursing workforce, reflecting a significant gender imbalance in the profession. This figure is reflective of other nations where the nursing workforce is also predominantly female. For example, in the United States, 9.6% of registered nurses are male (US Census Bureau, 2013), in the United Kingdom, 10.7% (Nursing and Midwifery Council, 2017), and in Australia, 11.8% (Nursing and Midwifery Board of Australia, 2019). By comparison, men

constitute ~21% of all nurses in Italy, 32% in Saudi Arabia, and 2% in China and Iceland (Demurtas, 2018; Li, 2018; Regan, 2012). This global gender imbalance confirms that the **social construction** of gender continues to shape the profession the same way it did when nursing was founded by Florence Nightingale (see Chapters 1 and 2).

Since men represent a small percentage of the global nursing workforce, a more diverse group of students needs to be recruited and retained if nursing is to survive. Yet, the nursing profession continues to maintain the status quo and appears uninterested in recruiting men into nursing. Nursing needs to be a stronger advocate for dispelling inequity within the discipline and making the profession more diverse, equitable, and inclusive; welcoming men and ethnically diverse individuals can be a start. To address the gender imbalance in nursing, one must examine the factors that influence the entry of men into this traditionally female-dominated profession.

Barriers to Men's Entry Into Nursing

One of the major barriers men face to entering the nursing profession is societal attitudes about work that is deemed appropriate for men versus women. Nursing is still not considered an appropriate career choice for men because it is associated with stereotypically feminine traits such as nurturing, gentleness, and caring. Men are expected to be strong and powerful and to hide their emotions. Male nurses have

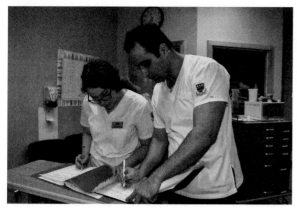

Student nurses completing documentation. (Marcia Porter, Memorial University Faculty of Nursing)

reported negative comments and discouraging reactions from others, including family members; these men undoubtedly had to be determined and committed to pursue a career in nursing.

Male nurses encountered similar reactions from other health care providers when medicine was still predominantly male. Indeed, such reactions were not uncommon within the profession of nursing itself; some female nurses tended to regard men who selected nursing as not "real men." Carnevale and Priode (2018) have highlighted the continuing challenges faced by men entering a profession that is viewed as feminine by both men and women and where roles and identity tend to support that view (Twomey & Meadus, 2016). Other difficulties faced by men who enter nursing include being perceived as gay and being questioned about why they chose nursing over medicine (Powers, Herron, Sheeler, & Sain, 2018).

Men were not readily accepted into nursing schools for many years. Initially, most of those who were accepted entered schools of nursing that were connected with mental hospitals because of the belief that men were physically more capable of dealing with violence. Strength was considered so important in psychiatric nursing that this specialty did not become a required part of basic nursing education in Canada until the 1950s and even the 1960s in some schools. Until the 1960s and 1970s, male nursing students were not permitted to study theory and practice in obstetric and gynecological nursing; they devoted that time to urologic nursing, caring for male patients only. Evans (2004) reported that differential barriers to residential accommodation, separate and weaker educational programs for male nursing students, and difficulty securing positions following graduation were historical deterrents to men's entry into the profession.

For many years, another barrier to the admission of men into nursing programs was an economic one, as nurses were poorly paid relative to those in other occupations. As a result, men who might have pursued nursing elected not to enter the profession because of the societal expectation that they be the "breadwinners." Male nurses who have higher ambitions for advancing their careers have sometimes been criticized for aspiring to senior positions as managers or administrators to earn enough to support a family (McMurry, 2011).

Discrimination Against Men in Nursing

Men have faced decades of discrimination in admission policies, nursing curricula, employment opportunities, and the regulation of nurses. Men have been frequently denied access to formal nursing education. During the 1960s, only 25 of the 170 diploma nursing schools in Canada accepted male applicants. Notably, the Victoria General Hospital in Halifax was one of the few to accept male applicants into their school of nursing. It is believed that male applicants were accepted because of the large number of sailors who used the hospital's services (McPherson, 2003). The small graduating class of 1899 from the hospital's school of nursing included two male graduates.

Male graduates of nursing programs in Canada found it difficult to obtain employment. Hospitals often refused to employ them, instead hiring lower-paid male orderlies and attendants. Schools of nursing did not employ male nursing instructors because it was deemed inappropriate for men to teach women how to nurse (Wedgery, 1966). Such biases maintained and perpetuated the status quo that men were anomalies in nursing, impacting their integration into the profession.

In the province of Quebec, restrictions on nursing practice were imposed on male registered nurses through discriminatory legislation; men could not register with the professional association, the Ordre des infirmières et infirmiers du Québec. In 1969, after years of lobbying by the Canadian Nurses Association and male nurses, Bill 89 was passed by the National Assembly of Quebec and the *Nurses Act* was amended: men were finally permitted to use nurse as a title and could register with the province.

In the Canadian Armed Forces, male registered nurses have experienced outright discrimination because of their gender. Men could not join the Nursing Division of the Canadian Armed Forces before 1967; female registered nurses could and were given nursing officer status, while men could be noncommissioned officers or work as medics or in other allied health care positions. Efforts to change this discriminatory policy were initiated in 1942 by the Registered Nurses Association of Ontario (RNAO). In 1956, the RNAO approved the formation of a Male Nurses Committee to promote recruitment of men into the profession and address other issues that affected men's participation within nursing. After a 25-year struggle, this committee along with the RNAO and the Canadian Nurses Association succeeded in changing the policy: men were finally allowed to join the Nursing Division of the Canadian military (Care, Gregory, English, & Venkatesh, 1996). Owing to these changes in military policy, Lieutenant Roy D. Field became the first male Armed Forces nurse to receive officer status in 1967.

RESEARCH FOCUS

This study explored the experience of being a male student in a female-dominated undergraduate baccalaureate program at three collaborative nursing school sites within one Atlantic province. Using a qualitative, phenomenological methodology, focus group interviews were conducted with 27 male student nurses who were in different years of a 4-year program, including several in the 2-year fast-track option. Five themes described male students' experience of being in the program: choosing nursing, becoming a nurse, caring within the nursing role, gender-based stereotypes, and visible/invisible. The theme "choosing nursing" reflected steps for seeking information about nursing and reasons for career choice. Common reasons identified by participants were job security, career mobility, and the opportunity to help others. The second theme, "becoming a nurse," involved interest, confidence, and satisfaction in completing the program. Support from family, friends, classmates, and faculty aided their journey. The third theme, "caring within the nursing role," represented men's expressions of caring associated with fear of accusations of sexual impropriety, and perceptions of patients, staff, and society of their role as a nurse. "Gender-based stereotyping" detailed how students in clinical areas believed they were perceived by nursing staff and patients. Several reported being seen as "doctors" and "muscle" who could lift or move patients and at times control potentially violent situations. The final theme, "visible/invisible," reflected their minority status and their experience of "standing out" because of their gender. Students disclosed that these perceptions impacted their recognition as a nursing student by patients, health professionals, and society. Findings revealed issues related to **gender bias** in nursing education, practice areas, and societal perceptions that nursing is not a suitable career choice for men. The most challenging experience for students was the maternal–child clinical rotation.

Source: Meadus, R. J., & Twomey, J. C. (2011). Men student nurses: The nursing education experience. *Nursing Forum*, *46*(4), 269–279.

Research on Men in Nursing

In his seminal review of research on men in nursing, Christman (1988), a staunch advocate for affirmative action to recruit men, found a dearth of studies on men in nursing and identified many inadequacies in the methods used and interpretation of results. In general, he found that study samples were small and not representative of the population being studied, an approach that can "result in sampling bias and incomplete knowledge of the phenomenon under study" (Christman, p. 198). Christman concluded: "If clarification of the male role in the nursing profession was a goal of the research done so far, then there are major shortcomings in both the research and the outcomes of research" (p. 202). He questioned the utility of studies that elicited opinion and argued against doing more of them. Instead, he suggested building on the beginnings of two studies by Brown and Stones (1972) and Holtzclaw (1981), both of which used standardized test batteries. He also emphasized obtaining larger multisite and more representative samples.

Some of Christman's concerns are still evident today in the published quantitative literature: study samples are small, and there is a paucity of international studies on men in nursing. Over the past 30 years, an abundance of both anecdotal and peer-reviewed research has been published on the topic of male nurses. Although limited in number, some studies address male nurses in practice, and a modest number of studies focus specifically on male students' educational experiences in undergraduate nursing programs. There is scant published literature on career satisfaction of male nurses and how caring is defined by these nurses in clinical practice.

In a review of research about men in nursing published 20 years after Chrisman's (1988) seminal work, O'Lynn and Tranbarger (2007) identified communication problems, reverse discriminatory practices, and gender-based barriers for male nursing students. These issues were discussed earlier in this chapter and have been documented in nursing history research. Later research has also investigated men's experiences as nursing students (see Research Focus Box, for example).

A great deal of literature is available on the recruitment of male nurses and the barriers they have experienced in choosing a nursing career. These barriers serve as a deterrent to men's entry into the profession: sexual stereotypes, public perception, value of nursing to society, images of nursing, organization and culture of nursing, lack of positive role models, and patient preference (O'Connor, 2015; Rajacich, Kane, Williston, & Cameron, 2013; Twomey & Meadus, 2016). However, despite their small representation in nursing and these barriers, some men continue choosing to enter the nursing profession: these men report satisfaction with career choice and have no hesitation in recommending nursing to others (Twomey & Meadus, 2016).

REVERSING THE GENDER IMBALANCE IN NURSING

There is no doubt that many factors have deterred men from entering and remaining in nursing and that some of the negative influences in society are slowly beginning to change. Factors such as cultural influences may serve to attract or discourage young people, particularly men, from choosing nursing as a career. The increasing number of Canadian immigrants coming from Asian and Latin American countries, where few men have chosen nursing as a profession, is one such factor. Another factor to consider is that many fields, such as medicine, dentistry, business, engineering, law, and pharmacy, are now available to women. As more women are attracted to these fields, there may well be a reverse effect of attracting more men to nursing; nursing has seen a gradual increase of men in its ranks over time (see Table 5.1), indicating a growing acceptance of men in the profession.

To attract more men to nursing, educators, professional nursing associations, and administrators must work together to correct the myths and overcome the barriers that deter men. Hospitals and other health care agencies and nursing schools need to use their publicity materials to portray men in the role of nurse to help change the public's perception of nursing. Twomey and Meadus (2016) cite examples of recruitment efforts that used posters downplaying feminine images of nursing and putting forward more masculine images that focused on men's abilities to do nursing. As a result of their study conducted in two large Canadian schools of nursing offering baccalaureate preparation, Dyck, Oliffe, Phinney, and Garrett (2009) recommended that nursing instructors be supported to develop "teaching strategies and approaches to better engage and avoid pressuring, privileging or alienating male students" (p. 653). Some of these classroom strategies include promoting a safe environment for all learners by not singling out male students and not assuming students' familiarity with feminine experiences. The RNAO offers a special interest group on men in nursing. This organization strives to educate the general public, nurses, and students about the profession and men in nursing. In these endeavours, the RNAO aims to strengthen the image of nursing across genders.

 APPLYING CONTENT KNOWLEDGE

Do you think that the profession has become more gender inclusive in its images of nursing? Search out specific websites related to nursing (i.e., schools of nursing, nursing unions, and the Canadian Nurses Association) to support your stance.

GENDER DIVERSITY AND LGBTQ2 ISSUES IN NURSING

Since the beginning of formalized nursing, nurses have been advocates for society's most vulnerable populations by addressing issues of health inequities. As the largest group of health professionals in Canada, nurses need to take action, adopt, advocate for, and create a culturally competent environment that is inclusive of LGBTQ2 patients and families. Several nurse scholars suggest that the health care needs of the LGBTQ2 populations are not being met, contributing to health inequities for this group. Further contributing to these health inequities is the health care system's alignment with historical notions of gender as defined by **heteronormativity** and **cisnormativity** (Carabez, Pellegrini, Mankovitz et al., 2015); for instance, the language around pregnancy birthing is still primarily oriented to serving **cisgender** women rather than **trans** (or **transgender**) or **nonbinary** individuals. These outdated gender norms are evident in the absence of gender-inclusive language and forms within health care organizations and registered nurses' lack of knowledge and education about gender identity and sexual orientation. LGBTQ2 individuals have reported negative experiences with health care providers, including **homophobia,** discrimination, hostility, and derogatory comments following disclosure of their sexual orientation and gender identity (Bonvicini, 2017; Dorsen, 2012). Such behaviours sustain the marginalization that many LGBTQ2 individuals have already experienced, leading them to delay or fail to seek health care.

In a systematic review of the top 10 nursing journals, Eliason, Dibble, and DeJoseph (2010) reported that nursing has failed in its "long-standing silence" on LGBTQ2 health issues. These authors issue a call for emancipatory efforts to challenge this silence in nursing and generate strategies for raising the visibility of LGBTQ2 patients and health care providers. The authors suggest that the prolonged silence has contributed to patient delays in seeking treatment, impaired nurse–patient communication, and a lack of knowledge of LGBTQ2 issues among health care providers. They recommend changes in all areas of nursing practice, research, education, and policy to redress this silence and to create broader diversity initiatives within nursing.

Jackman, Bosse, Eliason, and Hughes (2019) replicated the Eliason, Dibble, and DeJoseph (2010) systematic review, and completed a new systematic review of the top 20 nursing journals. These authors identified progress in nursing as slow. They reported that sexual and minority health research has received some attention but more work is needed to address the health needs of bisexual and transgender individuals in the nursing literature. These authors contend that the recommendations for nursing espoused by Eliason et al. are still pertinent today.

Similarly, in a qualitative study, Carabez, Eliason, and Martinson (2016) explored nurses' knowledge of the needs of transgender patients. The findings revealed nurses' discomfort and lack of knowledge about transgender people and their health care needs.

Several authors have argued that this prolonged silence has contributed to the invisibility of LGBTQ2 communities in health care (Harrell & Sasser, 2018; Goldberg, Rosenburg, & Watson, 2018; Shattell & Chinn, 2014). Furthermore, silence has contributed to inequities throughout the health care system that are fueled by stigma, discrimination, and lack of knowledge among health care providers. Between 2% and 10% of Canadians are estimated to self-identify as LGBTQ2 (Troute-Wood, 2015). The literature has also documented that this population is at higher risk of non-suicidal self-injury, suicidality, depression, and substance use compared with the general population (Green & Feinstein, 2012; Jackman, Honig, & Bockting, 2016; Lim, Brown, & Kim, 2014).

CASE STUDY

A 28-year-old patient named John Smith, who was assigned female at birth but self-identifies as a man, is admitted to the mental health unit with a possible diagnosis of acute anxiety. The patient has a history of not feeling well for about 5 months since taking a new position as assistant principal at a junior high school. John reports difficulty sleeping, pressure in the chest with shortness of breath, and an increased use of alcohol and tobacco.

Discussion questions:
1. Based upon the information, what fears might John have with respect to this hospital admission?
2. What strategies might the nurse use to create a climate of inclusion?
3. What strategies would the nurse use to build a therapeutic relationship with the patient?

CONCLUSION

Gender continues to exert a powerful influence on nursing. The foregoing discussion confirms that issues of gender pertain to both women and men. Although nursing has largely been characterized as feminine and thus a profession best suited for women, public attitudes are gradually shifting about the roles of men and women in society, the nature of nursing, and the kind of individuals required to provide high-quality nursing care (Anonson, Karkanis, & McDonnell, 2000). Nursing, in its association with feminism and support of equality, needs to advocate for equal

RESEARCH FOCUS

The purpose of the study was to understand the needs and concerns of older LGBT adults around aging and end-of-life care within the Ontario health care system. Using a qualitative approach, focus group interviews were conducted with 23 LGBT individuals ranging in age from 57 to 78 years. Thematic analysis revealed that participant experiences were reflected in an overall theme, "identifying as LGBT matters," and three associated subthemes: social connections and support, expectations for care, and staying out of the closet. Support from biological and nonbiological family members was deemed important. Owing to past experiences of stigma and discrimination, older LGBT adults had fears about social isolation. "Expectations of care" related to their fears around the lack of inclusiveness and heteronormative assumptions held by health care providers. Notably, participants reported being advocates for the rights of LGBT communities throughout their lives and having to continue that advocacy as they neared the last phase of life. "Staying out of the closet" characterized their fears and concerns about being open about their sexual orientation and identity. Participants acknowledged that feeling safe to disclose was key to their identity and freedom of sexual expression throughout aging and end-of-life.

Source: Wilson, K., Kortes-Miller, K., & Stinchcombe, A. (2018). Staying out of the closet: LGBT older adults' hopes and fears in considering end-of-life care. *Canadian Journal on Aging, 37*(1), 22–31.

participation of men in nursing. More recently, nursing has recognized the need to build a workforce that is more diverse in race, ethnicity, gender, and culture. Nursing should embrace diversity and commit to erasing gender stereotyping. Achieving this much-needed diversity would help nurses to provide patients with more culturally competent care. The nursing profession stands to gain much as it moves in the direction of a culturally diverse and gender-balanced workforce. However, the pace of change is likely to continue being slow and steady.

SUMMARY OF LEARNING OBJECTIVES

- Nursing has had a long and ambivalent relationship with the women's movement.
- The various philosophical views of feminism have perpetuated nursing as a gendered profession.
- Feminist research in nursing has helped to uncover the inequities faced by specific populations within the health care system and identified the need for change.
- To date, men remain a minority in nursing within Canada and worldwide.
- Nursing research has explored issues for male nurses in practice and male students completing undergraduate nursing programs. Several barriers have been identified that discourage men from choosing nursing as a career.
- Nursing has been largely silent on the issues facing LGBTQ2 populations with respect to accessing health care services. Efforts to make health care more inclusive and respectful are needed to address the marginalization experienced by LGBTQ2 communities.

CRITICAL THINKING QUESTIONS

1. Describe the impact of feminism on nursing over the past half century.
2. Why has nursing in modern times been practised primarily by women?
3. Are men able to pursue satisfying careers in nursing today?
4. What kinds of strategies are needed to develop best practices in working with LGBTQ2 communities?

REFERENCES

Anonson, J., Karkanis, A., & McDonnell, P. (2000). Recruiting nurses for the new millennium. *Canadian Nurse, 96*(5), 31–34.

Bonvicini, K. A. (2017). LGBT healthcare disparities: What progress have we made? *Patient Education and Counseling, 100*(12), 2357–2361. https://doi.org/10.1016/j.pec.2017.06.003.

Brown, R. G. S., & Stones, R. H. W. (1972). Personality and intelligence characteristics of male nurses. *International Journal of Nursing Studies, 9*(8), 167–177. https://doi.org/10.1016/0020-7489(72)90043-0.

Canadian Nurses Association. (2018). *Nursing statistics.* Retrieved from https://www.cna-aiic.ca/en/nursing-practice/the-practice-of-nursing/health-human-nursing/statistics.

Carabez, R., Eliason, M., & Martinson, M. (2016). Nurses' knowledge about transgender patient care: A qualitative study. *Advances in Nursing Science, 39*(3), 257–271. https://doi.org/10.1097/ANS.0000000000000128.

Carabez, R., Pellegrini, M., Mankovitz, A., et al. (2015). Does your organization use gender inclusive forms? Nurses' confusion about trans* terminology. *Journal of Clinical Nursing, 24*(21–22), 3306–3317. https://doi.org/10.1111/jocn.12942.

Care, D., Gregory, D., English, J., & Venkatesh, P. (1996). A struggle for equality: Resistance to commissioning of male nurses in the Canadian military, 1952–1967. *Canadian Journal of Nursing Research, 28*(1), 103.

Carnevale, T., & Priode, K. (2018). "The good ole' girls' nursing club": The male student perspective. *Journal of Transcultural Nursing, 29*(3), 285–291. https://doi.org/10.1177/1043659617703163.

Christensen, M. (2017). Men in nursing: The early years. *Journal of Nursing Education and Practice, 7*(5), 94–103. https://doi.org/10.5430/jnep.v7n5p94.

Christman, L. P. (1988). Men in nursing. In J. J. Fitzpatrick, R. L. Taunton, & J. Q. Benoliel (Eds.), *Annual review of nursing research* (pp. 193–205) (Vol. 6). New York, NY: Springer.

Demurtas, A. (2018). Icelandic nurses association to pay school fees for male nurse students. *Rekjavik Grapevine.* Retrieved from https://grapevine.is/news/2018/04/19/icelandic-nurses-association-to-pay-school-fees-for-male-nurse-students/.

Dixon Vuic, K. (2009). Review: Daring to care: American nursing and second-wave feminism. *Bulletin of the History of Medicine, 83*(1), 234–235. https://doi.org/10.1353/bhm.0.0174.

Dorsen, C. (2012). An integrative review of nurse attitudes towards lesbian, gay, bisexual, and transgender patients. *Canadian Journal of Nursing Research, 44*(3), 18–43.

Dyck, J. M., Oliffe, J., Phinney, A., & Garrett, B. (2009). Nursing instructors' and male nursing students' perceptions of undergraduate, classroom nursing education. *Nurse Education Today, 29*(7), 649–653. https://doi.org/10.1016/j.nedt.2009.02.003.

Eliason, M., Dibble, S., & DeJoseph, J. (2010). Nursing's silence on lesbian, gay, bisexual, and transgender issues: The need for emancipatory efforts. *Advances in Nursing Science, 33*(3), 206–218. https://doi.org/10.1097/ANS.0613e3181e63e49.

Evans, J. (2004). Men nurses: A historical and feminist perspective. *Journal of Advanced Nursing, 47*(3), 321–328. https://doi.org/10.1111/j.1365-2648.2004.03096.x.

Goldberg, L., Rosenburg, N., & Watson, J. (2018). Rendering LGBTQ+ visible in nursing: Embodying the philosophy of caring science. *Journal of Holistic Nursing, 36*(3), 262–271. https://doi.org/10.1177/0898010117715141.

Green, K., & Feinstein, B. (2012). Substance use in lesbian, gay, and bisexual populations: An update on empirical research and implications for treatment. *Psychology of Addictive Behaviours, 26*(2), 265–278. https://doi.org/10.1037/a0025424.

Gross, R. E. (2014). Relationship-based care: The influence of feminism on professional nursing. *Journal of Gynecologic Oncology Nursing, 24*(2), 21–27.

Harrell, B. R., & Sasser, J. T. (2018). Sexual and gender minority health: Nursing's overdue coming out. *International Journal of Nursing Studies, 79*, a1–a4. https://doi.org/10.1016/j./jnurstu.2017.12.002.

Holtzclaw, B.J. (1981). *The man in nursing: Relations between sex-type perceptions and locus of control.* Dissertation Abstracts International, 4202A. (University Microfilms No. 81-16, 752).

Im, E. (2010). Current trends in feminist nursing research. *Nursing Outlook, 58*(2), 87–96. https://doi.org/10.1016/j.outlook.2009.09.006.

Im, E. (2013). Practical guidelines for feminist research in nursing. *Advances in Nursing Science, 36*(2), 133–145. https://doi.org/10.1097/ANS.0b013e318290204e.

Jackman, K. B., Bosse, J. D., Eliason, M. J., & Hughes, T. L. (2019). Sexual and gender minority health research in nursing. *Nursing Outlook, 67*(1), 21–38. https://doi.org/10.1016/j.outlook.2018.10.006.

Jackman, K., Honig, J., & Bockting, W. (2016). Nonsuicidal self-injury among lesbian, gay, bisexual and transgender populations: An integrative review. *Journal of Clinical Nursing, 25*, 3438–3453. https://doi.org/10.1111/jocn.13236.

Li, Q. (2018). Numbers of men in nursing are rising in China. *Johns Hopkins Nursing.* Retrieved from https://magazine.nursing.jhu.edu/2018/06/numbers-of-men-in-nursing-are-rising-in-china/.

Lim, F. A., Brown, D. V., Jr., & Kim, S. M. J. (2014). Addressing health care disparities in the lesbian, gay, bisexual, and transgender population: A review of best practices. *American Journal of Nursing, 114*(6), 24–34. https://doi.org/10.1097/01.NAJ.0000450423.89759.36.

MacDonnell, J. A. (2014). Enhancing our understanding of emancipatory nursing: A reflection on the use of critical feminist methodologies. *Advances in Nursing Science, 37*(3), 271–280. https://doi.org/10.1097/ANS.0000000000000038.

McMurry, T. B. (2011). The image of male nurses and nursing leadership mobility. *Nursing Forum, 46*(1), 22–28. https://doi.org/10.1111/j.1744-6198.2010.00206.x.

McPherson, K. M. (2003). *Bedside matters: The transformation of Canadian nursing, 1900–1990.* Toronto, ON: University of Toronto Press.

Malka, S. G. (2007). *Daring to care: American nursing and second wave feminism.* Urbana and Chicago, IL: University of Illinois Press.

Nursing and Midwifery Board of Australia. (2019). *Nursing and midwifery regulation at work: Protecting the public in 2017/18.* Retrieved from https://www.nursingmidwiferyboard.gov.au/News/2019-03-07-profession-specific-report.aspx.

Nursing and Midwifery Council. (2017). *Annual equality, diversity and inclusion report 2017–2018.* Retrieved from https://www.nmc.org.uk/globalassets/sitedocuments/annual_reports_and_accounts/edi/annual-edi-report-2017-18.pdf.

O'Connor, T. (2015). Men choosing nursing: Negotiating a masculine identity in a feminine world. *Journal of Men's Studies, 23*(2), 194–211. https://doi.org/10.1177/10600826515582519.

O'Lynn, C. E. (2013). Men in nursing – it's not something new! In C. E. O'Lynn (Ed.), *A man's guide to a nursing career* (pp. 13–48). New York, NY: Springer.

O'Lynn, C. E., & Tranbarger, R. E. (2007). *Men in nursing: History, challenges and opportunities.* New York, NY: Springer.

Powers, K., Herron, E. K., Sheeler, C., & Sain, A. (2018). The lived experience of being a male nursing student: Implications for student retention and success. *Journal of Professional Nursing, 34*(6), 475–482. https://doi.org/10.1016/j.profnurs.2018.04.002.

Rajacich, D., Kane, D., Williston, C., & Cameron, S. (2013). If they do call you a nurse, it is always a "male nurse": Experiences of men in the nursing profession. *Nursing Forum, 48*(1), 71–80. https://doi.org/10.1111/nuf.12008.

Regan, H. (2012). Male nurses worldwide. *Realmanswork.* Retrieved from https://realmanswork.wordpress.com/2012/05/05/male-nurses-worldwide/.

Shattell, M. M., & Chinn, P. L. (2014). Nursing silent on LGBTQ health: Rebel nurses provide hope. *Archives of Psychiatric Nursing, 28*(1), 76–77. https://doi.org/10.1016/j.apnu.2013.11.002.

Strong-Boag, V. (2016). Women's suffrage in Canada. *The Canadian Encyclopedia.* Retrieved from https://www.thecanadianencyclopedia.ca/en/article/suffrage.

Sundean, L. J., & Polifroni, E. C. (2016). A feminist framework for nurses on boards. *Journal of Professional Nursing, 32*(6), 396–400. https://doi.org/10.1016/j.profnurs.2016.03.007.

Troute-Wood, T. (2015). Honouring sexual orientation and gender identity. *Canadian Nurse, 111*(1), 14–15.

Twomey, J. C., & Meadus, R. (2016). Men nurses in Atlantic Canada: Career choice, barriers, and satisfaction. *Journal of Men's Studies, 24*(1), 78–88. https://doi.org/10.1177/1060826515624414.

US Census Bureau. (2013). *Male nurses becoming more commonplace. Census Bureau Reports* (CB13-32). Retrieved from https://www. census.gov/newsroom/press-releases/2013/cb13-32html.

Wedgery, A. (1966). The will to match our opportunity. *The Canadian Nurse, 62*(6), 35–39.

Wilson, K., Kortes-Miller, K., & Stinchcombe, A. (2018). Staying out of the closet: LGBT older adults' hopes and fears in considering end-of-life. *Canadian Journal on Aging, 37*(1), 22–31. https://doi.org/10.1017/S0714980817000514.

Nursing Knowledge

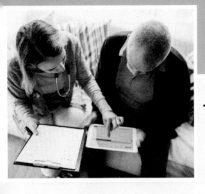

Theoretical Issues in Nursing in the Twenty-First Century: Nursing Theorizing as Everyday Practice

Victoria Smye

(e) http://evolve.elsevier.com/Canada/Ross-Kerr/nursing

LEARNING OBJECTIVES

After reading this chapter, you will be able to:
- Define nursing theory.
- Appreciate the place of early theorizing in nursing.
- Recognize the social, political, and historical factors shaping theory development in nursing.
- Explore notions of nursing ontology and nursing epistemology and their relationship to nursing theorizing.

- Identify key health care trends and challenges influencing the emergence of new forms of theoretical activity in nursing in Canada.
- Think about the role of theorizing in the everyday practice of nursing.

OUTLINE

KEY TERMS

big data
colonialism
competency
conceptual framework
cultural humility
data science
decolonization

deductive
dominant discourses
empiricism
epistemology
equity-oriented health care
heteronormativity
heuristic

human-factors research
indigenization
inductive hermeneutic
interpretive knowledge
liberalism
market economy
metaparadigm

neocolonial
neocolonialism
neoliberalism
omics
ontology
paradigm

praxis process
precision health care
reductionist
settler colonialism
spiritual
structural violence

structural and systemic
  factors
tacit knowledge
theorizing
welfare state
worldview

PERSONAL PERSPECTIVES

Research on the work of public health nurses (PHNs) in home visiting programs shows that PHNs positively influence maternal–infant attachment, improve parenting skills, reduce postpartum depression, improve infant nutrition, and increase the safety and quality of the home environment. Doane, Browne, Reimer et al. (2009) conducted a study analyzing in-depth interviews with PHNs who worked in home visiting programs. The researchers found that the way PHNs theorized, determined, and met their nursing obligations to "high-priority" families—and the way that the PHNs' taken-for-granted theorizing process was enacted as part of everyday practice—enabled the PHNs to be with families and create the desired outcomes. The following interview excerpt from this study by Doane, Browne, Reimer et al. (2009) provides an illustration:

Public Health Nurse (PHN): and she said I just can't handle my baby's crying any more. She said . . . I want to give my kids to someone else. And so I said okay, I can talk to a social worker and we can look at getting you some respite because I know you don't permanently want to give your kids to someone else but we all need a break sometimes and we can set this up for you. And we did. And she . . . so she had respite weekends for a period of time and I mean . . . if I had had to listen to that baby's crying all the time, I would have been the same place where she was! (PHN #17) (p. 97)

As the quote illustrates, nurse theorizing involves considering present and future implications simultaneously. As Doane, Browne, Reimer et al. (2009) noted, here the nurse had to manage multiple competing demands and the obligation to "do no harm." In this study, experienced nurses repeatedly described being able to respond to potentially at-risk situations in ways that were compassionate and respectful while still maintaining their focus on the safety of the family. This involved theorizing their obligations and making clinical decisions within the context of families' lives.

Similarly, in the author's (Smye) research in the area of Indigenous mental health, nurses' theorizing takes place in the context of often difficult circumstances. These situations can include the lack of safe housing for people being discharged from mental health institutions and the everyday impact of societal stigma, racism, and discrimination on people's health and well-being. As noted in the following interview excerpt, mental health nurses often have to navigate this complex terrain:

Nurse: And this guy [Indigenous] had just come out of a mental health institution where he had been for 11 months and he needed housing. He didn't talk but he would write on the walls with a felt pen . . . because of this, he only could get the lowest level housing—it was horrible. He lived with an obsessive–compulsive disorder and schizophrenia and had to move into this scuzzy hotel with bed bugs and rodents everywhere. It wasn't right. How could he ever get well? We worked with him for several months and advocated for better housing. We finally got him to write in pencil and eventually got him an improved level of housing, and when he got his new housing (a small but new apartment) the first thing he did was walk over to the wall and write "comfort" (in pencil).

In this case, the mental health nurse responded to this client's needs in the context of his living with a profound mental illness, which was also influenced by the everyday structural inequity (inadequate housing and poverty) he was exposed to. To respond appropriately, the nurse had to theorize their obligations as an advocate and be with the client in that obligation.

As Donaldson and Crowley (1978) have noted, nursing is defined by social relevance and value orientations rather than "empirical truths." Thus, the discipline must continually be reshaped in response to societal needs and scientific discoveries. Knowledge generation in nursing needs to be guided by a commitment to the fundamental problems that shape our world (Thorne, 2014). We need to ensure that, as nurses, our moral compasses are fully operational. To work in our full capacity as nurses, we need to be curious about and able to understand and then address the contextual features of people's lives—for example, attending to the determinants of people's health and well-being.

INTRODUCTION

Nursing has been described as the study of human health and illness processes (Thorne, Canam, Dahinten et al., 1998) as well as an inherent process of well-being, manifested by complexity and integration in human systems (Reed, 1997). The central paradox of nursing is that it is a professional-practice discipline at once so mundane that some of its technical aspects can be performed by almost anyone, yet so cognitively sophisticated and mysterious that its excellent application requires advanced education, extensive reflective clinical practice, and an ongoing commitment to inquiry. It is a discipline oddly situated between practice and academia (Hoeck & Delmar, 2018).

Nursing theory and **theorizing** has been the topic of much dialogue and debate over the past several decades. Nursing theory has been described as a **conceptual framework** (Dickoff, James, & Wiedenbach, 1968), a process of inquiry (Doane & Varcoe, 2005), and a set of concepts, definitions, and models; theories are derived from logical thinking and inductive reasoning (Adib-Hajbaghery & Tahmouresi, 2018). Nursing theories have also been proposed as philosophies of nursing (or at least closely related philosophical proclamations about nursing practice) (Edwards & Liaschenko, 2003; Kikuchi, 2004) and as nursing ontologies, where human action is understood as paramount (Flaming, 2004). In addition, nursing theorizing has been described as an ethical endeavour (Reed, 1989) because of its inescapable connection with the value choices, assumptions, and judgements of the theorist. Thus, nursing theory describes what is most characteristic of and fundamental to nursing practice. As Doane and Varcoe (2005) note, theory is always already practice. Therefore, everyday nursing practice is a critical site for theory development, and nursing theory, research, and practice are mutually interdependent and interactive (Dickoff, James, & Wiedenbach, 1968).

THE SOCIAL, POLITICAL, AND HISTORICAL CONTEXT OF THEORY DEVELOPMENT IN NURSING

Florence Nightingale (1946/1859) is often cited as the person responsible for formalizing the knowledge and practice of nursing into a profession, popularizing nursing for the modern era. As one of the discipline's early theorists, she rejected the traditional social role available to aristocratic women in Victorian times. Instead, she mobilized nurses to care for British soldiers injured in the Crimean War and subsequently created systems for the education of nurses and the delivery of nursing care (see Chapters 1 and 2 for more details). This was an age of considerable change within both society and science, bringing improved sanitation systems and systematic recording of clinical and public health data (de Graaf, Mossman, & Slebodnick, 1986). Recognizing that the epidemiological patterns of sickness and disease pointed to the need for public as well as individual health principles, Nightingale actively participated in a massive reform of the health care delivery system, shifting

🔁 RESEARCH FOCUS

A Theory of Maternal Engagement with Public Health Nurses and Family Visitors

The way in which maternal engagement with public health nurses and family is theorized is critical to nursing practice and research. Mothers of children at risk for developmental delays tend to be the most difficult to access and engage, and they commonly drop out of home visiting programs prematurely. In response to both practice and empirical knowledge, Jack, DiCenso, and Lofeld (2005) conducted a study of maternal engagement with public health nurses. Employing a grounded theory approach (a qualitative research methodology), they conducted record reviews and 29 in-depth interviews with 20 mothers receiving public health nurse and family visitor home visits. They found that mothers felt vulnerable and frequently powerless when they allowed the service providers into their homes. Mothers with at-risk children engage with public health nurses and family visitors through a basic social process of limiting family vulnerability, which has three phases: (1) overcoming fear; (2) building trust; and (3) seeking mutuality. The personal characteristics, values, experiences and actions of the public health nurse, family visitor, and mother influence the speed at which each phase is successfully negotiated and the ability to develop a connected relationship. The researchers concluded that public health nurses working with at-risk families need to identify client fears and perceptions related to home visiting and explain the role of public health nurses and family visitors to all family members. Given the importance that mothers place on the development of an interpersonal relationship, it is important for home visitors to continually assess the quality of their relationships with clients.

Source: Jack, S., DiCenso, A., & Lohfeld, L. (2005). A theory of maternal engagement with public health nurses and family visitors. *Journal of Advanced Nursing, 49*(2), 182–190.

the primary location of nursing from the private home to the hospital setting (Casteldine, 2007).

Over the following century, professional nursing evolved, its fortunes shifting with the sands of social change. For instance, during the periods between various feminist movements, nursing work was rendered invisible (as was all of women's work), and nurses' formal authority within health care decision making was eroded. In contrast, during wartime, the social status of nurses tended to be elevated and their contributions to key processes and decisions highly regarded. In the Nightingale tradition, many nurse leaders openly resisted and challenged the systems in which they operated, while others worked more quietly, using any available means to develop and expand nursing knowledge and practice for the benefit of patients and society (Libster, 2008). This quiet commitment to professional service by the larger community of nurses—catalyzed from time to time by an assertive and proactive leader willing to issue public challenges—characterized nursing until the conclusion of World War II.

When major advances in science and technology that had been developed for wartime purposes were redirected to society at large, health care and nursing were among the primary beneficiaries. The explosion of knowledge within all the health sciences during the 1950s and 1960s created a different climate for nursing. Nursing leaders were motivated to theorize and conceptualize the scientific basis of their practice and to distinguish the structure of nursing's knowledge from that of the more traditionally dominant health disciplines. In this context, it became increasingly important to conceptualize nursing and nursing science as disciplines with their own unique character and nature and not simply as applications of the knowledge generated by other disciplines. Nursing theory became the mechanism by which the discipline attempted to organize and understand the infinitely complex and dynamic body of knowledge, both borrowed and unique to nursing, that would be required for accountable, defensible, and excellent clinical practice (Beckstrand, 1978).

During the 1960s and 1970s, nursing theories, research, and education were shaped by the contextual features of health care and nursing education: the "increasing complexity of patient care, the relocation of nursing education from hospital-based diploma schools to colleges and universities, and the ongoing efforts of nurses to secure more professional autonomy and authority in the decades after World War II" (Tobbell, 2018, p. 63).

In a recent special edition of the journal *Nursing Research*, Callista Roy (2018), a prominent nurse theorist who developed the Adaptation Model of Nursing (Roy, 1970; Roy, 1975), described a "watershed event in nursing history": the publication of papers from three symposia on theory development in nursing by *Nursing Research* 50 years ago (p. 81). She explained that those papers "laid out the foundational ideas about the nature of nursing and nursing theory, and provided direction for the next 50 years of disciplinary knowledge development" (p. 81). The papers were reprinted in anthologies (Nicoll, 1986, 1992, 1997; as cited by Roy, 2018) and taken up widely by many nursing authors (e.g., Meleis, 2012; Walker & Avant, 2011).

Nursing theory and knowledge development in the late 1960s and early 1970s was in large part a response to the need for nursing to conceptualize the uniqueness of nursing practice knowledge and gain credibility as a professional discipline alongside medicine and scientific disciplines (Thorne, 1998). Donaldson and Crowley's (1978) definition of a professional discipline as "embod(ying) a knowledge base relevant to all realms of professional practice and which links, the past, present and future" (p. 117, cited in Grace, Willis, Roy, & Jones, 2016) continues to be as relevant today as it was at that time. According to Roy (2018), major contributions of theorizing in the twentieth century have included the maturing of the discipline, the clarification of the theoretical focus of nursing, and the development of a number of grand theories. During this time, "nursing," "persons," "environment," and "health" became the central concepts constituting the **metaparadigm** of nursing (Fawcett, 1984; Forchuk, Martin, Chan, & Jensen, 2005).

However, this nursing era was not without its challenges, including the ongoing critique and debate surrounding the metaparadigm concepts. Each theorist has their own perspective or **worldview** that has in turn shaped their beliefs, assumptions, and values and therefore their definitions of the **paradigm**s and metaparadigms of their discipline. These views underlie their behaviours and decisions. The paradigm debate was prominent in nursing research, education, and clinical practice for several decades. In their paper published in *Nursing Inquiry*, Thorne, Reimer-Kirkham, and Henderson (1999) recommended that nursing suspend the paradigm debate because it risked further inhibiting rather than fostering knowledge development. Thorne, Canam, Dahinten et al. (1998) also called on nurse theorists to come to the centre of these different positions by focusing on perspectives where they might find common ground rather than on issues where they became mired in paradigmatic debate; the authors' purpose was not to end this debate but rather create respectful dialogue. Thorne, Canam, Dahinten et al. (1998) proposed definitions that reflected common understandings and yet would permit a diverse range of perspectives, including the following definition of nursing and nursing practice:

Nursing is the study of human health and illness processes. Nursing practice is facilitating, supporting and assisting individuals, families, communities and/or societies to enhance, maintain and recover health, and to reduce and ameliorate the effects of illness. Nursing's relational practice and science are directed toward the explicit outcome of health-related quality of life within the immediate and larger environmental contexts. (p. 1265)

More recently, Jairath, Peden-McAlpine, Sullivan et al. (2018) shared their perspective on the relevance and current value of the nursing metaparadigm today. They discussed the ability of the metaparadigm to support shared meaning to advance knowledge; to define the domain, evaluate knowledge, and ask questions for knowledge discovery; and to support the design of research to obtain new data with knowledge-enhancing potential. The authors also suggested changes in the nursing metaparadigm. For example, they proposed "time" as a key concept that should be incorporated into the metaparadigm, given the temporal period inherent in considering and studying health across the lifespan. They also encouraged nurses to consider scientific advancements external to the discipline, such as expanded understandings of the environment that consider the sum of human environmental exposures over a lifetime. Another

---

RESEARCH FOCUS

An Example of Everyday Theorizing in Mental Health

Early in her career, Dr. Cheryl Forchuk, a now-distinguished university professor and researcher in mental health at Western University with years of clinical experience, tested Peplau's theory (Forchuk, 1994, 1995). This research was important to understanding the development of the therapeutic relationship, considered to be the crux of nursing by Peplau, and pointed to the need for research that specifically tested nursing theory. For example, in Forchuk's (1994, 1995) longitudinal study of 124 newly formed nurse–client dyads in mental health settings over a 6-month period, she found that almost one-third of hospitalized patients were discharged during what Peplau defined as the "orientation," or initial phase of treatment, before the therapeutic relationship had been established. Forchuk's findings reinforced the importance of the nurse–patient relationship and acknowledged that a therapeutic relationship with someone living with a chronic mental illness can take significant time to develop. Premature or early discharge can further complicate this challenge. Some of the questions raised from these findings have direct application to clinical practice, including the following (Forchuk, 1994, p. 536):

- What should or could be done about the number of clients discharged in orientation?
- Should hospitalizations be longer for the population with chronic mental illness to allow adequate time for the development of the orientation phase?
- Should staff somehow work more diligently or effectively in the limited time available to establish relationships?
- Should expectations be changed so that the development of the therapeutic relationship is not looked for but is relegated to community settings only?
- Should nurses provide care across in-patient and community situations to allow therapeutic relationships to develop?

Today, Forchuk has continued to use these findings to inform her research and theory development (e.g., Forchuk, Martin, Chan, and Jensen, 2005; Forchuk, Martin, Ouseley et al., 2013). This research has led to a deeper understanding of how theory actually works in practice. Many other mid-range theories exist. However, as Fawcett (1999) notes, it could be argued that the product of every nursing study represents a mid-range theory; theory, inquiry, and evidence are inextricably linked (Fawcett, Watson, Neuman et al., 2001).

Sources: Fawcett, J., Watson, J., Neuman, B., et al. (2001). On nursing theories and evidence. *Journal of Nursing Scholarship*, *33*(2), 115–119. https://doi.org/10.1111/j.1547-5069.2001.00115.x; Forchuk, C. (1994). The orientation phase of the nurse–client relationship. *Journal of Advanced Nursing, 20*, 532–537. https://doi.org/10.1111/j.1744-6163.1992.tb00384.x; Forchuk, C. (1995). Development of nurse–client relationships: What helps? *Journal of the American Psychiatric Nurses Association*, *1*(5), 146–153. https://doi.org/10.1177/107839039500100503; Fawcett, J. (1999). *The relationship of theory and research* (3rd ed.). Philadelphia, PA: F.A. Davis; Forchuk, C., Martin, M.-L., Chan, Y. L., & Jensen, E. (2005). Therapeutic relationships: From psychiatric hospital to community. *Journal of Psychiatric and Mental Health Nursing*, *12*, 556–564. https://doi.org/10.1111/j.1365-2850.2005.00873.x; Forchuk, C., Martin, M. L., Ouseley, S., et al. (2013). Integrating an evidence-based intervention into clinical practice: "Transitional Relationship Model." *Journal of Psychiatric and Mental Health Nursing, 20*(7), 584–594. https://doi.org/10.1111/j.1365-2850.2012.01956.x.

idea put forward was that basic concepts and patterns for knowledge development, including different approaches to communicate the relevance of nursing science to society, may need to undergo fundamental change if they are no longer viable; for example, there is a need for theorizing in nursing to include dialogue and examination of **omics** (Pierce & Henley, 2017), **big data** (e.g., Founds, 2018; Brennan & Bakken, 2015), and **data science** while ensuring their relevance in rapidly evolving and complex practice arenas.

During the 1960s, 1970s, and 1980s, a number of nursing "grand theories" and models emerged that provided for the articulation and testing of theories in practice and research. Grand theories are general concepts that pertain to the overall nature and goals of professional nursing. A grand theory is a synthesis of scholarly research, professional experience, and insights from theoretical pioneers. While there are many benefits to knowing and understanding grand theories, these constructions are often abstract and do not necessarily lend themselves to empirical testing or problems in specific nursing settings. For example, in the 1980s, Orem (Self-Care Deficit Theory), Roy (Adaptation Model), and Newman (Health as Expanding Consciousness) focused on the notions of "person" and Henderson (Nursing Need Theory) on the notion of "nursing" (Tobbell, 2018, p. 65).

However, more recently, some nursing scholars have argued against the relevance of grand theories. McGibbon, Mulaudzi, Didham et al. (2014) have argued that given their nature, grand theories are not generally applicable to practice and policy and the transformative change needed to address current issues in health care and nursing. For example, grand theories are not suitable for addressing health inequities experienced by people who face extreme marginalization (e.g., people with the lived experience of mental illness, poverty, or homelessness). These are not individual issues but rather are constituted and lived out within systems and structures that require redress.

During the 1960s, 1970s, and 1980s, middle- or midrange theories were also developed to make grand theories more concrete; these theories supported nursing interventions (Hoeck & Delmar, 2018). Mid-range nursing theories are narrower in scope than grand nursing theories and offer an effective bridge between grand nursing theories and nursing practice. Widely used mid-range nursing theories include Orlando's theory of the deliberative nursing process (Orlando, 1961), Peplau's theory of interpersonal relations (Peplau, 1952), Parse's theory of human becoming (Parse, 1992), and Watson's theory of human caring (Watson, 1979, 1990). The function of mid-range theory includes describing, explaining, or predicting phenomenon; thus, although also abstract, mid-range theories are testable by observation or experiment.

THE EPISTEMOLOGY AND ONTOLOGY OF NURSING AND THE INSEPARABILITY OF THEORY AND PRACTICE

Epistemology

Since the early 1960s, nursing has been in an era of theory construction, refinement, and systematic examination. Central to the advancement of nursing as a discipline and profession (Leininger, 1988) has been asking questions such as these: What characterizes the essential nature and essence of nursing? What constitutes the essential nature of nursing knowledge? What is different about nursing knowledge compared with that of other health disciplines?

Nursing **epistemology** is the "study of knowledge shared among the members of the discipline, the patterns of knowing and knowledge that develop from them, and the criteria for accepting knowledge claims" (Schultz & Meleis, 1988, p. 217). As a practice discipline, knowing in nursing is achieved in multiple ways through observation and experience in encountering the world and being in the world. Thus, knowing is a process, knowledge is a product, and knowing in nursing is about working on solutions that are important to the well-being of clients (Schultz & Meleis, 1988). According to Grace (2014), epistemological rigour in nursing requires that a theory accurately represent the phenomenon of concern, be philosophically sound, and can direct practice.

By now you will be familiar with Carper's (1978) foundational work on patterns of knowing: empirical, ethical, aesthetic, and personal knowing (Table 6.1). You also will be familiar with sociopolitical (White, 1995) and emancipatory knowing (Chinn & Kramer, 2011, 2015). Since Carper's work was first published, nursing has used this **heuristic**–conceptual framework as a conviction that the discipline needs to target multiple ways of knowing that are complementary to **empiricism**. Traditional empiricism is the idea that all knowledge originates from the senses—all concepts are about or are applicable to things that can be experienced; this is an approach to knowledge generation that is **deductive** and **reductionist** in nature. However, for some time, nursing scholars and researchers have noted the limitations of more traditional empiricism and argued for the inclusion of contemporary empiricism. In other words, contemporary empiricism values traditional empirical knowledge alongside **interpretive knowledge** to provide a context for the appropriate application of that knowledge (Giuliano, 2003). Contemporary empiricism provides the ability to bridge the gap between the *facts* of scientific knowledge and the *use* of scientific knowledge to facilitate the application of all types of nursing knowledge (Giuliano, 2003, p. 51). This has been an ongoing and important conversation in nursing: What constitutes empirical evidence in a discipline that is evidence based or informed?

TABLE 6.1   Patterns of Knowing in Nursing

Term	Definition	Example
Empirical knowing	Knowledge that is systematically organized into general laws and theories for the purpose of describing, explaining, and predicting phenomena of special concern to the discipline of nursing (Carper, 1978, p.14)—often referred to as the science of nursing (Chinn & Kramer, 2011, 2015). One way we employ this knowledge is through evidence-informed practice.	The Long-Term Care Best Practices Toolkit—This toolkit is informed by the empirical literature on person- and family-centered care, falls prevention and management, skin and wound care, continence care and bowel management, pain assessment and management, delirium, dementia and depression and responsive behaviours, prevention of abuse and neglect, alternative approaches to the use of restraints, oral care, and end-of-life care. (Registered Nurses' Association of Ontario, 2018)
Ethical knowing	This aspect of knowing focused on our nursing obligations, or "what ought to be done." Nurses apply standards, codes, and values to decide what is morally right; however, this application will not eliminate the necessity for moral choices. (Carper, 1978, p. 21)	The nurse is aware of the obligation to "do no harm" in the context of a patient refusing potentially life-sustaining treatment. The nurse considers "what ought to be done" in the context of conflicting values—the patient's right to refuse treatment and the obligation to "do no harm."
Aesthetic knowing	This aspect of knowing is often referred to as the art of nursing. It involves the creation of a singular, particular subjective expression of imagined possibilities or equivalent expression, not so easily put into words. (Carper, 1978)	Empathy and compassion are modes in the aesthetic pattern of knowing. We gain knowledge of another person's singular, particular, felt experience through, as one example, empathy.
Personal knowing	This is the knowledge of ourselves and what we have seen and experienced; this knowledge comes to us through ongoing observation and critical self-reflection. (Carper, 1978)	The nurse has admitted a patient to the delivery suite who has not had prenatal care. The patient also uses substances. The nurse reflects on their previous biases and assumptions related to pregnancy and substance use.
Sociopolitical knowing	This type of knowing enables the nurse to understand the political, social, and economic realities of persons (nurse and patient) and the profession of nursing (the profession as understood by society and the nurse and the nurse's understanding of society and its politics). (White, 1995)	A student nurse becomes acquainted with recent political events related to climate change and initiates a student committee in the school of nursing to connect with this issue.
Emancipatory knowing	The ability to critically reflect, recognize, and acknowledge social and political injustice or inequity; to realize that situations could be different; "to piece together complex elements of experience and context to change a situation as it is to a situation that improves people's lives." (Chinn & Kramer, 2011, p. 64)	A patient with a leg fracture is being discharged home from emergency; for this patient, home is the street. The nurse interrupts the discharge process and connects with the resources necessary to support safe discharge planning.

Sources: Carper, B. A. (1978). Fundamental patterns of knowing in nursing. *Advances in Nursing Science, 1*(1), 13–23; Chinn, P. L., & Kramer, M. K. (2011). *Integrated theory and knowledge development in nursing* (8th ed.). St Louis, MO: Mosby; Chinn, P. L., & Kramer, M. K. (2015). *Knowledge development in nursing theory and process* (9th ed.). St. Louis, MO: Elsevier; White, J. (1995). Patterns of knowing: Review, critique and update. *Advances in Nursing Science, 17*(4), 73–86; Registered Nurses' Association of Ontario. (2018). Long-term care toolkit best practices toolkit (2nd ed.). Retrieved from https://ltctoolkit.rnao.ca/.

CULTURAL CONSIDERATIONS

Indigenous Ways of Knowing

Some ways of knowing continue to be marginalized by Western epistemological perspectives, such as Indigenous ways of knowing (IWK) (Bourque Bearskin, Cameron, King, & Weber Pillwax, 2016; Stansfield & Browne, 2013). Although the nursing profession has drawn on diverse epistemological perspectives, content and teaching in nursing education in Canada and the United States has primarily been grounded in Western Eurocentric epistemological assumptions (Stansfield & Browne, 2013, p. 143). There are fundamentally different assumptions and processes underpinning IWK that the nursing learner needs to understand. As Marie Battiste (2008) notes, "Indigenous people's epistemology is derived from the immediate ecology; from people's experiences, perceptions, thoughts and memory, including dreams, visions, inspirations, and signs interpreted with the guidance of healers or elders" (p. 499, as cited in Stansfield & Browne, 2013, p. 144); it is an epistemology developed over thousands of years, yet it remains poorly represented within **dominant discourses** in health care (Stansfield & Browne, 2013, p. 144). While Indigenous knowledge and ways of knowing are diverse, spirituality is strongly interconnected with the physical, mental, and emotional domains across Indigenous belief structures. For example, the Midewiwin, also known as the Grand Medicine Society, is an ancient spiritual society that was once widespread among the Ojibwe (an Anishinaabe people) and many other Great Lakes tribes. In this society, Mides are considered healers and spiritual leaders, and the source of evidence is **spiritual** in nature.

Given the dominance of Western epistemologies and the heterogeneity and complexities associated with Indigenous knowing, learners will face challenges in learning about IWK, including its embeddedness in relational ways of being and the nonlinear and nondeterministic discourses associated with it (Stansfield & Browne, 2013, p. 144). For example, this kind of learning involves a predominance of "process" thinking as opposed to the "content" thinking favoured by a Western worldview (Duran & Duran, 2000, p. 91).

Learning about IWK also requires that those bringing IWK into the classroom give thoughtful attention to safe processes. Stansfield and Browne provide many recommendations regarding what constitutes safe processes (p. 149), including consultation, permission, and alignment with the intentions and principles of cultural safety—to name only a few. The Truth and Reconciliation Commission of Canada's (2015) Calls to Action document has provided principles and recommendations to guide the work of **decolonizing** and **indigenizing** within the realm of health professional education and health care.

Sources: Battiste, M. (2008). Research ethics for protecting Indigenous knowledge and heritage: Institutional and researcher responsibilities. In N. K. Denzin, Y. S. Lincoln, & L. T. Smith (Eds)., *Handbook of critical and Indigenous methodologies* (pp. 497–509). Thousand Oaks, CA: Sage Publications; Bourque Bearskin, L., Cameron, B. L., King, M., & Weber Pillwax, C. (2016). Mâmawoh Kamâtowin, "Coming together to help each other in wellness": Honouring Indigenous nursing knowledge. *International Journal of Indigenous Health, 11*(1), 18–33. Retrieved from https://doi.org/10.18357/ijih111201615024; Duran, B., & Duran, E. (2000). Applied postcolonial clinical and research strategies. In M. Battiste (Ed.), *Reclaiming Indigenous voice and vision* (pp. 86–100). Vancouver, BC: The University of British Columbia Press; Stansfield, D., & Browne, A. J. (2013). The relevance of Indigenous knowledge for nursing curriculum. *Journal of Nursing Education Scholarship, 10*(1), 143–151. https://doi.org/10.1515/ijnes-2012-0041; Truth and Reconciliation Commission of Canada. (2015). *Honouring the truth, reconciling for the future: Summary of the final report of the Truth and Reconciliation Commission of Canada.* Winnipeg, MB: Author.

Ontology

The word **ontology** is directly linked to philosophy. Nursing ontology describes what is most characteristic of and fundamental to nursing practice (e.g., Flaming, 2004). Ontology is the way of seeing and describing the whole (Reed, 1997), the "core of nursing" (Hoeck & Delmar, 2018, p. 2/10). Ontological descriptions explore the defining features or realities of being human; however, this is not to suggest that experience is an immutable state; rather, it is dynamic and shifting.

For several decades, nursing scholars have debated the theory–practice link. Nurses tend to avoid using the language of theory in practice unless mandated to do so (Liaschenko and Fisher, 1999). And sadly, as Doane and Varcoe (2005) note, educators tend to present theory as an abstract body of knowledge that is separate from the practice arena (p. 81). However, over the last two decades, there has been a call by some to move from an epistemological orientation in nursing education to an ontological orientation. As Dall'Alba and Barnacle (2007) note, when beginning with an ontological orientation, knowing becomes an embodied experience—it is situated within personal, social, historical, and cultural settings and experiences. Therefore, knowing is not merely intellectual but rather a way of thinking, making, and acting; it is a way of being.

RESEARCH FOCUS

Equity-Oriented Health Care

In three innovative research projects funded by the Canadian Institutes of Health Research (CIHR), nurse-led interprofessional teams of researchers defined and examined different approaches to **equity-oriented health care** (EOHC):

- Urban Aboriginal Health Care (UAHC), an ethnographic study of two primary health care clinics in British Columbia (2007–2011);
- EQUIP Primary Health Care, an intervention study in four primary health care clinics in British Columbia and Ontario (2011–2016); and
- EQUIP Emergency, an intervention study in three B.C. emergency departments (2016–2021; ongoing).

In UAHC, the researchers identified three key dimensions of EOHC:

1. Trauma and violence-informed care—Practices that shift beyond trauma-informed care to explicitly address the intersection and cumulative effects of interpersonal (e.g., child abuse, intimate partner violence) and structural (e.g., poverty, stigma) forms of violence on people's lives and health;
2. Culturally safe care—Practices that move beyond cultural sensitivity to explicitly address inequitable power relations, racism, discrimination, and ongoing impacts of historical and current inequities in health care encounters; and
3. Contextually tailored care—Services are tailored to the local communities and populations served, including the demographic, social, and community realities that vary with local politics, epidemiological trends,

and economic conditions (Browne, Varcoe, Wong et al., 2012; Browne, Varcoe, Lavoie et al., 2016).

In the EQUIP Primary Health Care project, the researchers studied the process of promoting the adoption of EOHC through staff education and organizational tailoring of their approaches to four key clinic contexts (i.e., patient population, organizational policies and priorities, community, and funding). The researchers also assessed the early impacts of this process for patients and staff (Indigenous and non-Indigenous) and organizations employing both qualitative and quantitative methods (a mixed-methods approach). The intervention was organized around the three key dimensions of EOHC, along with the development of 10 strategies to operationalize these dimensions and new indicators to monitor them. Informed by the findings of this project, harm reduction is now included as a key dimension of EOHC as part of contextually tailored care. Harm reduction focuses on introducing practices that mitigate harms related to substance use as well as historical, sociocultural, and political factors related to the responses to substance use (Browne, Varcoe, Ford-Gilboe et al., 2018; Ford-Gilboe, Wathen, Varcoe et al., 2018).

This mixed-methods study brought together different kinds of empirical knowledge to inform what constitutes effective equity-oriented practice in primary health care (Browne, Varcoe, Ford-Gilboe et al. 2018; Ford-Gilboe, Wathen, Varcoe et al., 2018). Thus, this research informed ongoing nursing theorizing regarding what constitutes the key dimensions of EOHC and how they might be applied in everyday practice.

Sources: Browne, A. J., Varcoe, C., Wong, S., et al. (2012). Closing the health equity gap: Evidence-based strategies for primary health care organizations. *International Journal for Equity in Health, 11*(59). https://doi.org/10.1186/1475-9276-11-59; Browne, A. J., Varcoe, C., Lavoie, J., et al. (2016). Enhancing health care equity with Indigenous populations: Evidence-based strategies from an ethnographic study. *BMC Health Services Research, 16*(1), 544. https://doi.org/10.1186/s12913-016-1707-9; Browne, A., Varcoe, C., Ford-Gilboe, M., et al. (2018). Disruption as opportunity: Impacts of an organizational-level health equity intervention in primary care clinics. *International Journal for Equity in Health, 17*, 154. https://doi.org/10.1186/s12939-018-0820-2; Ford-Gilboe, M., Wathen, N., Varcoe, C., et al. (2018). How equity-oriented health care impacts health: Key mechanisms and implications for primary health care practice and policy. *Millbank Quarterly, 96*(4), 635–671. https://doi.org/10.1111/1468-0009.12349.

For instance, universities are typically viewed as places where the knowledge and skills acquired can be decontextualized from the practice to which the knowledge and skills relate. In contrast to this view, Dall'Alba and Barnacle (2007) posit the notion of embodied knowledge and the *lived body* as central to professional practice and body–technology relations; that is, ontology and epistemology are interdependent

and thus inseparable. The increased use of technology is changing nursing practice, such as "nursing presence." Nursing presence has long been characterized by the need for a nurse to be physically present with a patient; however, new technologies are making it possible for nurses to interact with patients they have never met face to face. Therefore, nurses need to be mindful of what "presence" means in this context.

CASE STUDY
Home Care and the Palliative Patient

Carole is a home care nurse who has been visiting a family in a small rural community for the past 2 months. The primary focus of her visits, which usually last an hour, has been extensive wound care for 22-year-old Anna, a female client with advanced leukemia who is now palliative. Anna lives with her mother, Deirdre, 44; father, Alex, 45; and four brothers—Nick, 18, Carter, 16, Joel, 14, and David, 8. Anna's bed is set up in the family room, an open room adjacent to the kitchen and dining areas. She usually is sitting in a large recliner when Carole arrives on her visits, between 2:00 and 3:00 p.m. each day. Because of her condition, Anna must be moved very carefully, as her skin breaks down easily. Her wounds are now quite extensive; they are found primarily on the lower outer aspect of both legs and inner aspect of her right buttock. The most challenging issue is to keep the wounds clean and prevent them from becoming more extensive and infected.

Carole has noticed that Anna has become more agitated about being moved; generally, her parents assist Carole in this regard. Anna is usually in good spirits on these visits. Today, however, she is particularly annoyed with her mom, who is busy baking in the kitchen when Carole arrives. Deirdre works from home and usually busies herself when Carole visits. Anna quietly mentions to Carole that her mom moves her too quickly. Anna feels that her mom is not careful enough. She prefers when her dad moves her because he can lift her more easily. In addition, Anna complains that her mom replaces the soiled bandages on her legs incorrectly—at least not the way Carole does it.

Carole's Reflection

Carole is aware of several things simultaneously: the soiled bandages that require changing; Anna's vulnerability to further skin breakdown and infection; Anna's anxiety; and Deirdre's busy schedule and enormous workload. Carole is also aware of the transition this family is in during this challenging time and that Anna and her entire family are Carole's client.

Carole's Response

Initially, Carole found herself worrying about Anna's priority needs and what *should* be done first as well as being concerned about Deirdre's well-being and what she *should* say. However, as she began to busy herself with changing the bandages, Carole engaged Anna in a short discussion and then invited Deirdre over to see how the wounds were coming along. She then engaged Deirdre in general chitchat about how she was doing with her work, the home, the bandaging, medication administration, and so on. As Carole and Deirdre spoke, Carole was aware of their both becoming more at ease. She was also aware of Anna's demeanour, which had become more relaxed. Carole exhibited what we might describe as excellence in relational practice; she employed her skills alongside full engagement with her client (in this case, the family). By *being with* Anna and Deirdre and following their cues, Carole was able to navigate care. *Knowing* in this situation came alongside being. Carole was able to "think in action."

Sources: Benner, P., Hooper-Kyriakidis, P., & Stannard, D. (2011). *Clinical wisdom and interventions in acute and critical care: A thinking-in-action approach* (2nd ed.). New York, NY: Springer. Retrieved from http://lghttp.48653.nexcesscdn.net/80223CF/springer-static/media/samplechapters/9780826105738/9780826105738_chapter.pdf; Benner, P., Sutphen, M., Leonard, V., & Day, L. (2010). *Educating nurses: A call for radical transformation.* San Francisco, CA: Jossey-Bass.

THEORY AND ITS LINKAGE TO THE RELEVANCE AND UNIQUENESS OF NURSING PRACTICE

In their 2018 paper, Jairath, Peden-McAlpine, Sullivan et al. discuss the promise of "practice theory" for the discipline of nursing in today's world. Yet, they note that only a handful of nursing scholars have successfully explored nursing practice within the context of theory exploration. For example, early scholars Dickoff and James (1968/1986, 1968) brought four levels of theory to the nursing theory dialogue: (1) factor-isolating theory; (2) factor-relating theory; (3) situation-related theory; and (4) situation-producing theory. In their view, situation-producing theory is a practice-focused theory and thus the highest order of theory because of its focus on practice. From this perspective, theory is produced not just for the sake of theory development but to guide the shaping of reality; theory is inextricably tied to practice and to the discipline's professional purpose.

Jairath, Peden-McAlpine, Sullivan et al. (2018, p. 190) note three successful approaches to theory–practice inquiry, including (1) situation-producing theory (Dickoff, James, & Weidenbach, 1968, as cited in Jairath et al. 2018); (2) **inductive hermeneutic** approaches, whereby nurses' clinical practice and clinical reasoning are explored with the ultimate goal of theory generation (Benner, 2009, as cited by Jairath et al. 2018); and (3) an approach put forward by Rolfe entitled "nursing science of the unique" (Rolfe, 2006, as cited in Jairath et al. 2018), whereby each nurse–patient situation is considered to involve unique interactions, experiences, and situations that are different from all others. Using this third approach, nurse researchers generate informal theories about unique situations that demonstrate how they test hypotheses, and they experiment and modify theories in response to practice. "Nursing science of the unique" is also a means of uncovering the **tacit knowledge** of how nurses solve the most difficult problems of practice.

Consistent with the perspectives of Roy (2018), Jairath, Peden-McAlpine, Sullivan et al. (2018) also stress the importance of the knowledge development required for effective practice and the theories necessary to address the "social mandate" of nursing. They also argue that the challenge of integrating person-centered care and **precision health care** will not be possible unless **human-factors research** is employed alongside disciplinary pluralism (e.g., interprofessional collaboration). When human-factors research, which results in theory-driven interventions, is coupled with interprofessional collaboration, it ensures contextually relevant knowledge generation and person-centered, clinically efficacious actions that produce positive health outcomes.

An Example of Everyday Theorizing: Relational Inquiry and Culture

A few years ago, the author had the experience of teaching nursing theory to second-year undergraduate nursing students because we had been unable to find someone else to teach it. One of the students, whom I had come to know, told me upon entering the classroom on the first day of class that he would rather do almost anything other than take a nursing theory course—everyone within hearing distance (including myself) began to laugh; the reputation of the course had preceded me. The text had already been chosen, and this was only one of four sections of the course with a preset exam, so there would be no significant changes made to the course. However, this posed an interesting challenge.

As a nurse who had been in practice, primarily as a mental health nurse, for more than 20 years before coming into academia, I had learned that practice experiences played an integral role in the ongoing development of theory in my field (mental health). For many years, I had embraced a pragmatic understanding of theory. In keeping with this understanding, I was determined to bring theorizing to life for students in that classroom, regardless of the limitations posed. So, I introduced the students to the theorizing work of Doane and Varcoe (2005, 2010) and Doane and Brown (2010).

During the term, recent student practice experiences became central to the work in the classroom; together we relived them as situated in the everyday world and we theorized. For example, most student experiences were located in maternal health with new moms (and sometimes challenging breastfeeding experiences). Students grappled with several issues: anxious moms, defining "family," early discharge practices, and more. But fundamentally they struggled with how to take their minds off of what they *should* do and say (saying the "right" thing) and shift their thinking to "being with" in their doing. We discussed the theorists and their theories in the context of the everyday practice of these student nurses and, most importantly, we had a lot of fun doing it.

Pragmatism is derived from the Greek word meaning action, from which the words "practice" and "practical" are also derived (Doane & Varcoe, 2005, p. 82). As Doane and Varcoe explain, living a pragmatic process of theory development involves being grounded in immediacy, experience, and practice rather than living from a unified, fixed perspective (p. 83). Thus, "rather than being limited to an intellectual activity, theorizing is seen as an embodied, reflexive process of responsive action" (p. 83). A pragmatic process is a process of inquiry and choice (p. 83).

Doane & Varcoe (2005) bring a pragmatic understanding of theory to situation-producing theory (Dickoff & James, 1968) as a means to inquire into and question the "knowing" lived out in practice (p. 84). They contend that this knowing includes "theory development that may illuminate our action, guide and provide our action with meaning, and ultimately reshape reality" (p. 84). In this view, knowing and being are interdependent—as noted earlier, nursing's epistemology and ontology are intertwined.

For example, in their situation-producing theoretical work of "relational inquiry," and in striving towards "the ideals of compassion, equitable relations and the honouring of all life forms" (pp. 84–85), Doane and Varcoe (2005) retheorized "family" as a socially situated relational experience. Informed by research with women who had experienced violence, they made a shift from seeing family as a "configuration of people" to seeing family as constituted by experience and context. This is a profound shift. They found that nurses working with women in violent relationships often made statements such as "why doesn't she just leave," reflecting a notion of family as something we can simply leave. Decontextualizing the complex relational experience of both family and violence often led to the offering of very limited choices to women, culminating most commonly in advice to leave their partners.

In the words of Doane and Varcoe (2005), this limited theoretical perspective not only shapes nursing practice in a way "that significantly hinders nurses' understanding and responsiveness to women/families experiencing violence, but it also leaves in place and perpetuates the larger societal discourses and theories that limit the knowing and 'reality' of family and of violence" (p. 85). By examining the consequences of theories and ideas, these authors were able to evaluate the adequacy of those theories and ideas in everyday practice, with significant ramifications for practice (p. 86). They gradually retheorized their practice by taking a pragmatic stance, a process that involved seeking a deeper and more complex understanding of their focus of study and drawing on a wide range of theories and perspectives (p. 87). From their perspective and drawn from their experiences, situation-producing theory means that "reality is remade in every moment of nursing" (p. 88). And a pragmatic perspective of knowledge suggests that everyday nursing practice is a critical site for theory development: "action is integral to theory—it is simultaneously with, and the reason for, thinking" (p. 89).

Doane and Varcoe (2005) also note the shift they made to seeing culture as a relational experience; from this perspective, culture is dynamic. Instead of understanding the nurse as outside of the culture of the "other," the nurse shapes and participates in culture—"culture is happening as patients and nurses relate" (p. 88). As an example, when meeting with an Indigenous patient, the Euro-Canadian nurse enters into relationship within multiple and shifting cultures; relationship occurs within webs of power (and meaning) (e.g., the culture of health care, colonial and **neocolonial** Canadian culture [i.e., **settler colonialism**]). The theory–practice relation is a **praxis process**, that is, the process of enacting and embodying theory in practice. In their 2010 paper, Doane and Varcoe ask how closer attention to ontology might enhance theorizing in family nursing and health care, what it means to live theorizing as a "fluid uncertain process" (p. 136). They put forward the hope that attention to ontology coupled with an openness to engagement with *difference* might serve to enrich the nursing community and our disciplinary knowledge, where our differences serve as an opportunity for learning and growth.

Theorizing in the domain of *difference* and *culture* in nursing was led in large part by nursing scholar Madeleine

GENDER CONSIDERATIONS

In a 2018 CBC special report entitled "'We're going back into the closet': LGBTQ seniors wary of being 'out' in long-term care facilities," journalists Nick Purdon and Leonardo Palleja (2018) reported on the findings of interviews with gay and transgender seniors regarding their concerns about accessing long-term care: they expressed the fear they will need to hide their sexual orientation and fear about the care they would receive in those settings at a time of heightened vulnerability. In response to their lifelong experiences of homophobia and consequent stigma and discrimination, particularly in education and health care, several of the individuals interviewed have become advocates for education in health care. For example, one transgender man is working as a staff member and volunteer to help make providers in long-term care facilities aware of the discrimination faced by LGBTQ2 seniors.

However, regardless of their roles as advocates and spokespersons on this issue, they expressed fear of requiring care in long-term care settings. This fear is not without substance. For example, given stigma (societal and personal) and discrimination, the literature suggests that LGBTQ2 seniors in long-term care settings are more vulnerable to social isolation and depression than other seniors in those settings.

A study by Sussman, Brotman, MacIntosh et al. (2018) found that although LGBTQ2 inclusivity strategies are beginning to emerge in the Canadian long-term care sector, these strategies focus primarily on raising awareness for staff through the provision of one-time or ongoing training. While ongoing training at all levels is a good first step in engendering awareness of LGBTQ2 residents' fears of disclosure or discomfort in an environment that presumes heterosexuality or cisnormativity, comprehensive initiatives that create infrastructures to engage residents and families appear to support the movement from an environment of tolerance to one of solidarity and inclusion.

Many times, patients do not talk about their health concerns because they do not feel that their health care provider understands issues involving sexuality or gender identity. This lack of understanding can have unintended negative health outcomes. Nurses not only need to be aware of the issues of *difference* and *culture* as related to LGBTQ2 persons, they also need to be advocates for change.

Sources: Purdon, N., & Palleja, L. (2018, June 18). *"We're going back into the closet": LGBTQ seniors wary of being "out" in long-term care facilities.* CBC News. Retrieved from https://www.cbc.ca/news/canada/lgbtq-seniors-long-term-care-homes-discrimination-1.4721384; Sussman, T., Brotman, S., MacIntosh, H., et al. (2018). Supporting lesbian, gay, bisexual, and transgender inclusivity in long-term care homes: A Canadian perspective. *Canadian Journal on Aging, 37*(2), 121–132. https://doi.org/10.1017/S0714980818000077

Leininger (e.g., 1978, 1979, 1984, 1985, 1988), who developed the Culture Care Theory and what she called "transcultural nursing." This work was built upon by an array of nursing scholars who further conceptualized and critiqued notions of culture, cultural sensitivity, and cultural competence (e.g., Drevdahl, 2018) and added to this compendium on cultural safety (e.g., Aboriginal Nurses Association of Canada, 2009; Anderson, Reimer-Kirkham, Rodney et al., 2009; Browne, Varcoe, Smye et al., 2009; Browne & Varcoe, 2006; Ramsden, 1993, 2000; Reimer-Kirkham, Smye, Tang et al., 2002; Smye & Browne, 2002) and **cultural humility** (e.g., First Nations Health Authority, 2018; Yeager & Bauer-Wu, 2013).

We know that social determinants of health play a significant role in health status, yet the rising inequities in these determinants, along with poor access to health services for marginalized populations, is leading to increasingly poor health for many (Greenwood, de Leeuw, & Lindsay, 2018; Marmot & Allen, 2014; Marmot & Bell, 2016; Mikkonen & Raphael, 2010). In response, nursing theorizing in the domain of *difference* and *culture* has more recently shifted our attention from merely focusing on individual factors influencing health to **structural and systemic factors** (e.g., Drevdahl, 2018) such as racism and discrimination, poverty, **heteronormativity**, and **structural violence**. Structural and system factors have led some groups to experience longstanding social disadvantage and discriminations compared with others (e.g., people living with mental illness, substance use, or both; Indigenous peoples; and members of the LGBTQ2 community). More attention has been given, for instance, to the health inequities experienced by LGBTQ2 persons (e.g., Carabez, Pelligrini, Mankovitz et al., 2015; Klotzbaugh & Spencer, 2015).

👤 APPLYING CONTENT KNOWLEDGE

1. Who do you bring to practice? How is your "being" as a nurse shaped by how you know?
2. How does your practice reflect the essential place of nursing theorizing? For example, what kinds of issues arise in your everyday practice that create theorizing activity? Think for example about the ethical issues that arise in your everyday practice.

KEY HEALTH CARE TRENDS AND CHALLENGES AND THEORY DEVELOPMENT

Big Data and Information Technologies

Big data has been defined as the growth of digital information that cannot be comprehended or managed without computers and vast amounts of storage (Founds, 2018, p. 284). It is a large amount of data emerging from sensors (e.g., wireless sensors), novel research techniques, and abundant, ever-evolving information technologies. Big data is a metric of size, meaning that the data sets far exceed those commonly found. Therefore, these big data sets require new ways of managing data and new methods of analysis (Brennan & Bakken, 2015).

Big data and precision health care management (i.e., the use of information to sustain and enhance health and prevent the development of disease) is a growth industry (Galli, 2016, as cited in Founds, 2018). Nursing big data refers to the vast amount of data related to care and health, including the big data of hospital nursing, regional and local health service platforms, and big data based on nursing research or disease monitoring in large populations (Zhu, Han, Su et al., 2019, p. 230). (See Chapters 8 and 10.) There is no doubt that the knowledge work of nurses is data intensive (Ibrahim, Donelle, Sidani, & Regan, 2019; Sensmeier, 2016). As Booth (2016) notes:

Future nursing informaticians will also need to infuse their knowledge, skills and tacit experience into the analysis of massive databases and repositories of data. A by-product of increased digitization of healthcare has been the explosion in the volume, velocity and variety (i.e., big data) of all types of healthcare data being generated. Nursing informatics has a long history of data science in its knowledge base and definitions; drawing from this established foundation, further development of this skill set within the context of emerging healthcare practices and technologies will be important. This embedding of our classical data standards, knowledge, and values into new systems will ensure that the nursing role is recognized and represented in all future healthcare decision-making arising from the use of large-scale data analytics. (p. 67)

The past several decades have seen rapid parallel advances in nursing theory, nursing terminology, and nursing data in response to the need to explicate nursing's worldview in an era of rapid change in health care and technology (Monsen, Kelechi, McRae et al., 2018, p. 122). However, nursing theory and nursing terminology have remained separate (Matney, Brewster, Sward et al., 2011). "Missing from the theoretical discourse of nursing is the explicit notion that nursing data should express (operationalize) nursing theory. Likewise, nursing theory has often been underused in electronic health record (EHR) design and other applications generating data of interest to nurses" (Matney, Brewster, Sward et al., 2011, p. 122).

With the advent of electronic health records and increased use of technology, face-to-face assessment and embodied understanding of clients' lived bodies may be decreasing (Harrison, Kinsella, & DeLuca, 2019, p. 1/14). There is an immediate need for theory-based work to examine technologies and information management to ensure the creation of nursing-informed technologies and practice.

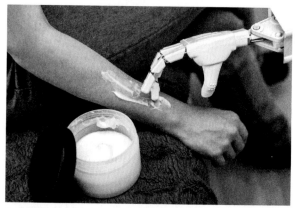

Can robots replace nurses? How can nurses remain relevant in a technologically advanced future? (istock.com/Miriam-doerr)

REGULATION, COMPETENCY-BASED EDUCATION, THE MARKET ECONOMY, AND "EVIDENCE-BASED" PRACTICE

Regulation

Public safety is a central focus in health care and nursing—an issue near and dear to nurse educators and researchers, policy decision makers, and regulators. The public safety mandate of nurse regulators is authorized through government legislation in each province and territory (e.g., the nursing profession in Ontario is regulated by the *Nursing Act, 1991* and the *Regulated Health Professions Act, 1991*). Under each piece of legislation are regulations, bylaws, and standards deemed to protect the public against harms that could result from professional misdeeds and malpractices; thus, regulatory bodies are inclined to serve the interests of the government from which they take their authority (see Chapter 21). As Rudge and Thorne (2013) have noted, this could have the effect of "orienting its priorities and policies in direct contradistinction to the expressed needs and values of the profession it self-regulates" (p. 187). This is not an indictment of regulation per se, but rather an important distinction to make when considering the profession's priority foci at this point in nursing's history. Alongside regulation, and tightly tied to it, is the notion of competency-based education.

Competency-Based Education

Competency has become a key concept in health professional education over the past four decades. Foth and Holmes (2017) have traced the competency-based movement to a period of broad transformation of Western societies from a **welfare state** to advanced **liberalism** (Browne, 2001) and a **market economy**. Although competence and competency are important for ensuring practice readiness, the authors argue that the preponderance of competency-based education and curriculum in nursing poses a threat to its professionalization. Nursing has become a marketable commodity that can be evaluated like any other commodity, and competency-based education now governs nursing knowledge. In Foth and Holmes' (2017) view, the concept of competency is both a "tool for transforming professional actions into technical and measurable terms" and a "political instrument redefining and governing professions" (p. 1), such as that used in approval processes by nursing regulatory bodies in Canada. Thus, the demands of clinical practice and hospital administrators as well as regulators bypass the question of unique nursing knowledge (Foth & Holmes, 2017, p. 7). This is not to suggest that we do not need to graduate competent practitioners, but rather that we are called to attend to the fundamental role of nursing and nursing theorizing.

Meleis (2012) has noted that with the focus on curriculum, nursing faculty (and thus nurses) have lost sight of the reasons for theory, that is, quality nursing practice and patient care (p. 49). As Kumagai (2014) wrote in relation to a recent movement to competency-based medical education, a reductionist approach that ignores the complexities of human behaviour and professional understanding runs the risk of neglecting the deep and reflective engagement with critical aspects of professional practice (p. 981). The interactions between an individual learner's personal worldview and new situations, ideas, and perspectives are considered critical factors in determining the extent of transformational learning.

Market Economy

Austin (2011) has pointed to market forces in health care as posing a real threat to professional nursing. Canadian health care has been restructured in the image of the marketplace to the detriment of the nurse–patient relationship and professional nursing practice. When care becomes a commodity, fundamental commitments to nursing codes of ethics (Canadian Nurses Association, 2017) and standards of practice—to nursing knowledge—are at risk. The dominant global forces of corporatism and commercialism are having a real impact. Unfortunately, to a great extent, cost effectiveness and efficiency have been taken up by nursing in the form of new managerialism (Beardwood, Walters, Eyles, & Franch, 1999). Sadly, that means that nurses' work is about tasks and productivity. We have "the object nurse of productivity, rather than the subject nurse who organizes care for patients" (Rudge, 2013, pp. 209–210). Nurses' practices have also become "increasingly instrumental and rationalized" (Ceci, Pols, & Purkis, 2017; as cited in Hoeck & Delmar, 2018, para 3). Managerial strategies in increasingly efficient and austerity-oriented models of health service delivery systems typically work to exert as much control as possible over the scope and decisional authority afforded to professional nursing practice (Rudge & Thorne, 2013).

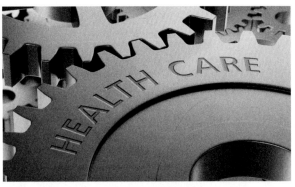

Nurses need to be curators of information. (istock.com/ Zerbor)

The impact of the new public management model was brought into sharp relief recently at a meeting with nursing leaders, where the leader of professional practice within an acute care setting said two things: nurses are "factory workers" and nurses are not interested in research. This was said in response to the efforts of those in the room to brainstorm models of practice education as a way to bring together academia and practice. Therefore, as Duncan, Thorne, and Rodney (2015) have noted, governance and nursing organizations in the twenty-first century must be intelligently informed and passionately motivated; nursing must, as Duncan, Rodney, and Thorne (2014) have suggested, attend relationally to issues of power and policy. Theorists and researchers must take up the critical questions associated with the regulatory and managerial cultures of our times and develop the knowledge that will allow us to sustain and enhance the power of the nursing profession in this century and beyond. As Karnick (2014) has noted:

> The discipline of nursing is on a slippery slope with regard to the ever increasing lack of nursing theory in its work. The misguided attempt to eliminate the use of nursing theory as the underpinning of practice is

> degrading nursing as a viable profession, ultimately affecting patient care. A clarion call to the discipline regarding the need for theory in research and practice is required. Nursing will soon become just another set of tasks rather than the profession needed by patients and their families. (p. 117)

Thorne and Sawatzky (2014) have also argued for an appreciation of the philosophical and theoretical nature of knowledge in nursing, a socially mandated discipline (p. 14), at a time when the vernacular of "evidence-based practice" governs health care alongside discourse around cost effectiveness and efficiency. They call attention to the inseparability of theory and practice. Thorne (2014) has also argued that the future of nursing is dependent on that core disciplinary knowledge to inform the nursing education of the next generation—including and beyond practice and what we study to an alignment with the "thinking structure" of the discipline—to keep us on the course of our "collective disciplinary mandate" (p. 2).

THE DECOLONIZATION OF COLONIAL INTELLECTUAL DEVELOPMENT IN NURSING

The Truth and Reconciliation Commission of Canada (TRC) was formed in response to the longstanding social and health inequities experienced by Indigenous peoples in Canada. The TRC spent 6 years travelling to all parts of Canada and heard from more than 6,500 witnesses. The TRC also hosted seven national events across Canada to engage the Canadian public, educate people about the history and legacy of the residential school system, and share and honour the experiences of former students and their families. The National Centre for Truth and Reconciliation at the University of Manitoba now houses all the documents collected by the TRC.

In June 2015, the TRC held a closing event in Ottawa and presented the executive summary of the findings contained in its multivolume final report. This included 94 Calls to Action (or recommendations) pertaining to child welfare, education, language and culture, health, and justice and directed at all levels of government to further the process of reconciliation between Canadians and Indigenous peoples. Multiple points of reconciliation, including rights and equity for Indigenous peoples, programs and services to foster respectful relationships with Indigenous peoples, and commemoration of Canadian heritage were included among these recommendations (Truth and Reconciliation Commission of Canada, 2015). Some of these recommendations can be directly addressed by the nursing profession, in particular three recommendations pertaining to health professional education.

In Canada, the needs most commonly identified by Indigenous peoples, as seen in their public statements and political processes, include self-determination, cultural preservation, and respect of their wholistic worldview (Hill & Wilkinson, 2014, p. 176). However, **colonialism** and **neocolonialism** and associated structures, processes, and practices continue to stand as a barrier to those aspirations, including the colonization of intellectual development in nursing (McGibbon, Mulaudzi, Didham et al., 2014). McGibbon, Mulaudzi, Didham et al. have pointed to the predominance of Western Eurocentric knowledge systems, including biomedicine, that underpin nursing's metaparadigm and grand theories. They have noted that the metaparadigm and grand theories, intended to lend credibility to nursing as an academic discipline and advance nursing knowledge in the context of the dominance of the medical profession, have failed to remain relevant. For example, they have argued that an uncritical adoption of the concepts of nursing, health, environment, and person puts the profession and its social mandate in serious jeopardy. The metaparadigm is grounded in a Western worldview underpinned by a focus on the individual (individualism) and largely inattentive to structures of oppression such as racism and managerial efficiency models in the delivery of nursing care. Currently, nursing is fully engaged with "discourses of management and market-driven healthcare reform based on the discipline of business, where profit is the ultimate goal" (p. 184). Nursing knowledge, closely tied to reductionist and empiricist foundations, obscures, for example, the root causes of inequities in health, including colonialism, neocolonialism, racism, and discrimination.

Instead, McGibbon, Mulaudzi, Didham et al. (2014) have argued for a decolonizing stance in which nursing creates a counternarrative, where nursing theory development is closely tied to nursing practice—where nurses unsettle, disrupt, and expose colonial ideologies, values, and structures embedded in nursing curricula, teaching methodologies, and professional development (p. 186). In the authors' view, it is not enough, for example, to simply enfold the concepts of racism and racialization into the metaparadigm concept of "environment," where they are at risk of being "hidden" (McGibbon & Etowa, 2009, p. 34);

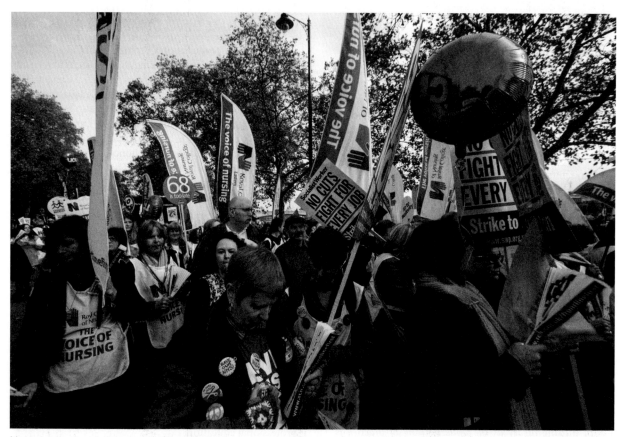

Nurses speak up. (istock.com/DavidCallan)

rather, nursing has an ethical responsibility to unearth and draw attention to the structural causes of health inequity. McGibbon, Mulaudzi, Didham et al. (2014) argue that **decolonization**, viewed as a discrete and peripheral concern in mainstream nursing, actually needs to be seen as a central path to urgently needed growth and transformation for the entire profession (p. 188).

In the context of **neoliberalism**, an increasingly corporate health care system, new public management and technologies, regulatory processes aligned with government legislation, and the context of building nation-to-nation relationships and reconciliation, we have before us very real challenges in nursing and health care in Canada. It is another historical juncture *and* a time of great opportunities. We have an opportunity to draw on the strength of our history and what we have learned from the pioneering work of early nursing scholars to address serious health inequities and other challenges. We need to have the courage to engage with theory and theorizing, research, and ongoing dialogue to produce counternarratives such as those put forward by so many of our nursing scholars in their current everyday theorizing work. These nursing scholars challenge us, for example, to think through the complexities associated with engaging relationally (e.g., Doane & Varcoe, 2005, 2010; Doane & Brown, 2011), addressing poverty, homelessness, and health inequity (e.g., Forchuk, Csiernik, & Jensen, 2011; Browne, Varcoe, Ford-Gilboe et al., 2018; Ford-Gilboe, Wathen, Varcoe et al., 2018), and responding to the burgeoning areas of growth such as digital health and technologies (e.g., Founds, 2018; Linnen, 2016; Sensmeier, 2016).

SUMMARY OF LEARNING OBJECTIVES

- Nursing's social mandate for the twenty-first century is health equity. Given its social mandate, nursing needs to be adaptive and flexible, stay attuned to the shifting health and social landscape, and remain relevant. As Duncan, Rodney, and Thorne (2014) have noted, we also need "full expression of the voice of the profession, both for the advancement of nursing practice and to unleash the profession's capacity to lead public policy and systems transformation" (p. 27). Foundational to this work is nursing theory and theorizing.
- Nursing theory describes what is most fundamental to nursing practice. Nursing is a professional practice discipline that involves the complex interplay of skills and abilities, critical thinking, and evidence-informed practice—nursing theory and theorizing are essential to maintaining this dynamism.
- Early theorists and scholars provided the foundation upon which we build nursing theory today. The early scholars and their debates set us on a path to inquiry as academics and professional practice, a professional orientation that would lead to and ensure transformative clinical practice, education, research, and policy and systems change.
- The metaparadigm acts as the scaffolding for the central concepts from which to build our theory and nursing knowledge: nursing, persons, environment, and health.
- Given that nursing is ever shifting, the metaparadigm may also need to shift. For example, nursing scholars have recommended more critical reflection on concepts such as time and the metaparadigm concept of "environment."
- Nursing's epistemology is the study of knowledge shared among the members of the profession, our pattern of knowing, and the criteria we set for accepting this as nursing knowledge. Knowing is a process, knowledge is a product, and knowing in nursing is about working on solutions that are important to the well-being of clients (client as individuals, families, communities, and populations) (Schultz & Meleis, 1988, p. 217).
- There are multiple ways of knowing and being: empirical, ethical, aesthetic, personal, sociopolitical, and emancipatory (Carper, 1978). There also are many other ways of knowing, including Indigenous ways of knowing; this understanding needs to inform nursing's everyday practice, theorizing, and knowledge development. For example, in this context, nursing needs to grapple with concepts such as decolonization and indigenization to meet its moral obligations and associated social mandate.
- The ontology of nursing is what is most characteristic of and fundamental to nursing. It is our embodied knowledge, our way of being.
- Everyday theorizing embedded in practice is essential to the work of nursing. Living a pragmatic process of theory development involves being grounded in the moment of the experience (i.e., practice) rather than coming to the experience from a unified, fixed perspective. For example, differences between people come to be seen as opportunities for learning—for deepening our relational engagement and understanding and the essential work of nursing.
- Practice, research, and theory are the cornerstones of the nursing profession: "Theory guided practice, in the form of practice theory, is the future of nursing" (Saleh, 2018, p. 18). As we progress into the twenty-first century, nurse scholars, scientists, researchers, and practitioners must place theory-guided practice at the core of nursing.

CRITICAL THINKING QUESTIONS

1. Why is it important to define nursing and engage with nursing theory?
2. What purpose do the four metaparadigm concepts play in shaping our understanding of nursing? How do you see their relevance for nursing today? What concept(s) might we consider adding to the metaparadigm given some of the challenges nursing is facing today?
3. How might nursing theory and theorizing inform how we manage big data, new technologies, regulation, managerialism, and some of the other key issues shaping nursing practice and education today?
4. How might nursing theorizing shape the next generation of nurses?

REFERENCES

Aboriginal Nurses Association of Canada. (2009). *Cultural competence and cultural safety in nursing education: A framework for First Nations, Inuit and Métis nursing.* Ottawa, ON: Author. Retrieved from https://www.cna-aiic.ca/~/media/cna/page-content/pdf-en/first_nations_framework_e.pdf.

Adib-Hajbaghery, M., & Tahmouresi, M. (2018). Nurse–patient relationship based on the Imogene king's theory of goal attainment. *Nurse Midwifery Studies, 7,* 141–144. https://doi.org/10.4103/2322-1488.235636.

Anderson, J. M., Rodney, P., Reimer-Kirkham, S., et al. (2009). Inequities in health and healthcare viewed through the ethical lens of critical social justice: Contextual knowledge for the global priorities ahead. *Advances in Nursing Science, 32,* 282–294. https://doi.org/10.4103/2322-1488.235636.

Austin, W. J. (2011). The incommensurability of nursing as a practice and the customer service model: An evolutionary threat to the discipline. *Nursing Philosophy, 12,* 158–166. https://doi.org/10.1111/j.1466-769X.2011.00492.x.

Beardwood, B., Walters, V., Eyles, J., & Franch, S. (1999). Complaints against nurses: a reflection of 'the new managerialism' and consumerism in health care? *Social Science and Medicine, 48,* 363–374. https://doi.org/10.1016/s0277-9536(98)00340-2.

Beckstrand, J. (1978). The notion of a practice theory and the relationship of scientific and ethical knowledge to practice. *Research in Nursing & Health, 1,* 131–136. https://doi.org/10.1002/nur.4770010306.

Booth, R. G. (2016). Informatics and nursing in a post-nursing informatics world: Future directions for nurses in an automated, artificially-intelligent, social-networked healthcare environment. *Canadian Journal of Nursing Leadership, 28*(4), 61–69. https://doi.org/10.12927/cjnl.2016.24563.

Brennan, P. F., & Bakken, S. (2015). Nursing needs big data and big data needs nursing. *Journal of Nursing Scholarship, 47*(5), 477–484. https://doi.org/10.1111/jnu.12159.

Browne, A. J. (2001). The influence of liberal political ideology on nursing science. *Nursing Inquiry, 8,* 118–129. https://doi.org/10.1046/j.1440-1800.2001.00095.x.

Browne, A. J., & Varcoe, C. (2006). Critical cultural perspectives and health care involving Aboriginal people. *Contemporary Nurse, 22,* 155–167. https://doi.org/10.5172/conu.2006.22.2.155.

Browne, A., Varcoe, C., Ford-Gilboe, M., et al. (2018). Disruption as opportunity: Impacts of an organizational-level health equity intervention in primary care clinics. *International Journal for Equity in Health, 17,* 154. https://doi.org/10.1186/s12939-018-0820-2.

Browne, A. J., Varcoe, C., Smye, V., et al. (2009). Cultural safety and the challenges of translating critically-oriented knowledge in practice. *Nursing Philosophy: An International Journal for Health Care Professionals, 10,* 167–179. https://doi.org/10.1111/j.1466-769X.2009.00406.x.

Canadian Nurses Association. (2017). *Code of ethics for registered nurses.* Ottawa, ON: Author. Retrieved from https://www.cna-aiic.ca/-/media/cna/page-content/pdf-en/code-of-ethics-2017-edition-secure-interactive.pdf?.

Carabez, R., Pelligrini, M., Mankovitz, A., et al. (2015). Never in all my years...": Nurses' education about LGBT health. *Journal of Professional Health, 31*(4), 323–329. https://doi.org/10.1016/j.profnurs.2015.01.003.

Carper, B. A. (1978). Fundamental patterns of knowing in nursing. *Advances in Nursing Science, 1*(1), 13–23. https://doi.org/10.1097/00012272-197810000-00004.

Casteldine, G. (2007). Florence Nightingale, a force to be reckoned with: The BJN over 100 years ago. *British Journal of Nursing, 16*(9), 525. https://doi.org/10.12968/bjon.2007.16.9.27242.

Chinn, P. L., & Kramer, M. K. (2011). *Integrated theory and knowledge development in nursing* (8th ed.). St. Louis, MO: Mosby.

Chinn, P. L., & Kramer, M. K. (2015). *Knowledge development in nursing theory and process* (9th ed.). St. Louis, MO: Elsevier.

Dall'Alba, G., & Barnacle, R. (2007). An ontological turn for higher education. *Studies in Higher Education, 32*(6). https://doi.org/10.1080/03075070701685130 679-669.

de Graaf, K. R., Mossman, C. L., & Slebodnick, M. (1986). Florence Nightingale: Modern nursing. In A. Marriner (Ed.), *Nursing theorists and their work* (pp. 65–79). St. Louis, MO: Mosby.

Dickoff, J., James, P. J., & Weidenbach, E. (1968). Theory in a practice discipline. *Nursing Research, 17,* 415–435. https://doi.org/10.1097/00006199-196811000-00014.

Dickoff, J., & James, P. J. (1968/1986). A theory of theories: a position paper. In L. H. Nicholl (Ed.), *Perspectives on nursing theory* (pp. 99–111). Glenview, IL: Scott, Foresman & Co.

Dickoff, J., & James, P. J. (1968). A theory of theories: a position paper. *Nursing Research, 17*(3), 197–203.

Donaldson, S. K. & Crowley, D. M. (1978). The discipline of nursing. *Nursing Outlook, 26*, 113–120.

Doane, G. H. & Varcoe, C. (2015). *How to nurse: Relational inquiry with individuals and families in change health care contexts.* Philadelphia, PA: Wolters Kluwer.

Doane, G. H., & Brown, H. (2011). Recontextualizing learning in nursing: Taking an ontological turn. *Journal of Nursing Education, 50*(1), 21–26. https://doi.org/10.3928/01484834-20101130-01.

Doane, G. H., & Varcoe, C. (2005). Towards compassionate action: Pragmatism and the inseparability of theory/practice. *Advances in Nursing Science, 28*(1), 81–90. https://doi.org/10.1097/00012272-200501000-00009.

Doane, G. H., & Varcoe, C. (2010). Boundaries and the culture of theorizing in nursing. *Nursing Science Quarterly, 32*(2), 130–137. https://doi.org/10.1177/0894318410362544.

Doane, G. H., Browne, A. J., Reimer, J., et al. (2009). Enacting nursing's obligations: Public health nurses' theorizing in practice. *Research for Theory and Practice: An International Journal, 23*(2), 88–106. https://doi.org/10.1891/1541-6577.23.2.88.

Drevdahl, D. J. (2018). Culture shifts: From cultural to structural theorizing in nursing. *Nursing Research, 67*(2), 146–160. https://doi.org/10.1097/NNR.0000000000000262.

Duncan, S., Thorne, S., & Rodney, P. (2015). Evolving trends in nurse regulation: What are the policy impacts for nursing's social mandate? *Nursing Inquiry, 22*(1), 27–38. https://doi.org/10.1111/nin.12087.

Duncan, S., Rodney, P., & Thorne, S. (2014). Forging a strong nursing future: Insights from the Canadian context. *Journal of Research in Nursing, 19*(7–8), 621–633. https://doi.org/10.1177/1744987114559063.

Edwards, D., & Liaschenko, J. (2003). On the quest for a theory of nursing. *Nursing Philosophy, 4*(1), 1–3. https://doi.org/10.1046/j.1466-769x.2003.00138.x.

Fawcett, J. (1984). The metaparadigm of nursing: Present status and future refinements. *Image, 16*(3), 84–87. https://doi.org/10.1111/j.1547-5069.1984.tb01393.x.

First Nations Health Authority. (2018). *It starts with me: FNHA's commitments to cultural safety and cultural humility.* Retrieved from http://www.fnha.ca/documents/fnha-policy-statement-cultural-safety-and-humility.pdf.

Flaming, D. (2004). Nursing theories as nursing ontologies. *Nursing Philosophy, 5*, 224–229. https://doi.org/10.1111/j.1466-769X.2004.00191.x.

Ford-Gilboe, M., Wathen, N., Varcoe, C., et al. (2018). How equity-oriented health care impacts health: Key mechanisms and implications for primary health care practice and policy. *Millbank Quarterly, 96*(4), 635–671. https://doi.org/10.1111/1468-0009.12349.

Forchuk, C., Csiernik, R., & Jensen, E. (2011). *Homelessness, housing, mental health, finding truths—Creating change.* Toronto, ON: Canadian Scholars Press.

Forchuk, C., Martin, M. L., Chan, L., & Jensen, E. (2005). Therapeutic relationships: From hospital to community. *Journal of Psychiatric and Mental Health Nursing, 12*, 556–564. https://doi.org/10.1111/j.1365-2850.2005.00873.x.

Foth, T., & Holmes, D. (2017). Neoliberalism and the government of nursing through competency-based education. *Nursing Inquiry, 24*. https://doi.org/10.1111/nin.12154.

Founds, S. (2018). Systems biology for nursing in the era of big data and precision health. *Nursing Outlook, 66*, 283–292. https://doi.org/10.1016/j.outlook.2017.11.006.

Galli, S. J. (2016). Toward precision medicine and health: Opportunities and challenges in allergic diseases. *The Journal of Allergy and Clinical Immunology, 137*(5), 1289–1300. https://doi.org/10.1016/j.jaci.2016.03.006.

Grace, P. J. (2014). Philosophies, models, and theories: Moral obligations. In M. R. Alligood (Ed.), *Nursing theory: Utilization & application* (5th ed., pp. 63–82). St. Louis, MO: Elsevier/Mosby.

Grace, P. J., Willis, D. G., Roy, S. C., & Jones, D. A. (2016). Profession at the crossroads: A dialog concerning the preparation of nursing scholars and leaders. *Nursing Outlook, 64*(1), 61–70. https://doi.org/10.1016/j.outlook.2015.10.002.

Greenwood, M., deLeeuw, S., & Lindsay, N. M. (2018). *Determinants of Indigenous peoples' health: Beyond the social* (2nd ed). Toronto, ON: Canadian Scholars Press.

Giuliano, K. (2003). Expanding the use of empiricism in nursing: can we bridge the gap between knowledge and clinical practice? *Nursing Philosophy, 4*, 44–52. https://doi.org/10.1046/j.1466-769x.2003.00111.x.

Harrison, H., Kinsella, A., & DeLuca, S. (2019). Locating the lived body in client-nurse interactions: Embodiment, intersubjectivity and intercorporeality. *Nursing Philosophy, 20*(2), e12241. https://doi.org/10.1111/nup.12241.

Hill, G., & Wilkinson, A. (2014). Indigegogy: A transformative Indigenous educational process. *Canadian Social Work Review, 31*(2), 175–193.

Hoeck, B., & Delmar, C. (2018). Theoretical development in the context of nursing—The hidden epistemology in nursing theory. *Nursing Philosophy, 19*. https://doi.org/10.1111/nup.12196.

Ibrahim, S., Donelle, L., Sidani, S., & Regan, S. (2019). Factors influencing Registered Nurses' intention to use health information technology in clinical practice: An integrative literature review. *Canadian Journal of Nursing Informatics, 1*(1). Retrieved from http://cjni.net/journal/?p=5981.

Jairath, N. N., Peden-McAlpine, C. J., Sullivan, M. C., et al. (2018). Theory and theorizing in nursing science: Commentary from the nursing research special issue editorial team. *Nursing Research, 67*(2), 188–193. https://doi.org/10.1097/NNR.0000000000000273.

Karnick, P. M. (2014). A case for nursing theory in practice. *Nursing Science Quarterly, 27*, 117. https://doi.org/10.1177/0894318414522711.

Kikuchi, J. (2004). Towards a philosophic theory of nursing. *Nursing Philosophy, 5*, 79–83. https://doi.org/10.1111/j.1466-769X.2004.00150.x.

Klotzbaugh, R., & Spencer, G. (2015). Cues-to-action in initiating lesbian, gay, bisexual, and transgender-related policies among magnet hospital chief nursing officers: A demographic assessment. *Advances in Nursing Science, 38*(2), 110–120. https://doi.org/10.1097/ANS.0000000000000069.

Kumagai, A. K. (2014). From competencies to human interests: Ways of knowing and understanding in medical education. *Academic Medicine, 89*(7), 978–983. https://doi.org/10.1097/ACM.0000000000000234.

Leininger, M. (1978). *Transcultural nursing concepts, theories and practices.* New York, NY: Wiley.

Leininger, M. (1979). *Transcultural nursing.* New York, NY: Mason.

Leininger, M. (1984). Transcultural nursing: An essential knowledge and practice field for today. *The Canadian Nurse, 80*(11), 41–45.

Leininger, M. (1985). Transcultural care diversity and universality: A theory of nursing. *Nursing and Health Care, 6*(4), 209–212.

Leininger, M. (1988). Leininger's theory of nursing: Cultural care diversity and universality. *Nursing Science Quarterly, 1*(4), 152–160.

Liaschenko, J., & Fisher, A. (1999). Theorizing the knowledge that nurses use in the conduct of their work. *Scholarly Inquiry for Nursing Practice, 13*(1), 29–41.

Libster, M. M. (2008). Elements of care: Nursing environmental theory in historical context. *Holistic Nursing Practice, 22*(3), 160–170. https://doi.org/10.1097/01.HNP.0000318025.37904.6c.

Linnen, D. (2016). The promise of big data: Improving patient safety and nursing practice. *Nursing, 46*(5), 28–34. https://doi.org/10.1097/01.NURSE.0000482860.31028.8f.

Marmot, M., & Allen, J. J. (2014). Social determinants of health equity. *American Journal of Public Health, 104*(SUPPL4), S517–S519. https://doi.org/10.2105/AJPH.2014.302200.

Marmot, M., & Bell, R. (2016). Social inequalities in health: a proper concern of epidemiology. *Annals of Epidemiology, 26*(4), 238–240. https://doi.org/10.1016/annepidem.2016.02.003.

Matney, S., Brewster, P. J., Sward, K. A., et al. (2011). Philosophical approaches to the nursing informatics data–information–knowledge–wisdom framework. *Advances in Nursing Science, 34*, 6–18. https://doi.org/10.1097/ANS.0b013e3182071813.

McGibbon, E., Mulaudzi, F. M., Didham, P., et al. (2014). Toward decolonizing nursing: the colonization of nursing and strategies for increasing the counter-narrative. *Nursing Inquiry, 21*(3), 179–191. https://doi.org/10.1111/nin.12042.

McGibbon, E., & Etowa, J. (2009). *Anti-racist health care practice.* Toronto, ON: Canadian Scholars Press.

Meleis, A. (2012). *Theoretical Nursing Development and Progress* (5th ed). Philadelphia, PA: Lippincott William & Wilkins, Wolters Kluwer.

Mikkonen, J., & Raphael, D. (2010). *Social Determinants of Health: The Canadian Facts.* Toronto, ON: York University School of Health Policy and Management.

Monsen, K. A., Kelechi, T. J., McRae, M. E., et al. (2018). Nursing theory, terminology, and big data: Data-driven discovery of novel patterns in archival randomized clinical trial data.

Nursing Research, 67(2), 122–132. https://doi.org/10.1097/NNR.0000000000000269.

Nightingale, F. (1946/1859). *Notes on nursing: What it is and what it is not.* Philadelphia, PA: Lippincott.

Orlando, I. J. (1961). *The dynamic nurse–patient relationship: Function, process, and principles.* New York, NY: G. P. Putnam's Sons.

Parse, R. (1992). Human becoming: Parse's theory of nursing. *Nursing Science Quarterly, 5*(1), 35–42. https://doi.org/10.1177/089431849200500109.

Peplau, H. E. (1952). *Interpersonal relations in nursing.* New York, NY: G. P. Putnam's Sons.

Pierce, J. D., & Henley, S. J. (2017). Omics in nursing science. *Nursing Research, 66*(20), 61–62. https://doi.org/10.1097/NNR.0000000000000205.

Ramsden, I. (1993). Kawa whakaruruhau: Cultural safety in nursing education in Aotearoa, New Zealand. *Nursing Praxis in New Zealand, 8*(3), 4–10.

Ramsden, I. (2000). Cultural safety/Kawa whakaruruhau ten years on: A personal overview. *Nursing Praxis in New Zealand, 15*(1), 4–12.

Reed, P. (1989). Nursing theorizing as an ethical endeavor. *Advances in Nursing Science, 11*(3), 1–9. https://doi.org/10.1097/00012272-198904000-00005.

Reed, P. (1997). Nursing: the ontology of the discipline. *Nursing Science Quarterly, 10*(2), 76–79. https://doi.org/10.1177/089431849701000207.

Reimer-Kirkham, S., Smye, V., Tang, S., et al. (2002). Waiting for the field: Rethinking cultural safety. *Research in Nursing and Health, 25*, 222–232. https://doi.org/10.1002/nur.10033.

Roy, C. (1970). Adaptation: a conceptual framework for nursing. *Nursing Outlook, 18*(3), 42–5.

Roy, C. (1975). A diagnostic classification system for nursing. *Nursing Outlook, 23*, 90–94.

Roy, C. (2018). Key issues in nursing theory: Developments, challenges and future directions. *Nursing Research, 67*(2), 81–92. https://doi.org/10.1097/NNR.0000000000000266.

Rudge, T. (2013). Desiring productivity: Nary a wasted moment, never a missed step! *Nursing Philosophy, 14*, 201–211. https://doi.org/10.1111/nup.12019.

Rudge, T., & Thorne, S. (2013). Editorial: Tightening the reins on nursing practice. *Nursing Inquiry, 20*(3), 187. https://doi.org/10.1111/nin.12047.

Saleh, U. S. (2018). Theory guided practice in nursing: An editorial. *Journal of Nursing Research Practice, 2*(1), 18.

Schultz, P. R., & Meleis, A. I. (1988). Nursing epistemology: Traditions, insights, questions. *Journal of Nursing Scholarship, 20*(4), 217–221. https://doi.org/10.1111/j.1547-5069.1988.tb00080.x.

Sensmeier, J. (2016). Understanding the impact of big data on nursing knowledge. *Nursing Critical Care, 11*(2), 11–13. https://doi.org/10.1097/01.CCN.0000480755.60698.ff.

Smye, V., & Browne, A. J. (2002). 'Cultural safety' and the analysis of health policy affecting Aboriginal people. *Nurse Researcher: The International Journal of Research Methodology in Nursing and Health Care, 9*(3), 42–56. https://doi.org/10.7748/nr2002.04.9.3.42.c6188.

Thorne, S. (2014). What constitutes core disciplinary knowledge? *Nursing Inquiry, 21*(1), 1e2. https://doi.org/10.1111/nin.12062.

Thorne, S., & Sawatzky, R. (2014). Particularizing the general: Sustaining theoretical integrity in the context of an evidence-based practice agenda. *Advances in Nursing Science, 37*(1), 5–18. https://doi.org/10.1097/ANS.0000000000000011.

Thorne, S., Canam, C., Dahinten, S., et al. (1998). Nursing's metaparadigm concepts: disimpacting the debates. *Journal of Advanced Nursing, 27*, 1257–1268. https://doi.org/10.1046/j.1365-2648.1998.00623.x.

Thorne, S., Reimer-Kirkham, S., & Henderson, A. (1999). Ideological implications of paradigm discourse in nursing research, education and practice theory. *Nursing Inquiry, 6*(2), 123–131. https://doi.org/10.1046/j.1440-1800.1999.00016.x.

Tobbell, D. (2018). Nursing's boundary work: Theory development and the making of nursing science, ca. *1950-1980. Nursing Research, 67*(2), 63–73. https://doi.org/10.1097/NNR.0000000000000251.

Truth and Reconciliation Commission of Canada. (2015). *Honouring the truth, reconciling for the future: Summary of the final report of the Truth and Reconciliation Commission of Canada.* Winnipeg, MB: Author.

Walker, L., & Avant, K. (2011). *Strategies for theory construction in nursing* (5th ed.). New York, NY: Prentice Hall.

Watson, J. (1979). *Nursing: The philosophy and science of caring.* Boston, MA: Little, Brown.

Watson, J. (1990). Caring knowledge and informed moral passion. *Advances in Nursing Science, 13*(1), 15–24. https://doi.org/10.1097/00012272-199009000-00003.

White, J. (1995). Patterns of knowing: Review, critique and update. *Advances in Nursing Science, 17*(4), 73–86. https://doi.org/10.1097/00012272-199506000-00007.

Yeager, K. A., & Bauer-Wu, S. (2013). Cultural humility: Essential foundation for clinical researchers. *Applied Nursing Research, 26*(4), 251–256. https://doi.org/10.1016/j.apnr.2013.06.008.

Zhu, R., Han, R., Su, Y., et al. (2019). The application of big data and the development of nursing science: A discussion paper. *The International Journal of Nursing Sciences, 6*, 229–234. https://doi.org/10.1016/j.ijnss.2019.03.001.

Thinking Philosophically in Nursing

Tammie R. McParland

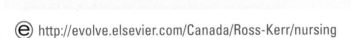

http://evolve.elsevier.com/Canada/Ross-Kerr/nursing

LEARNING OBJECTIVES

After reading this chapter, you will be able to:
- Understand, from a historical perspective, the development of how nursing has been conceptualized.
- Distinguish between scientific and philosophical conceptions of nursing.
- Identify the philosophical basis and implications for nursing's ways of thinking on creating a sound conception of nursing and increasing nursing knowledge.
- Articulate what philosophical thinking in nursing demands of the inquirer.
- Identify pivotal assumptions and values that promote or impede philosophical thinking in nursing.
- Identify creative ways to advance philosophical thinking in nursing and one's own responsibility in this activity.

OUTLINE

KEY TERMS

borrowed theories
conceptions of (the nature of) nursing
epistemological
nursing body of knowledge

nursing theories
philosophical thinking
scientific theories
translational gap or relevance gap

PERSONAL PERSPECTIVES

Laurie is a registered nurse who is pursuing a master's in nursing. In her class on the development of nursing knowledge and the identity of nursing, she has an assignment to ask her peers what philosophical framework guides their nursing actions. Laurie is surprised and somewhat flustered when most of her peers indicate that they do not think or feel that a philosophy for nursing makes any difference in their day-to-day work with their patients. One peer tells her that "philosophy belongs in the ivory tower, not the weeds." Laurie wants to bring this perspective up in class for discussion, but first she wants to understand where this conception of nursing might have come from and how she can articulate to her peers why a sound philosophical basis should underlie nursing.

INTRODUCTION

During the last 40 years of the twentieth century, many in the nursing profession were involved in an ambitious enterprise: to base the development of a body of nursing knowledge on **conceptions of the nature of nursing**. The result of this enterprise was presented in the form of **nursing theories**, conceptual models, and frameworks that were intended to help nurses explain the uniqueness of their work. Today, in the first two decades of the twenty-first century, buzzwords that reflected that endeavour, such as "conceptual models of nursing" or "grand nursing theories," are not heard as often in undergraduate studies. These terms have been replaced by new buzzwords such as evidence-based practice and knowledge transfer. This is reflective of a new enterprise: to base nursing practice on predominantly scientific evidence. As this new "scientific-focused" enterprise has come to the foreground, the earlier "conceptually based" one has receded into the background. Concomitantly, nurses have become less concerned about specifying the nature of nursing and of nursing knowledge and developing a body of nursing knowledge. Risjord (2010, as cited in Theodoridis, 2017) argues that either a **translational gap** or a **relevance gap** exists which causes nurses to focus more on generic science-knowledge rather than nursing-knowledge in their professional practice. A translation gap pertains to the understanding and use of theories in the practice of nursing, while a relevance gap is more concerned with the importance (relevance) of nursing knowledge and theory to the practice of nursing.

If nurses continue to feel a lack of concern for a conception of the nature of nursing knowledge and its use in practice, will the nursing profession lose itself before it finds itself? Does a lack of concern for the relevance of conceptions of nursing mean that the profession should revive its earlier enterprise? The purpose of this chapter is to suggest another option: by engaging in philosophical thinking, nurses can develop a clear, coherent, and comprehensive philosophical conception of the nature of nursing on which to base their nursing knowledge.

BASING NURSING KNOWLEDGE ON CONCEPTIONS OF NURSING

The work to base the development of a body of nursing knowledge on conceptions of the nature of nursing began in the late 1960s in response to a problem identified by nurse educators (Smith & Parker, 2015). In the absence of knowledge about the nature of nursing, nurse educators were unable to determine what to include in a nursing curriculum as the **nursing body of knowledge**. Thinking that the problem could be solved by developing conceptions of the nature of nursing, nurse scholars set about developing them (Kikuchi, 1997).

When the enterprise to create a nursing body of knowledge was initiated during the 1950s, 1960s, and 1970s, science and "logical thought" reigned supreme, and nurses' preparation to do research was primarily scientific in nature. This was due to the societal value of scientific knowledge; consequently, the scientific method was the educational focus of many of the nurse educators who were teaching nursing at the time (Smith & Parker, 2015). As a result, conceptions of the nature of nursing were erroneously assumed to be scientific rather than philosophical in nature, and there was a tendency to derive or borrow them from one or another scientific theory from disciplines such as psychology, physiology, and sociology; to characterize them by the levels and ranges attributed to sociological theories (such as grand, middle, and micro); and to assign purposes to them as per basic **scientific theories** (i.e., to describe, explain, and predict).

Initially, the enterprise went well. For the most part, nurses eagerly adopted the various conceptions that were put forward. Soon, however, as the conceptions began to be labelled variously as conceptual models of nursing, conceptual nursing frameworks, and nursing theories, confusion set in about the nature of the conceptions. Were they models, frameworks, or theories (Kikuchi, 1997)? Did they really explain what nurses do and what nursing is?

The nursing conceptions that began being developed (including identifying the nursing knowledge being used) were based on **borrowed theories** (i.e., scientific theories) or philosophical theories. These were considered to be nursing science and thus were increasing the confusion nurses felt about what made up nursing conceptions. It did not help that the methods used to develop the conceptions were not always explicitly stated, and validation to help explain the theories was difficult to carry out. Skepticism about the worth of these nursing conceptions grew, fueled by nurses' complaints that they were difficult to understand, too abstract, and far removed from the particulars of everyday practice. By the 1990s, the conceptions were being characterized as useless, impractical, and unnecessary (Thorne, 2003). This perception remains in practice today in some educational sectors that focus primarily on the practical aspects of nurse education. Part of the desire to have a baccalaureate degree was because of the breadth and depth requirement to foster critical thinking and analysis. To accomplish this requirement, most nursing baccalaureate degrees include courses on nursing theories or thinking philosophically in their curriculum.

👤 APPLYING CONTENT KNOWLEDGE

Why do you think that nurses continue to be willing to do their activities of "nursing" without being guided by a clear, coherent, and comprehensive conception of what nursing might be?

THE DOWNFALL OF CONCEPTIONS OF NURSING: ITS AFTERMATH AND IMPLICATIONS

In their heyday, the existing conceptions of nursing were used as a basis for courses taught in nearly every undergraduate and graduate nursing program in Canada and the United States. That is no longer the case: many schools of nursing have dropped these conceptions of nursing from their curricula. Yet, Chinn (2001) has called for their reinstatement, warning that if nurses do not learn to apply these conceptions of nursing and continue to take on "doctoring" activities (such as task-focused activities that are biomedical in nature, and actions such as treatments and medicine delivery), nursing will find itself once again serving as a handmaiden to doctoring, as the call of nursing has yet to be responded to in a serious manner. Further, as nurses' confidence in the power and necessity of conceptions of nursing has decreased, so too has their concern about specifying the nature of nursing and of nursing knowledge and developing a body of nursing knowledge.

For example, nurses tend not to base their research on any conception of nursing (Kikuchi, 2003a; Spear, 2007). In the nursing theoretical literature on evidence-informed practice development, little or no mention is made of basing nursing practice on a conception of nursing or of developing a specific body of nursing knowledge. The literature used is usually a compilation of the most relevant and validated research—of which nursing, by virtue of its focus on both science and art, may have less evidence. This leaves a space for non-nursing evidence to become a part of the practice while discouraging nursing-based and conceptualized information.

In the document *Toward 2020: Visions for Nursing*, prepared for the Canadian Nurses Association, Villeneuve and MacDonald (2006) have said that by the year 2020, registered nurses should be doing much of what general practitioners currently do (pp. 4–5). Further, registered nurses should be acting as coordinators, educators, consultants, and advocates in the health care system, leaving the provision of direct nursing care mainly to others. Also, they asserted the necessity of fluid professional boundaries and of not focusing on profession-specific activities such as the development of nursing research. Villeneuve and MacDonald also forecasted that by 2020, generic terms will have replaced profession-specific terms such as "nursing diagnosis" and "nursing care plans." It is interesting that conceptions of nursing and of nursing knowledge are not mentioned in the document and none are identified as underpinning their work. Rather, the efficient use of human health care resources drives the forecasted scenarios, and the care part of nursing is left to others. A compelling argument can be made for the impact of the removal of caring activities from the nursing profession. Nursing's connection with care and caring is both a noun and an adjective (Adams, 2016).

Today, as 2020 has arrived, the roles that nurses could occupy—as identified by the authors of the "Toward 2020" document—are in place in the health care system. But these roles are not as plentiful as hoped and are often occupied by non-nursing staff. For the most part, nurses still work within a biomedical model in acute care settings (Canadian Institute for Health Information [CIHI], 2019), and the nursing profession remains in a position that is still subservient to medicine. Although nursing has made strides, the recent increased use of physician assistants rather than uptake of nurse practitioners (despite their expanded role) is an example of the fallout that can occur when a profession does not engage in purposeful exploration of that profession's raison d'être. By not articulating a strong and clear conception of nursing in their document, Villeneuve and MacDonald have suggested a good health human resource strategy but not necessarily a good nursing one.

Today, in line with the call by Villeneuve and MacDonald for registered nurses to be more fluid and less focused on profession-specific activities, fewer registered nurses work in community or long-term care or other nontraditional areas even though the number of professional nurses working in Canada has increased. The higher number of nurses belongs proportionally to the category of licensed or practical registered nurses. Two levels of nursing professionals are still a reality in Canada. Chapter 17 discusses where nurses work and with what type and percentage of the population.

If nurses remain unconcerned about specifying the nature of nursing and of nursing knowledge and developing a body of nursing knowledge, then nursing stands in great danger of losing itself and not meeting its potential as a profession but rather the needs and requirements of other professions, particularly those of physicians and "doctoring." As Gottlieb and Gottlieb (2007) have reiterated, if nursing is to become a profession in its own right and to provide the kind of care that the public deserves, it must differentiate itself and develop its own body of knowledge. Further, it must differentiate itself as a profession that complements rather than competes with other professions. Chinn and Kramer (2015) have identified that knowledge creation specific to nursing must be viewed through the contexts of values and resources. Values include individual (self), professional (discipline), and societal. Resources can also be viewed from the contexts of individual (such as education, cognitive style, and innate talents of individual members of the profession), professional (the practice traditions, experiences, language, and methodologies used to create knowledge), and societal (that which is available to support knowledge creation and provided by the broader community, such as funding to create knowledge through research).

The need for the nursing profession to attend to these matters is brought home by White, Oelke, Besner et al.'s (2008) study of how Western Canadian nurses perceived their scopes of practice. In their study, the authors found that the practice and morale of all groups of nurses (registered nurses, licensed practical nurses, and registered psychiatric nurses) were being negatively affected by unclear intraprofessional and interprofessional scopes of practice. Based on their findings, White, Oelke, Besner et al. (2008) stated that

> clearly defining and articulating the role of nurses, and clarifying what is unique to nursing practice and what is shared with other healthcare professionals, pose ignificant challenges to the profession at this time. We must be able to describe nursing practice in terms of the knowledge and principles that underpin nurses' roles. If nurses are unable to explain the theoretical basis for their practice, they may find themselves unable to articulate what motivates their actions. It is difficult indeed to document accountability for one's practice

> without an explanatory framework within which to evaluate practice. (p. 54)

So, then, ought the profession begin to revive the enterprise of developing a body of nursing knowledge using extant conceptions of nursing?

ANOTHER WAY FORWARD

Aside from the problems mentioned earlier, the aforementioned enterprise—to base the development of a body of nursing knowledge on conceptions of the nature of nursing—has serious foundational problems of an **epistemological** nature that make it an untenable option. One such problem is the assumption that conceptions of the nature of nursing should be developed using scientific means. Another problem is the adherence to the idealist thought that reality conforms to the mind—that the world and all that exists in it are a reflection of the mind. Consequently, conceptions of the world and all that exists in it are characterized as ideologies; as such, they lie in the realm of taste and are beyond the realm of reason, argumentation, and questioning. The conceptions of the world are chosen on the basis of preference and become dominant by might rather than by reason (Adler, 1990; Kikuchi, 2003b).

If one cannot revive this enterprise nor avoid specifying the nature of nursing and of nursing knowledge, what options remain? A sound option would be for the nursing profession to get its bearings by reaffirming the truth of the following philosophical proposition, upon which the enterprise of the 1960s was based: developing a conception of the nature of nursing is necessary to define a body of knowledge as a body of nursing knowledge. However, to avoid the previously discussed foundational problems of that enterprise, it must proceed on a different footing: it must be based on the moderate realist tenets that (1) the mind conforms to reality, (2) philosophical thought focuses on that which is immaterial (i.e., the nonphenomenal, and therefore, nonobservable), and (3) philosophical knowledge is attainable in the form of probable truth, or truth beyond a reasonable doubt (Adler, 1965; Maritain, 1959). On that footing, a conception of nursing would be developed by thinking philosophically about aspects of nursing that are nonphenomenal or nonobservable (e.g., toward the end goal of nursing practice). In contrast, a conception of nursing developed using scientific means is a conception of the phenomenal or observable aspects of nursing as they existed at the time of observation (Kikuchi, 1997). As Smith and Parker (2015) have maintained, defining nursing only by what can be seen or done is problematic. The functions of our practice as nurses differ depending on where we work and what that context entails.

THINKING PHILOSOPHICALLY IN NURSING

Philosophical thinking, or philosophizing, entails asking questions about the nature of that which exists and happens in the world and about what humans ought to seek and do. In the pursuit of truth, as answers are proposed, ever more penetrating questions are asked and answered in a contingent, logical, and rational manner (Adler, 1965; Phenix, 1964). For example, suppose we were asked, "What is good nursing care?" In attempting to answer it, we would likely soon find ourselves having to answer more basic and penetrating questions such as "What is the nature of that which is good?" As the dialogue proceeds, we will likely find that "good" has been defined in a moral sense (as that which is morally sound) and in an artistic sense (as that which is artistically sound). We will then have to consider whether by "good nursing care" we are referring to nursing care that is good in the moral sense, in the artistic sense, or in both senses. Sooner or later, we are apt to come face to face with such questions as these:

- What is the nature of nursing?
- What is the nature of care or caring?
- What is the nature of the nurse–patient relationship?
- What is the nature of human beings?

These are all philosophical questions. As such, they can be answered only by philosophizing. However, as Pieper (1952) reminds us, philosophizing entails more than just asking and answering philosophical questions. He cautions that if we ask and answer questions in the absence of wonder, we are not genuinely philosophizing. In this case we are operating as technicians, treating philosophizing as a skill that can be acquired in the way that we can acquire any skill. Philosophizing is indeed a matter of skill, but only in a skeletal sense. Principles and rules for asking and answering questions that have the capacity to deepen our understanding of the world (e.g., asking questions that call for other than a "yes" or "no" answer) can be learned or taught, but to think philosophically we must acquire such skills within the context of wonder. It is wonder that will give our question asking and answering its philosophical character of "searching for the truth" (Pieper, 1952, p. 103).

Pieper describes the philosophical act, or philosophizing, as "a full, personal attitude which is by no manner of means at the sole disposal of the ratio" (p. 18). In other words, reason alone cannot dictate the philosophical act because another attitude toward the world is necessary—one of "standing in wonder" before the world as it exists and longing to understand it. This approach to the world is the exact opposite of one more familiar to us: relating to things only from the perspective of our pragmatic interests so that we ask questions only for the purpose of determining

how to use them to our advantage or to solve a problem. According to Pieper (1952):

To philosophize is to act in such a way that one steps out of the workaday world . . . the world of work, the utilitarian world, the world of the useful, subject to ends . . . a world in which there is no room for philosophy or philosophizing. (pp. 70–71)

Pieper (1952) emphasizes that in stepping out of, or transcending the workaday world, we do not leave it behind us nor consider it as nonessential. Rather, the opposite is the case. We back away from the usual way of looking at the things of our everyday lives—of our workaday world—to see them for what they ultimately are. We cannot, however, merely tell ourselves to step out of the workaday world. It is not that simple. Pieper says that a shock, one that stuns and shakes us, is necessary to "pierce the dome that encloses the . . . workaday world" (pp. 72–73). It is comparable to the spiritual awakening that one experiences on coming face to face with something that inspires awe, such as the birth of a baby. It can happen when we encounter questions of the sort that Socrates posed—questions with the capacity "to strip things of their everyday character" (p. 98) so that we realize we do not know of what we speak and are no longer as complacent as we were. Because his questions had this effect, Socrates "compared himself . . . to an electric fish that gives a paralyzing shock to anyone who touches it" (p. 98). In the nursing world, the question mentioned earlier—"What is good nursing care?"—holds the potential to have this kind of effect on nurses who think they know the answer only to find that the opposite is the case.

The shock that stirs us from our complacency is described by Pieper (1952) as wonder, for wonder moves and shakes us to the point where "the ground quakes beneath [our] feet, [our] whole spiritual nature, [our] capacity to know . . . is threatened" (p. 101). He attributes this effect to the fact that "wonder signifies that the world is profounder, more all-embracing and mysterious than the logic of everyday reason had taught us to believe" (p. 102). Although wonder is often said to be the beginning of philosophy, Pieper (1952) asserts:

Wonder is not just the starting point of philosophy . . . [but also its] lasting source . . . The inner form of philosophizing is virtually identical with the inner form of wonder . . . To wonder is not merely not to know; it means to be inwardly aware and sure that one does not know, and that one understands oneself in not knowing. And yet it is not the ignorance of resignation. On the contrary, to wonder is to be on the way, in via; it certainly means to be struck dumb, momentarily, but equally it means that one is searching for the truth. (p. 103)

Given the essential role of wonder in philosophizing, it is clear that if nurses are to philosophize, they must develop their own sense of wonder. But that is easier said than done. Wonder is an innate human capacity that, like any other innate capacities, can be developed to the degree to which we possess it; moreover, wonder should be developed under beneficial circumstances to be expressed holistically (Adler, 1978; Pieper, 1952). However, the circumstances under which nurses are educated and practise are still such that they impede rather than facilitate not only the development of wonder, but also the kind of questioning that wonder engenders.

 APPLYING CONTENT KNOWLEDGE

What do you think it will take for nurses to realize that they need to think philosophically, and not just scientifically, in nursing?

IMPEDIMENTS TO WONDERING AND PHILOSOPHIZING IN NURSING

Most of the impediments to the development of nurses' capacities to wonder and philosophize have been, and continue to be, built into the nursing curricula. Hockey (1990), a British nurse, asserts that basic nursing programs, including the baccalaureate, "are too tightly packed with essential information and the crucially important measures to ensure safe practice, to allow critical enquiry into everyday phenomena, which must be the essence of philosophy" (p. 49). Similarly, Levine (1995), an American nurse, eloquently states:

> Nursing is a humanitarian enterprise. The emphasis placed on scientific and technical knowledge is indispensable to the development of the craft—but it is imperfectly achieved without the intellectual skills that are the special province of the humanities . . . Racing through curricula which seek to be all-inclusive, there is seldom time for courses in philosophy or literature, or history or music . . . [Consequently,] nurses . . . do not have the language and reading and thinking skills that are the basis of a liberal education. This failure . . . ultimately limits the depth and meaning of the profession itself. (p. 19)

Dellasega, Milone-Nuzzo, Curci et al. (2007) agree. Given the unprecedented rate at which scientific and technological knowledge is now becoming available and being included in nursing curricula, they assert that it is more urgent than ever for nursing students to be exposed to the humanities and engage in the liberal thought that is a cornerstone of an academic education. This thought is echoed by Chinn and Kramer (2015), who state that nursing education has moved away from a focus on theory and philosophy and more toward traditional empirics to ensure that focus of the curriculum is the content required to meet regulatory standards. As it stands today, university degrees of nursing are expected to meet approval standards indicating that the curriculum is delivering content that will make for a safe and knowledgeable practitioner for three types of agencies: the national accrediting body for schools of nursing that indicate excellence in nurse education (i.e., the Canadian Association of Schools of Nursing); the provincial and territorial regulatory bodies to which the nurse will be accountable (called entry-to-practice competencies); and university- or ministry-specific requirements, such as individual institutional accountability frameworks that are mandated by either the academic senate or the government ministry responsible for the institution's funding envelope (e.g., the requirement of the Ministry of Training, Colleges, and Universities in Ontario that universities engage in academic quality assurance activities. Failure to do so may result in a fine for the institution or, in the worst-case scenario, impact the funding to the institution from the government).

Stinson (1990), a Canadian nurse, related the near-exclusive emphasis of nursing curricula on scientific knowledge and inquiry to another concern: the lack, in Canada and elsewhere, of nursing faculty who are adequately prepared in philosophy and history. Although the number of faculty with such preparation is increasing, it continues to be insufficient: Stinson has stated that "there is often a lack of due recognition and support given to the few who are adequately prepared in such areas" (p. 3). This remains a problem even into the second decade of the new millennium and is compounded by an impending shortage of nurses. In Canada, 22% of nurses (all levels) are currently over 55 years old, and the growth rate of the profession is the slowest it has been in 5 years (1.0% now versus 2.2% in 2014) (CIHI, 2019). While the age of nurses has declined, the type of nursing education paints a concerning picture from a philosophical perspective. The largest increase in the nursing workforce is among licensed or registered practical nurses; they grew four times the number of registered nurses and twice the number of registered psychiatric nurses (CIHI, 2019). This particular nursing workforce is educated in 1- or 2-year programs in a college or technical school setting, where practical is emphasized over theoretical and content is largely technical and skills-based knowledge.

The Canadian Nurses Association website has indicated that there may be as many as 60, 000 vacancies for nurses by 2022 (Canadian Nurses Association, 2020). The looming impact of retirees and recent health care spending cuts have created a situation where philosophical thinking is not emphasized as extensively as it might be at the baccalaureate level. The reason why is that focusing on philosophical thinking may be too expensive and take too much away from the "required" content that readies the practitioner to "hit the ground running." The lack of health care spending and lack of time to develop philosophical thinking skills have created a reactive situation in the practice setting: nurses must operate with an "every nurse for themselves" mentality to accomplish all that is required in a shift to meet the health care needs of those whose care they are entrusted with. The inability to be intentional in action, as a result of thoughtful and deep thinking about what one is doing and believes to be true, can lead to a decline in satisfaction with one's work and increased moral conflict and distress.

The seriousness of these problems was reflected in Levine's (1995) early description of nursing faculty who had never studied philosophy and thought of it merely "as the preamble to the curriculum required for accreditation by the National League for Nursing" (p. 21) in the United States, or, in Canada, by the Canadian Association of Schools of Nursing. Levine maintains that, in outnumbering faculty schooled in philosophy, those without formal philosophical education are able to perpetuate the notion that philosophy is what they have produced: "a mundane listing of 'We believe . . .'" (p. 21).

Another continuing impediment to the development of nurses' capacities to wonder and philosophize is apparent in Hockey's (1990) declaration that "by and large, philosophy tends to be a fringe subject in nursing courses . . . and so-called philosophical pronouncements are often little more than disguised policy statements, dictated by exigencies and need rather than developmental thought" (p. 49). Here, Hockey is bringing our attention to both the fringe status of philosophy in nursing programs and an ever-increasing problem: the mere pragmatic concerns of special-interest groups, including those of political bodies, dictating what the preparation of nurses, and what adequate nursing care, shall entail. In Canada, this plays out where the increase in the number of nursing education seats is seen in the licensed practical nurse, or practice sector, and not in the university sector.

By responding as they have to the demands of political and economic factions, universities are fast becoming part of the workaday world. Half a century ago, Pieper (1952) expressed concern that the workaday world "is becoming our entire world and threatens to engulf us completely . . . [to the point where] philosophy—inevitably—becomes more and more distant, strange and remote; [and] even assumes the appearance of an intellectual luxury" (p. 71). It would appear that Pieper had every reason to be concerned. Increasingly, university students are choosing their courses and careers almost purely for pragmatic reasons. Wonder and inquisitiveness are taking a back seat to acquiring the content-related knowledge needed to be successful in their health care roles. Similarly, faculty members' choices of research projects and careers are being driven more by what the universities reward (e.g., large grants from prestigious funding sources and publications in renowned journals) than by intellectual matters. Unfortunately, graduate students are being socialized by their faculty mentors to do likewise (Meleis, 2001). Within such a climate, philosophical endeavours that are driven by a sense of wonder, take considerable time to complete, and can be undertaken without large grants are not seen as desirable and thus fare poorly.

As the study by Maben, Latter, and Macleod Clark (2007) revealed, the climate of the practice setting is not any better. Historically, nurses have been taught to follow the directions of "authorities" (e.g., other health care providers, particularly physicians) and not to ask questions. Recognizing the ominous potential consequences of nurses continuing to behave in that manner, the nursing profession is encouraging nurses to become independent thinkers. However, with other professionals still tending to view them mainly as receivers and implementers of their orders and with the current lack of clarity about the nature of nursing practice, nurses find it tough to question the directions of "authorities." They discover that doing so usually results in negative consequences (e.g., they are reprimanded). Consequently, nurses are apt to question authority only if serious harm is likely to follow from their not doing so. Otherwise, nurses tend to be acquiescent and to carry out the orders of other health care providers even if, in so doing, nursing care is compromised.

For example, to get patients to a particular place at a particular time as ordered, nurses still tend to hurry them through their meals or baths, or skip these entirely. The ongoing financial cutbacks to health care and shortage of health care providers are making it harder than ever for nurses to do otherwise or to stand back and reflect on what is happening (Rankin & Campbell, 2006). This situation has not improved in the time since Maben, Latter, and Macleod Clark (2007) published their study. Currently, the crisis in "hallway health care" in acute care settings and the decline of the registered nurse in acute, community, and long-term care facilities have impacted the culture of wondering and philosophizing that is the cornerstone of a self-determining discipline (Registered Nurses Association of Ontario, 2016). Berg and Seeber (2016) argue that the motivation for "fast knowledge," job-related skills, and immediate payoff makes courses that prioritize reflective, critical

RESEARCH FOCUS

This essay explores Springer and Clinton's (2017) analysis of the corporatization of academia due to the encroachment of capitalist interests into the daily work of the university. Although this analysis is specific to graduate education, it can be extrapolated to undergraduate education. The focal shift of the university to the "preponderance of business interests, the increasing dependence of universities on industry funding, cults of efficiency, research intensivity and the pursuit of profit so prevalent in today's corporatized university shrinking funding dollar" (p. 1) has negatively impacted the ability of universities to engage in philosophical thinking. Corporatization is thus eroding the philosophy, values, and free speech that underpin any type of postsecondary education, including nursing education.

A key tenet of a university mission is to allow, and even invite, critical discourse to engage members in free exploration of the world and one's place in it. In becoming a "liberated human spirit" (p. 2), a commitment must be made to asking and discussing deep and potentially disturbing questions. Springer and Clinton lament the demise of this goal due to the involvement of corporate entities and the devaluing of the creation of the liberated human spirit so valued by the university. This is due to the influence of the "forced transformation of academics from intellectuals, teachers, and mentors, to competitive adversaries, positioning themselves to claim academic territory and a share of research funds" (Springer & Clinton, 2017, p. 2).

The authors identify where nursing education has played a role in this transformation through financial backing or support from business interests. They give several examples of circumstances where the "corporatization" of the university, and specifically nursing education, is troubling. They imply that nursing is complicit in the trend owing to the university's acceptance of funds in exchange for giving naming rights to pharmaceutical companies or other health care companies for laboratories, nursing units, or research funding attached to a particular disease or condition. This affects the integrity of the research done at the university.

The concerns espoused by the authors with respect to the impact of corporatization on nursing relate to the impact on the ability to engage in critical thinking and analysis of the current situation in nursing. The lack of an ability to engage in deep philosophical thinking ultimately "undermine(s) critical reflection on the discipline of nursing and its future contribution to health and wellness" (Springer & Clinton, 2017, p. 4).

As a closing suggestion to the profession, the authors advise that without engaging in a "thoughtful examination of the effects of corporatization on how we are preparing nurses, we risk not only a (re)shaping of the profession going forward, but also, and more importantly, diminishing human health and well-being" (Chinn, 2013; Springer & Clinton, 2018; p. 6). Springer and Clinton encourage schools of nursing to not lose sight of the true purpose of educating students to become nurses.

Sources: Chinn, P. (2013). *Making time for dialogue* [web log post]. Retrieved from http://ansjournalblog.com/2013/10/making-time-for-dialogue/. Springer, R. A., & Clinton, M. E. (2017). "Philosophy Lost": Inquiring into the effects of the corporatized university and its implications for graduate nursing education. *Nursing Inquiry*, 24(4), e12197. https://doi.org/10.1111/nin.12197.

thinking, and self-development less desirable, especially when those courses require close and intense reading of philosophical articles and texts (Springer & Clinton, 2017).

Clearly, the circumstances under which nurses are learning and practising are not conducive to wondering and philosophizing. Changing them, however, will not be a simple matter, mainly because of the special-interest groups that have a vested interest in maintaining the status quo. For example, by preserving society's current conception of nursing work as work requiring little more than some practical skills and a willingness to follow directions, governments and employers can keep nursing education and health care costs down while other health care providers continue to have passive nursing staff do their bidding. The increase in the numbers of health care providers who receive less education but have a scope of practice that is similar to the baccalaureate-prepared registered nurse impacts the ability of the profession to engage in thoughtful and deep philosophical discourse. If nurses are not taught to think and discuss philosophically and are then given a workload micromanaged by government by virtue of penalties for long wait times—or are replaced by a less educated body of health care providers—the result is not conducive to professional knowledge development. For example, in Ontario, a recent letter from Christine Elliott, Deputy Premier and Minister of Health and Long-Term Care, outlined an expansion of the scope of practice of registered practical nurses to include skills currently within the purview of registered nurses (Elliott, 2019).

Given these current circumstances, how is the nursing profession to develop a sound philosophical conception of nursing and of nursing knowledge? The answer lies in wisely using a once scarce but now growing nursing resource: nurses who are developing their capacities to think philosophically despite the existing impediments to wondering and philosophizing in nursing.

TOWARD A SOUND PHILOSOPHICAL NURSING BASIS

Against all odds, philosophical thought is starting to increase, maybe even flourish, in nursing. This change is largely thanks to nurse educators' recent recognition that not just a knowledge of research methods but also an understanding of their philosophical underpinnings is required to develop nursing science (Chinn & Kramer, 2015). Chinn and Kramer also identify the recent change in the vernacular of evidence-based to evidence-informed practice and assert that it broadens the ways of knowing inherent in nursing theory as being more than what comes from the evidence only. The evolution of the baccalaureate entry-to-practice requirement as the standard across most of Canada supports a broader and deeper education in nursing that creates opportunities for the development of thinking philosophically earlier in a nurse's career. With courses on the philosophy of nursing science being included in most if not all doctoral nursing programs, a growing (albeit still small) number of nurses are managing to develop their philosophical capacities and helping to increase awareness of the need for nurses to wonder and philosophize about their profession and discipline. The increase in seats in postgraduate education in Canada is also a positive step toward philosophical thinkers starting to lead the way (see Table 7.1). These scholars are participating in philosophical discussions at conferences and online and contributing substantively to the nursing literature. More philosophical conferences are opening up, as are themes within conferences related to philosophical thinking.

In the 1980s, few papers of a philosophical nature appeared in nursing journals. Today, such papers appear regularly in such prestigious nursing journals as the *Journal of Advanced Nursing* and *Nursing Inquiry*. Also, with the growing interest in nursing philosophy, the *Canadian Journal of Nursing Research* devoted issues in 1995 and 2000 to the topic "Philosophy/Theory." In 1999, the journal *Scholarly Inquiry for Nursing Practice* published a special issue entitled "Philosophy of Nursing: Emerging Views." Then, in 2000, the journal *Nursing Philosophy* was established; it will celebrate its twentieth anniversary in 2020. Moreover, books pertaining specifically to nursing philosophy have become more available. Building on this availability are works by Dahnke and Dreher (2015), Forss, Ceci, and Drummond (2013), and Suzie Hesook Kim (2015).

The growing literature on philosophical nursing knowledge has been helpful in creating an atmosphere conducive to wondering and philosophizing in nursing. So, too, have infrastructures such as the Unit for Philosophical Nursing Research (uPNR), established in 1988 at the University of Alberta (previously called the Center for Philosophical Nursing Research), and the International Philosophy of Nursing Society (IPONS), established in the United Kingdom in 2003. The nursing philosophy conferences organized by the uPNR, the IPONS, and institutions such as Laval University are helping to meet nurses' needs to come together and philosophize. In 2016, Laval, the IPNR, and the IPONS brought together two nursing philosophy conferences, the 20th International Philosophy of Nursing Conference and the 12th Philosophy in the Nurse's World Conference, to jointly discuss the past, present, and future contributions of nursing philosophy to the discipline and practice of nursing (Dallaire & Krol, 2018). It resulted in a special issue of the journal *Nursing Philosophy* with articles from presentations at the conference.

While there are still few nurses who are now thinking philosophically, it is getting to the point where removal of the impediments to wondering and philosophizing and the development of a sound philosophical conception of nursing and of nursing knowledge are no longer fantastical goals. Consequently, at this time, we (the profession) would do well to begin thinking about what we could be doing to work toward these goals. We need to think about

TABLE 7.1 **Postgraduate Nursing Seats in Canadian Universities**		
	2012	**2018**
Master's degree	775	1111
Doctoral degree	84	95

Source: Canadian Association of Schools of Nursing. (2017/2018). *Registered nurse education in Canada statistics.* December 2019. Ottawa, ON: Author. Retrieved from https://www.casn.ca/wp-content/uploads/2019/12/2017-2018-EN-SFS-DRAFT-REPORT-for-web.pdf.

RESEARCH FOCUS

Several authors have written on the subject of philosophy and the conceptions of nursing. The following are some research articles that explore philosophy in nursing.

Bruce, Rietze, and Lim (2014) explore concerns about the relevance of philosophy to nursing in its everyday actions. They discuss the relevance of philosophy to the value of critical thinking and reflection and how it impacts individual nurses. The article closes with a call for more research and understanding of the interdependence of both the practical and philosophical perspectives of nursing to move the profession forward.

Garrett's (2014) book explores the history of the development of scientific and philosophical thought and relates them to nursing practice and knowledge creation. He also explores why a sound grounding in nursing philosophy and science are needed to support nursing practice.

A philosophical examination by Reimer-Kirkham, Varcoe, Browne et al. (2009) of their attempts (as Canadian nurse researchers) to translate their work in critical inquiry raises questions about whether and how disparate philosophical stances can be accommodated.

Thoun, Kirk, Sangster-Gormley, and Young (2019) explore three philosophies of truth (correspondence, pragmatism, and coherence) and how these theories facilitate or impede nursing knowledge creation. The authors make a recommendation as to which theory best embraces the diversity and ideals to which nursing as a professional discipline aspires.

Sources: Bruce, A., Rietze, L., & Lim, A. (2014). Understanding philosophy in a nurse's world: What, where and why? *Nursing and Health, 2*(3), 65–71. https://doi.org/10.13189/nh.2014.020302; Garrett, B. (2014). *Science and modern thought in nursing: Pragmatism and praxis for evidence-based practice.* Toronto, ON: Northern Lights Media; Reimer-Kirkham, S., Varcoe, C., Browne, A. J., et al. (2009). Critical inquiry and knowledge translation: Exploring compatibilities and tensions. *Nursing Philosophy, 10*, 152–166. https://doi.org/10.1111/j.1466-769X.2009.00405.x; Thoun, D. S., Kirk, M., Sangster-Gormley, E., & Young, J. O. (2019). Philosophical theories of truth and nursing: Exploring the tensions. *Nursing Science Quarterly, 32*(1), 43–48. https://doi.org/10.1177/0894318418807945

how to develop more nurses who can truly do what Smadu (2007), a past president of the Canadian Nurses Association, asks: "As nurses we need to lead the discussions about what nursing is, in language that is clear, forthright and complete—neither minimizing nursing work, nor taking for granted that others know what we are and do" (p. 3). Here, we would do well to bear in mind that this endeavour is not a simple one to execute, given the growth of diverse philosophical stances among nurses. While generative, it has also made for challenging dialogue (Reimer-Kirkham, Varcoe, Browne et al., 2009).

Finally, it would be unrealistic to expect that all nurses would do all the work necessary to develop a sound philosophical basis for nursing. A more realistic expectation is that nurses would contribute to that development in whatever ways they can. For example, those with the necessary philosophical preparation could take responsibility for the project and do the in-depth philosophical analysis, while those without such preparation could contribute in their own ways (e.g., by sharing their thoughts regarding those aspects of the scope of nursing practice that need to be clarified). Dialoguing together, each group could benefit from the expertise of the other with regard to insights gained as well as the development of their capacities to wonder and philosophize.

 APPLYING CONTENT KNOWLEDGE

1. At what stage of their education should nurses be introduced to philosophical inquiry?
2. Can a case be made for not introducing nurses to philosophical inquiry? Why or why not?

CONCLUSION

With the need for a sound philosophical conception of nursing and of nursing knowledge, the path that has been cleared thus far to advance philosophical thought in nursing is very encouraging. Indeed, it is remarkable, given the impediments to wondering and philosophizing that continue to exist both within and outside of nursing educational and practice settings. Or as recently stated by Thoun, Kirk, Sangster-Gormley, and Young (2019), "nursing is what nursing believes" (p. 47). Much more work lies ahead if the profession is not to lose itself before it finds itself, because there are already signs that the nursing profession may be on the way to becoming an amorphous entity.

SUMMARY OF LEARNING OBJECTIVES

- The quest to conceptualize nursing knowledge began in the 1960s, when nurse educators began to identify what constituted nursing education and could be included in the nursing curriculum.
- Scientific conceptions of nursing are based on the worldview that all aspects of nursing can be explained through scientific theories and be expanded or explained through experimentation, observation, or description. Philosophical conceptions of nursing are those that help to explain the nature of nursing itself and nursing practice. They have been called conceptual models of nursing, conceptual nursing frameworks, or nursing theories. They do not seek to prove or discover one truth—as does scientific thinking—but they do seek to understand both the uniqueness and the commonality of knowledge inherent in nursing.
- A philosophical way of thinking in nursing should be approached from a point of wonder about what is inherent in nursing as a professional discipline. It is not grounded in empirical thinking, but in thinking that is expansive and is outside the "workday," or everyday world.
- Thinking philosophically requires one to think outside their sphere of work and everyday existence and consider such questions as "What is nursing?," "What is caring?,"

and "What does it mean to be human?" Philosophical thinking leads to a deeper understanding of the essence of nursing outside the actions and outcomes of nursing.
- Impediments to thinking philosophically in nursing exist in the nursing curriculum and in the practice environment. Education focuses on preparing students to be practice ready; the practice environment does not encourage philosophical thinking because the work environment suffers from staff shortages and insufficient beds. The corporatization of universities also compromises the ability of philosophical thinking to occur. Promotion of philosophical thinking includes developing the baccalaureate entry-to-practice requirement, increasing the number of postgraduate nursing seats, increasing the number of philosophical journals and articles being published, as well as increasing the number of nursing philosophy conferences.
- Creative ways to advance philosophical thinking include partnerships between nursing practice and nursing scholars. All nurses should reflect upon their relationship to what they came to know about nursing and how this translates into their daily practice and engagement in the art and science of nursing. It is a lifelong journey of discovery.

CRITICAL THINKING QUESTIONS

1. What is an essential difference between a conception of nursing developed using scientific means and one developed using philosophical means based in moderate realism?

2. What are some fundamental implications of grounding nursing practice in a conception of nursing based on idealism? Based in moderate realism?

3. What differentiates thinking philosophically from critical thinking?

REFERENCES

Adams, L. Y. (2016). The conundrum of caring in nursing. *International Journal of Caring Sciences, 9*(1), 1–8.

Adler, M. J. (1965). *The conditions of philosophy.* New York, NY: Dell.

Adler, M. J. (1978). *Aristotle for everybody.* New York, NY: Macmillan.

Adler, M. J. (1990). *Intellect: Mind over matter.* New York, NY: Macmillan.

Berg, M., & Seeber, B. (2016). *The slow professor. Challenging the culture of speed in the academy.* Toronto, ON: University of Toronto Press, Scholarly Publishing Division.

Canadian Association of Schools of Nursing. (2019). *Registered Nurses Education in Canada Statistics 2017–2018.* Retrieved from: https://www.casn.ca/wp-content/uploads/2019/12/2017-2018-EN-SFS-DRAFT-REPORT-for-web.pdf.

Canadian Institute for Health Information. (2019). *Nursing in Canada, 2018: A lens on supply and workforce.* Ottawa, ON: Author.

Canadian Nurses Association. (2020). Elimination Canada's RN shortage. News Release. May 2009. Retrieved from: https://www.cna-aiic.ca/en/news-room/news-releases/2009/eliminating-canadas-rn-shortage.

Chinn, P. L. (2001). Where is the nursing in nursing education? [Editorial]. *Advances in Nursing Science, 23,* v–vi.

Chinn, P. L., & Kramer, M. K. (2015). *Knowledge development in nursing: Theory and process* (9th ed.). St. Louis, MO: Elsevier.

Chinn, P. (2013). *Making time for dialogue* [web log post]. Retrieved from http://ansjournalblog.com/2013/10/making-time-for-dialogue/.

Dahnke, M. D., & Dreher, H. M. (2015). *Philosophy of science for nursing practice: Concepts and application.* New York, NY: Springer.

Dallaire, C., & Krol, P. (2018). Revisiting the roots of nursing philosophy and critical theory: Past, present and future. [Editorial]. *Nursing Philosophy, 19*(1). https://doi.org/10.1111/nup.12204.

Dellasega, C., Milone-Nuzzo, P., Curci, K. M., et al. (2007). The humanities interface of nursing and medicine. *Journal of Professional Nursing, 23*, 174–179. https://doi.org/10.1016/j.profnurs.2007.01.006.

Forss, A., Ceci, C., & Drummond, J. S. (2013). *Philosophy of nursing: 5 Questions.* Copenhagen, Denmark: Automatic Press/VIP.

Garrett, B. (2014). *Science and modern thought in nursing: Pragmatism & praxis for evidence-based practice.* Toronto, ON: Northern Lights Media.

Elliott, C. (2019, June 13). *Letter to College of Nurses of Ontario to change scope of practice for Registered Practical Nurses.* Retrieved from https://rnao.ca/sites/rnao-ca/files/Scope_of_Practice_letter_-_CNO.pdf.

Gottlieb, L. N., & Gottlieb, B. (2007). The developmental/health framework within the McGill Model of Nursing: "Laws of nature" guiding whole person care. *Advances in Nursing Science, 30*, E43–E57. https://doi.org/10.1097/00012272-200701000-00013.

Hockey, L. (1990). The philosophical underpinnings of doctoral education. In P. A. Field (Ed.), *Advancing doctoral preparation for nurses: Charting a course for the future* (pp. 45–53). Edmonton, AB: Faculty of Nursing, University of Alberta.

Kikuchi, J. F. (1997). Clarifying the nature of conceptualizations about nursing. *Canadian Journal of Nursing Research, 29*(1), 97–119.

Kikuchi, J. F. (2003a). Nursing theories: Relic or stepping stone? *Canadian Journal of Nursing Research, 35*(2), 3–7.

Kikuchi, J. F. (2003b). Nursing knowledge and the problem of worldviews. *Research and Theory for Nursing Practice, 17*, 7–17. https://doi.org/10.1891/rtnp.17.1.7.53167.

Kim, H. S. (2015). *The essence of nursing practice: Philosophy and perspective.* New York, NY: Springer.

Levine, M. E. (1995). Discourse: On the humanities in nursing. *Canadian Journal of Nursing Research, 27*(2), 19–23. Retrieved from https://cjnr.archive.mcgill.ca/article/view/1276/1276.

Maben, J., Latter, S., & Macleod Clark, J. (2007). The sustainability of ideals, values, and the nursing mandate: Evidence from a longitudinal qualitative study. *Nursing Inquiry, 14*(2), 99–113. https://doi.org/10.1111/j.1440-1800.2007.00357.x.

Maritain, J. (1959). *The degrees of knowledge* (G.B. Phelan, Trans.). New York, NY: Charles Scribner's Sons.

Meleis, A. I. (2001). Scholarship and the R01 [Editorial]. *Journal of Nursing Scholarship, 33*, 104–105.

Phenix, P. H. (1964). *Realms of meaning.* New York, NY: McGraw-Hill.

Pieper, J. (1952). *Leisure: The basis of culture* (A. Dru, Trans.). New York, NY: Pantheon Books.

Rankin, J. M., & Campbell, M. L. (2006). *Managing to nurse: Inside Canada's health care reform.* Toronto, ON: University of Toronto Press.

Registered Nurses' Association of Ontario. (2016). *Mind the safety gap in health system transformation: Reclaiming the role of the RN.* Toronto, ON: Author.

Reimer-Kirkham, S., Varcoe, C., Browne, A. J., et al. (2009). Critical inquiry and knowledge translation: Exploring compatibilities and tensions. *Nursing Philosophy, 10*, 152–166. https://doi.org/10.1111/j.1466-769X.2009.00405.x.

Smadu, M. (2007). We must use our voices and speak up about nursing. *The Canadian Nurse, 103*(2), 3.

Smith, M. C., & Parker, M. E. (2015). Nursing theory and the discipline of nursing. In M. C. Smith, & M. E. Parker (Eds.), *Nursing theories and nursing practice* (4th ed.). Philadelphia, PA: F. A. Davis.

Spear, H. J. (2007). Nursing theory and knowledge development: A descriptive review of doctoral dissertations. *2000–2004. Advances in Nursing Science, 30*, E1–E14. https://doi.org/10.1097/00012272-200701000-00010.

Springer, R.A., & Clinton, M.E. (2017). 'Philosophy Lost': Inquiring into the effects of the corporatized university and its implications for graduate nursing education. *Nursing Inquiry, (24)*e, 12197. https://doi.org/10.1111/nin.12197.

Stinson, S. M. (1990). Prologue. In P. A. Field (Ed.), *Advancing doctoral preparation for nurses: Charting a course for the future* (pp. 1–5). Edmonton, AB: Faculty of Nursing, University of Alberta.

Theodoridis, K. (2017). Nursing as concrete philosophy. Part I: Risjord on nursing knowledge. *Nursing Philosophy, 19*(1–8), e-12205. https://doi.org/10.1111/nup.12205.

Thorne, S. (2003). Theoretical issues in nursing. In J. C. Ross-Kerr, & M. J. Wood (Eds.), *Canadian nursing: Issues and perspectives* (4th ed, pp. 116–134). Toronto, ON: Mosby.

Thoun, D. S., Kirk, M., Sangster-Gormley, E., & Young, J. O. (2019). Philosophical theories of truth and nursing: Exploring the tensions. *Nursing Science Quarterly, 32*(1), 43–48. https://doi.org/10.1177/0894318418807945.

Villeneuve, M., & MacDonald, J. (2006). *Toward 2020: Visions for nursing.* Ottawa, ON: Canadian Nurses Association.

White, D., Oelke, N. D., Besner, J., et al. (2008). Nursing scope of practice: Descriptions and challenges. *Canadian Journal of Nursing Leadership, 21*(1), 44–57. https://doi.org/10.12927/cjnl.2008.19690.

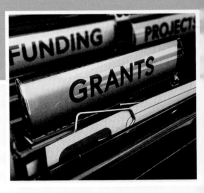

8

Nursing Research in Canada

Lynn McCleary

e http://evolve.elsevier.com/Canada/Ross-Kerr/nursing

LEARNING OBJECTIVES

After reading this chapter, you will be able to:
- Describe the development of Canadian nursing research.
- Describe the challenges and benefits of conducting research in teams.
- Describe the development of patient and service user stakeholder engagement in nursing research.
- Explain and critique changes in funding for nurse researchers.
- Compare externally funded and unfunded nursing research.
- Describe the role of nursing organizations and nurse leaders in the development of nursing research in Canada.
- Explain the impact of changes in research policy related to strategic funding and knowledge mobilization on Canadian nursing research.
- Examine factors that impact sustainability of the nursing research enterprise in Canada.
- Describe factors that influence the ability of the profession to demonstrate the impact of nursing research.

KEY TERMS

infrastructure support
interdisciplinary research
knowledge transfer
knowledge translation
knowledge mobilization

multidisciplinary research
Research Chair
research dissemination
transdisciplinary research

PERSONAL PERSPECTIVES

What draws nurses to be researchers? Maybe you will catch the research bug like they did. Maybe you already have. The author asked Canadian nurse researchers and PhD students about the experiences that made them catch the research bug. Common responses were curiosity, motivation to make a difference in practice, having fun with early exposure to research through graduate studies or as a research assistant, realizing that their research could contribute to nursing, and encouragement from professors. Here is what they said:

> Even though I took a research course as an undergraduate student, I was nonchalant about research. A professor who showed me the connection between clinical problems and research supported me in an undergraduate research project that inspired me to pursue graduate studies and, eventually, research.

> To be able to make little changes that would impact nursing and nurses positively and improve patient care.

> My master's supervisor encouraged me to apply to a PhD program. I wasn't sure about continuing as an advanced practice nurse. I wasn't sure what a nurse researcher did, but I wanted to improve care for patients and working conditions for nurses, so I applied. That got me doing research.

> When I did my first study, I gained insight into the thoughts and feelings of participants. I realized I could make a difference by sharing their stories.

> I think it's mainly my passion and insatiable thirst for learning that makes me love research because it allows me to explore, discover, and ponder questions deeply. Plus, I get to do this with a team of people who share the same passion!

> A professor told me I should publish a literature review I did about a clinical question when I was a masters student.

> Being a research assistant when I was an undergraduate student showed me the impact research could have. Plus, it was fun.

> The public health unit where I worked hired a social work student to evaluate a nursing program. I thought, "Why am I explaining nursing practice so someone else can evaluate our practice? Nurses need to develop the evidence that supports what we do." I'd been planning to go to grad school since my fourth year of undergrad and this made it clear to me.

THE EVOLUTION OF CANADIAN NURSING RESEARCH

The evolution of nursing research in Canada is linked to developments in the profession of nursing, the establishment of nursing journals and nursing research journals to disseminate research findings, developments in graduate nursing education, and availability of funding for nursing research. Key events in the evolution of nursing research in Canada are summarized in Table 8.1.

Research in nursing developed gradually as the pool of nurses with research expertise slowly grew. This development paralleled the evolution of graduate education in nursing, because graduate education is where research skills are learned and honed. As part of their education, graduate students are taught research methods and conduct research to fulfill thesis requirements. Master's nursing education programs prepare graduates to critique and synthesize research, conduct quality improvement research, and collaborate in research (Canadian Association of Schools of Nursing [CASN], 2014c). Doctoral nursing education prepares graduates to independently obtain funding for research, conduct research, and disseminate research findings (CASN, 2014b). Following the establishment of graduate programs in nursing, Canadian nursing research activities increased in scope and number.

Few Canadian universities offered master's degrees before the early 1980s. But as of 2019, 29 universities offered master's degrees in nursing, with more graduate nursing programs being proposed. The first funded doctoral program began at the Faculty of Nursing, University of Alberta, in January 1991. From 1991 to 2007, another 14 doctoral programs were established in Canadian universities. Opportunities for graduate education are now available across Canada, with 19 doctoral nursing programs, some of which offer online and distance learning options.

The lack of a Canadian doctoral program in nursing until 1991 forced nurses to be resourceful and to find alternative ways to develop research skills. These alternatives included entering doctoral programs in nursing in other countries, most notably the United States, and completing doctoral programs in other disciplines, most often sociology, psychology, education, and anthropology. The development of Canadian doctoral programs in nursing gave nurses expanded options to pursue graduate programs. It also resulted in the development of postdoctoral research fellowships for PhD graduates, something that was virtually unknown in Canadian nursing before 1991. Postdoctoral research fellows are employed by established researchers, typically for 1 or 2 years. They gain additional knowledge and skills to prepare them to be successful researchers, including knowledge about specialized research methods,

TABLE 8.1	Timeline of the Evolution of Nursing Research in Canada
Year	Event
1900	First US nursing journal, *American Journal of Nursing*
1905	First Canadian nursing journal, *Canadian Nurse*
1908	Canadian Nurses Association (CNA) established
1942	Canadian Association of University Schools of Nursing established (later renamed the Canadian Association of Schools of Nursing [CASN])
1952	First US nursing research journal, *Nursing Research*
1959	First Canadian publicly funded graduate program, a 1-year diploma in nursing service administration, established at University of Western Ontario
1962	Canadian Nurses Foundation (CNF) established by CNA to support research and education
1969	First Canadian nursing research journal, *Nursing Papers* (renamed *Canadian Journal of Nursing Research* in 1984)
1971	Canada's first national nursing conference in Ottawa, sponsored by The University of British Columbia and funded by the National Health Research and Development Program (NHRDP)
1971	First Canadian centre for nursing research established at McGill University, funded by Health and Welfare Canada
1970s	Establishment of nursing research journals *Research in Nursing and Health*, *Advances in Nursing Science*, *Image: Journal of Nursing Scholarship*, and *The Western Journal of Nursing Research* (founded by Canadian nurse Pamela Brink)
1978	Kellogg National Seminar on Doctoral Preparation for Canadian Nurses organized by the CNA, CNF, and CASN and funded by the W.K. Kellogg Foundation
1982	Alberta Foundation for Nursing Research established and funded by the government of Alberta
1983	First International Nursing Research Congress in Madrid, Spain
1985	Publication of first nursing research textbook by Canadian authors, *Nursing research: The application of qualitative approaches*
1986	Second International Nursing Research Congress held in Alberta, Canada
1987	Canadian Nursing Research Group established as a result of a meeting at the 1986 International Nursing Research Conference
1989	First career awards for nurse researchers from NHRDP and the Medical Research Council of Canada (MRC) awarded to three nurse researchers
1991	*Qualitative Health Research* journal founded by Canadian nurse Janice Morse
1992	First PhD nursing program in Canada established at the University of Alberta
1993	National consensus conference on Nursing Minimum Data Set sponsored by CNA
1994	Mandate of MRC changed from funding biomedical research only to funding all health research
1997	Dissolution of Alberta Foundation for Nursing Research as provincial funding ends
1998	International Institute for Qualitative Methodology established at University of Alberta by Janice Morse
1999–2009	Nursing Research Fund established by Government of Canada and administered by the Canadian Health Services Research Foundation (CHSRF; $25 million over 10 years)
2000	NHRDP and MRC dissolved; Canadian Institutes of Health Research (CIHR) formed
2000	Miriam Stewart, University of Alberta, appointed as inaugural Scientific Director, CIHR Institute of Gender and Health
2001	Dorothy Pringle, University of Toronto, appointed as inaugural chair of Institute Advisory Board, CIHR Institute of Aging
2002	Tier 1 Canada Research Chair awarded to Annette O'Connor, University of Ottawa, in Health Care Consumer Decision Support
2003–2008	Nursing Care Partnership Program, a $2.5 million grant from the CHSRF, awarded to CNF to support clinical nursing research over a 5-year period
2003	Nancy Edwards, University of Ottawa, appointed to Governing Council of CIHR
2012	Social Sciences and Humanities Research Council of Canada (SSHRC) stops funding health-related research

TABLE 8.1	Timeline of the Evolution of Nursing Research in Canada (*Cont*)
Year	**Event**
2018	SSHRC expands funding to include health-related research projects with a focus on social sciences and humanities
2019	CIHR announces funding competition for six Indigenous Research Chairs in Nursing

Sources: Bottorff, J. L., DiCenso, A., Doran, D., et al. (2011). Does nursing research have a future? *Canadian Nurse, 107*(4), 14; Coyte, P. C., Wise, L. M., & Motiwala, S. S. (2008). *An evaluation of the Nursing Research Fund: Lessons to date and recommended next steps.* Ottawa, ON: Canadian Health Services Research Foundation; Pasieka, D. E. (2017). *A history of the evolution of nursing research in the Faculty of Nursing, University of Alberta from 1980 to 1998.* Edmonton, AB: University of Alberta. Retrieved from https://era.library.ualberta.ca/items/ff9c2e3f-3bb7-4cec-bb58-3acfdcceea14; ResearchNet. (2019). *Canadian Institutes of Health Research Chair: Indigenous Research Chairs in Nursing.* Retrieved from https://www.researchnet-recherchenet.ca/rnr16/vwOpprtntyDtls.do?all=1&masterList=true&org=CIHR&prog=3033&resultCount=25&sort=program&type=EXACT&view=currentOpps&language=E; Stinson, S. M., Lamb, M., & Thibaudeau, M.-F. (1990). Nursing research: The Canadian scene. *International Journal of Nursing Studies, 27*(2), 105–122. https://doi.org/10.1016/0020-7489(90)90065-q; Wilson, T. (2017). *Research grants at SSHRC: An overview.* Retrieved from https://www.queensu.ca/urs/sites/webpublish.queensu.ca.urswww/files/files/SSHRC%20Tim%20Wilson%20Presentation%2012%20Sep%202017.pdf.

grant writing skills, and **research dissemination** skills, including writing for publication. These positions are funded through research grants held by the supervising researcher or by awards to the postdoctoral fellow from research funding organizations.

Research Conducted in University and College Faculties and Schools of Nursing

Most nursing research is conducted by university professors whose jobs are primarily focused on research. More recently, college faculty have also begun to engage in research. At most universities, 40% of a professor's time is allocated to research and writing and 40% to teaching. The rest of their time (20%) is spent working on committees, doing administration, and contributing to organizations outside the university. In some universities, there are two kinds of nursing professors: one type primarily conducts research and teaches graduate students, while the other primarily teaches undergraduate students. In these positions, those with more responsibility for research may spend up to 80% of their time doing research, whereas those who primarily teach undergraduate students have little time for research.

Nursing professors in colleges face unique challenges in conducting research. Traditionally, colleges were seen as an alternative to universities, and their mandate was to provide vocational training and prepare graduates for employment, with limited engagement in research. Consistent with global trends, colleges now award some baccalaureate degrees either independently or in collaboration with universities. This change was coincidental with the decision to make baccalaureate education a nursing entry-to-practice requirement, a move that required the establishment of nursing degree programs in colleges in collaboration between colleges and universities. In contrast to universities, research tends to be a less important part of the mandate of colleges. College faculty have less **infrastructure support** for research; do not generally hold PhD degrees, which would prepare them to independently conduct research; and must devote most of their work time to teaching, leaving them without as much time for research (Duncan, Mahara, & Holmes, 2014; Skolnik, 2016). This situation is similar to the experience of university nursing faculty in the 1980s, when most full-time professors had less than 10% of their time allocated to research (O'Connor & Bouchard, 1991).

However, nursing faculty in colleges with nursing degree programs are expected to conduct research, and colleges must therefore find ways to support their nursing faculty to do research. Standards set by the CASN (2014a) for accreditation of baccalaureate nursing education programs include expectations that colleges and universities provide infrastructure support for research and that faculty engage in scholarship, including research, that results in peer-reviewed publications or presentations. The Canadian Association of Schools of Nursing (CASN) offers courses and webinars on nursing scholarship and research for nursing professors (CASN, n.d.). Various strategies to support faculty research have been implemented at colleges and universities that have less infrastructure support for research. Implementing these strategies requires leadership from college administrators. Strategies include supporting professors to obtain PhD degrees, conducting research collectively within a nursing program, engaging in small-scale research in the local community, engaging in knowledge translation activities, engaging in research about nursing education, and mentorship from university nursing professors who have research expertise (Duncan, Mahara, Holmes et al., 2014).

 APPLYING CONTENT KNOWLEDGE

Consider differences in the history of nursing research at colleges and universities. What accounts for these differences? As colleges make the transition to offering degree programs in collaboration with universities, how will this influence nursing research?

Nursing research impressively grew from a small endeavour at just a few universities to a broad-based and better-financed undertaking. With more faculty becoming qualified at the doctorate level to undertake research and a greater availability of funding, nursing research at universities entered a new era in the 1980s and 1990s. Nursing faculty had access to vastly increased amounts of funding in the 1990s and early 2000s (Clarke, 2009; Coyte, Wise, & Motiwala, 2008), a far cry from the bleak levels of research funding reported in the 1960s (Griffin, 1971).

Nursing Research in Health Care Agencies

In the 1980s, nursing research at health care agencies took off as the importance of nursing research to health care was recognized and more research funding became available. Many large teaching hospitals appointed nursing researchers to plan and conduct research within the nursing department; these researchers often toiled alone. By the end of the 1980s, research activities were having a significant impact on nursing practice, and the research programs and spirit of inquiry that had evolved were the envy of many, including other professions. Mutually beneficial collaborations developed between nursing researchers at health care agencies and those at universities. Joint appointments of researchers to these organizations facilitated the investigation of nursing research problems. This collaborative work undoubtedly resulted in important developments in the nature of the research questions asked and the quality of the research effort.

By the early 1990s, many hospital-based nursing research positions were phased out or significantly changed in response to reduced government spending. The remaining positions were reconfigured to emphasize evaluation and quality improvement duties on a hospital-wide basis. This drastically decreased research involvement by hospital nurses for several years. When funding of hospital-based nursing research resumed in the late 1990s, research had shifted from a discipline-based endeavour to a multidisciplinary one. Academic health centres established **multidisciplinary research** divisions for research administration and support. Some of these centres included nurse scientists, who were expected to conduct large-scale clinical research. See Box 8.1 for an example and a description of one such nurse researcher. Today,

---

BOX 8.1   Nurse Scientist

Dr. Kathy McGilton is a Senior Scientist at KITE, the research division of the Toronto Rehabilitation Institute. She conducts research about the care of people who have cognitive impairment, with a focus on identifying and testing the effectiveness of interventions and models of care delivery. One of her studies used a patient-centred rehabilitation model of care as an effective approach to providing rehabilitation following hip fracture. Decline in functioning and the ability to perform activities of daily living is too common among older adults following hip fracture. Rehabilitation is important to prevent this decline. Patients who have dementia are often deemed ineligible for rehabilitation. Dr. McGilton and her colleagues developed a model of rehabilitation for hip fracture that includes approaches tar-geting people who have dementia. They received a CIHR research grant to conduct their study. The researchers compared the outcomes for 73 patients who had received the new model of care with the outcomes of 76 patients who received the usual care. The two groups did not differ in terms of mobility at discharge. However, patients who received the new model of care, including those who had cognitive impairment, were more likely to be discharged home. A subsequent study investigating 6-month outcomes provided further evidence that patients who have cognitive impairment can benefit from rehabilitation following a hip fracture. In fact, functional impairment prior to the hip fracture was more strongly associated with poor outcomes than cognitive impairment was.

Sources: McGilton, K. S., Chu, C. H., Naglie, G., et al. (2016). Factors influencing outcomes of older adults after undergoing rehabilitation for hip fracture. *Journal of the American Geriatrics Society, 64*, 1601–1609. https://doi.org/10.1111.jgs.14297; McGilton, K. S., Davis, A. M., Naglie, G., et al. (2013). Evaluation of patient-centred rehabilitation model targeting older persons with a hip fracture, including those with cognitive impairment. *BMC Geriatrics, 13*, 136. https://doi.org/10.1186/1471-2318-13-136.

GENDER CONSIDERATIONS

Accounting for Nonbinary Youth in Nursing and Health Research

Dr. Hélène Frohard-Dourlent and colleagues, who research vulnerable youth, tell the story of administering a questionnaire to high school students and being repeatedly asked by the students why there were only two options for sex instead of multiple options for gender. At the same time, the research team was analyzing data from the first Canadian Trans Youth Health Survey, in which 41% of the 923 youths surveyed identified as having a nonbinary gender.

These experiences led the team to reflect on nursing and health research methods and prompted them to issue a call for health researchers to become more gender inclusive in their research. Failure to do so would risk perpetuating the health inequities and discrimination experienced by gender minority persons in their encounters with the health care system. Frohard-Dourlent and colleagues have suggested that researchers consider nonbinary gender identities at all stages of the research process. For example, these considerations include purposefully being inclusive of diverse genders when recruiting participants, distinguishing between sex and gender in data collection, developing validated inclusive measures of gender identity, thinking about how to analyze data in relation to sex and gender, and using appropriate knowledge dissemination strategies.

Source: Frohard-Dourlent, H., Dobson, S., Clark, B. A., et al. (2017). "I would have preferred more options": Accounting for nonbinary youth in health research. *Nursing Inquiry, 24*(1), 1–9. https://doi.org/10.1111/nin.12150.

some health centres and hospitals continue to employ nurse researchers with PhDs who support evidence-informed practice initiatives, conduct small-scale studies, and engage nurses in research.

Breadth of Nursing Research

As noted previously, in the absence of Canadian master's and doctoral nursing programs, many nurses received their graduate education within the social sciences. Others embarked on graduate studies at a faculty of education or studied epidemiology at a faculty of medicine. Rarely, some nurses undertook graduate studies in the biological sciences. Wherever nurses studied, their early research training socialized them to the ways and topics of interest of other disciplines, including the research methods common to those fields. It is that exposure to a breadth of research methods that accounts for the tremendous diversity in research methods used by Canadian nursing researchers and the respect within the nursing profession for the value of all research methods in advancing knowledge.

Common topics for nursing research have evolved, corresponding to changing trends in the nursing profession and trends in health care. For example, in the 1970s, during the early years of the development of nursing research in Canada, the profession was concerned with nursing education. As a result, most research focused on nursing education and, later, on nursing theory. In the 1980s, research about clinical practice began to increase (Pasieka, 2017). Developments in the profession continue to influence the topics of nursing research. For example, the advent of high-fidelity simulation led to research about its use in nursing education and continuing education, as shown in Figure 8.1. The methods and approaches used by nurse researchers to conduct research with different populations are also influenced by social and health care trends. For example, as described in the Gender Considerations box, evidence about the health inequities experienced by

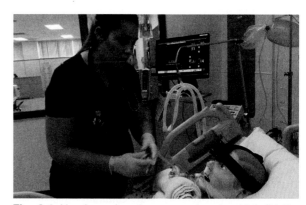

Fig. 8.1 Nursing education research using high-fidelity simulation and video recording. In Dr. Karyn Taplay's research, simulation patients are equipped with video cameras mounted near their eyes. Students view videos of themselves providing care to patients as a way to gain insight into the patient experience of nursing care. (K. Taplay and K. Tryer)

gender minority persons, as well as growing awareness of gender diversity in society and within the health care system, means that nurses are called on to include non-binary genders in health research (Frohard-Dourlent, Dobson, Clark et al., 2017).

Research Teams

Most nursing researchers work with research teams that might include other nursing professors, researchers from other professions or disciplines, clinicians and mangers employed by health care agencies, policy makers, and stakeholders in the research. Research team members are often located at different universities. **Transdisciplinary research** teams are more likely to receive research funding than are teams with one profession or discipline; the expectation is that bringing together diverse approaches and ways of thinking to address complex problems is more likely to yield solutions (Grigorovich, Fang, Sixsmith et al., 2019). To be successful, these large and complex research teams require careful planning, time to establish working relationships between researchers with different backgrounds, and regular communication between team members.

Stakeholders are people who may affect or influence the research process, be affected by outcomes of the research, or have an interest in the research. Stakeholders can include nurses and others who may use the findings, patients and care partners, health care agencies, and other organizations. Research funding agencies often expect research teams to engage stakeholders, not as research participants but as advisors, collaborators, and partners who contribute to decisions about research design, conducting research, and disseminating findings. Meaningfully engaging stakeholders in decisions about research improves the relevance, quality, and impact of the research and supports the dissemination of research findings beyond academia (Phoenix, Nguyen, Gentles et al., 2018). See Figure 8.2.

Patient and service user engagement in research is a recent development. Researchers use various approaches to include patients and service users, and the effectiveness of these different methods are still being evaluated (Black, Strain, Wallsworth et al., 2018; Forsythe, Carman, Szydlowski et al., 2019). The potential benefits of patient engagement include refined and more relevant research questions, patient-centred and culturally appropriate interventions, selection of relevant and less burdensome outcomes and measures, improved recruitment and participant engagement processes, and selection of acceptable methods for data collection (Forsythe, Heckert, Margolis et al., 2018). Challenges with patient engagement include the effort that it takes to build research team relationships; training patient and service user collaborators; researcher

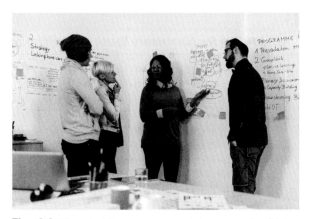

Fig. 8.2 Stakeholder engagement in research. Stakeholders may be in engaged at any point in the research process, from design through to data collection, data analysis, and dissemination of research findings. (iStock.com/Drazen_)

discomfort with sharing control of the research; clarifying the difference between patient engagement and participation in research, particularly participation in qualitative research; a tendency for tokenism in research instead of meaningful engagement; the time and cost of patient engagement; and the feasibility of patient engagement with limited research funding (Black, Strain, Wallsworth et al., 2018; Brett, Staniszewska, Mockford et al., 2014; Doria, Condran, Boulos et al., 2018). See Box 8.2 for an example of patient engagement activities.

Patient engagement methods are similar to the qualitative research methods valued in nursing, such as participatory action research, focus groups, interviews, and partnership. Given nurse researchers' expertise in these methods and their understanding of the methods' value, nursing is well situated to adopt patient engagement in research and contribute to knowledge about the best ways to engage patients and stakeholders.

👤 APPLYING CONTENT KNOWLEDGE

The iCAN-ACP research team engaged the Canadian Patient Advisors Network in their national, multi-year study of end-of-life experiences of older adults with serious illnesses (see Box 8.2). The Canadian Patient Advisors Network supports patient advisors to be involved in the health care system and as partners in research. How does patient and stakeholder involvement in research compare with patient and stakeholder involvement in decisions about the health care system? (See Chapter 11 for details.)

BOX 8.2 Patient Engagement in a Multifaceted Pan-Canadian Study

The iCAN-ACP study is a 3-year national study that is introducing and evaluating advance care planning tools in primary care, long-term care, and acute care settings. The study is funded by the Canadian Frailty Network. Thirty-two researchers from various health professions, five international collaborators, and many research staff and students are involved in the study; three teams of researchers and partners are focused on each setting, and a fourth team is focused on access to advance care planning for diverse populations. In this study, the lead researchers defined a "patient advisor" as a patient, family member, or volunteer who provides insights and input from the family perspective to help ensure that the patient perspective and experience is explicitly included in the research. Patient advisors in the study are expected to consider the research from the patient perspective with the aim of ensuring that the work is relevant to patients. The patient advisors speak from their own experiences or perspectives; they are not expected to speak on behalf of others' experiences. Some of the strategies for patient and consumer stakeholder engagement in this study include:

- Consulting and partnering with the Canadian Patient Advisors Network, an independent organization of people who act as patient and family advisors for health care organizations and health care research, when the study was being planned and on an ongoing basis;
- Appointing three patient advisors to the overall research team, with subteams engaging in patient engagement strategies that suit their context;
- Patient advisors participating in regular meetings of the research leaders and in annual national meetings of the entire research team;
- Allocating time at research team meetings for team members to get to know each other and learn about the potential roles of the patient advisors;
- Consulting with patient and family councils at research sites;
- Including a patient advisor at one site in data collection and in qualitative data analysis discussions;
- Asking patient advisors for feedback and input into interpretation of findings prior to publication and dissemination of findings; and
- Consulting with patient advisors about knowledge translation products and activities.

FUNDING NURSING RESEARCH

Nursing researchers seek research funding in four primary areas: conducting research, infrastructure (space and equipment) for conducting research, research training, and salary support for the researcher (career research awards). Historical overviews of the kinds of nursing research conducted over the years by governments, service agencies, professional associations, and university researchers were first presented in Ottawa in 1971 at the inaugural Canadian national conference on nursing research (Griffin, 1971; Imai, 1971; Poole, 1971). These overviews documented that most nursing research studies had been undertaken since 1965. Some studies were funded by a variety of sponsoring agencies, but most were self-funded. That is, conducted by graduate students or by faculty without the financial assistance of research grants (Griffin, 1971). Funding for nursing research only became readily available once Health Canada's National Health Research Development Program (NHRDP) incorporated funding in its terms of reference. Until then, there were few sources of funding for nursing research other than the limited resources of the Canadian Nurses Foundation (CNF) and those of private foundations and charitable organizations.

The NHRDP was a government agency that funded public health and health services research. It was the main source of federal funding for nursing research and nursing scholarships until the late 1990s. At the time, the other source of funding for health-related research was the Medical Research Council of Canada (MRC), which had a budget eight to nine times the size of the NHRDP's. However, nurses were largely unsuccessful in obtaining funding from the MRC, which limited its funding to biomedical research (Stinson, Lamb, & Thibaudeau, 1990). In addition to the NHRDP, most funding to nurse researchers was provided by provincial ministries of health and other provincial ministries, with smaller amounts of funding from the federal Social Sciences and Humanities Research Council of Canada (SSHRC), foundations such as the Heart and Stroke Foundation, local agencies, and the MRC. Unfunded research was common: about 40% of research projects conducted by nurses at Canadian universities in the late 1980s were unfunded (O'Connor & Bouchard, 1991).

Canadian nurses have struggled to obtain an equitable share of external research support. The process used by research funding agencies to distribute grant funds is complex. Researchers who need financial support to complete a research project must apply to an appropriate funding agency, and the topic must fit the agency's funding priorities. The researcher prepares a detailed application describing their research and the qualifications, expertise, and experience of the research team. Most decisions at agencies that fund research are arrived at with input from other researchers. Funding agencies strike review committees of researchers from various disciplines that have been funded by the agency. Initially, this created a catch-22 for nurse funding applicants, as there were too few previously funded nurse researchers to be on review committees and share their perspectives on the research questions and methods, some of which were less familiar to review committees (e.g., qualitative methods).

Lack of representation on review committees at least partly explained the lower funding success rates for nurses. However, other factors also contributed to the challenges nurses experienced in obtaining research funding: lack of experience with and skill in crafting research funding applications; lack of research and publication experience; lack of fit between nursing research questions and the mandates of the funding agencies; and gender bias affecting female applicants. While gender bias remains an issue with funding agencies, such that female applicants for research funding are less likely to be successful (Tamblyn, Girard, Qian et al. 2018; Witteman, Hendricks, Straus, &

Tannenbaum, 2019), many of the other challenges were overcome as the expertise of nurse researchers grew. Nurses regularly participate in research funding review committees, there is more openness to various research methodologies, and nurses successfully compete for research funding.

Most applications for research funding are unsuccessful. For example, the Canadian Institutes of Health Research (CIHR) Project Grants are awarded for research studies that take about 4 years to complete, with an average budget of about $170,000 per year. Of 2,484 applications in the fall 2018 competition, 371 (15%) were funded (Canadian Institutes of Health Research [CIHR], n.d.). Funding rates are higher from SSHRC, between 21% and 54%, depending on the type of research competition (Social Sciences and Humanities Research Council of Canada, n.d.). Between 2013 and 2018, the success rate for open grants at CIHR was 14.2%. The success rate for applications with a nurse as the lead applicant was 12.5%. For applications with a nurse as a lead applicant or co-applicant, it was 15.5%. Of all open grants, 1.7% were led by a nurse and 6.9% had a nurse as a research team member. Between 2013 and 2018, 143 nurses were lead applicants of 235 funded CIHR open grants and 567 nurses were lead applicants or co-applicants of 828 funded open grants (personal communication, CIHR, 2020).

🔖 RESEARCH FOCUS

Dr. Janice Morse arrived in Canada in 1982 from New Zealand via the United States to begin her career as a nursing researcher at the University of Alberta. She held graduate degrees in both anthropology and nursing. Her training in anthropology helped her to shape the research questions she posed and the research methods she used to address those questions. She primarily used qualitative research methods to study *comfort*—a topic of central concern to nursing. Her plan was to study comfort from various perspectives, including those of nurses, patients, and families, to develop a theory that would guide research and nursing practice.

When she sought funding for her research, her methods were heavily criticized by biomedical reviewers who were unfamiliar with this research approach. She faced the same criticisms locally and nationally and was unable to secure major funding that would provide financial support for her research and students. When the MRC and NHRDP development grants were established to encourage nursing research in Canada, Morse was one of the award recipients. Receiving this grant increased her

eligibility for other major Canadian research funding. With the broadening of the mandate of the MRC/CIHR in the late 1990s and the infusion of more public funds into research, Morse applied for and received additional grants.

Morse has made significant contributions to the development of qualitative research. Her research ingenuity has led to improved scientific methods and analyses. Students around the world have used her research methods books (Morse & Field, 1995; Richards & Morse, 2006) to learn about qualitative research. Canadian nursing researchers who received training in Morse's lab went on to address their own questions related to nursing.

Janice Morse is one of many of the early generation of Canadian nurse researchers who helped to shape the nursing research landscape. The path of many of these researchers was similar to that taken by Morse. Thanks to the efforts of these pioneers in nursing research, the current and next generation of Canadian nurse researchers will have better access to funding, enabling them to continue advancing nursing knowledge.

Sources: Morse, J. M., & Field, P. A. (1995). *Qualitative research methods for health professionals.* Thousand Oaks, CA: Sage Publishing; Richards, L., & Morse, J. M. (2006). *README FIRST for a user's guide to qualitative methods.* Thousand Oaks, CA: Sage Publishing.

Much of nurses' current success with obtaining research funds can be attributed to the Canadian Nurses Association (CNA), the CNF, the CASN, and nurse leaders. These organizations and individuals lobbied governments to provide more funding to nurse researchers and to support the development of research expertise within the nursing profession (Clarke, 2009; Stinson, Lamb, & Thibaudeau, 1990). In response to the CNA's advocacy efforts, the MRC established the Working Group on Nursing Research in 1982. Final recommendations in the report of the Working Group in 1985 referred to the need to designate funds for nursing research within the MRC's structure and the need to assist in creating opportunities for the establishment of doctoral nursing programs across the country. In 1989, the MRC and NHRDP created a jointly funded program to develop nursing research capacity through competitive funding for 5-year career support awards. For the duration of the 10-year program, 17 nurses at nine universities received funding that allowed them to devote 80% of their time to research. These nurses went on to be highly successful in their research careers, increased the credibility of nursing research, and contributed to the growth of nursing research expertise through their mentorship of graduate students (Canadian Health Services Research Foundation, 2008; Clarke, 2009).

In 1994, the federal government announced that the mandate of the MRC would be broadened to include health research. The MRC was transformed into CIHR in 2000. The resulting new programs of this agency and its 13 institutes resulted in increased funding of nursing research projects and the integration of nursing research into mainstream health research in Canada. For the first time, the full range of research methods suitable for health research questions were proposed and funded. CIHR funding of nursing research rose from $2.3 million in 2000 to $11.6 million in 2005 (Gottlieb, 2007). Nurses have served in leadership positions at CIHR (see Table 8.1) and are represented on research funding review committees.

In 1999, the federal government established the Nursing Research Fund (NRF), budgeting $25 million for nursing research over 10 years. The impetus for this decision came from the CNA, which had lobbied extensively for a dedicated source of funding for the development of nursing research. The association envisioned that the MRC program would serve as the model for the NRF program, by funding salaries of researchers and supporting their research project costs. When the government gave the Canadian Health Services Research Foundation (CHSRF) the responsibility for administering funds from the NRF, a model of funding emerged that displeased many in the nursing community. The mandate of the CHSRF, which was health services research, did not represent the broad research interests

of nurses, particularly those engaged in clinical research. Whereas the NRF had at first appeared to be a positive development for nursing research, it now seemed to be inaccessible to many nursing researchers who worked in fields outside the CHSRF mandate. The other issue was that the CHSRF required the applicant to obtain partnership funding equal to 60% of the request, which was difficult, and sometimes impossible, to procure. Many researchers, even those who fit the health services mandate of the CHSRF, were discouraged from applying because of the partnership funding requirement.

After several years of lobbying, CHSRF transferred funding to the CNF in 2003 for support of clinical nursing research, creating the Nursing Care Partnership Program (NCP). Like the NRF, the NCP required partnership funding. This program provided $500,000 per year in funding between 2003 and 2009. An evaluation conducted when the NCP ended in 2009 concluded that the program had successfully increased research capacity among nurses, leading many NCP recipients to establish successful careers after they had secured career awards and grants (Coyte, Wise, & Motiwala, 2008). The evaluators commented that the program ended just as it got momentum. They recommended a 25-year vision for a continuation of the program, noting a need for more training awards for junior faculty, support for smaller institutions without established research programs, and more funding for clinical nursing research.

🔍 APPLYING CONTENT KNOWLEDGE

The availability of funding for nursing research has changed over the years. What implications has this had for Canadian nursing? How have changes in federal support affected nursing research and efforts to build nursing knowledge?

In the 1990s, Canadian researchers experienced a funding boom thanks to lobbying by researchers across disciplines and the economic and political climate of the time. Several new research foundations or agencies were created in addition to the NRF and CHSRF. The Canadian Foundation for Innovation was established in 1997 to fund research infrastructure that would build research capacity at universities, research hospitals, and research institutes. The fund supports the equipment, buildings, laboratories, and databases required to conduct research. The **Canada Research Chairs** program was launched in 2000 to help universities and research hospitals recruit and retain top researchers and thus become world-class centres of research and research training. The Canada Research Chairs program continues today. Chair awards are for a period of 7 to 10 years and

BOX 8.3   Annette O'Connor, Trailblazing Nurse Researcher

Dr. Annette O'Connor, Emeritus Professor at the University of Ottawa, was awarded a Tier 1 Canada Research Chair in Health Care Consumer Decision Support in 2002 (University of Ottawa Faculty of Health Sciences, n.d.). When Dr. O'Connor began her research, there was little formal support available for patients facing health care decisions and uncertainty about the risks, benefits, and potentially conflicting outcomes of different treatments. Yet patients must often ask themselves difficult questions— Should I take hormone replacement therapy? Would a lung transplant be right for me? Should I have this therapy for my cancer?—to arrive at a decision. Patient decision aids are designed to support and streamline the process of shared decision making. Shared decision making is defined as a process of health care providers "interacting with patients in arriving at value-based choices when options have features that patients value differently" in order to arrive at the best decision for the patient; it involves

sharing "personalized information on options, outcomes, probabilities, and scientific uncertainties, and patients communicating the personal value or importance they place on benefits versus harms" (O'Connor, Llewellyn-Thomas, & Flood, 2004, pp. 63–64).

Dr. O'Connor's research and leadership has been instrumental in building patient decision support as a new field of study. She developed and tested a measure of decisional conflict, developed theoretical models of decision support, conducted randomized controlled trials of patient decision aids, and was part of an international group that established standards for patient decision aids. She is a trailblazer who has had many firsts in her research career, including a systematic review of trials of decision aids, a national survey of Canadian patients' needs for decision-making support, trials of skill development for health coaches, and the first Canadian study implementing shared decision making in nursing.

Sources: University of Ottawa Faculty of Health Sciences. (n.d.). *Annette M. O'Connor.* Retrieved from https://health.uottawa.ca/people/oconnor-annette-m; O'Connor, A. M., Llewellyn-Thomas, H. A., & Flood, A. B. (2014). Modifying unwarranted variations in health care: Shared decision making using patient decision aids. *Health Affairs,* 23(Suppl. 2). https://doi.org/10.1377/hlthaff.var.63.

are renewable. At any given time, there are 1,800 Canada Research Chair holders. Nurses are among the past and current Chair holders (Government of Canada, 2019). Chairs enable researchers to devote their time to research and graduate student training. Annette O'Connor, Emeritus Professor at the University of Ottawa, was the first nurse recipient of a Tier 1 Canada Research Chair (see Box 8.3).

The development of new funding sources resulted in the increased funding of nursing research. The amount of funding held by nurses tripled between 1998 and 2001 (Pringle, 2006). By 2000, times were good for nursing research, and nurses were optimistic about the future of nursing research (Edwards, DiCenso, Degner et al. 2002). Since the 2000s, however, federal funding for research has been decreasing, impacting the availability of health research funding. In 2017, an advisory panel reported that federal research funding had been steadily decreasing since 2008 and that Canada, which had previously been a top performer in research output, had significantly slipped compared with other OECD countries (Advisory Panel for the Review of Federal Support for Fundamental Science, 2017). Nurse researchers are now feeling the pinch of reduced research funding. As the number of nurses and others conducting health research continues to rise, there is increased competition for a smaller pool of funds, leaving more researchers without funding.

UNFUNDED RESEARCH AND NURSING SCHOLARSHIP

A significant amount of nursing research is either unfunded or funded through small grants from small agencies or the researcher's university. A critique of unfunded and small-scale research is that such studies may be less likely to build new nursing knowledge. There is a concern that nurses conduct too many small-scale studies that do not build on each other. Furthermore, small-scale studies do not have sufficient resources to establish causal associations or the effectiveness of interventions. However, unfunded research can provide evidence of the feasibility of a research approach or method and increase chances of funding for larger-scale follow-up studies. Unfunded research also contributes to research training: thesis research conducted by graduate students is often unfunded. Quality improvement research in agencies contributes to improved processes and patient outcomes.

According to Thorne (2014a), with research funds diminishing, nurse researchers need to be creative about how they do meaningful work. For instance, nurse researchers can conduct smaller-scale but still-important research studies that advance nursing knowledge. Funded research is not the only way to build nursing knowledge. The CASN position statement on scholarship among

TABLE 8.2	**Boyer's Domains of Scholarship**	
Domain	**Description**	**Example**
Scholarship of discovery	Builds new knowledge through basic and applied research Builds scientific basis for nursing	Peer-reviewed grants, publications, and presentations of research findings
Scholarship of teaching	Develops teaching methods and materials Builds knowledge about teaching and learning Methods include research, evaluation, theorizing, philosophizing, and integrating knowledge across disciplines	Peer-reviewed grants, publications, and presentations Creating and disseminating teaching and instructional resources
Scholarship of integration	Builds new knowledge by analyzing and synthesizing original scholarship across disciplines and professions	Publication of a textbook, textbook chapter, or literature review Policy analysis Creation of a new health program
Scholarship of application	Builds knowledge with a community for use by the community Builds knowledge about application of knowledge in practice	Peer-reviewed funding for practice innovation or knowledge translation Publication of evaluation of practice innovations

Source: Canadian Association of Schools of Nursing. (2013). *Position statement: Scholarship among nursing faculty.* Retrieved from https://www.casn.ca/position-statements/.

nursing faculty endorses Boyer's model of scholarship in four overlapping and interrelated domains, as shown in Table 8.2 (CASN, 2013). According to this statement, the activities must be documented to be considered scholarship, and the product or result of the scholarship must be peer reviewed and publicly disseminated for critique and replication. Some of this scholarship can be conducted without funding. Furthermore, important activities of theorizing and philosophizing about nursing for the development of nursing knowledge do not necessarily depend on funding (Grace, Willis, Roy et al., 2016; Thorne, 2019).

ADVOCACY FOR NURSING RESEARCH

The upturn in research funding in the 1990s demonstrated the benefits of a united voice when advocating for nursing research. In 2002, the Office of Nursing Policy at Health Canada brought together policymakers and researchers to consider the future of nursing research in Canada. They recommended creating the Canadian Consortium for Nursing Research and Innovation (CCNRI), which was a collaboration of key nursing organizations (including the CASN) that continued until 2011. Among its priorities were advocating for research funding (Health Canada, 2006). The consortium commissioned a report on the status of nursing research in Canada to determine nursing research capacity and productivity (Jeans, 2008).

In 2011, nurse members of the Canadian Academy of Health Sciences raised an alarm about the future of

nursing research. They noted that an increased number of researchers were competing for a diminishing pool of research funds, resulting in lower rates of research funding, decreased availability of career support awards, and threats to the quality of PhD education and training for the next generation of nurse researchers (Bottorff, DiCenso, Doran et al., 2011). The Canadian Academy of Health Sciences called on national nursing organizations to develop a strategic plan that would address threats to support for nursing research. Whereas these organizations had successfully influenced support for nursing research in the past, there has been no concerted public response to this call for action.

Who Sets the Agenda?

Historically, research was exclusively investigator driven, meaning that researchers decided what research questions needed to be asked based on their knowledge of the field. In the 1970s, the NHRDP introduced strategic funding priorities, allocating a significant portion of its research funding budget to the strategic priorities that were important to federal and provincial health departments. The earliest strategic health research priorities were in the areas of aging and HIV/AIDS. Other Canadian funding agencies followed suit. In the 1990s, strategic funding priorities were promoted by the federal government to improve accountability for research funds and increase the impact of the government's investment. In the same way that citizens and stakeholders are now involved in research, there

RESEARCH FOCUS

Engaging Patients and the Public to Identify Priorities for Dementia Research in Canada

Consulting with stakeholders can better align research aims with the priorities of people who experience health conditions and the people who care for them. The purpose of the Canadian Dementia Priority Setting Partnership was to engage people with dementia, their family and friends, and professional care providers in identifying priorities for dementia research. With funding from the Alzheimer Society of Canada, a steering group led a three-stage consultation process. In the first stage, 1,217 participants completed an online survey, identifying 79 research questions about living with dementia as well as the prevention, treatment, and diagnosis of dementia. The 79 questions were categorized, merged, and summarized, then checked against existing research evidence. The second stage involved another online survey, with 249 participants, and a focus group consisting of persons with

dementia, who identified 23 of the 79 research questions as high priority. In the final stage, 30 participants, including 7 persons with dementia and 5 care partners of persons with dementia, attended a 2-day workshop to identify the top 10 priorities for dementia research in Canada. This study demonstrated the enormous value of engaging stakeholders in setting research priorities. As one workshop participant with lived experience of dementia stated:

The process of breaking down the types of projects and the numbers made a project of this size and magnitude so easy. In spite of the fact each of us probably had our own pet project that we would have liked to put forward, or a private agenda, there was none of that. (Canadian Dementia Priority Setting Partnership, 2017, p. 4)

Sources: Bethell, J., Pringle, D., Chambers, L. W., et al. (2018). Patient and public involvement in identifying dementia research priorities. *Journal of the American Geriatrics Society, 66*(8), 1608–1612. https://doi.org/10.1111/jgs.15453; Canadian Dementia Priority Setting Partnership. (2017). *Canadian dementia research priorities: Report of the Canadian Dementia Priority Setting Partnership.* Toronto, ON: Author. Retrieved from https://alzheimer.ca/en/Home/Research/Canadian-dementia-priority-setting-partnership.

is now a trend toward citizen and stakeholder engagement in setting research priorities. For example, lay members are appointed to governing bodies of research funding agencies, and public consultations are held for strategic planning and identification of research priorities. An example is the Canadian Dementia Priority Setting Partnership, described in the Research Focus box (Bethell, Pringle, Chambers et al., 2018).

The strategic funding policy affects all federal research funding. Critics have argued that this policy has resulted in the underfunding of investigator-driven research and the hampering of knowledge generation. The combination of decreased funds, proportionately less funding for investigator-driven research, and an increased number of researchers led to the amount of investigator-driven funding per Canadian researcher decreasing by 35% between 2006 and 2013 (Advisory Panel for the Review of Federal Support for Fundamental Science, 2017). For nursing and other professions, this has meant less control within the profession over the production of new knowledge for the profession.

The setting of strategic priorities by funding agencies was the first step in a new direction in research policy. Some of the directions set by funding agencies and other organizations had a beneficial impact on health research. One example is the focus on **interdisciplinary research** and transdisciplinary research. Granting agencies now favour interdisciplinary and, more recently, transdisciplinary

approaches to research, funding research by teams of researchers across disciplines and professions (e.g., social sciences, nursing, and engineering). This change had the effect of changing the focus from discipline-based to patient-based research. As Thorne (2014b) has pointed out, nurse researchers need to build knowledge that is core to nursing and that will inform interdisciplinary health care. The trend towards interdisciplinary research means that it is difficult for nurse researchers to obtain funding for research questions that are specific to nursing. Some Canadian nurse researchers have found that including a nursing theory or focusing on a problem that is specific to nursing in a grant application is like "the kiss of death," rendering the application unfundable. This limitation diminishes the ability of the profession to build knowledge that is core to the profession (Grace, Willis, Roy et al., 2016; Thorne, 2014b).

APPLYING CONTENT KNOWLEDGE

Imagine that you were asked to advise funders on priorities for health research and nursing research. What would that experience be like? What could the funders do to make sure that your experience as a student was heard? What would you tell them?

KNOWLEDGE MOBILIZATION

Another change in research funding policy that is affecting how nursing research is conducted and the kind of research being funded is the emphasis on **knowledge transfer** and **knowledge translation** (or **knowledge mobilization**) to nonacademics. Granting agencies have concluded that one reason research was not sufficiently impacting the health of Canadians was that researchers were not effectively disseminating their findings to policymakers, the public, and practitioners (referred to as "knowledge users" by research funding agencies). Most researchers have long believed that their target audience is other researchers. Moreover, researchers have typically shared their research findings by publishing articles in peer-reviewed journals or presenting their work at academic or professional conferences. Publishing and presenting research findings are still a vitally important part of the research process. But funders now expect researchers to actively share findings with nonacademic audiences in ways that make it easy for them to adopt research findings into practice. In many cases, research findings must also be shared in ways that are meaningful to the public.

The Canadian Foundation for Healthcare Improvement (formerly the CHSRF) has a strong focus on knowledge transfer, particularly to policymakers and practitioners. It also has several funding initiatives to train researchers on knowledge transfer, to train health care executives and managers on using research, and to build partnerships between researchers and policymakers. CIHR, SSHRC, and charitable funding agencies (e.g., Heart and Stroke Foundation, Alzheimer Society of Canada) require that research grant applications include knowledge dissemination plans. The knowledge dissemination plan depends on the target audience of the research findings. Research plans must identify who the potential users of the research are and the best ways to reach various types of knowledge users. Knowledge dissemination to nonacademic knowledge users after the completion of a study can include live and archived webinars, presentations, op-ed publications in newspapers, plain language reports, policy briefs, and social media. Another approach to knowledge translation, called integrated knowledge translation, involves engaging knowledge users in the process of designing and conducting the research and sharing the findings.

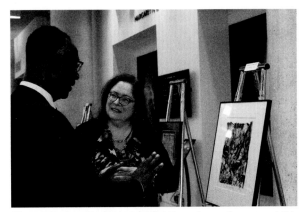

Fig. 8.3 Knowledge mobilization through art exhibitions. Dr. Sheila O'Keefe-McCarthy discusses an artist's visual interpretation of the experience of prodromal cardiac symptoms at a public art exhibit. (Brock University, Colleen Patterson)

Dr. Sheila O'Keefe-McCarthy and her research team interviewed women about their experiences of cardiac symptoms and used their findings to develop a screening scale for cardiac prodromal symptoms (O'Keefe-McCarthy & Guo, 2014). In addition to developing the screening scale, Dr. O'Keefe-McCarthy created poems based on the themes that arose in the interviews and the women's stories. She then engaged artists to create visual images in response to the poetry. The poems and visual art have been presented and displayed at nursing conferences, in practice settings, and at a public exhibition (Figure 8.3).

The emphasis on knowledge transfer means that nurse researchers must develop this expertise and collaborate with or hire knowledge transfer experts. Graduate students and postdoctoral fellows are expected to learn these skills as part of their research training. CIHR provides support for knowledge transfer training. For example, the Summer Program in Aging, offered by the Institute of Aging, is a competitive-admittance 1-week program that includes knowledge translation training. CIHR has funding for standalone knowledge translation activities. SSHRC has funding for research in partnership between researchers and community-based agencies that use research findings, where the agencies identify research questions that are important to them and are active in the research process.

As part of the policy of improving the uptake of research findings, federal funding agencies now require that some research findings be published as open access, either in journals that do not require a subscription to access research articles or in journals that provide open access to some articles. This policy is a reaction to the high cost of journal subscriptions and lack of access to journals by people who are not in

 APPLYING CONTENT KNOWLEDGE

What strategies do you think researchers should use to ensure that knowledge from research is accessed and used by nurses and nursing students?

academic settings. Open-access journal publication typically requires that researchers pay fees from their research grants. Fees can go up to $5,000 (US dollars), but the typical range is between $2,000 and $3,000 per publication. University libraries are developing low-cost, open-access platforms as an alternative to journals with high publication fees.

 APPLYING CONTENT KNOWLEDGE

Do you think publicly funded research findings should be free to access? Who should pay to publish research findings? What difference would this make for nurses?

GROWTH AND SUSTAINABILITY OF THE NURSING RESEARCH ENTERPRISE

The tremendous growth of nursing research in Canada since the 1980s can be attributed to more nurses earning their PhDs; an increased capacity to train graduate students and postdoctoral fellows, making it possible for nurses to successfully compete for research funding; and an increased availability of funding for applied health research. As discussed, decreases in government research funding over the past decade are affecting nurse researchers. A challenge for nursing will be to sustain these achievements and continue the growth of nursing research.

Faculty Shortage

The current shortage of North American nursing faculty is predicted to worsen (American Association of Colleges of Nursing [AACN], 2019; Vandyk, Chartrand, Beké et al., 2017). The lack of nursing faculty has implications for nursing research and the capacity to train and prepare future nurse researchers at the doctoral level. In 2018, in the United States, 7.9% of faculty positions requiring a doctoral degree were vacant (AACN, 2019). As shown in Figure 8.4, the number of nurses in Canada with PhD degrees has increased dramatically over the past decade (Canadian Institute for Health Information, 2018). However, there are not enough nurses graduating with PhD degrees to fill current and predicted vacancies, as many faculty members will retire in the coming decade (Vandyk, Chartrand, Beké et al., 2017). In Canada, 60% of nursing professors are over age 55 (CASN, 2014d). Similarly, in the United States, 60% of nursing professors in the workforce as of 2016 are expected to retire by 2025 (AACN, 2019).

What has led to the shortage of nursing faculty who can conduct research? To begin with, a limited number of people graduate with PhD degrees in a given year. Of these PhD graduates, not all will fill empty faculty positions. In fact, many PhD students already have faculty positions (Vandyk, Chartrand, Beké et al., 2017), including faculty at colleges that have transitioned to offering baccalaureate education. Furthermore, not all PhD graduates take up positions in academia. A doctoral degree is increasingly required for senior nursing leadership positions in health care agencies and in government or professional organizations, where salaries may be higher than in academia. The deans of Canadian nursing education programs have noted that there are limited financial incentives for nurses to move from clinical to academic positions; as a result,

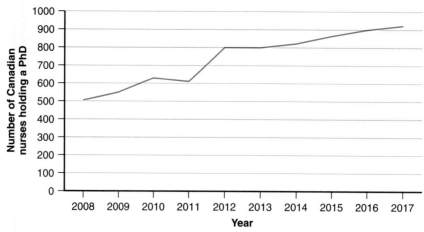

Fig. 8.4 Growth in the number of Canadian registered nurses holding PhD degrees from 2008 to 2017. (**Source:** Canadian Institute for Health Information. (2018). *Regulated nurses 2017*. Ottawa, ON: Author. Retrieved from https://www.cihi.ca/en/regulated-nurses-2017)

many nurses choose to pursue graduate-level education to become nurse practitioners rather than master's degrees that lead to a PhD (Vandyk, Chartrand, Beké et al., 2017).

With the planned introduction of Doctor of Nursing Practice (DNP) education in Canada, more nurses who in the past would have pursued PhD education might instead choose DNP education in preparation for advanced clinical practice. However, the DNP degree does not prepare graduates to conduct research. Some nurse researchers have expressed concern that any growth of DNP programs may threaten the capacity to educate and train future nurse researchers if faculty in PhD programs are stretched to also contribute to DNP programs.

Nursing faculty typically have a shorter career after completing their PhD education compared with professors in other disciplines because of the many years nurses spend in clinical practice or administration before pursuing PhD education. A trend toward more nurses entering graduate studies immediately or shortly after completing their baccalaureate degrees may eventually have an impact on increasing the number of PhD-educated nurses in the workforce.

A continued nursing faculty shortage would lead to an insufficient number of faculty to supervise and train PhD students and postdoctoral fellows. A lack of faculty who can teach at the PhD level translates to a lack of faculty to supervise, train, and instruct undergraduate and master's students. Nursing researchers have expressed concern that this shortage may lead to a redistribution of faculty workload to meet teaching needs, with more time allocated to teaching and hence less time for research (Vandyk, Chartrand, Beké et al., 2017). Proposed solutions include increasing funding for PhD education, drawing on health professionals outside of academia to teach, and hiring faculty with degrees and research related to nursing, such as epidemiology, pathophysiology, or policy (AACN, 2019). Some nurse education leaders surveyed by Vandyk and colleagues (2017) have expressed strong opinions against the idea of hiring faculty who are not nurses. Currently, many Canadian nursing faculties would not hire a professor who lacks graduate nursing education, let alone one who is not a nurse.

Research by Nurses Who Have Not Completed PhDs

Another way to grow nursing research in the face of a looming shortage of PhD-educated nurses at colleges and universities is to support research by nurses in practice, particularly research by advanced practice nurses (see Research Focus box). This approach presents several challenges. Although these positions typically include an expectation of doing research, requirements for clinical service and to support clinical staff make it difficult to have time for research. Research grants are more challenging to obtain when the researcher does not have a PhD degree. A master's education prepares nurses to collaborate on research teams but does not necessarily prepare them to independently design and conduct research (CASN, 2014c); hence, ongoing mentorship and support are required.

RESEARCH FOCUS

Examining the Nurse Practitioner Role in Nonspecialized Palliative Care Practice

Many people who would benefit from palliative care do not receive it. Nurse practitioners (NPs) have been proposed as a way to fill this gap in care. Little is known about how NPs who are not palliative care specialists integrate palliative care into their work with clients with chronic life-limiting conditions. Carmel Collins, a nurse practitioner who specializes in palliative care in St. John's, Newfoundland and Labrador, and Dr. Sandra Small, a professor at Memorial University, conducted a descriptive qualitative study to learn more about the role of NPs who provide palliative care (Collins & Small, 2019). Collins interviewed 19 NPs who were not palliative care specialists and did not work in palliative care settings. Participants described NPs as being "ideally suited" for providing palliative care, stating that there was a "perfect fit" between the NP role and the requirements of palliative care. This fit was associated with their autonomy, their scope of practice, the fact that NPs are present in many settings where palliative care is appropriate, and their ability to be present with patients and families. NPs who had no experience providing palliative care thought that they did not have enough specialized knowledge to provide it. NPs who did have experience providing palliative care thought that this experience gave them the confidence to continue providing palliative care. The findings suggest that by providing continuing education in palliative care and access to consultation from palliative care experts, NPs can incorporate palliative care into their clinical settings, thereby providing palliative care to patients who might not otherwise have access to it.

Source: Collins, C. M., & Small, S. P. (2019). The nurse practitioner role is ideally suited for palliative care practice: A qualitative descriptive study. *Canadian Oncology Nursing Journal, 29*(1), 4–9. https://doi.org/10.5737/2368807629149

Harbman, Bryant-Lukosius, Martin-Misener et al. (2017) reported on an academic–practice partnership designed to support advanced practice nurses to conduct research. The partnership included advanced practice nurses, hospital administrators, and researchers; the support consisted of a 3-month research course designed for the advanced practice nurses, one-to-one mentorship from PhD-educated university professors, and guaranteed release time from supervisors to participate in the education. The advanced practice nurses reported improved knowledge, skills, and confidence related to evidence-based practice and research. They engaged in quantitative, qualitative, and mixed-design research studies and quality improvement research.

However, even with support, it can be very difficult to find the time to engage in research. Landeen and colleagues evaluated supporting advanced practice nurses' research in the Hope Research Community of Practice project (Landeen, Kirkpatrick, & Doyle, 2017). A community of practice is a group of people with a common interest who share experiences, expertise, and support with each other to learn and apply their learning (Landeen, Kirkpatrick, & Doyle, 2017). Two facilitators who had PhDs supported a community of practice that began with seven members, four of whom continued to be involved over the 13 months of the project. The group held monthly 3-hour seminars for 12 months, discussing all aspects of the research process. Funding was available to pay for research expenses such as participant reimbursement, transcription, and equipment and software for data analysis. The researchers found that 12 months was not long enough to complete the research projects. Six months after the seminars ended, one project was completed, one was at the data analysis stage, and two had recruitment challenges and were still in the process of collecting data. Participants felt more confident about conducting research. The most significant barrier was finding time to engage in the research. As a participant described, "It's not an easy thing to add research in. You really have to protect the time. And, of course, I struggled with that, and I wasn't the only one" (Landeen, Kirkpatrick, & Doyle, 2017, p. 131).

Training and Mentorship of Nurse Researchers

Having an established track record as a researcher increases one's chances of obtaining research funding (Cleary, Sayers, & Watson, 2016). Grant reviewers judge an applicant's potential to successfully complete research and disseminate findings based on the applicant's research experience and demonstrated success with funding and publishing. For new researchers, past funding may include scholarships and grant funding, such as small grants to support dissertation research.

A research career can be started by volunteering or working on a research team as an undergraduate student, presenting at professional and research conferences while an undergraduate or graduate student, or revising an academic paper for publication in a peer-reviewed journal. There is a snowball effect of early success as a student, whereby PhD students who have published in peer-reviewed journals are more likely to receive graduate awards and postdoctoral fellowships. Nursing graduate students compete with students in other disciplines for doctoral and postdoctoral fellowships. In many non-nursing disciplines, students complete thesis research as part of their undergraduate and graduate education and thus are more likely to have published than nursing students. By contrast, nursing students tend to complete practice-based master's education with no requirement for thesis research and even less opportunity to publish.

Additional training and mentorship beyond PhD studies is required to establish a career in nursing research, especially with increased competition for diminishing research funds (Cleary, Sayers, & Watson et al., 2016; Happell & Cleary, 2014; Nowell, Norris, Mrklas et al., 2016). The training and mentorship to develop skills such as grant writing, knowledge mobilization, supervision of graduate students, and publication can be obtained through formal postdoctoral training or through mentorship from more experienced researchers. For nurses who are new professors, they can find mentors within their university or seek mentorship from collaborators at other universities.

The NRF, described earlier, supported the development of research capacity in nursing through training awards to master's and doctoral students; postdoctoral awards that allowed new faculty to devote time to establishing their research; regional training centres; and Nursing Research Chairs. The Nursing Research Chair program provided 10 years of funding for the chairholders, including funding for training programs; mentorship; and funding for graduate students, postdoctoral fellows, and junior faculty associated with the Research Chairs. This program had positive effects on the research funding and publications of students, fellows, and junior faculty. For example, as the Advanced Practice Nursing Research Chair at McMaster University, Dr. Alba DiCenso successfully increased the capacity and expertise of nurse researchers to study the impact of advanced practice nurses (Bryant-Lukosius, DiCenso, Israr et al., 2013). Twenty-five graduate students studying at North American universities as well as three junior faculty and two postdoctoral fellows participated in the program. The program resulted in funding for 48 research studies and significant dissemination of research findings, including 787 conference presentations, 236 publications, and 21 book chapters. Other Research Chair holders were similarly successful in launching the research careers of students associated with their programs (Coyte, Wise, & Motiwala, 2008).

APPLYING CONTENT KNOWLEDGE

Consider the support and mentorship needs of new researchers and advanced practice nurses. What kinds of support do these nurses need? Is it possible for advanced practice nurses to conduct research, and should they?

THE IMPACT OF NURSING RESEARCH

It is almost impossible to accurately measure the effects of research in practice professions, including nursing. This has long been a challenge in health research. The lack of convincing evidence of the impact of health research was part of the impetus for research policy changes calling for more citizen engagement in research and funding targeted to government-determined priority topics. A further challenge in nursing has been identifying outcomes that are most likely to be affected by nursing and consistently measuring them.

Bibliometrics and Altmetrics

Many academics quantify the impact of research within a discipline by counting the number of times one publication is cited in another publication and calculating the resulting impact. Journals report this as an "impact factor," a measure of how frequently articles published in the journal are cited in subsequent publications. The h-index quantifies the impact of a researcher's publications. These kinds of measures are called bibliometrics. Databases such as Web of Science, Scopus, and Google Scholar provide the h-index. Hack and colleagues examined the publication records and the h-index of Canadian university nursing faculty in 2010 and again in 2019 (Hack, Bell, Plohman et al., 2019; Hack, Crooks, Plohman et al., 2010). They found a significant increase in the h-index of the most-cited nurse researchers.

Social media is increasingly being used by researchers to share their findings with other academics, practitioners, and the general public. Journals and researchers are also engaging with social media, sharing links that direct their followers to research websites with plain language summaries or to the journal. There is some evidence that health care providers think social media influences their practice and that promotion on social media increases the number of times abstracts are accessed (Borgmann, Dewitt, Tsaur et al., 2015; Thoma, Murray, Huang et al., 2018). Social media may be more effective for brief messages about research findings and less effective at enticing readers to download and read full articles (Thoma, Murray, Huang et al., 2018).

The use of social media for research dissemination has given rise to altmetrics. This new way of measuring research impact is an alternative to the traditional bibliometrics, namely impact factor and h-index. Altmetrics are based on any kind of use of an electronic source (i.e., articles on journal websites). For example, downloads, tweets, shares, likes, posts, Wikipedia citations, bookmarks, and more (Bornmann, 2014). There is a time lag between the publication of research and the publication of new research citing it, whereas research can show up in electronic sources much more quickly. Nurse researchers will likely be increasingly expected to use social media to disseminate their research, and altmetrics will become a more accepted method of measuring research impact (Smith & Watson, 2016).

Bibliometrics and altmetrics are indicators of knowledge transfer. Bibliometrics and, increasingly, altmetrics are used to evaluate researchers as part of hiring and promotion decisions at universities and decisions about research funding. They are, at best, an indirect indicator of potential impact on nursing practice.

Demonstrating the Impact of Nursing Using Standardized Data

As described in detail in Chapter 10, problems have long existed with using standardized data to document the impact of nursing on patient outcomes. The term "minimum data set" (MDS) refers to standardized data that are extracted from all patient records. There are versions of MDS data for hospitals, home care, and long-term care, including items like admitting diagnosis, surgeries performed, complications, discharge diagnosis, cause of death, and so on. MDS data are used by planners, policymakers, and researchers to understand and make decisions about health services. These data are valuable and can be used to examine some indicators of quality nursing care (Estabrooks, Knopp-Sihota, & Norton, 2013). When combined with other data, MDS data can be used to examine the impact of, for instance, nursing staffing mixes and staffing levels on mortality rates or symptoms (Boscart, Sidani, Poss et al., 2018; Estabrooks, Hoben, Poss et al., 2015). However, the MDS was not designed to capture information about nursing problems, nursing interventions, or nursing contributions to patient care. See the next Research Focus to read about the work of Carol Estabrooks and colleagues.

Beginning in the early 1990s, nurses have persisted in doing work to determine what should be included in a nursing MDS and to implement standardized collection of nursing data. This work continues amidst a lack of harmonized electronic data collection in Canadian health care settings (White, Nagle, & Hannah, 2017). An example of this work is the Health Outcomes for Better Information and Care (HOBIC) project in Ontario (Institute for

RESEARCH FOCUS

Dying in a Nursing Home: Treatable Symptom Burden and Its Link to Modifiable Features of Work Context

Residents of long-term care homes experience a high rate of distressing symptoms during their last year of life. Ameliorating these symptoms would improve residents' quality of life and decrease health care costs. Dr. Carole Estabrooks and colleagues used the Resident Assessment Instrument-Minimum Data Set (RAI-MDS 2.0) data, which are routinely collected in long-term care homes, to examine relationships between symptom burden, resident dementia diagnosis, and organizational characteristics of work environments in 36 Canadian long-term care homes (Estabrooks, Hoben, Poss et al., 2015). Organizational context included factors such as leadership, culture, team interactions, resources, and organizational slack. The researchers found a high prevalence of dyspnea, pain, delirium, use of antipsychotics, and challenging behaviour.

The prevalence of these symptoms was higher closer to the time of death. Some symptoms were more prevalent for residents with dementia than among those without dementia, some were less prevalent for residents with dementia, and some were equally likely regardless of dementia diagnosis. Residents in long-term care homes with more positive work environments were less likely to experience dyspnea, pain, and urinary tract infections. These long-term care homes also had higher rates of delirium and challenging behaviour and lower rates of potentially inappropriate antipsychotic use. The researchers concluded that it is possible to optimize the organizational characteristics and culture of long-term care homes and that such enhancements would have a positive impact on suboptimal care in the last year of life.

Source: Estabrooks, C. A., Hoben, M., Poss, J. W., et al. (2015). Dying in a nursing home: Treatable symptom burden and its link to modifiable features of work context. *Journal of the American Medical Directors Association, 16*(6), 515–520. https://doi.org/10.1016/j.jamda.2015.02.007.

Clinical Evaluative Sciences, 2016). The project involves collecting standardized clinical information that is relevant to the work of nursing and other health professionals in acute care, complex-continuing care, home care, and long-term care settings. HOBIC provides a rich source of data for nursing research. For example, Woo and colleagues used the HOBIC database to examine the prevalence and incidence of pressure ulcers and the association between pressure ulcers, patient factors such as functional status and symptoms, and type of health care setting (Woo, Sears, Almost et al., 2017). They found that the prevalence of pressure ulcers varied by type of health care setting.

The prevalence rate in complex-continuing care settings (22.6%) was more than twice the rate in acute care (10.2%) and long-term care (8.4%) settings, leading the researchers to question whether resources and staffing in complex-continuing care fit the needs of patients. About one-third of patients who developed pressure ulcers in long-term care homes did so within 1 week of discharge from acute care settings, suggesting that skin damage occurred in hospital. These data presented an opportunity for improved nursing care with respect to preventing pressure ulcers. The Canadian-HOBIC project has been built on the original HOBIC program (Canadian Nurses Association, n.d.).

SUMMARY OF LEARNING OBJECTIVES

- Nursing research development in Canada is linked to the development of the profession, including nursing education, professional organizations, and professional journals.
- The establishment of master's and doctoral nursing programs in Canada gave nurses the opportunity to train as researchers.
- Nursing professors are expected to conduct research. University faculty have more time and support for research than college faculty, but strategies are being implemented to support research at colleges.

- Research by nurses in health care agencies is less common than it once was. Nurses associated with research institutes in large teaching hospitals conduct large-scale research studies.
- Diversity in the graduate education of nurses before PhD programs in nursing were introduced has resulted in nursing research encompassing many different research methods.
- The topic and focus of nursing research are influenced by trends in the profession, trends in health care, and research funding policy.

- Nursing research teams often include researchers from other disciplines, knowledge users, and stakeholders. Bringing diverse approaches to complex problems should make it more likely that those problems are solved. This approach adds complexity to the research process.
- Engaging patients and service users in the process of determining research priorities, planning research, conducting research, and knowledge mobilization is endorsed in research policy. This is seen as a strategy to improve the relevance, quality, and impact of research. Approaches are similar to some qualitative research methods.
- In the early years of Canadian nursing research, most studies were unfunded. The first major federal funder of nursing research was the NHRDP. The MRC, a larger funding organization, focused on funding biomedical research, not nursing research. Research funds became more available to nurse researchers in the 1990s and early 2000s, when the CIHR was established and the NCP was funded by the federal government.
- Lack of nursing representation in research funding organizations and on research grant review committees was initially a problem for research funding. Nurses are now among the leaders at CIHR and volunteer on grant review committees of major funding organizations.
- Since the early 2000s, government funding for research has been decreasing at the same time as the number of researchers has been increasing, resulting in more competition for research funding and impacting all health research, including nursing.
- Unfunded research is still common. It can contribute to nursing scholarship and advancing nursing knowledge. Small, unfunded studies do not have enough resources to establish evidence of the effectiveness of interventions.
- Canadian nursing associations and nurse leaders lobbied for support for nursing research, including support to develop more nurses with research expertise

and funding for nursing research. Their advocacy was instrumental in achieving research policy changes and major funding to develop Canadian nursing research in the 1990s. There is a continuing need for advocacy.
- Government research funding policies favour strategic funding of research that addresses topics that are priorities to governments. By affecting what kind of research will be funded, this policy affects the kind of research nurses conduct and the topics of their research.
- Research funding policies that require knowledge mobilization and knowledge translation on the part of the researcher are intended to increase the likelihood of research having an impact on Canadians' health. Nurse researchers have increased their knowledge translation skills and include knowledge translation experts on their research teams. Nursing research findings are increasingly likely to be published in open-access formats.
- A growing shortage of nursing faculty in North America is a result of too few nurses graduating with PhD degrees, the short time to retirement of many current faculty, the appeal of nonacademic jobs in health care or government for master's and doctoral graduates, the appeal of advanced practice degrees, and the introduction of DNP education. This shortage may lead to increased demands to teach and less time for research.
- Advanced practice nurses in health care settings can potentially conduct nursing research, but face challenges such as lack of resources and support to build research skills and a lack of commitment from employers.
- Bibliometrics and altmetrics are an indicator of knowledge transfer—of research findings being read or discussed—but they do not necessarily indicate that research is being used.
- Research demonstrating the impact of nursing is facilitated and influenced by nurses' efforts to develop standardized collection and recording of data on patient outcomes.

CRITICAL THINKING QUESTIONS

1. Why has nursing research in Canada changed over the years?
2. Consider the difference between funded and unfunded research. Of the nursing research studies you have read in peer-reviewed journals, which ones reported external funding and which did not? How did funded and unfunded studies compare?
3. Advocacy by nursing organizations was important for building capacity for nursing research in Canada. What

nursing research issues do you think Canadian nursing organizations (CNA, CNSA, and CASN) and provincial nursing associations should be engaged with? Which organizations include nursing research in their mandates?
4. What are the implications of strategic research funding for nursing? Is it possible to reconcile the trends for strategic funding, citizen engagement, and interdisciplinary research with the need to develop core nursing knowledge through research?

5. Select a nursing research article referred to in this chapter. Look up the altmetrics and bibliometrics for your chosen article on the journal website and on Web of Science, Google Scholar, or Scopus. What is the difference between altmetrics and bibliometrics? Which are most important, and why?

6. Write a job posting for a nurse researcher. Include all the educational requirements and skills that you would expect the successful applicant to have.

REFERENCES

American Association of Colleges of Nursing. (2019). *Fact sheet: Nursing faculty shortage*. Retrieved from www.aacnnursing. org/news-information/research-data.

Advisory Panel for the Review of Federal Support for Fundamental Science. (2017). *Investing in Canada's future - Executive summary*. Retrieved from http://www.sciencereview. ca/eic/site/059.nsf/eng/home.

Bethell, J., Pringle, D., Chambers, L. W., et al. (2018). Patient and public involvement in identifying dementia research priorities. *Journal of the American Geriatrics Society*, *66*(8), 1608–1612. https://doi.org/10.1111/jgs.15453.

Black, A., Strain, K., Wallsworth, C., et al. (2018). What constitutes meaningful engagement for patients and families as partners on research teams? *Journal of Health Services Research and Policy*, *23*(3), 158–167. https://doi. org/10.1177/1355819618762960.

Borgmann, H., Dewitt, S., Tsaur, I., et al. (2015). Novel survey disseminated through Twitter supports its utility for networking, disseminating research, advocacy, clinical practice and other professional goals. *Journal of the Canadian Urological Association*, *9*, E713–E717. https://doi.org/10.5489/cuaj.3014.

Bornmann, L. (2014). Do altmetrics point to the broader impact of research? An overview of benefits and disadvantages of altmetrics. *Journal of Informetrics*, *8*(4), 895–903. https://doi. org/10.1016/j.joi.2014.09.005.

Boscart, V. M., Sidani, S., Poss, J., et al. (2018). The associations between staffing hours and quality of care indicators in long-term care. *BMC Health Services Research*, *18*(1), 1–7. https://doi.org/10.1186/s12913-018-3552-5.

Bottorff, J. L., DiCenso, A., Doran, D., et al. (2011). Does nursing research have a future? *Canadian Nurse*, *107*(4), 14.

Brett, J., Staniszewska, S., Mockford, C., et al. (2014). Mapping the impact of patient and public involvement on health and social care research: A systematic review. *Health Expectations*, *17*(5), 637–650. https://doi.org/10.1111/j.1369-7625.2012.00795.x.

Bryant-Lukosius, D., DiCenso, A., Israr, S., et al. (2013). Resources to facilitate advanced practice nursing outcomes research. In *Outcome assessment in advanced practice nursing* (3rd ed., pp. 313–338). New York, NY: Springer.

Canadian Association of Schools of Nursing. (n.d.). *Scholarship*. Retrieved from: http://cnei-icie.casn.ca/our-programs/ continuing-education-course/scholarship/.

Canadian Association of Schools of Nursing. (2013). *Position statement: Scholarship among nursing faculty*. Retrieved from https://www.casn.ca/position-statements/.

Canadian Association of Schools of Nursing. (2014a). *CASN accreditation program standards*. Retrieved from https://www. casn.ca/accreditation/accreditation-program-information/.

Canadian Association of Schools of Nursing. (2014b). *National nursing education framework: Doctoral*. Retrieved from https://www.casn.ca/education/education-home/.

Canadian Association of Schools of Nursing. (2014c). *National nursing education framework: Master's*. Retrieved from https://www.casn.ca/education/education-home/.

Canadian Association of Schools of Nursing. (2014d). *Registered nurses education in Canada statistics: 2012–2013*. Retrieved from http://casn.ca/wp-content/uploads/2014/12/2012-2013-SFS-FINAL-report-revised.pdf.

Canadian Health Services Research Foundation. (2008). *Nursing research in Canada: A status report*. Retrieved from http:// www.cfhi-fcass.ca/migrated/pdf/nursingrescapfinalreport_ eng_finalb.pdf.

Canadian Institute for Health Information. (2018). *Regulated nurses 2017*. Retrieved from https://www.cihi.ca/en/regulated-nurses-2017.

Canadian Institutes of Health Research. (n.d.). *Project grants: Fall 2018 results*. Retrieved May 28, 2019, from http://www.cihr-irsc.gc.ca/e/51312.html.

Canadian Nurses Association. (n.d.). *C-HOBIC Canadian health outcomes for better information and care project*. Retrieved May 30, 2019, from https://c-hobic.cna-aiic.ca/about/default_e.aspx.

Clarke, S. P. (2009). Funding for nursing scholarship, research, and capacity-building: an interview with Dr. Dorothy Pringle. *Canadian Journal of Nursing Research*, *41*(1), 41–45.

Cleary, M., Sayers, J., & Watson, R. (2016). Essentials of building a career in nursing research. *Nurse Researcher*, *23*(6), 9–13. https://doi.org/10.7748/nr.2016.e1412.

Coyte, P. C., Wise, L. M., & Motiwala, S. S. (2008). *An evaluation of the Nursing Research Fund: Lessons to date and recommended next steps*. Ottawa, ON: Canadian Health Services Research Foundation.

Doria, N., Condran, B., Boulos, L., et al. (2018). Sharpening the focus: Differentiating between focus groups for patient engagement vs. qualitative research. *Research Involvement and Engagement*, *4*(1), 6–13. https://doi.org/10.1186/s40900-018-0102-6.

Duncan, S. M., Mahara, S., & Holmes, V. (2014). Confronting the social mandate for nursing scholarship—One school of nursing's journey. *Nursing Education*, *1*(1). https://doi. org/10.17483/2368-6669.1018.

Edwards, N., DiCenso, A., Degner, L., et al. (2002). Burgeoning opportunities in nursing research. *Canadian Journal of Nursing Research*, *32*(4), 139–149.

Estabrooks, C. A., Knopp-Sihota J. A., & Norton P. G. (2013). Practice sensitive quality indicators in RAI-MDS 2.0 nursing. *BMC Research Notes*, 0-5. https://dx.doi.org/10.1186/1756-0500-6-460.

Estabrooks, C. A., Hoben, M., Poss, J. W., et al. (2015). Dying in a nursing home: Treatable symptom burden and its link to modifiable features of work context. *Journal of the American Medical Directors Association, 16*(6), 515520. https://doi.org/10.1016/j.jamda.2015.02.007.

Forsythe, L., Heckert, A., Margolis, M. K., et al. (2018). Methods and impact of engagement in research, from theory to practice and back again: Early findings from the Patient-Centered Outcomes Research Institute. *Quality of Life Research, 27*(1), 17–31. https://doi.org/10.1007/s11136-017-1581-x.

Forsythe, L. P., Carman, K. L., Szydlowski, V., et al. (2019). *Patient engagement in research: Early findings from the Patient-Centered Outcomes Research Institute. Health Affairs (Project Hope), 38*(3), 359–367. https://doi.org/10.1377/hlthaff.2018.05067.

Frohard-Dourlent, H., Dobson, S., Clark, B. A., et al. (2017). I would have preferred more options": Accounting for non-binary youth in health research. *Nursing Inquiry, 24*(1), 1–9. https://doi.org/10.1111/nin.12150.

Gottlieb, L. (2007). Canadian nursing scholarship: A time to celebrate, a time to stand guard. *Canadian Journal of Nursing Research, 39*(1), 5–10.

Government of Canada. (2019). *Canada Research Chairs Chairholders.* Retrieved from http://www.chairs-chaires.gc.ca/chairholders-titulaires/index-eng.aspx.

Grace, P. J., Willis, D. G., Roy, C., et al. (2016). Profession at the crossroads: A dialog concerning the preparation of nursing scholars and leaders. *Nursing Outlook, 64*(1), 61–70. https://doi.org/10.1016/j.outlook.2015.10.002.

Griffin, A. (1971). *Nursing research in Canadian universities.* National Conference on Research in Nursing Practice, Ottawa, ON.

Grigorovich, A., Fang, M. L., Sixsmith, J., et al. (2019). Defining and evaluating transdisciplinary research: Implications for aging and technology. *Disability and Rehabilitation: Assistive Technology, 14*, 533–542. https://doi.org/10.1080/1743107.2018.146361.

Hack, T. F., Bell, A., Plohman, J., et al. (2019). Research citation analysis of Canadian nursing academics: 9-year follow-up. *Journal of Advanced Nursing, 75*(6), 1141–1146. https://doi.org/10.1111/jan.13977.

Hack, T. F., Crooks, D., Plohman, J., et al. (2010). Research citation analysis of nursing academics in Canada: Identifying success indicators. *Journal of Advanced Nursing, 66*(11), 2542–2549. https://doi.org/10.1111/j.1365-2648.2010.05429.x.

Happell, B., & Cleary, M. (2014). Research career development: The importance of establishing a solid track record in nursing academia. *Collegian, 21*(3), 233–238. https://doi.org/10.1016/j.colegn.2013.04.005.

Harbman, P., Bryant-Lukosius, D., Martin-Misener, R., et al. (2017). Partners in research: Building academic–practice partnerships to educate and mentor advanced practice nurses.

Journal of Evaluation in Clinical Practice, 23(2), 382–390. https://doi.org/10.1111/jep.12630.

Health Canada. (2006). *Nursing issues: Research.* Retrieved from https://www.canada.ca/en/health-canada/services/health-care-system/reports-publications/nursing/issues-research.html#a7.

Imai, H. R. (1971). *Association and research activities.* National Conference on Research in Nursing Practice, Ottawa, ON.

Institute for Clinical Evaluative Sciences. (2016). *Health Outcomes for Better Information and Care (HOBIC) acute care in Ontario 2014.* Toronto, ON. Retrieved from http://www.ices.on.ca/Research/Research-programs/Health-System-Planning-and-Evaluation/HOBIC.

Jeans, M. E. (2008). *Nursing research in Canada: A status report.* Retrieved from https://www.cfhi-fcass.ca/migrated/pdf/nursingrescapfinalreport_eng_finalb.pdf%0A%0A.

Landeen, J., Kirkpatrick, H., & Doyle, W. (2017). The Hope Research Community of Practice: Building advanced practice nurses' research capacity. *Canadian Journal of Nursing Research, 49*(3), 127–136. https://doi.org/10.1177/0844562117716851.

Nowell, L., Norris, J. M., Mrklas, K., et al. (2016). Mixed methods systematic review exploring mentorship outcomes in nursing academia. *Journal of Advanced Nursing, 73*(3), 527–544. https://doi.org/10.1111/jan.13152.

O'Connor, A. M., & Bouchard, J. L. (1991). Research activities in Canadian university schools and faculties of nursing for 1988-1989. *Canadian Journal of Nursing Research, 23*(1), 57–65.

O'Keefe-McCarthy, S., & Guo, S. (2014). Development of the Prodromal Symptoms-Screening Scale (PS-SS): Preliminary validity and reliability. *Canadian Journal of Cardiovascular Pain, 26*(2), 10–18.

Pasieka, D.E. (2017). *A history of the evolution of nursing research in the Faculty of Nursing, University of Alberta from 1980 to 1998.* University of Alberta. Retrieved from https://era.library.ualberta.ca/items/ff9c2e3f-3bb7-4cec-bb58-3acfdcceea14.

Phoenix, M., Nguyen, T., Gentles, S. J., et al. (2018). Using qualitative research perspectives to inform patient engagement in research. *Research Involvement and Engagement, 4*(1), 1–5. https://doi.org/10.1186/s40900-018-0107-1.

Poole, P. E. (1971). Research activities conducted or sponsored by government or service agencies. National Conference on Nursing Practice, Ottawa, ON.

Pringle, D. (2006). Realities of Canadian nursing research. In M. McIntyre, E. Thomlinson, & C. McDonald (Eds.), *Realities in Canadian nursing* (2nd ed., pp. 262–281). Philadelphia, PA: Lippincott, Williams & Wilkins.

Skolnik, M. L. (2016). Situating Ontario's Colleges between the American and European models for providing opportunity for the attainment of baccalaureate degrees in applied fields of study. *Canadian Journal of Higher Education, 46*(1), 38–56.

Smith, D. R., & Watson, R. (2016). Career development tips for today's nursing academic: bibliometrics, altmetrics and social media. *Journal of Advanced Nursing, 72*(11), 2654–2661. https://doi.org/10.1111/jan.13067.

Social Sciences and Humanities Research Council of Canada. (n.d.). *Competition statistics*. Retrieved May 28, 2019, from http://www.sshrc-crsh.gc.ca/results-resultats/stats-statistiques/index-eng.aspx.

Stinson, S. M., Lamb, M., & Thibaudeau, M.-F. (1990). Nursing research: The Canadian scene. *International Journal of Nursing Studies, 27*(2), 105–122. https://doi.org/10.1016/0020-7489(90)90065-Q.

Tamblyn, R., Girard, N., Qian, C. J., et al. (2018). Assessment of potential bias in research grant peer review in Canada. *CMAJ, 190*(16), E489–E499. https://doi.org/10.1503/cmaj.170901.

Thoma, B., Murray, H., Huang, S. Y. M., et al. (2018). The impact of social media promotion with infographics and podcasts on research dissemination and readership. *Canadian Journal of Emergency Medicine, 20*(2), 300–306. https://doi.org/10.1017/cem.2017.394.

Thorne, S. (2014a). Toward rediscovering unfunded research. *Canadian Oncology Nursing Journal, 24*(3), 141–143.

Thorne, S. (2014b). What constitutes core disciplinary knowledge? *Nursing Inquiry, 21*(1), 1–2. https://doi.org/10.1111/nin.12062.

Thorne, S. (2019). The study of nursing. *Nursing Inquiry, 26*(1), e12282. https://doi.org/10.1111/nin.12282.

Vandyk, A., Chartrand, J., Beké, É., et al. (2017). Perspectives from academic leaders of the nursing faculty shortage in Canada. *International Journal of Nursing Education Scholarship, 14*(1), 286–297. https://doi.org/10.1515/ijnes-2017-0049.

White, P., Nagle, L., & Hannah, K. (2017). Adopting national nursing data standards in Canada. *Canadian Nurse, 113*(3), 18–22.

Witteman, H. O., Hendricks, M., Straus, S., & Tannenbaum, C. (2019). Are gender gaps due to evaluations of the applicant or the science? A natural experiment at a national funding agency. *The Lancet, 393*(10171), 531–540. https://doi.org/10.1016/S0140-6736(18)32611-4.

Woo, K. Y., Sears, K., Almost, J., et al. (2017). Exploration of pressure ulcer and related skin problems across the spectrum of health care settings in Ontario using administrative data. *International Wound Journal, 14*(1), 24–30. https://doi.org/10.1111/iwj.12535.

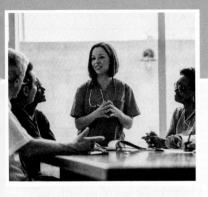

Knowledge Translation and Evidence-Informed Practice

Lynn McCleary

ⓔ http://evolve.elsevier.com/Canada/Ross-Kerr/nursing

LEARNING OBJECTIVES

After reading this chapter, you will be able to:

- List the elements of evidence-informed nursing practice.
- Explain the significance of evidence-informed practice for nursing.
- Analyze the evolution of evidence-informed nursing practice.
- Describe the knowledge-to-action and innovation and diffusion models of the use of research evidence and practice change.
- Explain how filtered sources of evidence increase nurses' access to evidence for practice.

- Describe three types of sources of filtered evidence for nursing practice.
- Describe historical and current programs to reduce barriers to evidence.
- Explain the six steps in the action cycle of the knowledge-to-action process model.
- Describe the roles of administrators, advanced practice nurses, staff nurses, educators, and researchers in evidence-informed nursing practice.
- Describe the stakeholders in evidence-informed practice and their roles.

OUTLINE

KEY TERMS

competencies
filtered research evidence
meta-analysis
opinion leader

policy
research synopses
systematic review

 PERSONAL PERSPECTIVES

It all started at the public health nurses' team meeting during a discussion of activities to mark World Breastfeeding Week. A nurse talked about having attended a conference and learning about organizations that were implementing new practices to support breastfeeding. Another talked about having heard that breastfeeding rates were low in their region. After the meeting, the two nurses confirmed that breastfeeding rates in their region were inconsistent with Health Canada recommendations and they approached their manager. With support from the manager and director, the nurses led a committee that reviewed breastfeeding research evidence as well as current practices, resources, and supports in the health unit. They talked to a leader from another organization where breastfeeding rates were higher. Based on their research, the nurses recommended implementing certain recommendations in the Registered Nurses' Association of Ontario (RNAO) Breastfeeding Best Practice Guidelines (Dennis, Semenic, Abbass-Dick et al., 2018). The director assigned the quality assurance manager to work with the nurses on the project plan. As part of the new public health unit initiative, the nurses would need to update policies, develop new approaches to including family members in breastfeeding education, update in-service education for nurses, modify new-hire orientation and training, and assign a nurse to work with the local breastfeeding peer-support organization. The manager and director regularly checked in on the progress of the new initiative and provided necessary resources.

INTRODUCTION

The research process does not end with the publication of research findings. It continues with the use of research in nursing practice to improve patient care. Much has been written about the challenges of translating research findings into practice. Despite this extensive work, the rate of uptake of research into practice is slow, and practices that have been shown to be ineffective, or worse, harmful, continue (Melnyk, 2017). All health professions are being encouraged to improve "evidence-informed" practice. A central issue is the need to make the use of research findings a natural part of practice, supported by health care systems. Achieving and sustaining evidence-informed practice is a complex issue that must be addressed in all aspects of nursing.

In the past, to ensure that research was incorporated into the everyday practice of nurses, the research had to be part of nurses' knowledge base. Nurses were expected to know almost everything they needed to be able to provide good care. A "good nurse" was one who always knew what to do in any situation. Nurses were expected to learn everything they needed to know in their formal training and education. What they learned in the classroom was put into practice through the service they supplied to their training institutions. With this combination of instruction and practice, most senior nursing students were expected to take charge of a hospital unit and function almost as well as veteran nurses. However, ever-expanding new knowledge means that it is impossible to acquire all the knowledge needed to provide care. Research and technological development can make the knowledge gained in undergraduate education obsolete. Now, nurses must strive to develop skills for lifelong learning, including the skills needed to find new knowledge and evaluate its quality.

WHAT IS EVIDENCE-INFORMED PRACTICE?

Evidence-informed nursing practice is "the ongoing process that incorporates evidence from research, clinical expertise, client preferences and other available resources to make nursing decisions about clients" (Canadian Nurses Association, 2010, p. 3). Other similarly defined terms are evidence-based practice and evidence-informed decision making (DiCenso, Guyatt, & Ciliska, 2005; Yost, Thompson, Ganann et al., 2014). Figure 9.1 illustrates the four components of evidence-informed nursing. As described by DiCenso and colleagues, patient preferences are central to the process and can be influenced by their values, clinical condition, past experiences, family, financial resources, health insurance, and understanding of their options (DiCenso, Guyatt, & Ciliska, 2005). Using

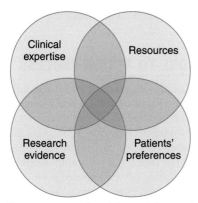

Fig. 9.1 Components of evidence-informed practice. **Source:** DiCenso, A., Cullum, N., & Ciliska, D. (1998). Implementing evidence-based nursing: Some misconceptions. *Evidence-Based Nursing, 1*(2), 38–40. (As adapted from Haynes, R. B., Sackett, D. L., Gray, J. A. M., et al. (1996). Transferring evidence from research into practice. I. The role of clinical care research evidence in clinical decisions. *ACP Journal Club, 124,* 14–16).

the best research evidence means using the most methodologically sound and relevant research about particular assessments, therapies, or management strategies. Clinical expertise is the nurse's use of clinical skills, drawing on past experiences. Finally, the availability of resources influences practice. For example, managers must weigh the benefits of staffing models, equipment, and supplies against cost and budget, meaning that some best evidence may not be implemented. The demonstrated benefits of evidence-informed practice include better patient outcomes, improved safety, decreased morbidity and mortality, and decreased health care costs (Brower & Nemec, 2017).

Evidence-Informed Practice: A Goal for Nursing

Striving to achieve evidence-informed practice is a major goal for nursing, one that is expressed in provincial and territorial standards of nursing practice as well as the Canadian Nurses Association (CNA) *Code of Ethics* (Canadian Nurses Association, 2017). All Canadian nursing professional associations include evidence-informed practice on their websites as a priority. Evidence-informed practice **competencies** are part of the entry-to-practice competencies of provincial nursing regulators in Canada. For example, the Nova Scotia College of Nursing (2013) uses a variation of the definition of evidence-informed care as one of the competencies that new nurses are expected to use when providing nursing care. The Ontario College of Nurses requires that nurses entering practice use

"evidence-informed decision-making to develop health care plans" (College of Nurses of Ontario, 2014, p. 7). In professional documents and publications, many terms are used to refer to aspects of evidence-informed practice, which can be confusing. The terms "knowledge transfer," "knowledge translation," and "research utilization" are sometimes used synonymously with evidence-informed practice. Research utilization seems too narrow, as some knowledge that could be used in practice is not research based. As described in Chapter 8, knowledge translation involves getting research evidence into the hands of practitioners and policymakers, but it does not ensure that the evidence is taken up into practice.

The Evidence-Informed Practice Movement

Although the term "evidence-informed practice" is relatively recent, the issue has been around since the eighteenth century (Mackey & Bassendowski, 2017). Florence Nightingale was the first nurse to advocate for a type of practice that today would be referred to as evidence-informed. For example, using evidence from careful observation and experimentation, considering the effect of patient characteristics on treatment outcomes, and advocating for statistical methods to control for patient differences when comparing institutional death rates were practices implemented by Nightingale in the 1800s and are components of evidence-informed practice today (Brower & Nemec, 2017; Mackey & Bassendowski, 2017).

The modern evidence-informed practice movement is considered to have started in the 1970s. At that time, a large nursing research utilization project was being carried out in the United States (Conduct and Utilization of Research in Nursing [CURN]) (Horsley, Crane, & Bingle, 1978). Yet it is the Scottish physician Archie Cochrane who is regarded as a pioneer of the modern evidence-informed practice movement. He observed that health care providers were not able to gain access to the evidence needed to provide good care. Cochrane was subsequently funded by the National Health Service in the United Kingdom to make research evidence accessible. He believed that preparing reviews and summaries of research in all areas of health care and making them readily available would put evidence within reach of practitioners. This led to the formation of the Cochrane Collaboration, an affiliation of clinician-researchers who generate reviews of research in various areas of health care and maintain them in databases that are available to practitioners and the public. Cochrane Canada is one of 14 international Cochrane Centres. Many health care profession organizations are partners in Cochrane Canada, including the CNA and the RNAO (Cochrane Canada, 2019), and Canadian nurses publish Cochrane reviews.

⚡ RESEARCH FOCUS

Effectiveness of Sucrose for Analgesia in Newborn Infants Undergoing Painful Procedures

Painful procedures are common for infants in neonatal intensive care units. Approaches to prevent or relieve this pain vary and are often not used. Many studies have tested the administration of oral sucrose, with or without a pacifier, prior to and during painful procedures. The researchers in this study conducted a Cochrane review of the efficacy of sucrose for analgesia. In addition to efficacy, the researchers were interested in determining whether differences, if they existed, depended on the use of a pacifier and whether this intervention was safe. Seventy-four randomized controlled trials were included in the review. The researchers found that there was compelling high-quality evidence of effectiveness as an analgesic at heel lance, venipuncture, and intramuscular injections. There was no difference between oral sucrose only and a pacifier dipped in sucrose. Sucrose was not effective for pain from circumcision. Evidence about the effectiveness of sucrose for other painful procedures was limited. Sucrose was not associated with adverse effects.

Source: Stevens, B., Yamada, J., Ohlsson, A., et al. (2017). Sucrose for analgesia in newborn infants undergoing painful procedures. *The Cochrane Collaboration, 2016*(7), 1–254. https://doi.org/10.1002/14651858.CD001069.pub5

The term "evidence-based medicine" was coined in the early 1990s by David Sackett and colleagues at McMaster University (Mackey & Bassendowski, 2017). Initially, the term referred to the use of research evidence in concert with clinical expertise, with the concept of patient preference added later (Brower & Nemec, 2017). DiCenso and colleagues explicitly included another concept—health care resources—in their definition of evidence-based nursing (DiCenso, Cullum, & Ciliska, 1997; see Figure 9.1). The evidence-informed practice movement has been embraced by many practice disciplines, including nursing, and by government agencies. The Canadian government has made a significant investment in evidence-informed practice through policies of research funding agencies that emphasize knowledge mobilization (see Chapter 8) and through support of organizations and agencies that focus on knowledge mobilization. The government has also invested in technology to support evidence-informed practice. These inducements have been effective in moving the Canadian health care system and health care professions, including nursing, towards evidence-informed practice.

KNOWLEDGE-TO-ACTION PROCESS

The process of moving research knowledge into practice is described in the Knowledge-to-Action Framework devised by Graham and colleagues and adopted by the Canadian Institutes of Health Research (Canadian Institutes of Health Research [CIHR], 2016; Graham, Logan, Harrison et al., 2006). The model has two components: (1) the generation and tailoring of new knowledge for users and (2) a cycle of actions to adopt and sustain the use of that knowledge in practice (Figure 9.2).

ENHANCING ACCESS TO EVIDENCE

With millions of health research publications released annually, health care providers are unable to read everything that relates to their practice area, no matter how small the field. Archie Cochrane argued that it is not the volume of available research but practitioners' access to it that is the problem. As described in Chapter 8, researchers are increasingly including clear messages about practice implications in their communication about research findings. However, another challenge with accessing the primary research literature is that researchers often present findings in tentative terms and discuss results as they relate to theory and the need for further inquiry. Researchers may use standard research jargon and emphasize methodological or statistical issues instead of implications for practice. Although sometimes appropriate among researchers, it can be difficult to discern the relevance to nursing practice of findings in published research studies. Many strategies that have been developed to enhance evidence-informed practice are intended to increase the accessibility of research evidence.

The inner funnel of the knowledge-to-action process model (see Figure 9.2) represents the process of reviewing, appraising, collating, and summarizing findings from individual studies to come up with practice recommendations. The products of this process are known as **filtered research evidence**. Filtered evidence lessens practitioners' workloads. Practitioners do not have to find and appraise unfiltered primary research studies. Several sources of filtered evidence are available, including:

1. **Research synopses** of studies that have been appraised for their validity;
2. **Systematic reviews** and **meta-analyses;**
3. Practice guidelines; and
4. Computerized decision-support systems linked to evidence-informed guidelines.

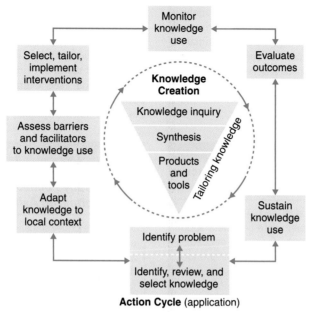

Fig. 9.2 Knowledge-to-action process model. **Source:** Adapted from Graham, I. D., Logan, J., Harrison, M. B., et al. (2006). Lost in knowledge translation: Time for a map? *The Journal of Continuing Education in the Health Professions, 26*(1), 13–24. https://doi.org/10.1002/chp.47

These sources are arranged in a hierarchy, with synopses placed at the bottom of the hierarchy. When valid sources higher on the hierarchy are available, it is not necessary to seek sources lower on the hierarchy. For example, a high-quality practice guideline would be preferred over a systematic review (Alper & Haynes, 2016; DiCenso, Bayley, & Haynes, 2009). Reliable sources of filtered evidence must be chosen to ensure that the best evidence is found, and knowledge users should assess the quality of the process used to create the filtered evidence (DiCenso, Guyatt, & Ciliska, 2005). There are challenges associated with filtered evidence. One, it can become outdated, forcing knowledge users to seek evidence lower on the hierarchy. Two, producing and updating high-quality sources of filtered evidence is time consuming and costly.

Synopses of Individual Studies and Systematic Reviews

One way to help practitioners gain access to research is by enlisting experienced researchers to evaluate published articles or systematic reviews and prepare a summary for practitioners. These synopses of individual articles or individual systematic reviews can ease the practitioner's load. The journal *Evidence-Based Nursing* uses this approach, as do a number of online databases such as BMJ Best Practice, ACP Journal Club, DARE (Database of Abstracts of Reviews of Effectiveness), and Embase. Online subscriptions to many of these sources make it possible for nurses to receive synopses of evidence in their practice fields.

Systematic Reviews

Another approach to making evidence available to practitioners is the systematic review, whereby researchers employ a rigorous method to review the primary research on a specific topic. Strategies are used to surmount biases that can arise during the various stages of a systematic review. Although these methods were originally developed for randomized controlled trials, they are also used for nonrandomized quantitative research (Ciliska, DiCenso, & Guyatt, 2005) and for qualitative research (often referred to as a meta-synthesis) (Patterson, Thorne, & Canam, 2001).

The stages of a systematic review include posing the question, finding the research, applying inclusion and exclusion criteria, abstracting the data, assessing the results, and having the analysis approved by peers (Ciliska, DiCenso, & Guyatt, 2005). In some systematic reviews, the data from a number of studies may be combined and reanalyzed through a process referred to as a **meta-analysis**. The advantage of a meta-analysis is that data from small-sample studies can be combined to give a better estimate of the effect of a treatment than that which could be obtained from individual studies. The meta-analysis also produces a concise, reader-friendly statement of conclusions about particular interventions, saving the practitioner much work.

RESEARCH FOCUS

Does Continuing Education Result in Practice Change?

Continuing education meetings and workshops are commonly used to update health care providers about new research evidence. However, nurse educators who provide these workshops sometimes wonder about how much influence these sessions have on practice. Some people think it is most efficient to provide information succinctly through a lecture with some examples, while others think it is better to have more active and interactive learning. Forsetlund and colleagues conducted and updated a Cochrane systematic review of 81 studies and found that these continuing education workshops can improve practice (Forsetlund, Bjorndal, Rschidian et al., 2012). Workshops that combined interactive learning and lectures were more effective than workshops with just lectures or just interactive learning. However, lectures and workshops were not likely to be effective on their own when complex behaviour change was required. In this case, additional strategies to support practice change are needed.

Source: Forsetlund, L., Bjorndal, A., Rschidian, A., et al. (2012). Continuing education meetings and workshops: Effects on professional practice and health care outcomes. *Cochrane Database of Systematic Reviews, 2009*(2). https://doi.org/10.1002/14651858.CD003030.pub2

The Cochrane Collaboration website contains systematic reviews on many topics. It also includes a record of reviews conducted and published outside of the collaboration. Quality systematic reviews that have been peer reviewed can also be located in health care journals. Many systematic reviews have been completed on topics of interest to nurses, as well as by nurses.

An important source of systematic reviews for evidence-informed nursing practice is the Joanna Briggs Institute (JBI) in Adelaide, Australia. The first North American JBI Centre of Excellence was established at

Queen's University in 2004. Several other Canadian universities are among the 70 universities and educational institutions around the world that make up the Joanna Briggs Collaboration. The JBI supports and facilitates syntheses of research evidence through the Joanna Briggs Collaboration (see Cultural Considerations box.) JBI publishes two journals, *JBI Evidence Synthesis* and *JBI Evidence Implementation*.

CULTURAL CONSIDERATIONS

Joanna Briggs Systematic Review of Culturally Focused Interventions for Hospitalized Asian Minority Patients

Nurses are professionally obligated to provide culturally competent care. A significant proportion of Canadians are from Asian cultures or are Asian immigrants, and understanding ways to improve culturally competent care for this segment of the population is important. Alfred and colleagues conducted a Joanna Briggs systematic review of interventions to improve access to cultural preferences of adult Asian hospitalized patients living in countries where they are a minority (Alfred, Ubogaya, Chen et al., 2016). The researchers found many publications that seemed as though they might be relevant. But after careful review, only three studies provided both an intervention and information about patient satisfaction, including a Canadian study. Interventions in the three studies were multifaceted, with different combinations of interventions in each study. Interventions included Chinese services (e.g., social workers, cultural interpreters), Chinese meals, Chinese signage, cultural training for staff, a Chinese unit with Chinese decorations, and language translation reference tools. Findings suggested that these services were associated with more patient satisfaction with communication, pain management, and treatment. The review noted that all of the included studies used descriptive methods, and thus it was not possible to make conclusions about the effectiveness of the interventions.

Source: Alfred, M., Ubogaya, K., Chen, X., et al. (2016). Effectiveness of culturally focused interventions in increasing the satisfaction of hospitalized Asian patients. *JBI Database of Systematic Reviews and Implementation Reports, 14*(8), 219–256. https://doi.org/10.11124/JBISRIR-2016-003048

Clinical Practice Guidelines

The clinical practice guideline is another useful document for nurses. The guidelines consist of reviews of evidence that culminate with clinical recommendations. Because the clinical practice recommendations are only as good as the guideline, the guideline itself needs to be evaluated. Who participated in the development of the guideline (experts, clinicians, consumers)? Who is sponsoring the guideline (industry, a special-interest group, government, or non-governmental agency)? Is the description of the method comprehensive (including the search for evidence)? Has the guideline been peer reviewed?

There are several online sources for clinical guidelines. The National Guideline Clearinghouse in the United States and The National Institute for Health and Care Excellence in the United Kingdom are reliable sources that can be accessed free of charge. They contain many relevant clinical guidelines. The RNAO website includes nursing best practice guidelines. Specialized nursing clinical guidelines may be published in journals or available through websites. For example, the Hartford Institute for Geriatric Nursing ConsultGeri website includes evidence-informed practice protocols and clinical practice tools for gerontological nursing.

REMOVING SOME BARRIERS TO EVIDENCE

Because of the importance of evidence-informed practice to nursing, governments invested in developing new approaches to help nurses. These initiatives included providing access to resources and developing continuing education programs related to evidence-informed practice. Several of these initiatives were launched in the 1990s and early 2000s, when evidence-informed practice was a funding priority for the federal government and some provincial governments. These programs, such as the SEARCH Canada program in Alberta, the Nursing Chairs programs of the Canadian Health Services Research Foundation (see Chapter 8), and the Centre for Health Evidence at the University of Alberta, included education and support for evidence-informed practice. The NurseOne website of the CNA was available to CNA members and nursing students. It was a portal linking users to many free resources for evidence-informed practice as well as e-journals and e-books. It also included access to resources such as the Cochrane database, ACP Journal Club, and links to other resources for evidence-informed practice. It was replaced by the MyCNA platform, which is more focused on resources internal to the CNA as well as providing access to e-books through Proquest Ebook Central.

RNAO Nursing Best Practice Guidelines

The RNAO Nursing Best Practice Guidelines is a long-standing program developed in 1999 with funding from the Ontario government. It creates clinical guidelines and healthy workplace environment guidelines that are of interest to Canadian nurses. The 50 guidelines can be accessed through an app, which makes them available at or near the bedside. A toolkit and other resources for implementing guidelines are also available through this program. The associated Best Practice Spotlight Organization initiative, established in 2003, supports organizations that implement multiple RNAO guidelines.

 APPLYING CONTENT KNOWLEDGE

Many of the formal programs designed to improve access to knowledge about and for evidence-informed nursing practice were disbanded. What are the potential implications of losing these programs? Do you think that these programs are still needed?

SPREAD OF NEW KNOWLEDGE: INNOVATION AND DIFFUSION

Rogers (2003) provided a useful framework for viewing the process of adopting research into practice. He refers to the new knowledge generated from research as the "innovation" and the process of implementing the innovation as "diffusion." Diffusion of an innovation (new knowledge) occurs in five stages: awareness (or knowledge), persuasion, decision, implementation, and adoption (Rogers, 2003). According to Rogers, diffusion is a process of moving an innovation from an idea to a reality in practice. The process starts with the discovery of the innovation, and then moves on to the communication channel—the means by which the innovation is shared. Another element is the time it takes for an individual to move from the point of discovery to the adoption or rejection of the innovation. A social system is a particular set of interrelated units that jointly engage in problem solving to accomplish a common goal. The social system influences implementation of the innovation. This complex process occurs every time a potential adopter considers a new idea, and it includes forming an attitude, whether positive or negative, about the idea; experimenting with the idea; and finally, choosing to adopt or reject the idea.

Researchers estimate that it takes 8 to 15 years from the time new knowledge is created until the time it is used in practice (Dobbins, Ciliska, Estabrooks et al. 2005). The development of one innovation (penicillin) and its diffusion illustrate this complex process (Box 9.1). Understanding how individuals decide to adopt (or not adopt) new knowledge is useful when planning evidence-informed practice initiatives.

BOX 9.1   The Spread of an Innovation

The story of Sir Alexander Fleming's 1928 discovery of the first antibiotic agent, penicillin, is fairly well known. However, the story of how penicillin came to be used is not.

During World War I, Fleming noticed that many soldiers died from relatively minor wounds that became infected. He began to search for a means of preventing such deaths—an antibacterial agent. Fleming, bemoaning the extra work he had had to do since his lab assistant's departure, considered a stack of Petri dishes that had yet to be cleaned. There was something strange about one dish, however. A mould had grown on the dish and killed the *Staphylococcus aureus* that had been growing there before.

Fleming isolated the "mould juice," naming it "penicillin," and proceeded to publish papers and give lectures about its virtues. No one seemed to care. Fleming received no fame and fortune for his discovery. People could understand cleaning and sterilizing a wound, but injecting people with mould to cure infection did not make sense. Fortunately, one man listened.

A former student of Fleming's, Cecil Paine, was intrigued by Fleming's paper and began to experiment with penicillin. Although the experiments worked—he successfully treated two cases of eye infection—Paine did not disseminate his results. He did, however, discuss his work with Professor Howard Florey.

In 1938, Florey was conducting bacteriology research when Fleming's work was again brought to his attention. Florey was rather indifferent, but his colleague Ernst Chain was fascinated by penicillin. In their experiments, the two established both that penicillin could combat infections and that it was safe to use on humans. The scientific community began to take notice. Then World War II broke out; once again, wounded soldiers would die of infections. In 1941, Florey and an assistant moved to the United States from Europe to continue the research and development of penicillin. There, they developed a method by which penicillin could be produced in far greater quantities. By the end of the war, enough penicillin was produced per year to treat 7 million patients. Deaths due to infection dropped dramatically among soldiers, while hospital patients were quickly and effectively cured of ailments like strep throat, scarlet fever, and various venereal diseases.

Fleming was finally acknowledged when, in 1943, along with Howard Florey, he was knighted and later, in 1945, when he received the Nobel Prize alongside Florey and Chain. Though he is widely credited with penicillin's discovery, it took Florey and Chain to turn his discovery into a safe, usable medicine.

The chain of discovery, dissemination, uptake of knowledge, and development of production methods took nearly 30 years.

PUTTING EVIDENCE INTO ACTION

The action cycle of the knowledge-to-action process model (see Figure 9.2) describes the application of knowledge into practice. It can be used to plan for practice change and the adoption of new evidence in health care organizations or among groups of health care providers. Advance practice nurses and nurse educators are often in a position to use this model to lead evidence-informed practice initiatives. The application of new evidence into practice involves six actions, beginning at the bottom of the circle, where new filtered knowledge exits the inner circle of knowledge creation. The double-headed arrows in the model indicate that cycling can occur back and forth between the actions. Although "sustaining knowledge use" is indicated as the last step, it must be planned for from the beginning of the process.

Identify New Evidence

As with Rogers' (2003) model, the first step in the action cycle is awareness of new knowledge or evidence. This new information could be the result of learning something new or the result of new evidence being sought in response to a problem. For example, as described in the Personal Perspectives box at the beginning of this chapter, practices to support breastfeeding changed because nurses became aware of new knowledge and identified a problem, resulting in their reviewing the evidence. The need for practice change and new evidence could be identified by many different people: nurses at the point of care, nurse leaders, administrators, stakeholders such as patients or academic partners, or policymakers and funders.

APPLYING CONTENT KNOWLEDGE

Thinking about nursing practices in your clinical courses, have you noticed problems where new evidence is needed? What approaches could nurses in your clinical settings use to find evidence?

Adapt Knowledge to Local Context

Throughout the process of moving new evidence into practice, such as implementing practice recommendations from systematic reviews or implementing practice guidelines, one must consider the local context of where the practice change is occurring. As a first step, recommendations may be adapted to take into account differences between settings where the evidence or guidelines were created and the culture, resources, and capacity of the local context of implementation (Harrison, Graham, Fervers et al., 2013; Wang, Norris, & Bero, 2018). Formalized processes for adapting guidelines have been developed, but many of these processes have not been formally evaluated (Wang, Norris, & Bero, 2018). To ensure that the adapted recommendations are valid, the process should be systematic and should include stakeholders in the practice, including those who will support practice change and practitioners.

Guideline adaptation may be done within an organization that wants to use the guideline. For example, a team leading an evidence-informed practice initiative could adapt the guideline. This team would usually be led by an advanced practice nurse and may include other practice experts. Guideline adaptation may also be done by groups of experts, for the benefit of practitioners in contexts that are different from where the guideline was developed.

It may be tempting to forge ahead with practice change to save time and because of the perceived cost of engaging stakeholders. However, it is worthwhile to invest upfront in listening to nurses explain how adopting new evidence relates to their practice context. Failure to consider the local context can lead to the failure of practice change initiatives (Wang, Norris, & Bero, 2018).

Assess Barriers and Facilitators to Knowledge Use

Barriers to knowledge use and the adoption of new evidence can be grouped into four categories: the nature of the new evidence and practice; the organization; the environment; and the individuals who will be changing their practice (Dobbins, Ciliska, Estabrooks et al., 2005). Any of these factors or a combination of them can determine whether or not the new knowledge is adopted. Table 9.1 contains examples of factors that influence the adoption of new knowledge. Barriers and facilitators that are internal to the nurse include attitudes and knowledge about the new evidence, perceived usefulness and relevance of the new evidence, and perceived congruence between the new evidence and the practice context. Most barriers and facilitators are outside the control of individual nurses; for example, equipment, space, time, workload, availability of continuing education, support from supervisors, and

TABLE 9.1 What Influences the Adoption of New Knowledge?

Category	Characteristic
Innovation or knowledge	The innovation is an improvement
	It is acceptable to nurses
	It is easy to understand
	It can be tried on a small scale first
	It can be evaluated
Organization	Structure of the organization (size, number of departments, number of managers, number of services)
	The value the organization places on research
	Success of communication
	Support of research by leadership and resources
Environment	Location—urban or rural
	Financial resources of the region
	Peer pressure to adopt the knowledge
	Degree of competition for resources
	Reputation of the organization compared with those of others in the region
Individual (the nurse)	Attitudes to research
	Ability to make changes to practice

Source: Dobbins, M., Ciliska, D., Estabrooks, C., et al. (2005). Changing nursing practice in an organization. In A. DiCenso, G. Guyatt, & D. Ciliska (Eds.), *Evidence-based nursing: A guide to clinical practice* (pp. 3–19). St. Louis, MO: Mosby.

patient perceptions and attitudes about the practice. The assessment of barriers and facilitators is used to decide what strategies should be used to implement the new knowledge in practice.

The innovation and diffusion model (Rogers, 2003) explains why some people are relatively quick to adopt new knowledge or change practice, whereas others may not adopt the new practice or wait a long time to adopt it. Rogers classified people in relation to their likelihood of adopting a particular innovation. A very small number of people would be classified as innovators who are often sources of new information. They are comfortable with risk when it is uncertain whether a new innovation will be beneficial. They can accept failure when new innovations are not successful. Early adopters are among the first to try a new idea. They can be **opinion leaders** and role models for adopting new practices. Most people fall into the category of the early majority or the late majority. The early majority are those who are deliberate and more cautious about practice change than early adopters are. The late majority are more skeptical about new ideas and need to be convinced by others who have successfully adopted the new practice that it is safe to do so. Finally, the last to adopt new knowledge are classified as laggards, who may have more to lose if the practice change fails and are thus more cautious about change.

CASE STUDY

Assessing Barriers and Facilitators to Knowledge Use

Six home care agencies in Eastern Ontario implemented 15 evidence-informed oncology symptom management guides (Ludwig, Bennis, Carley et al., 2017). As part of the process, the implementation team interviewed and surveyed managers, supervisors, nurse educators, and clinical nurses about their opinions of the guides, how they would need to be adapted, and potential barriers and facilitators to nurses' using them in the agencies. The purpose was to use this information to adapt the guides and to determine approaches to overcome barriers and take advantage of facilitators. Numerous barriers and facilitators were identified. The implementation team organized information about barriers and facilitators to using the guides in four categories: (1) practice guide factors (e.g., layout of the guide did not leave enough space for comments, the guides were in a user-friendly format, relationship to other practices); (2) nurse-level factors (e.g., lack of awareness of the guides, need to learn how to use the guides, adaptability of the guides, and the perception of whether the guide would improve practice); (3) client-level factors (e.g., concern that clients might find the detailed assessments irritating); and (4) organization-level factors (e.g., capacity to train nurses on use of the guides, the potential to incorporate in current documentation). This information was used to identify strategies to successfully implement the guidelines in practice. These strategies include adding training to the orientation of new nurses and making the guides part of the electronic documentation system.

Source: Ludwig, C., Bennis, C., Carley, M., et al. (2017). Managing symptoms during cancer treatments: Barriers and facilitators to home care nurses using symptom practice guides. *Home Health Care Management & Practice, 29*(4), 224–234. https://doi.org/10.1177/1084822317713011

Select, Tailor, and Implement Interventions to Support the Use of New Knowledge

Many strategies can be used to support practice change and the use of new knowledge in practice. Table 9.2 contains

TABLE 9.2   Evidence-Informed Practice Intervention Strategies

Strategy	Example
Education	Presentations, coaching, printed education materials
Audit and feedback	Data about the extent to which specific evidence-informed practices are applied in practice are collated, and the results are shared with practitioners
Local opinion leaders	Influential nurses or resource nurses who deliberately influence others' practice
Patient-mediated interventions	Educating patients about evidence related to their clinical condition
Organizational-level interventions	Changing professional role responsibilities, changing skill mix among nursing staff, enhancing team communication
Integrating new knowledge in organizational processes	Automated patient-specific reminders, integrating clinical pathways in documentation systems, restructuring clinical records

Source: Davies, B., Rothwell, D., McAuslan, D., et al. (2012). *Toolkit: Implementation of best practice guidelines* (2nd ed.). Toronto, ON: Registered Nurses' Association of Ontario.

a summary of strategies. The evidence about which strategies are most effective is developing, but what is known is that multiple strategies are needed (Davies, Rothwell, McAuslan et al., 2012). Continuing education alone does not ensure that new knowledge will be used. Recalling the extent to which factors outside of the individual nurse can act as barriers to using new knowledge, this situation makes sense. However, there is still a tendency to provide in-service education with an expectation that it will result in the adoption of new practices. Support from supervisors and leaders is required throughout the process (Bornbaum, Kornas, Peirson et al. 2015; Gifford, Squires, Angus et al., 2018).

Monitor Knowledge Use and Evaluate Outcomes

Monitoring knowledge use and evaluating outcomes are overlapping activities. The plan for monitoring and evaluation should be in place early in the process of implementing evidence-informed practice change initiatives. Results can be used to modify implementation strategies and to fine-tune plans for sustaining practice change. Monitoring knowledge use includes examining processes (e.g., number of nurses that attended education about the new practice, the extent to which knowledge and skills changed as a result of the education, engagement of nurses with coaches and mentors) as well as structures to support the new practice (e.g., embedding the practice in policy, changing documentation). Evaluating the outcome means assessing the outcomes for staff and clients (e.g., improved pain scores, decreased prevalence of skin breakdown). This is the same approach used in quality improvement (see Chapter 12).

APPLYING CONTENT KNOWLEDGE

Think about the clinical settings where you have been. How are data about nursing practices collected? To what extent is research evidence embedded in policies and procedures?

Sustain Knowledge Use

Without concerted efforts, people tend to fall back to old ways of doing things. One definition of sustainability is "when new ways of working and improved outcomes become the norm" (Maher, Gustafson, & Evans, 2010, p. 6). Sustainable knowledge use means that "not only have the process and outcome changed, but the thinking and attitudes behind them are fundamentally altered and the systems surrounding them are transformed as well. In other words, the change has become an integrated or mainstream way of working rather than something 'added on'" (Maher, Gustafson, & Evans et al., 2010, p. 6). Factors that influence sustainability are summarized in Table 9.3. Sustainability depends on the success of earlier steps in the action cycle and advance planning. Engagement of senior leaders and clinical leaders in the organization, such as administrators, nursing managers, and clinical educators, is vitally important (Gifford, Squires, Angus et al., 2018; Maher, Gustafson, & Evans et al., 2010). Senior leaders must therefore be deeply involved in the process and use their influence to remove barriers to sustaining evidence-informed practices. Furthermore, clinical leaders who are respected understand and promote particular evidence-informed practices, take responsibility to overcome barriers, and actively support change (Maher, Gustafson, & Evans et al., 2010).

NURSING ROLES IN KNOWLEDGE TRANSLATION AND EVIDENCE-INFORMED PRACTICE

Clearly, knowledge translation and achieving evidence-informed practice are complex processes. Who is responsible for this complex set of activities? In addition to researchers, there is the need for nurses working in administration, education, and clinical practice to have specific and critical responsibilities that may best be realized

TABLE 9.3	Factors That Influence Sustainability
Element	**Component Factor**
Process	Benefits beyond helping patients are evident to and experienced by nurses and other stakeholders (e.g., decreased duplication of efforts, improved workflow)
	Evidence is perceived as credible by nurses and stakeholders
	The new practice is adaptable and does not depend on one person or group of people to keep it going
	There is a system to monitor progress and communicate results to stakeholders
Staff	Staff are involved from the beginning and throughout the change process
	Staff are supported to become confident with new evidence-informed practices
	Staff share ideas about and experience with the practice change, and these ideas influence the process
	Senior leaders visibly demonstrate and communicate their support of the new practice and use their influence to overcome barriers
	Extensive involvement of clinical leaders in supporting the practice change
Organization	The new practice fits with the organization's culture and strategic priorities, and sustaining the new practice is a priority
	Infrastructure supports sustained evidence-informed practice
	Staff have education and confidence to enact the new practice
	The evidence-informed practice becomes part of policies and procedures, and there are appropriate spaces, equipment, and supplies

Source: Maher, L., Gustafson, D., & Evans, A. (2010). *Sustainability model and guide.* NHS Institute for Innovation and Improvement. Retrieved from https://improvement.nhs.uk/resources/Sustainability-model-and-guide/

through collaborative partnerships. Although interdisciplinary collaboration is often needed, partnerships within nursing are the crucial first steps.

Administrators

Organizations that support evidence-informed practice infuse their corporate philosophy, mission, vision, and strategic plan with this sentiment. At the senior management level, nursing administrators are responsible for ensuring that the philosophy, mission, vision, and strategic plan are integrated into daily operations. Administrators contribute to an evidence-informed practice culture by ensuring that nursing policies and procedures are based on nursing research findings; developing job descriptions for staff that include evidence-informed practice competencies; and making infrastructure support available (e.g., evidence-informed practice mentors like advanced practice nurses and clinical educators, access to library resources) (Melnyk, 2014).

At the operational level, nursing unit managers anchor organizational efforts for evidence-informed practice. They are responsible for establishing a climate that encourages inquiry and change, where nurses feel free to question practice and have the time and resources to read and critique research and research syntheses. Other nurse manager activities to support evidence-informed practice include participation in evidence-informed practice initiatives; modeling evidence-informed decision making; managing resources; supporting collaboration, including evidence-informed competencies in staff hiring and performance appraisals; celebrating nurses' engagement in research and evidence-informed practice; and removing barriers to evidence-informed practice (Melnyk, 2014; Shuman, Ploutz-Snyder, & Titler, 2018). Increasing attention is being directed to supporting nurse managers' gaining competencies for leadership of evidence-informed practice, with some indication that there is room for improvement (Shuman, Ploutz-Snyder, & Titler, 2018). Training and education to improve nurse managers' knowledge, skills, and attitudes about evidence-informed practice and their leadership role in evidence-informed practice is being developed and evaluated (Shuman, Ploutz-Snyder, & Titler, 2018).

Staff Nurses

Ultimately, it is staff nurses who incorporate research into their practice. Staff nurses have important roles throughout the knowledge-to-action process: they raise questions that lead to research; identify new research evidence; collaborate in research, thus contributing to the practice utility of research (see information about stakeholder involvement in Chapter 8); and collaborate in planned evidence-informed practice initiatives. Registered nurses are expected to find and critique nursing and other health

research, be knowledgeable about research related to health issues, use an evidence-informed approach to providing care, and collaborate to support the use of research findings in practice (College of Nurses of Manitoba, 2018). A survey of over 2,000 nurses in 19 US health care systems found that there were substantial deficits in nurses' evidence-informed practice competencies (Melnyk, Gallagher-Ford, Zellefrow et al., 2018). Strategies to improve evidence-informed practice competencies of staff nurses include mentorship, continuing education, involvement in research, and involvement in evidence-informed practice initiatives.

Educators

Other partners in evidence-informed nursing practice are nursing educators, those who teach in academic settings, and those who instruct nursing staff in the clinical area. Collaboration between nurses in academic settings and in practice settings for conducting research has become more common (see Chapter 8). These same collaborative partnerships can be used to enhance evidence-informed nursing practice. For example, academic-based nurses who have cross-appointments in practice settings participate in evidence-informed practice initiatives. Their knowledge and access to university libraries and graduate students can contribute to successful practice-change initiatives.

Educators also develop and deliver nursing curricula, preparing new nurses for evidence-informed practice. While nursing education emphasizes the importance of evidence-informed practice, there is variability in educational approaches. Most health disciplines have taught emerging practitioners to approach learning new knowledge the same way they have taught researchers. This process involves a lengthy search of unfiltered research evidence, reading many articles, integrating the findings into a coherent piece, and then forming conclusions that can be applied. This approach helps students to improve analytic skills and develop the information literacy needed for evidence-informed practice, but there has been less attention on learning to access and critique filtered evidence. An integrative literature review concluded that undergraduate nursing education effectively instills positive attitudes about using research and evidence-informed practice, but improvements are needed in terms of students' confidence to use research for evidence-informed practice (Ryan, 2016). Integrating evidence-informed practice assignments in clinical courses has been suggested as a way to improve competency for evidence-informed practice (Horntvedt, Nordsteien, Fermann et al., 2018). Melnyk and colleagues developed a set of 13 evidence-informed practice competencies for registered nurses that can be used by educators to evaluate curricula (Melnyk, Gallagher-Ford, Long et al., 2014).

Clinical educators in health care facilities, who are responsible for continuing education and in-service education for nursing staff, have a significant role to play in offering programs designed to enhance evidence-informed nursing competencies. Returning to the survey of over 2,000 nurses in the United States—where nurses showed substantial deficits in evidence-informed practice competencies—we once again see that nurses who reported having access to mentorship for evidence-informed practice had higher levels of competencies; this research reinforces the importance of clinical educators and advanced practice nurses (Melnyk, Gallagher-Ford, Zellefrow et al., 2018). Clinical educators are often responsible for providing education about new evidence-informed practices and must be knowledgeable about the most effective ways to do so.

Researchers

Nurse researchers are prominent in the relatively new field of implementation science that grew out of the evidence-informed practice movement. Implementation science is the study of methods to achieve evidence-informed practice. This research includes developing theories and models of evidence-informed practice as well as developing and testing approaches to improve evidence-informed practice. For example, Carole Estabrooks, a professor at the University of Alberta, has held a Canada Research Chair in Knowledge Translation since 2005. She has an extensive research program and has trained many graduate students who now have their own knowledge translation research programs. She leads Translating Research in Elder Care (TREC), a research program that includes a multi-site longitudinal study of research use in Canadian long-term care homes. TREC has thus far published 77 journal articles (Translating Research in Elder Care, 2019) and made significant contributions to knowledge about evidence-informed nursing practice.

Advanced Practice Nurses

Clinical nurse specialists and nurse practitioners are known as advanced practice nurses (APNs). They play an important role in facilitating evidence-informed practice. Several APN competencies relate to evidence-informed practice, in addition to the role of the APN in conducting research (Box 9.2). To facilitate evidence-informed practice, APNs need to be knowledgeable about change theory and knowledge translation theory. Effective facilitators are perceived as credible and trustworthy. They have clinical expertise and expertise in coaching, mentoring, and educating. They are encouraging and positive about change. They have good networking and communication skills and are able to lead

---

⚡ RESEARCH FOCUS

The Importance of Clinical Educators in Research Use

This study from Carole Estabrooks' TREC research program was based in the PARiHS framework of research use, which specifies that three factors influence evidence-informed practice: the evidence, facilitation, and practice context. Knowing that clinical educators have a positive influence on evidence-informed practice in hospitals, the researchers wanted to know whether this was the case in long-term care (LTC) homes. The authors mentioned some notable differences between hospitals and LTC homes, namely that most direct care in LTC homes is provided by health care aides monitored by regulated health care providers and that nurse educator roles are embedded within other nursing roles in a variety of ways in LTC homes. The researchers conducted a cross-sectional survey of 3,873 care aides from 294 units in 91 LTC homes in Western Canada. They found that health care aides' research use was positively associated with facilitation (frequency of contact with a clinical educator or someone who brings new ideas), unit leadership, supportive work culture, and being on a unit where data are issued to evaluate care quality. The relationship between research use and facilitation depended on unit-level leadership. In units where leadership was low, facilitation had a stronger association with research use; it compensated for the lower effects of leadership on research use. There was a similar finding for unit culture, such that facilitation had a stronger association with research use where there was a less supportive work culture. The effect of facilitation on research use was enhanced in units that were more likely to use data to evaluate quality, such that there was synergy between facilitation and evaluation practices. The researchers concluded that clinical educators have a positive effect on the evidence-informed practice of health care aides in LTC homes and that the magnitude of this effect is influenced by other factors that affect research use.

Source: Lo, T. K. T., Hoben, M., Norton, P. G., et al. (2018). Importance of clinical educators to research use and suggestions for better efficiency and effectiveness: Results of a cross-sectional survey of care aides in Canadian long-term care facilities. *BMJ Open, 8*(7), 1–9. https://doi.org/10.1136/bmjopen-2017-020074

teams (Cranley, Cummings, Profetto-McGrath et al., 2017; Melnyk, Gallagher-Ford, Long et al., 2014).

Knowledge Brokers

Knowledge brokers play an intermediary role between researchers and research users. This role is relatively new in health care. It can be a standalone role, where knowledge brokering is the person's sole responsibility, or it can be incorporated into other roles (e.g., as part of the advanced practice nursing role). The role varies, but it can encompass three types of activities: (1) involvement in research and application of research; (2) facilitating exchange between researchers and knowledge users, including decision makers and practitioners, to support evidence-informed practice; and (3) building capacity for evidence-informed practice (Cranley, Cummings, Profetto-McGrath et al., 2017). Other specific tasks that knowledge brokers engage in that support nurses' evidence-informed practice include searching for and retrieving research evidence; synthesizing research findings and creating tailored knowledge products; identifying opportunities for evidence-informed practice; providing education and training related to evidence-informed practice; evaluating practice change; and supporting sustainability (Bornbaum, Kornas, Peirson et al., 2015). There is no specific education for the role. The effect of knowledge brokers on evidence-informed practice is still being evaluated (Bornbaum, Kornas, Peirson et al., 2015; Cranley, Cummings, Profetto-McGrath et al., 2017). In the meantime, it is becoming a more common role.

STAKEHOLDERS IN BEST PRACTICE

Nurses and other health care providers are not the only stakeholders in evidence-informed practice. Manufacturers, policymakers, media, and the public are also stakeholders.

Industry

In health care, new knowledge often means that new products and drugs become available. Hence, one of the earliest stages of achieving best practice is the exchange of

RESEARCH FOCUS

Promoting Best Practices to Prevent and Manage Incontinence-Associated Dermatitis

Allison D'Hondt and Esther Coker (2019), two advanced practice nurses at a complex continuing care hospital in Hamilton, Ontario, led an evidence-informed practice project to standardize the nursing approach to preventing and managing incontinence-associated dermatitis (IAD). IAD causes pain, discomfort, infection, and pressure ulcers. Ulcers are difficult to distinguish from pressure injuries as well as difficult and costly to treat. Prevalence of IAD was determined by adding an IAD assessment to the routine yearly audit of pressure injuries. The researchers found that 22% of patients had signs of IAD, and of these, 26% had a documented care plan to address IAD. D'Hondt and Coker started by engaging staff nurses to create new skin care guidelines. The nurses identified several challenges with prevention and management of IAD, including inconsistent preferences for and use of skin products and nonspecific documentation. A care protocol linked to the severity of IAD was developed, specifying which products to use for cleansing and which products to use for protecting the skin. A representative from the product manufacturer participated in education about the correct use of products. The protocol was trialed on one unit before being implementing in the rest of the hospital so that the protocol could be revised based on staff feedback. Effectiveness will be evaluated by reassessing prevalence of IAD.

Source: D'Hondt, A., & Coker, E. (2019). *Promoting best practices to prevent and manage incontinence-associated dermatitis.* Canadian Gerontological Nursing Association 20th Biennial Conference, Calgary, AB.

knowledge between the research laboratory and the manufacturer so that products can be developed, marketed, and distributed. However, simply making products available does not guarantee their use, nor are all new products or drugs as effective as manufacturers' advertising claims. An evidence-informed approach to selecting products and supplies is needed.

The pharmaceutical industry is highly engaged in knowledge transfer. Once a product has been developed, the pharmaceutical industry invests heavily in advertising so that the product will be used (and profits will be made). The target advertising audience is typically physicians, pharmacists, and hospitals and, where permitted, the public, as a strategy for indirectly influencing physicians to prescribe their products.

Evidence-Informed Policymaking

One outcome of the evidence-informed practice movement is the evidence-informed **policy** movement. A goal of the health care system is to ensure that practice is the best that can be achieved with safe, effective, and cost-efficient interventions. One of the best ways to achieve this goal is to make sure that health care policy decisions are based on the best evidence. Nevertheless, few policy decisions could be defined as evidence-informed. This ought not to be a surprise, because policymaking is a complex matter in which research evidence is only one of many influencing factors.

Breast cancer screening illustrates some of that complexity (Gray, 1998). The US National Institutes of Health (NIH) convened a consensus conference to look at the evidence for or against routine mammography screening of women aged 40 to 49. Based on the evidence, the panel recommended that screening of women before 50 years of age was not necessary, a recommendation that was consistent with those made in Canada and the United Kingdom. Led by the *New York Times*, the press launched a vicious attack on the NIH experts, whom they accused of killing American women. This hyperbole attracted the attention of Congress, which applied pressure to the National Cancer Institute (NCI). Members of the NCI Advisory Board subsequently overruled the Consensus Panel decision, recommending payment for routine mammographic screening for women in the United States beginning at age 40. They opted for values over evidence. A similar process occurred 10 years later (Deppen, Aldrich, Hartge et al., 2012). In 2009, the US Preventative Service Task Force revised their recommendations based on new systematic reviews that found overdiagnosis through screening among young women. The task force continued to recommend routine screening after age 50 and recommended that regular screening before this age should be an individual decision. Again, the media questioned the recommendation, and

legislators maintained funding for routine screening mammograms for women under age 50.

The Role of the Public

The public is community members (including patients and their families) and the media. These groups, which have a powerful influence on the use or nonuse of health care therapies and practices, are often the groups that are most disadvantaged when it comes to dealing with science and evidence. The public lacks technical knowledge about research and health disciplines. They trust researchers and health care providers to supply them with unbiased, accurate information.

As the example about mammography demonstrates, community members and the media have important roles in making decisions about what interventions will be available or used. They can push an innovation into the marketplace or pull it back into obscurity. In 2002, the media reported early results from one study about adverse events associated with combined progesterone–estrogen hormone replacement therapy (Health Canada, 2004). Women taking any kind of hormone replacement therapy abandoned their drugs virtually overnight, without medical supervision. In another historic case, the public successfully pushed to have an innovation made available that practitioners were not convinced was safe or efficacious (Box 9.3).

An Example of the Adoption of Poor Evidence

In the late 1990s, rumours had been circulating about a possible link between the vaccine for measles, mumps, and rubella (MMR) and the development of autism in children. Then, a fatally flawed British study was published in *The Lancet* in 1998 (Wakefield, Murch, Anthony et al., 1998). A group of 12 children had been selected to participate in a study because they had two syndromes: bowel symptoms and autistic-like behaviour (there was no control group). The children ranged in age from 3 to 10 years. Parents were asked to recall whether the onset of behavioural symptoms occurred after vaccination. The potential for recall errors and biased responses was high. Some parents had to think back a long way, and all parents knew they were participating in a study about the link between autism and MMR vaccination.

The tone of the *Lancet* article suggested a relationship between these syndromes and MMR vaccination even though the authors said, "We did not prove an association between measles, mumps and rubella vaccine and the syndrome described." In the last paragraph of the article, the researchers said, "Onset of symptoms was after measles, mumps, and rubella immunisation." When the article was released, the media picked it up as a potentially hot story given recent rumours and parents' natural fears about their children. At a press conference, the lead researcher stepped

BOX 9.3 The Public Push

At the beginning of the 1800s, Joseph Priestley tested the effects of various gases on animals and humans, measuring their therapeutic effects. At the same time, an American chemist named Humphrey Davey conducted a series of experiments to determine the effects of inhaling different quantities of gases, including oxygen, hydrogen, nitrous oxide, and carbon dioxide. He noted the power of nitrous oxide to calm the pain of a bad toothache and headache. At the time, nitrous oxide was primarily used as an attraction at travelling shows; patrons could choose to inhale the gas and experience its effects—euphoria and laughter. On one occasion, a group of patrons, who accidentally inhaled too much of the gas, went into a deep sleep.

Following one such exhibition, a dentist named Horace Wells supposed that nitrous oxide could be used to suppress pain during tooth extraction. He believed in this proposition so strongly, in fact, that in 1844, he extracted one of his own teeth while under the influence of nitrous oxide. He was subsequently embarrassed when, at a public demonstration, his "anaesthetized" patient cried out in pain—perhaps he had not used a high enough dose.

At around the same time, the American surgeon William Crawford Long was experimenting with the use of ether as an anaesthetic. His experiments, performed largely on himself and his assistants, culminated in the first use of anaesthesia for surgery. In March 1842, he removed a tumour from the neck of a patient. The patient had been anaesthetized with ether and felt no pain whatsoever. Long did not make this information public. However, in 1846, eminent surgeon John Warren held a public demonstration, much as Wells had. His presentation went far better, though, as the patient anaesthetized with ether felt no pain when a tumour was surgically removed from his cheek. People began to take note of anaesthetics.

At the time, ether was held in far higher esteem than nitrous oxide. Nitrous oxide was, after all, essentially a sideshow attraction at travelling circuses, known more for its ability to induce laughter than its effectiveness at reducing pain. Ether, on the other hand, was already in common use as a medical agent—though not yet as an anaesthetic.

In 1847, Wells travelled to the Académie de médecine in Paris to propose the use of nitrous oxide and ether as anaesthetics. Wells' work, combined with news of the surgery performed by Dr. Warren, prompted a debate at the Académie de médecine and the academies of sciences. While some doctors were quick to praise the virtues of anaesthesia, others, most notably Dr. François Magendie, fought against it. How were surgeons to work without the cries of the patient to guide them? How would an unconscious patient know when the surgeon was making mistakes or being too heavy handed?

Despite these objections, news of anaesthesia soon found its way into the press. The public avidly supported the idea of painless surgery, and the press catalyzed their hopes. The public's impatience, bolstered by continuing accounts of the wonders of anaesthesia, led to enormous pressure on the scientific community. Thus, both ether and a new substance, chloroform, were quickly incorporated into standard surgical practice.

outside the limits of the research and announced that MMR should not be given to children.

The story received worldwide attention and created confusion and fear. Shocking details about the research emerged for many years afterward. Wakefield, the lead investigator, was accused of taking money to find a link between MMR and autism—the money was alleged to have come from a legal group that wanted to sue the drug manufacturer. He was also accused of wanting to discredit the MMR vaccine so that he could develop his own vaccine. The research did not receive peer review to determine whether it had adhered to ethical guidelines, a step that could have uncovered the financial relationship and other conflicts of interest. Whether or not these conflicts of interest influenced data analysis is unclear; however, the data were incorrectly interpreted to suggest a link between MMR and autism. As the controversy grew, Wakefield's coinvestigators and *The Lancet* distanced themselves from the research. Eventually, Wakefield faced a disciplinary hearing before the medical association. *The Lancet* published its regrets and retracted the article, and other medical journals published position statements in an attempt to offset the negative effects of the news stories.

The result of the media attention was a significant drop in MMR vaccinations as well as outbreaks of measles and measles-related deaths. Much effort has been made to overcome this misinformation, and its impact has diminished. However, it is still present in social media and continues to impact vaccine hesitancy (Jang, Mckeever, Mckeever et al., 2019). There are evidence-informed guidelines to support nurses' work with parents who are hesitant about childhood vaccination (MacDonald, Desai, Gerstein et al., 2018). This is an example of invalid research that should not have been published and should never have influenced practice or behaviour. It is also an example of how misinformation sticks (Gould, 2017) and how valuable nurses' roles are in using evidence-informed practice to overcome misinformation.

APPLYING CONTENT KNOWLEDGE

The example of the adoption of poor evidence (MMR and autism) and the discussion about influenza immunization raise questions about what nurses can and should do when these situations arise. What are the responsibilities of the individual nurse and of nursing associations when the adoption of poor evidence threatens public health?

SUMMARY OF LEARNING OBJECTIVES

- Evidence-informed nursing practice means using research evidence and clinical evidence, considering client preferences and available resources. It results in improved outcomes for patients and the health care system.
- Nursing professional associations and nursing practice regulators prioritize evidence-informed practice.
- Although the term evidence-informed nursing practice is relatively new, advocating for use of research in nursing practice is not new.
- The evidence-informed practice movement in medicine and health care influenced the development of knowledge about evidence-informed nursing practice, and the larger evidence-informed practice movement was influenced by nursing and nurse leaders.
- The knowledge-to-action process model includes two components, generating knowledge and adopting that knowledge into practice.
- Accessibility of new knowledge to practitioners is enhanced through the creation of knowledge products that filter evidence—such as synopses, systematic reviews, practice guidelines, and computerized decision-support systems—so that practitioners do not have to read and critique the primary research to answer their practice questions and achieve evidence-informed practice.
- Sources of filtered evidence include the Cochrane database of systematic reviews, the Joanna Briggs Collaboration, and the RNAO.
- Many of the programs to improve evidence-informed nursing practice that were established in the 1990s and 2000s were disbanded when they were no longer a priority for government funders. The RNAO practice guideline program continues.
- According to Rogers' Diffusion of Innovation Framework, the process of new ideas being adopted into practice is complex and can take years. The process involves individuals and groups of people becoming aware of the knowledge, being persuaded to use it, deciding to use it, beginning to implement it, and adopting it fully into their practice. The social system in which knowledge is adopted influences the process.
- The decision to implement new knowledge into nursing practice can be initiated by learning about new evidence

for practice through the recognition of a problem and the resulting search for knowledge to solve the problem.
- Successful adoption of new evidence-informed practices is influenced by the local context, and evidence-informed practice recommendations and guidelines may need to be adapted to the local context, either formally or informally.
- Barriers and facilitators to adopting new knowledge may be internal to the nurse or external to the nurse, in the practice environment. People vary in their willingness and ability to take risks and adopt new knowledge into their practice.
- The choice of strategies to support practice change depends on identifying barriers and facilitators to the new evidence-informed practice. Multiple strategies are often required, and support from supervisors and leaders throughout the process is essential.
- Monitoring and evaluating a new evidence-informed practice involves assessing processes, structures, and outcomes.
- Sustaining new evidence-informed practice should be planned for early in the change process. It is vitally important that senior leaders and clinical leaders actively support the new practices in to achieve sustained practice change.
- Administrators and managers support evidence-informed nursing practice by developing their personal competencies for such practice and by leading to ensure that it becomes part of organizational culture. These efforts include participating in evidence-informed practice initiatives, ensuring that the organization has policies and procedures that are based on nursing research, incorporating evidence-informed competencies into job descriptions and performance appraisals, providing infrastructure support, celebrating evidence-informed practice achievements, and removing barriers to evidence-informed practice.
- Nursing staff participate throughout the knowledge-to-action cycle and ultimately are the ones who implement evidence-informed practice.
- Educators in colleges and universities collaborate in evidence-informed nursing practice in health care organizations. They determine the curricula that then

influence the extent to which graduating nurses achieve evidence-informed practice competencies.
- Clinical educators and advanced practice nurses play an important role in facilitating evidence-informed practice. In addition, advanced practice nurses must be able to contribute to the development and appraisal of filtered evidence.
- Knowledge brokers are a relatively new addition to health care. They may be involved in research and application of research in practice, facilitating exchange between researchers and knowledge users, and building capacity for evidence-informed practice.

- Manufacturers of new medications and products promote the use of their products, and an evidence-informed approach to decisions about product use is needed.
- Health care policies at the health system level are influenced by evidence and other factors.
- Public attitudes about new evidence influence policy and practice. The media and community members do not have the same competencies for appraising evidence as nurses do. Nurses must use their evidence-informed practice knowledge and skills to counteract misinformation and misunderstanding about research.

CRITICAL THINKING QUESTIONS

1. Describe factors that influenced the development of evidence-informed nursing practice in Canada.
2. Imagine that you are planning to implement new evidence about postoperative pain management in nursing practice at a hospital. How would you involve nursing staff through the action stage of the knowledge-to-action process?
3. Compare the roles of managers and advanced practice nurses in achieving evidence-informed nursing practice.

REFERENCES

Alper, B. S., & Haynes, R. B. (2016). EBHC pyramid 5.0 for accessing preappraised evidence and guidance. *Evidence-Based Medicine, 21*(4), 123–125. https://dx.doi.org/10.1136/ebmed-2016-110447.

Bornbaum, C. C., Kornas, K., Peirson, L., et al. (2015). Exploring the function and effectiveness of knowledge brokers as facilitators of knowledge translation in health-related settings: A systematic review and thematic analysis. *Implementation Science, 10*(1), 1–12. https://doi.org/10.1186/s13012-015-0351-9.

Brower, E. J., & Nemec, R. (2017). Origins of evidence-based practice and what it means for nurses. *International Journal of Childbirth Education, 32*(2), 14–19.

Canadian Institutes of Health Research. (2016). *Knowledge translation.* Retrieved from http://www.cihr-irsc.gc.ca/e/29418.html.

Canadian Nurses Association. (2010). *Evidence-informed decision-making and nursing practice.* Ottawa, ON. Retrieved from https://www.cna-aiic.ca/-/media/nurseone/pagecontent/pdf-en/evidence-informed-decision-making-and-nursing-practice.pdf.

Canadian Nurses Association. (2017). *2017 Edition code of ethics for registered nurses.* Ottawa, ON: Author. Retrieved from https://www.cna-aiic.ca/html/en/Code-of-Ethics-2017-Edition/files/assets/basic-html/page-1.html#.

Ciliska, D., DiCenso, A., & Guyatt, G. (2005). Summarizing the evidence through systematic reviews. In A. DiCenso, G. Guyatt, & D. Ciliska (Eds.), *Evidence-based nursing: A guide to clinical practice* (pp. 235–244). St. Louis, MO: Elsevier Mosby.

Cochrane Canada. (2019). *Cochrane Canada partners.* Retrieved from https://canada.cochrane.org/partners-0.

College of Nurses of Manitoba. (2018). *Entry-level competencies for Registered Nurses.* Retrieved from https://www.crnm.mb.ca/support/resources.

College of Nurses of Ontario. (2014). *Entry-level competencies for Registered Nurses.* Retrieved from https://www.cno.org/globalassets/docs/reg/41037_entrytopracitic_final.pdf.

Cranley, L. A., Cummings, G. G., Profetto-McGrath, J., et al. (2017). Facilitation roles and characteristics associated with research use by healthcare professionals: A scoping review. *BMJ Open, 7*(8), 1–18. https://doi.org/10.1136/bmjopen-2016-014384.

Davies, B., Rothwell, D., McAuslan, D., et al. (2012). *Toolkit: Implementation of best practice guidelines* (2nd ed.). Toronto, ON: Registered Nurses' Association of Ontario.

Dennis, C.-L., Semenic, S., Abbass-Dick, J., et al. (2018). *Breastfeeding-promoting and supporting the initiation, exclusivity, and continuation of breastfeeding for newborns, infants, and young children.* Toronto, ON: Registered Nurses' Association of Ontario. Retrieved from https://rnao.ca/bpg/guidelines/breastfeeding-promoting-and-supporting-initiation-exclusivity-and-continuation-breast.

Deppen, S. A., Aldrich, M. C., Hartge, P., et al. (2012). Cancer screening: The journey from epidemiology to policy. *Annals of Epidemiology, 22*(6), 439–445. https://doi.org/10.1016/j.annepidem.2012.03.004.

DiCenso, A., Bayley, L., & Haynes, R. B. (2009). Accessing preappraised evidence: Fine-tuning the 5S model into a 6S model. *EBN, 12*(4), 99–101. https://dx.doi.org/10.1136/ebn.12.4.99-b.

DiCenso, A., Cullum, N., & Ciliska, D. (1997). *Implementing evidence-based nursing: Some misconceptions, 1*(2), 9–17. https://dx.doi.org/10.1136/ebn.1.2.38.

DiCenso, A., Guyatt, G., & Ciliska, D. (Eds.). (2005). *Evidence-based nursing: A guide to clinical practice*. St. Louis, MO: Mosby, Inc.

Dobbins, M., Ciliska, D., Estabrooks, C., et al. (2005). Changing nursing practice in an organization. In A. DiCenso, G. Gyatt, & D. Ciliska (Eds.), *Evidence-based nursing: A guide to clinical practice* (pp. 172–204). St. Louis, MO: Mosby.

Gifford, W. A., Squires, J. E., Angus, D. E., et al. (2018). Managerial leadership for research use in nursing and allied health care professions: A systematic review. *Implementation Science, 13*, 1–23. https://dx.doi.org/10.1186/s13012-018-0817-7.

Gould, K. A. (2017). Vaccine safety: Evidence-based research must prevail. *Dimensions of Critical Care Nursing, 36*(3), 145–147. https://doi.org/10.1097/DCC.0000000000000250.

Graham, I. D., Logan, J., Harrison, M. B., et al. (2006). Lost in knowledge translation: Time for a map? *The Journal of Continuing Education in the Health Professions, 26*(1), 13–24. https://doi.org/10.1002/chp.47.

Gray, J. A. M. (1998). Evidence based policy making. In A. Haines, & A. Donald (Eds.), *Getting research findings into practice*. London, UK: BMJ Books.

Harrison, M. B., Graham, I. D., Fervers, B., et al. (2013). Adapting knowledge to local context. In S. E. Straus, J. Tetroe, & I. D. Graham (Eds.), *Knowledge translation in health care* (pp. 110–120). Toronto, ON: John Wiley & Sons. https://doi.org/10.1002/9781118413555.ch10.

Health Canada. (2004). *It's your health: Benefits and risks of hormone replacement therapy (estrogen with and without progestin)*. Retrieved from http://www.hc-sc.gc.ca/iyh-vsv/med/estrogen_e.html.

Horntvedt, M. E. T., Nordsteien, A., Fermann, T., et al. (2018). Strategies for teaching evidence-based practice in nursing education: A thematic literature review. *BMC Medical Education, 18*(1), 1–11. https://doi.org/10.1186/s12909-018-1278-7.

Horsley, J. A., Crane, J., & Bingle, J. D. (1978). Research utilization as an organizational process. *The Journal of Nursing Administration, 8*(7), 4–6.

Jang, S. M., Mckeever, B. W., Mckeever, R., et al. (2019). From social media to mainstream news: The information flow of the vaccine-autism controversy in the US, Canada, and the UK. *Health Communication, 34*(1), 110–117. https://doi.org/10.1080/10410236.2017.1384433.

MacDonald, N., Desai, S., Gerstein, B. et al. (2018). *Working with vaccine-hesitant parents: An update*. Retrieved from https://www.cps.ca/en/documents/position/working-with-vaccine-hesitant-parents.

Mackey, A., & Bassendowski, S. (2017). The history of evidence-based practice in nursing education and practice. *Journal of Professional Nursing, 33*(1), 51–55. https://doi.org/10.1016/j.profnurs.2016.05.009.

Maher, L., Gustafson, D., & Evans, A. (2010). *Sustainability model and guide. NHS Institute for Innovation and Improvement*. Retrieved from https://improvement.nhs.uk/resources/Sustainability-model-and-guide/.

Melnyk, B. M. (2014). Building cultures and environments that facilitate clinician behavior change to evidence-based practice: What works? *Worldviews on Evidence-Based Nursing, 11*(2), 79–80. https://doi.org/10.1111/wvn.12032.

Melnyk, B. M. (2017). The difference between what is known and what is done is lethal: Evidence-based practice is a key solution urgently needed. *Worldviews on Evidence-Based Nursing, 14*(1), 3–4. https://doi.org/10.1111/wvn.12194.

Melnyk, B. M., Gallagher-Ford, L., Long, L. E., et al. (2014). The establishment of evidence-based practice competencies for practicing registered nurses and advanced practice nurses in real-world clinical settings: Proficiencies to improve healthcare quality, reliability, patient outcomes, and costs. *Worldviews on Evidence-Based Nursing, 11*(1), 5–15. https://doi.org/10.1111/wvn.12021.

Melnyk, B. M., Gallagher-Ford, L., Zellefrow, C., et al. (2018). The first U.S. study on nurses' evidence-based practice competencies indicates major deficits that threaten healthcare quality, safety, and patient outcomes. *Worldviews on Evidence-Based Nursing, 15*(1), 16–25. https://doi.org/10.1111/wvn.12269.

Nova Scotia College of Nursing. (2013). *Entry-level competencies for Registered Nurses*. Retrieved from https://www.nscn.ca/professional-practice/practice-standards/entry-level-competencies.

Patterson, B. C., Thorne, S. E., & Canam, C. (2001). *Meta-study of qualitative health research: A practical guide to meta-analysis and meta-synthesis*. Thousand Oaks, CA: Sage Publications.

Rogers, E. M. (2003). *Diffusion of innovations* (5th ed.). New York, NY: Free Press.

Ryan, E. J. (2016). Undergraduate nursing students' attitudes and use of research and evidence-based practice—an integrative literature review. *Journal of Clinical Nursing, 25*(11–12), 1548–1556. https://doi.org/10.1111/jocn.13229.

Shuman, C. J., Ploutz-Snyder, R. J., & Titler, M. G. (2018). Development and testing of the Nurse Manager EBP Competency Scale. *Western Journal of Nursing Research*(2), 175–190.

Translating Research in Elder Care. (2019). *Translating research in elder care: Our publications*. Retrieved from https://trecresearch.ca/resources/publications.

Wakefield, A., Murch, S., Anthony, A., et al. (1998). Ileal-lymphoid-nodular hyperplasia, non-specific colitis, and pervasive developmental disorder in children. *The Lancet, 351*, 637–641 (Retraction published February, 2010, *The Lancet, 375*, 445).

Wang, Z., Norris, S. L., & Bero, L. (2018). The advantages and limitations of guideline adaptation frameworks. *Implementation Science, 13*(1), 1–13. https://doi.org/10.1186/s13012-018-0763-4.

Yost, J., Thompson, D., Ganann, R., et al. (2014). Knowledge translation strategies for enhancing nurses' evidence-informed decision making: A scoping review. *Worldviews on Evidence-Based Nursing, 11*(3), 156–167. https://doi.org/10.1111/wvn.12043.

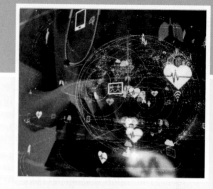

10

Nursing Informatics and Digital Health

Margaret Ann Kennedy

(e) http://evolve.elsevier.com/Canada/Ross-Kerr/nursing

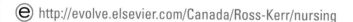

LEARNING OBJECTIVES

After reading this chapter, you will be able to:

- Describe the evolution and progression of digital health and nursing informatics.
- Describe the practice of nursing informatics and the competencies necessary to practice in contemporary digital health environments.
- Describe the role of key agencies in the Canadian health information management domain.
- Describe how standardized nursing languages represent nursing practice in the health care system.
- Describe how nursing data science offers new ways of understanding past, current, and future health information to support future health care and nursing practice.

- Describe how Canada and leading Canadian health care organizations are progressing in the adoption of digital health and how nurses' roles are evolving across care boundaries.
- Describe the various ways in which nurses can be active in nursing informatics communities.
- Describe how provincial and federal legislation guide the privacy and protection of personal health information in Canada.

OUTLINE

KEY TERMS

artificial intelligence	mHealth	practice-based evidence
clinical information systems	nursing data science	robotics
clinical intelligence	nursing data standards	smart devices
digital health	nursing informatics	standardized data
eHealth	ontology	telehealth
gamification	personalized medicine	uHealth
gross domestic product	portals	virtualization

 PERSONAL PERSPECTIVES

Your community has experienced a sudden upsurge in teen deaths as a result of suicide and accidental drug overdoses. Your health care organization, local public health, and teen advocacy groups have held several strategic meetings and have agreed to partner to develop a new teen mental health initiative that will include multiple digital tools. A call has gone out for staff who are interested in participating in the design and development of the new program resources. This new suicide prevention and mental health and addictions program will be anchored with a patient portal, several mobile applications, and a community network. Your unit manager has invited you to participate in the consultations and design team.

Consider what kinds of information should be included on the portal, and what kinds of applications could be designed to support crisis intervention, prevention goals, and improved health outcomes. What key design principles should be flagged to optimize teen engagement with the various tools?

EVOLUTION OF TECHNOLOGY AND DIGITAL HEALTH

Over the past several decades, Canada, like many other nations, has witnessed a dramatic shift in how health care is conceptualized, informed, and delivered. Emerging trends have evolved into drivers that we now take for granted—things like evidence-informed practice, consumer health, a movement towards health for all, and more balanced partnerships between consumers and health care providers. At the same time, technology has infiltrated everyday life in ways that were impossible to imagine only a few short years ago. The ways in which we can instantly access information, track our personal interests, hobbies, and biometric values, and communicate with each other and the world has shifted not only how we perceive the world but our expectations of every industry, including health care.

Health care continues to expand the application of technology—through **clinical information systems** and electronic health records (EHRs), **artificial intelligence**, nanotechnology, **robotics**, **personalized medicine**, mobile apps, **portals**, **virtualization**, **gamification**, and more—to all manner of health care services across the care continuum, transforming manual and paper-based management of health care into **digital health**. Health care providers can deliver care remotely through direct or virtual care such as **telehealth**, **smart devices**, and other emerging technologies. The era of **eHealth** (health services mediated or delivered by electronic means), **mHealth** (health services mediated or delivered by mobile technologies), and **uHealth** (ubiquitous technology in health care) has made it clear that innovation will become the hallmark of this generation of health care leaders and information technology designers. Likewise, the array of possibilities will continue to expand opportunities for and increase demands on health care providers to integrate innovation into practice.

Innovation also demands that health care providers maintain a clear-eyed sense of value in regard to the dazzling expanse of technological innovations. The technological gymnastics that are possible as a consequence of current levels of digital innovation offer meaningful value only insofar as they help to optimize health outcomes or support professional practice. In the absence of delivering at least one of these two values, innovation becomes superfluous. More than ever, nurses and health care providers need to recognize and advocate for these two values to be embedded in every innovation and in every practice change that is precipitated by technological innovation.

Practice will continue to evolve and transform as increasingly sophisticated technologies enable greater access and flexibility to deliver quality health care to every person, regardless of geographic location or location on the health care continuum. The challenge becomes integrating digital innovations into clinical practice so as to preserve the caring, holistic approach of nursing while capitalizing on the benefits of digital innovation to extend appropriate and cost-effective care to all persons. Nurses are ideally positioned and uniquely qualified to take on this role of leading for quality, value, and meaningful transformation.

Pressures on Health Care Systems

The significant changes in social and cultural characteristics around the world are in turn placing enormous demands on health care systems. The World Health Organization (WHO) has provided insight into the startling shifts in ageing and accompanying noncommunicable disease burden we can expect to see in the future. Between 2019 and 2050, the proportion of persons over age 65 is projected to almost double from approximately 9% to 16%, and the number aged 80 and older will triple to 426 million (United Nations, 2019). The WHO (2019a) reported the sharpest increase in projected lifespan between 2000 and 2015, with an increase of 5 years in average life expectancy.

Canada is also experiencing similar demographic shifts. In 2019, Canada's population was estimated at 37,238,595 (World Population Review, 2019). The highest proportion of the population was aged 60 to 64 years, and Statistics Canada (2016) reported that citizens aged 65 and over outnumbered the proportion of children below age 15 for the first time in Canada's history.

This widely acknowledged expansion in our aging population will have a significant impact on social infrastructure and health care provision. The main health burdens for older persons stem from noncommunicable diseases, including cardiovascular diseases, cancers, respiratory diseases, and diabetes (WHO, 2015, 2019b). The Canadian Institute for Health Information (CIHI) (2018) forecasted that Canada would spend $6,839 on health care for every person in Canada. As illustrated in Figure 10.1, this will total an expenditure of $253 million on health care, which is 11.3% of the national **gross domestic product;** the growth of total health expenditures is expected to rise by 4.2% (CIHI, 2018). Further, the CIHI observed that while the top three health expenses are hospitals (28.3%), drugs (15.7%), and physicians (15.1%), spending on drugs will grow faster than the categories, at 3.2% per year (Figure 10.2). Thus, there is an imperative to find solutions that support cost-effective management of health care expenses and delivery.

As these historic demographic shifts are occurring, technology embeddedness has become a global phenomenon and a ubiquitous factor in almost every aspect of life in Canada. The management of health information through the use of electronic technologies has rapidly developed since the first computers were developed in the 1950s and 1960s and continued to expand in clinical applications into the 1980s (Hannah, Ball, & Edwards, 2006, p. 28). The introduction of the computer for use by organizations and individuals, as well as the rapid expansion of computing power over just a few decades, has led to extensive automation of basic operations in health care agencies and

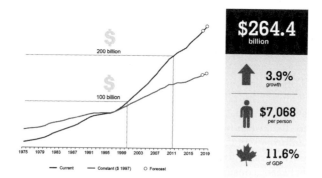

Fig. 10.1 Projected health care spending in 2018. (**Source:** Canadian Institute for Health Information. (2019). National health expenditure trends, 1975 to 2019. Ottawa, ON: Author.)

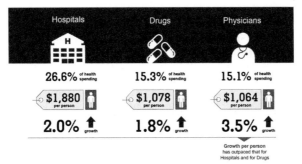

Fig. 10.2 Canadian health care costs per capita. (**Source:** Canadian Institute for Health Information. (2019). National health expenditure trends, 1975 to 2019. Ottawa, ON: Author.)

in management of clinical processes at the unit and institution level.

In some instances, health care crises have tragically illustrated the impact of gaps in health information. The well-known 2003 severe acute respiratory syndrome (SARS) epidemic is a prime example, whereby 44 Canadians died and the speed of infection and fragmented access to patient health information was a significant obstacle to rapid treatment (Branswell, 2013; M. Pearce, personal communication, August 30, 2017). The *Naylor Report* (Naylor, Girard, Mintz et al., 2015) involved a comprehensive investigation of the SARS epidemic in Canada. The authors issued numerous recommendations to strengthen the health care system in Canada, specifically by improving the management of health information through the adoption of digital health information, the meaningful use of digital health information, secure digital access for patients to their own information, the development of virtual care, greater interoperability to enable measurement and analytics, and a national strategy for innovation to optimize Canada's digital health benefits.

We have already witnessed the significant social and cultural transformation brought on by the emergence of eHealth. Digital systems are providing unprecedented opportunities to rapidly access information at the point of care (e.g., pharmaceutical and other types of authoritative databases, laboratory values, and best practice guidelines); document nursing and health care practice; exchange information across the continuum of care; and support health care outcomes and professional practice through clinical decision-support tools. The WHO (2017) has defined eHealth as "the use of information and communication technologies (ICT) for health." The services and activities implicated in eHealth address the full spectrum of health priorities, such as providing direct care to patients, research and education, health care administration, and public health surveillance.

Current information management applications support the range of business needs for most organizations, including patient scheduling and transfer, billing and financial management, diagnostic imaging, lab reporting, order-entry applications, prescribing and pharmacy management, inventory and materials management, staff scheduling and utilization, clinical information systems (documenting patient care), and clinical decision-support tools. Many systems vendors offer sophisticated applications that integrate tools for all units in a single or multi-site health care facility. Many areas of the country are adopting such systems, as administrators have recognized the immense benefits of making health care information readily accessible to care providers regardless of location within or outside the health care facility.

Amid the rapid expansion of technologies into all aspects of contemporary health care, however, Hannah (2005) has noted that "the issues for nurses are no longer computers or management information systems, but rather information and information management. The computer and its associated software are merely tools to support nurses as they practice their profession" (p. 48). This observation remains true today, and perhaps is of even greater importance. It is imperative that nurses be actively engaged in developing systems that support professional practice and attentive to the content of information systems rather than the technology itself (Hannah, 2005). This transition in focus away from the necessary but basic skills of using a computer to intentionally managing information is significant. Hannah's observation has continued rising in importance as technology use and adoption has escalated: nurses have had to become more proactive and intentional about the presence of nursing in organizational technology decisions and making the best use of information to strengthen health care outcomes and improve professional practice.

⊕ CULTURAL CONSIDERATIONS

Using Technology to Advance a Nursing Leadership Project: Mentorship to Support Community Health Nursing Certification in Indigenous Communities

Jacquelyn MacDonald and Heather MacDonald, from the First Nations and Inuit Health Branch (FNIHB) at Indigenous Services Canada, co-led a project that used technology to provide mentorship to nurses in Indigenous communities in Atlantic Canada. They explained that nursing leadership is essential for innovation and advancing information technology within health care organizations across Canada. Nursing leadership is especially important in the field of public health because nurses are the largest group of providers in the community and are ideally positioned to promote healthy behaviours, monitor health trends, and react quickly to changing needs. There are 33 First Nations and 5 Inuit communities across four provinces in Atlantic Canada; these Indigenous communities represent Mi'kmaq, Maliseet, Inuit, and Innu. This study illustrates how technology was used to support a nursing leadership project for nurses working at the community level in these Indigenous communities.

Many Indigenous communities have become actively involved in implementing eHealth initiatives. However, the evolution toward this active use of digital health has been long and, at times, challenging. In order to understand digital health in Atlantic First Nations communities, it is necessary to understand the development of connectivity. In 1999, when Atlantic Canada's First Nation Help Desk (ACFNHD) was started in Membertou First Nation in Nova Scotia, all the schools had only dialup connections to access the Internet (28 Kbps). This speed stands in contrast to the current high-speed or fibre optic networks that move enormous amounts of information at speeds measured in gigabytes or terabytes. Contemporary communication and digital health applications, including videoconferencing and others, minimally require the robust infrastructure of Internet protocol connectivity. Every Atlantic First Nation community now has videoconferencing capabilities that connects to the ACFNHD network, and more than 75 units are connected to ACFNHD videoconferencing infrastructure. Most communities have multiple videoconferencing units that serve health and education clients; the use of videoconferencing infrastructure enables health services to be delivered regardless of geographical location, referred to as telehealth. Several communities have also instituted videoconferencing in their band offices and other administrative buildings.

The FNIHB at Indigenous Services Canada has had a longstanding role supporting nurses who work in First Nations communities. Each First Nation community operates public health programs from a community health centre facility, which consists of a variety of health care providers and support staff. Many First Nations and Inuit communities are remote or isolated, represent small populations, and are served by community health centres. The core public health programs are comparable to provincial programs, and services are delivered on reserve to the local population. Program examples include maternal child health, immunization, communicable disease control, and home and community care.

The purpose of the project was to develop a mentorship model to support community health nurses working in Indigenous communities to achieve their Canadian Nurses Association (CNA) specialty practice certification (community health nursing certification, or CCHN(c)). Evidence has shown that specialty nursing practice certification has a positive impact on both patient and organizational outcomes. Despite this recognized value, the number of nurses in the Atlantic provinces with community health nursing certification is lower than the national average.

The project involved 10 nurses from different jurisdictions working in seven of the 38 First Nations and Inuit communities in Atlantic Canada. The objectives of the project included raising awareness of the value of competency-based specialty practice, providing nursing mentorship opportunities using technology, fostering a robust community of practice as a vehicle for peer support and education, and using the CNA's specialty practice certification exam blueprint to structure the education.

The project's co-leads, Jacquelyn MacDonald and Heather MacDonald, generated support for the project from a number of key partners. Support was provided by the FNIHB Atlantic region, CNA, Canadian Nurses Foundation, Community Health Nurses of Canada, Dorothy Wylie Health Leaders Institute, First Nations communities, and ACFNHD. Building and strengthening relationships with the CNA and CNF was important for the successful implementation of this initiative in the Atlantic region. Enabling strategic partnerships is also essential to scaling up this work to support nurses nationally.

Using videoconference technologies, the nurses established a virtual community of practice study group consisting of guest presenters and collaborative partnerships. The project had five phases (preplanning, facilitation, implementation, certification exam writing, and evaluation) and various steps in a mentorship model that was co-created between the project leaders and participants. The co-leaders created a survey with questions to address study group participants' learning needs and preferences. The co-facilitators for this project wanted to better understand the core pillars for a mentorship model and the educational needs of nurses wishing to obtain this national specialty certification. To co-create this model, they wanted to hear from community health and home care nurses firsthand. The information collected in the survey was meant to help in the design and structure of the mentorship study group format. It was designed with a grassroots approach for the mentorship model.

The leadership project met the stated goals and objectives in the 12-month time frame, and feedback was extremely positive. All participants who wrote the certification exam were successful in achieving their CNA specialty certification in community health nursing with a 100% pass rate. The nurses celebrated their achievements at the 2017 Atlantic Nursing Professional Development and Networking Session in Halifax, Nova Scotia, which was hosted by the Mi'kmaq Confederacy of Prince Edward Island.

Successful use of technology was based on the fact that all communities had the essential videoconferencing equipment, training, and network capability. The videoconferencing technology was an interactive way for nurses to exchange knowledge on a regular basis over a 4-month period, review nursing competencies, review exam questions, and support one another through the study review. This approach had a huge impact, as the model created a sustainable community of practice for the nurses.

This project was designed to support nurses working in First Nations and Inuit communities in the Atlantic region, but the co-leads believe that it can be successfully applied more widely in their region and onto a national platform. As a result of the project's success, they were invited by the CNA certification group to develop a draft collaborative model with the CNA for use by other specialty groups interested in creating mentorship opportunities. Additionally, project leaders received an invitation to share the mentorship project with the International Council of Nurses' Nursing Now 2020 campaign to highlight successful initiatives happening in Indigenous communities.

Jacquelyn MacDonald and Heather MacDonald thank the community health nurses from across the Atlantic provinces who joined them on this journey to advance Indigenous health in rural, remote, and isolated communities.

NURSING INFORMATICS

Nurses have always been knowledge workers, transforming data and information into a coherent clinical understanding of the patient and their unique health needs. However, managing vast amounts of diverse information related to patient demographics and clinical needs, diagnostic results, and planned or active treatment regimes, in addition to coordinating community supports, represents only a portion of the work performed by nurses on a daily basis in Canada and around the globe. These information management activities are increasingly supported by technology, and new ways to approach information management are challenging previous ways of knowing and doing. Continuing to implement linear, paper-based processes in digital environments will not deliver the full value and potential benefits that digital health offers (Remus, 2016). Nursing as a discipline needs a critical reset on its perspective on information management and professional practice, and this will require vision as well as specific skills and knowledge. This is where nursing informatics comes into focus, a field with an essential role to play in shaping the future of nursing in contemporary digital environments.

Similar to the progression of technological innovation, definitions of **nursing informatics** have evolved from a primary focus on technology itself to a more information and practice focus. The Nursing Informatics Special Interest Group of the International Medical Informatics Association (IMIA-NI) formally adopted a new nursing informatics definition at the General Assembly meetings in Helsinki on June 28, 2009:

> *Nursing informatics science and practice integrates nursing, its information and knowledge and their management with information and communication technologies to promote the health of people, families and communities worldwide.* (IMIA-NI, 2009, para. 2).

Since the IMIA-NI definition was published, other definitions have arisen to illustrate specific dimensions of digital health, including connected health, cost, accessibility, and integration of information in nursing practice; although there is no single definition of nursing informatics, many commonalities exist. The CNA defines nursing informatics as "the practice and science of integrating nursing information and knowledge with technology to manage and integrate health information. The goal of nursing informatics is to improve the health of people and communities while reducing costs" (Canadian Nurses Association [CNA], 2019).

Canada has played a significant and ongoing role in the definition and advancement of nursing informatics across the profession of nursing. The first text on nursing informatics was published in 1984 by Dr. Marion Ball from the United States and Dr. Kathryn Hannah from Canada (Ball & Hannah, 1984). Since that time, collaborations with the CNA, the Canadian Nursing Informatics Association (CNIA), the Canadian Association of Schools of Nursing (CASN), and nursing informatic leaders such as Dr. Kathryn Hannah, Dr. Lynn Nagle, Peggy White, Dr. Dorothy Pringle, Dr. Sylvie Jette, Dr. Leanne Currie, Dr. Elizabeth Borycki, and others have made significant contributions to the proliferation of academic and applied texts, peer-reviewed journals, conferences, and educational programs and online resources, all directed at preparing nurses to capitalize on applying technology to its optimal potential.

As digital health information management is increasingly embedded in nursing practice and care delivery settings, nursing informatics has become less of a "specialty practice" and more of a foundational skill required by all nurses, which is aligned with the CNA e-Strategy (CNA, 2006a). The CNA (2017a) and the CNIA have jointly declared that

nursing informatics competencies are essential for nurses in all roles to function in complex, contemporary health-care environments. Moreover, there is a need to have nurses with a specialization in informatics

to support decision-making relevant to the profession's use of information and technology in digitally connected health environments. (p. 2)

In 2015, the CASN released its seminal document on core nursing informatics competencies (Canadian Association of Schools of Nursing, 2015). These competencies were identified and validated by nursing informatics leaders from across Canada, Canadian nursing regulators, and the deans and directors of Canadian schools of nursing with membership in the CASN. This broad endorsement and adoption of the minimum competencies for nurses entering the practice of nursing reflects the importance of formalizing the use of digital technologies in professional practice as distinct from the common social uses of technology. In summary, nurses who have developed the key competencies in nursing informatics are described as being able to use "information and communication technologies to support information synthesis in accordance with professional and regulatory standards in the delivery of patient/client care." Three individual competency statements were developed, each with multiple accompanying indicators of achievement (Table 10.1).

As noted in the CASN competencies document, nursing students are expected to bring a number of foundational

TABLE 10.1 CASN Nursing Informatics Entry-to-Practice Competencies for Registered Nurses

Competency	Competency Statement	Indicator
Information and Knowledge Management	Uses relevant information and knowledge to support the delivery of evidence-informed patient care	Accesses and appraises online literature and resources supporting clinical judgement Analyses, interprets, and documents pertinent nursing data and patient data using standardized nursing and other clinical terminologies (e.g., ICNP, C-HOBIC, SNOMED-CT, etc.) to support clinical decision making and nursing practice improvements Assists patients and their families to access, review, and evaluate information they retrieve using Information Communication Technologies (ICTs) (i.e., current, credible, and relevant) and leverage ICTs to manage their health (e.g., social media sites, smart phone applications, online support groups, etc.) Describes the processes of data gathering, recording and retrieval, in hybrid or homogenous health records (electronic or paper), and identifies informational risks, gaps, and inconsistencies across the health care system Articulates the significance of information standards (i.e., messaging standards and standardized clinical terminologies) necessary for interoperable electronic health records across the health care system Articulates the importance of standardized nursing data to reflect nursing practice, to advance nursing knowledge, and to contribute to the value and understanding of nursing Critically evaluates data and information from a variety of sources (including experts, clinical applications, databases, practice guidelines, relevant websites, etc.) to inform the delivery of nursing care

TABLE 10.1   CASN Nursing Informatics Entry-to-Practice Competencies for Registered Nurses (*Cont.*)

Competency	Competency Statement	Indicator
Professional and Regulatory Accountability	Uses ICTs in accordance with professional and regulatory standards and workplace policies	Complies with legal and regulatory requirements, ethical standards, and organizational policies and procedures (e.g., protection of health information, privacy, and security)
		Advocates for the use of current and innovative ICTs that support the delivery of safe, quality care
		Identifies and reports system process and functional issues (e.g., error messages, misdirections, device malfunctions, etc.) according to organizational policies and procedures
		Maintains effective nursing practice and patient safety during any period of system unavailability by following organizational downtime and recovery policies and procedures
		Demonstrates that professional judgement must prevail in the presence of technologies designed to support clinical assessments, interventions, and evaluation (e.g., monitoring devices, decision-support tools, etc.)
		Recognizes the importance of nurses' involvement in the design, selection, implementation, and evaluation of applications and systems in health care
Information and Communication Technologies (ICTs)	Uses ICTs in the delivery of patient and client care	Identifies and demonstrates appropriate use of a variety of ICTs (e.g., point-of-care systems, electronic health records, electronic medical records, capillary blood glucose monitoring, hemodynamic monitoring, telehomecare, fetal heart monitoring devices, etc.) to deliver safe nursing care to diverse populations in a variety of settings
		Uses decision-support tools (e.g., clinical alerts and reminders, critical pathways, web-based clinical practice guidelines, etc.) to assist clinical judgment and safe patient care
		Uses ICTs in a manner that supports (i.e., does not interfere with) the nurse–patient relationship
		Describes the various components of health information systems (e.g., results reporting, computerized provider order entry, clinical documentation, electronic medication administration records, etc.)
		Describes the various types of electronic records used across the continuum of care (e.g., EHR, EMR, PHR, etc.) and their clinical and administrative uses
		Describes the benefits of informatics to improve health systems and the quality of interprofessional patient care

Source: Canadian Association of Schools of Nursing (2015). *Nursing informatics: Entry-to-practice competencies for registered nurses.* Ottawa, ON: Author.

skills to their undergraduate education such as the basic use of devices (including but not limited to desktop and laptop computers, mobile devices, and printers) and the use of intranet and extranet. Additionally, students are expected to develop skills in the use of an operating system, electronic communication, multimedia, word processing and presentations, networking applications, and use of technology to support self-directed learning. Supports are typically available through the nursing programs and university information technology services if necessary.

As a result of the vision of and commitment by nurse leaders and practitioners, there has been considerable progress in nursing informatics in Canada and internationally; however, more work needs to be done to fully achieve the benefits of seamless, interoperable digital health. A broad range of efforts are underway to ensure that nursing informatics continues to grow and evolve in Canada. One key initiative to support this continued growth is the support for ongoing graduate work and research. A group of Canadian nursing informatics leaders recognized the need to support ongoing scholarship advancing nursing competency and digital health. To that end, a partnership with the CNF was created in 2014 to establish an annual scholarship supporting a Canadian nurse pursuing graduate studies in informatics in Canada. The Dr. Kathryn J. Hannah Nursing Informatics Scholarship, awarded annually through the CNF, is the first scholarship of its kind in Canada dedicated specifically to nursing informatics. The first scholarship was presented in 2016 and will continue to support Canadian nurse informaticists.

CANADIAN HEALTH INFORMATION MANAGEMENT

Internet connectivity is widely available across Canada. According to Statistics Canada (2017), Canadians tend to view the Internet as a tool that helps connect people, saves time, and helps inform decisions. Canadians are increasingly comfortable using technology to support their health care, becoming knowledgeable consumers in the process. See Box 10.1, Figure 10.3, and Figure 10.4 to learn more about Canadians' use of the Internet and relationship with technology.

BOX 10.1   Internet Use in Canada

Statistics Canada (2017) has reported that "nearly all Canadians under the age of 45 use the Internet every day." The rates of Internet use steadily decline between 45 and 75 years of age, with less than half of Canadians over age 75 using the Internet daily. Internet use rates are consistently high across the provinces, but variation does exist. Alberta has the highest percentage of Internet users (94%), while New Brunswick has the lowest rate (86%). Statistics Canada has reported that the top devices owned by Canadians include smartphones (76%), laptop computers (71%), and tablets (54%).

Source: Statistics Canada. (2017). *The Internet and digital technology.* Retrieved from https://www150.statcan.gc.ca/n1/pub/11-627-m/11-627-m2017032-eng.htm.

Several key organizations are advancing digital health and the collection and dissemination of health information in Canada, and nurses require a working knowledge of them. The Canadian Institute for Health Information

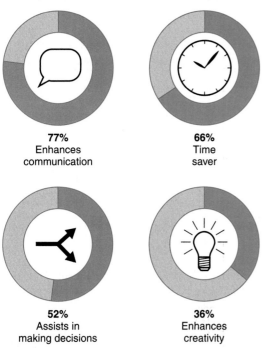

Fig. 10.3 Canadians' perspectives on technology. (**Source:** Statistics Canada. (2017, November 14). The Internet and digital technology. Retrieved from https://www150.statcan.gc.ca/n1/pub/11-627-m/11-627-m2017032-eng.htm.)

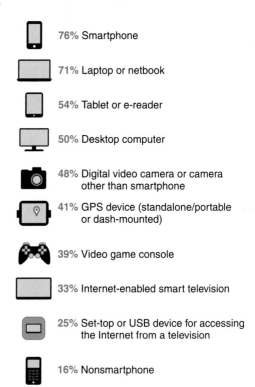

Fig. 10.4 Top 10 devices owned by Canadians. (**Source:** Statistics Canada. (2017, November 14). The Internet and digital technology. Retrieved from https://www150.statcan.gc.ca/n1/pub/11-627-m/11-627-m2017032-eng.htm.)

(CIHI) is a national independent nonprofit that records and disseminates essential data and analysis on Canada's health system and the health of Canadians (CIHI, 2019a). The CIHI collects extensive data on health care services and spending, health human resources, and population health from hospitals, regional health authorities, governments, and physicians. They also maintain an extensive array of national databases (Table 10.2) on everything from organ replacement and surgical day procedures to the workforce trends of health care providers. The CIHI provides access to reports and databanks to Canadians and generates benchmarking analyses and reports to inform reporting organizations on the status of care. The CIHI (2019a) provides critical leadership on a broad scope of topics, including data quality, specific data standards, methodologies for data analysis, and coding and classification.

Canada Health Infoway is another key contributor to advancing Canada's digital health landscape. It is a federally funded, independent nonprofit whose primary focus is the development of secure, integrated, and patient-centred EHRs (Canada Health Infoway [CHI], 2018). Infoway acts as a funding partner to each province to enable the development and adoption of core infrastructure (i.e., client registry, provider registry, laboratory test results, diagnostic images, drug information, and clinical reports and immunizations). Infoway has played a crucial role in the development of a national blueprint for digital health transformation and the development and adoption of necessary health information standards. This mandate has largely been fulfilled, as all provinces have completed the implementation of core digital health foundations (Table 10.3). Infoway has demonstrated the significant adoption and use of digital health

				Availability of Preliminary Data	
Data Holding	**Types of Care/ Professions**	**Most Current Year Available**	**Next Data Release**	**Data Requests**	**Reports for Participating Organizations**
Hospital Care					
Discharge Abstract Database (DAD)	Inpatient day surgery	2018–2019	July 2020	Yes	Monthly
National Ambulatory Care Reporting System (NACRS)	Emergency department visits, day surgery, and outpatient clinics	2018–2019	July 2020	Yes	Monthly
Hospital Morbidity Database (HMDB)	Inpatient day surgery	2018–2019	Nov. 2020	—	—
National Rehabilitation Reporting System (NRS)	Inpatient rehabilitation	2019–2020	Aug. 2020	Yes	Quarterly
Continuing Care Reporting System (CCRS)	Hospital continuing care	2019–2020	Sept. 2020	Yes	Quarterly
Community Care					
Continuing Care Reporting System (CCRS)	Residential care	2019–2020	Sept. 2020	Yes	Quarterly
Home Care Reporting System (CCRS)	Home care	2019–2020	Sept. 2020	Yes	Quarterly
Specialized Care					
Hospital Mental Health Database (HMHDB)	Inpatient	2018–2019	Mar. 2021	—	—

TABLE 10.2   Canadian Institute for Health Information Database Holdings

(Continued)

TABLE 10.2   Canadian Institute for Health Information Database Holdings (*Cont.*)

Data Holding	Types of Care/ Professions	Most Current Year Available	Next Data Release	Availability of Preliminary Data	
				Data Requests	Reports for Participating Organizations
Ontario Mental Health Reporting System	Inpatient	2019–2020	Aug. 2020	Yes	Quarterly
Canadian Organ Replacement Register (CORR)	Dialysis transplant	2018	Sept. 2020	Yes	—
National Trauma Registry (NTR)	Specialized care	2012–2013	—	—	—
Ontario Trauma Registry (OTR)	Specialized care	2018–2019	July 2020	—	—
Canadian Joint Replacement Registry (CJRR)	Specialized care	2018–2019	Aug. 2020	Yes	—
Medical Imaging Technology Database (MITDB)	Specialized care	2012	—	—	—
Canadian Multiple Sclerosis Monitoring System (CMSMS)	Specialized care	2015–2016	—	Yes	—
Pharmaceuticals					
National Prescription Drug Utilization Information System (NPDUIS)	—	2019	Sept. 2020	Yes	After each submission
Patient Experience					
Canadian Patient Experiences Reporting System (CPERS)	Acute care inpatient	2017–2018	—	—	In development
Patient Safety					
National System for Incident Reporting (NSIR)	—	—	—	—	After each submission
Health Workforce					
National Physician Database (NPDB)	Physicians	2017–2018	Sept. 2020	—	—
Scott's Medical Database (SMDB)	Physicians	2018	July 2020	—	—

TABLE 10.2 Canadian Institute for Health Information Database Holdings (*Cont.*)

Data Holding	Types of Care/ Professions	Most Current Year Available	Next Data Release	Availability of Preliminary Data	
				Data Requests	Reports for Participating Organizations
Health Workforce Database (HWDB)	Audiologists	2017	Fall 2020	Yes	Annually
	Chiropractors	2017	Fall 2020	Yes	Annually
	Dental assistants	2017	Fall 2020	Yes	Annually
	Dental hygienists	2017	Fall 2020	Yes	Annually
	Dentists	2017	Fall 2020	Yes	Annually
	Dietitians	2017	Fall 2020	Yes	Annually
	Environmental public health professionals	2017	Fall 2020	Yes	Annually
	Genetic counsellors	2017	Fall 2020	Yes	Annually
	Health information management professionals	2017	Fall 2020	Yes	Annually
	Licensed practical nurses	2018	Spring 2021	Yes	Annually
	Medical laboratory technologists	2017	Fall 2020	Yes	Annually
	Medical physicists	2017	Fall 2020	Yes	Annually
	Medical radiation technologists	2017	Fall 2020	Yes	Annually
	Midwives	2017	Fall 2020	Yes	Annually
	Occupational therapists	2018	June 2021	Yes	Annually
	Opticians	2017	Fall 2020	Yes	Annually
	Optometrists	2017	Fall 2020	Yes	Annually
	Paramedics	2017	Fall 2020	Yes	Annually
	Pharmacists	2018	June 2021	Yes	Annually
	Pharmacy technicians	2017	Fall 2020	Yes	Annually
	Physician assistants	2017	Fall 2020	Yes	Annually
	Physiotherapists	2018	June 2021	Yes	Annually
	Psychologists	2017	Fall 2020	Yes	Annually
	Registered nurses and nurse practitioners	2018	Spring 2021	Yes	Annually
	Registered psychiatric nurses	2018	Spring 2021	Yes	Annually
	Respiratory therapists	2018	Fall 2020	Yes	Annually
	Social workers	2018	Fall 2020	Yes	Annually
	Speech-language pathologists	2018	Fall 2020	Yes	Annually

(Continued)

TABLE 10.2 Canadian Institute for Health Information Database Holdings (*Cont.*)

Data Holding	Types of Care/ Professions	Most Current Year Available	Next Data Release	Availability of Preliminary Data	
				Data Requests	Reports for Participating Organizations
Spending					
National Health Expenditure Database (NHEX)	—	2019	Oct. 2020	—	—
Canadian Management Information System Database (CMDB)	—	2018–2019	Mar. 2021	Yes	Annually
Canadian Patient Cost Database (CPCD)	—	2017–2018	Fall 2021	—	—
International Comparisons					
Organisation for Economic Cooperation and Development (OECD)	—	2018	June 2020	—	Annually
Commonwealth Fund (CMWF)	—	2019	Feb. 2021	—	Annually
Access and Wait Times					
Wait Times	Acute care	2018	July 2020	—	Annually

Source: Canadian Institute for Health Information. (2020). *Data holdings.* Retrieved from https://www.cihi.ca/en/access-data-and-reports/make-a-data-request/data-holdings.

TABLE 10.3 Progress on Canada's Core Health Information Infrastructure

Program	Target	% of Target
Diagnostic Imaging	Provide access to shared digital images in ~80% of Canada's acute care public hositpals	100%
Drug Information Systems	Electronically capture and store ~75% of dispensed medication information	100%
	Provide ~50% of retail pharmacies with access to patients' medication profiles	100%
Laboratory Information Systems	Capture, store, and share 75% of laboratory test result information in Canada	100%
Client Registry	Uniquely identify 99% of all Canadians	100%
Provider Registry	Uniquely identify 100% of Canadian physicians	100%
Integrated Electronic Health Record (iEHR)	Provide 50% of Canada's acute care public hospitals with the capability of viewing and updating electronic health information about their patients	100%
	Provide at least 25% of all eligble practising clinicians, including family physicians, specialists, nurses, and pharmacists, with the capability of viewing and updating electronic health information about their patients	100%

Source: Canada Health Infoway. (2015). *The path of progress: Infoway annual report 2014–2015* (p. 7). Retrieved from https://www.infoway-inforoute.ca/en/component/edocman/resources/i-infoway-i-corporate/annual-reports/2771-annual-report-2014-2015.

tools by Canadians, a trend that is generating significant benefits (Figure 10.5). The organization has estimated that $30 billion in efficiencies and savings have been generated through Canada's investments in digital health.

While Infoway's overall mission to accelerate the progression of digital health in Canada has remained stable, their efforts are now being refined to drive clinical value and meaning from the investments to date and support more sophisticated digital functionality to further maximize efficiencies and benefits. Looking forward, Infoway is focused on three efforts: operating and maintaining PrescribeIT, a multijurisdictional e-prescribing service to strengthen prescribing, medication reconciliation, and the monitoring of prescribing patterns across Canada; expanding the use of telehealth and telehomecare; and linking Canadians to their personal health information through a new program called ACCESS 2020. Information about ACCESS 2020 is available on the Infoway website.

 CULTURAL CONSIDERATIONS

Digital Health for Indigenous Communities

Three main areas are currently important in the use of digital health for Indigenous communities: remote and rural access, reflection of traditional ways of being and knowing, and data sovereignty.

Remote Access

Many Indigenous communities are located far from urban centres and can only be accessed by plane, boat, or extended travel. In the past, health care providers would intermittently travel to communities. However, recent advances in virtual care have enabled remote synchronous delivery (at a distance, but at the same time) of primary health care services. For example, a primary care provider (nurse practitioner or physician) might schedule one day a week for virtual care visits. In this instance, the local registered nurse facilitates the visit using remote devices such as a digital stethoscope or digital otoscope. In addition, emergency visits previously required medical evacuation services so that the person needing care could be seen by a health care provider. Using virtual care, on-call emergency consultations can happen via video communication. As a result, not only can virtual care prevent delays in treatment, but the patients no longer require lengthy travel for basic primary care. Many remote Indigenous communities still have telecommunication access via satellite alone; although access is improving, many remote areas do not have broadband access projects. Increased attention is required to ensure that all Indigenous communities have equitable access to technologies to support the delivery of health care.

Reflection of Traditional Ways of Being and Ways of Knowing

Traditional ways of being and knowing are often not reflected in health care software. Indeed, most health care software was originally designed to support billing. In a time of reconciliation and cultural revitalization as part of the Truth and Reconciliation Commission of Canada recommendations, software developers need to pay more attention to ensuring that health care software can capture traditional ways of being and knowing. One of the first systems to do so was recently designed by First Nations for First Nations, the Mustimuhw Community Electronic Medical Record (cEMR) (pronounced moose-tee-mook) (Mustimuhw Information Solutions Inc., n.d.). This software includes traditional healing practices as part of the data that might be collected. Incorporating traditional ways of healing and knowing into electronic medical records and care plans is another positive step towards reconciliation.

Indigenous Data Sovereignty

Finally, data sovereignty is an issue of growing concern for all Canadians. In the context of Indigenous communities, data sovereignty refers to principles of ownership, control, access, and possession (OCAP) of all data. The OCAP principles originated in reference to First Nations communities' asserting jurisdiction over their own data in the context of research. But this has grown to a broader conversation about data sovereignty in all contexts. Indigenous communities are increasingly using technologies for health care, prompting the question of who owns the health care data about Indigenous peoples. This question is being asked throughout Canada and internationally (Kukutai & Taylor, 2016) and may take some time to sort out. Nurses working in all sectors need to understand how technologies used for health care can enhance health for Indigenous peoples in Canada, but also how technologies can create additional barriers.

Sources: Kukutai, T., & Taylor, J. (Eds.). (2016). *Indigenous data sovereignty: Toward an agenda.* Canberra, Australia: ANU Press. Retrieved from https://press-files.anu.edu.au/downloads/press/n2140/pdf/book.pdf; Mustimuhw Information Solutions Inc. (n.d.). *Mustimuhw Community Electronic Medical Record (cEMR) System.* Retrieved from https://www.mustimuhw.com/solutions/software-solutions/mustimuhw-community-electronic-medical-record-cemr-system/.

An estimated

$30 billion

in benefits since 2007 from
foundational investments
(connected health
information, telehealth
and telehomecare, drug
information systems,
diagnostic imaging, and
physician and ambulatory
clinic electronic medical
records). An increase of
$4.5 billion in the past year.

In 2019, **7 in 10 Canadians** can access
some of their personal health information electronically
(up from 2 in 10 in 2015). **3 in 10** can access multiple
parts of their record in a single solution.

81%

satisfaction
rate among
Canadians
who use virtual
care services.

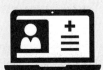

More than

40,000

Canadians
have been enrolled
in telehomecare
programs since 2010.

An estimated

210,000

**health care
professionals**
access clinical
information
integrated into their
point-of-care systems.

More than

1 million

**telehealth
consultations**
in 2018, an increase of more
than 500% since 2010.

More than
**$420 million in
avoided expenses**
and more than
**280 million km
in travel saved**
by using telehealth to access
specialized care such as for mental
health and stroke patients in rural
and remote communities.

Fig. 10.5 Advances in Canadian health care. (**Source:** Canada Health Infoway. (2019). *Annual report 2018–2019: A new day in health care is coming. Toronto,* ON: Author. Used with the permission of Canada Health Infoway.)

STANDARDIZED NURSING DATA

There is a longstanding need to make nursing visible in a meaningful way (Clark & Lang, 1992; CNA, 2000; Hannah, Ball, & Edwards, 2006; Graves & Corcoran, 1989; Werley, 1988). In their timeless position on nursing visibility and representation, Clark and Lang (1992) noted that "if we cannot name it, we cannot control it, finance it, teach it, research it, or put it into public policy" (p. 109). Hannah, Ball, and Edwards (2006) contextualized this issue in Canada by noting that nurses' contributions to Canadian health care were not recorded in institutional or national databases representing essential elements of care provision. This approach effectively rendered nursing invisible in terms of its impact on health outcomes and prevented the expression of authority from which nurses could exert control over their own practice and influence systemic health care decision making. The perspective advanced by Clark and Lang (1992), Hannah, Ball, and Edwards (2005), and other informatics pioneers was that in order to give nursing visibility, the nursing profession needs a standardized language to reflect what nursing is and what nursing does.

While this historical perspective may seem outdated, it has actually gained both impact and momentum as technology has become an essential platform of digital health and contemporary health care delivery. The need for standardization is critical in terms of tracking care and outcomes and to enable comparative analytics that inform health care decisions. Although the progression of EHRs across Canada continues, the fact that nursing data is not regularly abstracted and formally included in discharge summaries for inclusion at the national level remains a persistent concern. In 2016, a group of nursing informatics experts, increasingly concerned about the lack of standardized nursing data and lack of progress on this agenda, established the National Nursing Data Standards Symposium. This event, hosted annually at the Lawrence S. Bloomberg Faculty of Nursing, University of Toronto, brings together nursing leaders from administration, practice, policy, education, and research as well as contributors and partners such as CIHI, Infoway, CASN, Canadian Patient Safety Institute, Accreditation Canada, and others (Nagle & White, 2018). Cosponsored by the CNA, CIHI, and Infoway, the symposium recognizes that standards are essential for nursing and digital health.

White, Nagle, and Hannah (2017) have observed that despite the significant progress in eHealth across Canada, little effort has been made to unify the approaches that guide electronic clinical documentation and **nursing data standards**. As organizations focus on establishing their own unique format and content for assessments, critical opportunities to harmonize documentation across the health care system are being missed. As Nagle and White noted, "healthcare still struggles with a lack of shareable, comparable data" (2018, p. 7). Compounding this challenge is a lack of understanding by most clinicians about how the information captured in the information system is actually used, or how much potential exists to generate greater insight and meaning from this data. "Collect once, use many times" is a key theme in the discussion around standards. Figure 10.6 illustrates the spectrum of uses of standardized data.

REPRESENTING NURSING DATA AND NURSING PRACTICE

In Canada, the process of working toward capturing nursing data was initiated in the early 1990s by the Alberta Association of Registered Nurses at a national conference to generate consensus on the Canadian Nursing Minimum Data Set (CNA, 1993). The Canadian version of a national minimum data set is recognized as Health Information: Nursing Components (HI: NC) and enjoys consensus on patient status, nursing interventions, patient outcomes, nursing intensity, and nurse identifier (CNA, 2000; Hannah, 2005). The CNA (2000) described HI: NC as the "most important pieces of data about the nursing care provided to the patient during a health care episode" (p. 5). Hannah (2005) summarized these data as follows:

- *Patient status* is broadly defined as a statement on the patient's overall health and for which nurses provide care;
- *Nursing interventions* reflects the specific nursing activities delivered to patients based on a nursing assessment of the patient's status;
- *Patient outcome* is the patient's status postintervention and is considered a consequence of the intervention;
- *Nursing intensity* reflects the level of nursing expertise or resourcing required to deliver effective care; and
- *Primary Nurse Identifier* is a single, unique lifetime identification number for each individual nurse. This identifier is independent of geographic location (province or territory), practice sector (e.g., acute care, community care, public health), and employer.

It is essential to have **standardized data** for trending, comparison, and analysis (Hannah, White, Nagle et al., 2009). Many specific languages and taxonomies have been created

| • Health policy
• Legislation
• Research | **National**
Comparative disease incidence, prevalence, trends, resource utilization |

Data collected, abstracted, aggregated, analyzed

| • Health policy
• Legislation
• Health system performance
• Funding
• Public reporting
• Research | **Regional/Jurisdictional**
Disease incidence and prevalence, outcome, cost of care, resource utilization |

Data collected, abstracted, aggregated, analyzed

| • Safety & quality
• Resource management
• Funding
• Accreditation
• Public reporting
• Research | **Organization/Sector**
Case volumes, outcomes, cost of care, resource utilization |

Data collected, abstracted, aggregated, analyzed

| • Safety & quality
• Accountability
• Outcomes
• Evidence | **Individual/CMG**
Assessments, interventions, outcomes, provider, hours of care, adverse events, cost of care |

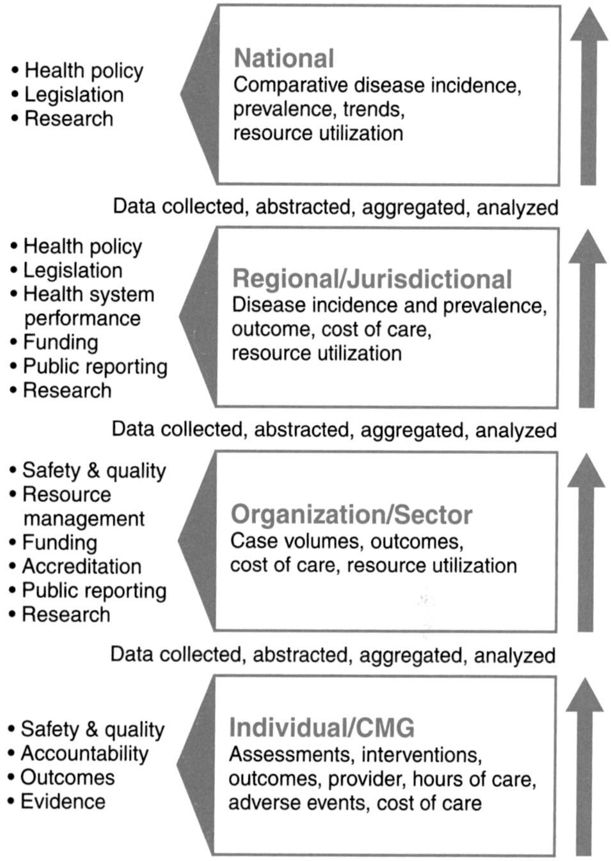

Fig. 10.6 Uses of standardized data in nursing. (**Source:** Nagle, L. M., & White, P. (2015). Towards a Pan-Canadian strategy for nursing data standards. Unpublished white paper.)

in attempts to present nursing data in standardized ways. The North American Nursing Diagnosis Association, the Omaha Classification System, the Clinical Care Classification, the Nursing Intervention Classification, and the Nursing Outcome Classification have all attempted to quantify nursing into standardized formats according to the various foci of the given taxonomy or classification system (Table 10.4).

In an effort to represent nursing in a standard unified way, the International Council of Nurses (ICN) established the International Classification for Nursing Practice (ICNP) (International Council of Nurses [ICN], 2019a). The ICNP is "an international standard that enables nurses to document their practice, regardless of geographical location, practice setting, or language, and allows for comparison of standardized data". The ICNP evolved through several iterations to its current state of development, which is available as a freely accessible, interactive browser (ICN, 2019b).

TABLE 10.4 Standardized Nursing Terminologies

Terminology	Year Introduced	Nursing-Specific Items From the Nursing Minimum Data Set				Focus
		Nursing Diagnosis	Nursing Interventions	Nursing Outcomes	Nursing Intensity	
NANDA*	1992	X				Comprehensive
Nursing Interventions Classification (NIC)*	1992		X			Comprehensive
Nursing Outcomes Classification (NOC)*	1997			X		Comprehensive
Omaha	1992	X	X	X		Comprehensive
Clinical Care/Home Care Classification System (CCC /HCCC)	1992	X	X	X		Home care/community care
Perioperative Nursing Data Set (PNDS)	1997	X	X	X		Perioperative care
International Classification for Nursing Practice (ICNP)	2000	X	X	X		Comprehensive
SNOMED CT	1999	X	X	X		Comprehensive
SNOMED CT Nursing Activities Subset		X				Comprehensive
Logical Observation Identifiers, Names and Codes (LOINC)	2002	X				Comprehensive
Alternate Billing Concepts	2000		X			

*Must be used together to cover assessment, interventions, and outcomes.
Sources: Thede, L., & Sewell, J. (2012). *ANA recognized nursing terminologies.* Retrieved from http://dlthede.net/Informatics/Chap16Documentation/anarecterm.html; Tastan, S., Linch, G. C. F., Keenan, G. M., et al. (2014). Evidence for the existing American Nurses Association-recognized standardized nursing terminologies: A systematic review. *International Journal of Nursing Studies, 51*(8), 1160–1170. https://doi.org/10.1016/j.ijnurstu.2013.12.004.

Many nurses from countries around the world assisted in the evaluation of terms and coding structures, and they collaborated with the ICN to develop the ICNP and generate numerous translations. With a network of research and development centres around the globe, including two in Canada, the ICNP continues to develop content and implementation maturity. A number of catalogues dedicated to specific nursing practice areas are available to facilitate the adoption of the ICNP in clinical information systems (ICN, 2019c; Table 10.5).

The seven axes that support the ICNP are action, client, focus, judgement, location, means, and time. Terms are combined to create nursing diagnoses, nursing interventions, and nursing outcomes. Similar to previous versions, both nursing diagnoses and nursing outcome statements must contain a term from the focus axis and the judgement axis and may include terms from additional axes as needed to fully describe the phenomenon of attention. Nursing interventions must include a term from the action axis and the target axis and may include additional terms from other axes as necessary.

Nurses have further recognized the need to establish standards governing nursing data and have participated in developing international nursing models and terminologies to support a standardized approach to nursing representation and communication. A key example of standards upholding nursing data is the ISO 18104 standard and its subsequent adoption in Canada (Hannah, 2005, p. 50; International Organization for Standardization, 2014). The ISO *Health informatics: Categorial structures for representation of nursing diagnoses and nursing actions in terminological systems* sets forth the relationships between nursing diagnoses and nursing interventions to ensure a consistent **ontology** between nursing reference terminologies and interface terminologies—essentially to support interoperability. In accordance with ISO practices, ISO 18104 was subjected to review in 2013 to ensure it was updated for continued relevance and guidance; it recently completed a

TABLE 10.5 International Classification for Nursing Practice (ICNP) Catalogues

ICNP Pre-Coordinated Nursing Diagnosis/ Outcomes & Interventions
ICNP Diagnosis/Outcomes
ICNP Interventions
ICNP Catalogues
Community Nursing
Dementia Care
Disaster Nursing
Nursing Care of Children with HIV and AIDS
Nursing Outcome Indicators
Paediatric Pain Management
Palliative Care
Partnering with Individuals and Families to Promote Adherence to Treatment
Prenatal Nursing Care
Equivalency Tables
ICNP to SNOMED CT Equivalency Table for Diagnosis and Outcome Statements
ICNP to CCC Equivalency Table for Nursing Diagnoses
ICNP Catalogues in Progress
Hospitalized Adult Mental Health Client
Hospitalized Paediatric Client
Post-Surgical Total Hip Replacement
Pressure Ulcer Prevention
Special Care Nursery

Source: ICN. (2019). *ICNP catalogues.* Retrieved from https://www.icn.ch/what-we-do/projects/ehealth-icnp/about-icnp/icnp-catalogues.

public review before final approval. Through involvement in ISO, SNOMED International, and other nursing informatics associations, Canada continues to contribute to this essential standard and to ensure that any revisions or additions represent Canadian nursing needs.

Further, Canada Health Infoway, in consultation with various health care groups, adopted SNOMED CT (Systematized Nomenclature of Medicine – Clinical Terms) as the terminology for use in the pan-Canadian EHR. SNOMED International and the ICN have a collaborative agreement that enables cross-mapping of ICNP terms into SNOMED CT to ensure that nursing data are accurately and effectively captured, and that terms are cross-mapped to provide comprehensive documentation. With regular releases, SNOMED CT is the most comprehensive terminology in the world, reporting 352,567 terms as of the January 31, 2020 release (SNOMED International, 2020).

The Canadian Health Outcomes for Better Information and Care (C-HOBIC) builds on the original Health Outcomes for Better Information and Care (HOBIC) project in Ontario and has included multiple standardized clinical terminologies and assessment tools, including ICNP, SNOMED CT, and interRAI (Canadian Health Outcomes for Better Information and Care [C-HOBIC], n.d.). The specific nursing-sensitive outcomes targeted for implementation in C-HOBIC include functional status, therapeutic self-care (or readiness for discharge), symptom management (pain, nausea, fatigue, dyspnea), and patient satisfaction (C-HOBIC, n.d.). In Canada, the collection of data about nursing practice and outcomes, and the representation of that data, provides a rich research opportunity to use standardized documentation.

 CULTURAL CONSIDERATIONS

eStigma

While informatics is a topic of increasing importance and interest, researchers and social advocates are paying increased attention to more socially conscious aspects of technology and its impact on people. This box on eStigma presents the master's research of Kelly Davison from The University of British Columbia. Her critical examination of the social impact of both subtle and explicit stigmatizing processes, designs, and philosophies in technology presents a unique opportunity to challenge assumptions and implicit biases and advocate for the adoption of more inclusive and empowering approaches to the design, use, and implementation of digital technologies.

The manner in which information and communication technologies (ICT) and the data they produce interact with marginalizing or empowering social phenomena is not well understood and requires thoughtful consideration. ICTs are created and designed by social beings, with specific biases that may contribute to social marginalization or may influence power and privilege. If we treat ICT design as static rather than malleable, we may unwittingly internalize this bias, enable institutional prejudice, and miss a critical opportunity to address health inequities for our patients.

eStigma—stigma that is enacted or enabled through the design and use of ICTs in the context of society—is an emerging concept that has important implications for health care informatics practice. In particular, ICTs and the data they produce need to be connected to the social justice agenda (Taylor, 2017) and ought to be used to

(Continued)

🌐 CULTURAL CONSIDERATIONS (*Cont.*)

address inequities in vulnerable and stigmatized popula-tions. Nurses, as clinicians who are expected to incorpo-rate ICTs into their skilled practice on a daily basis, and who provide care to vulnerable and stigmatized populations, are in a unique position to advocate for changes in ICT design and ICT-enabled practices that facilitate health equity. In a recent review of the literature on stigma, ICTs, and sexual and gender diversity, three main themes arose that demon-strate or may contribute to eStigma: the social impacts of technology, data visibility and invisibility, and institutional-ized prejudice. The following table summarizes some key points to consider.

Theme	Issue(s)	Overcoming the issue(s)
Social impacts of technology	Health inequities arise from complex systems and are a key priority for global health and operational research	Technology can support the principle of universality and can also enable exclusion. ICTs can facilitate equity through antidiscrimination or inequity through discrimination
Data (in) visibility	Through the creation of visibility of data about certain populations, we can learn how stigma impacts important outcomes such as life expectancy	Routine collection of data about vulnerable and stigmatized populations is paramount to addressing health inequities that are worsened by data invisibility
	Marginalizing social constructs, such as representing gender as a static binary, are hard-coded into ICTs and the databases that constitute them. This institutionalized prejudice squelches representation of gender diversity in the data and has many negative downstream impacts	Equity-informed design is required to establish data structures that appropriately reflect diversity
Institutionalized prejudice	Health care culture may not be psychologically safe for vulnerable and stigmatized persons and may itself be a barrier to access. ICTs contribute to this culture	Creating health care cultures that celebrate diversity and equity can improve outcomes. ICTs contribute to this culture
	Patients may be made to feel marginalized or invisible if fundamental truths about them (i.e., their sexual orientation) are not honoured in ICT design	Thoughtfully designed ICTs can override cultural barriers that impact health equity and improve outcomes
	Bias created by data invisibility threatens the validity, reliability, and generalizability of research results	Implementing diversity in data(bases) can help ensure that important advancements in research (e.g., genomics) are accurate and equitable
	The impact of ICTs on mediating or moderating marginalizing social processes does not seem to be widely considered in the global evidence pertaining to vulnerable and stigmatized persons and populations	Rhetoric around health inequities is well developed, and equity is contextualized by deep-seated power issues. Routine institutional data rarely captures complexities of reality. Planners require appropriate data to produce tools to address health inequities
	There is a dearth of literature examining the potential harms of ICTs in health care	The risk of publication bias should be considered

Source: Taylor, L. (2017). What is data justice? The case for connecting digital rights and freedoms globally. *Big Data & Society.* https://doi.org/10.1177/2053951717736335

NURSING DATA SCIENCE

As technology expands across the health care system, the volume of information is increasing exponentially. Data is being generated at unprecedented rates from a wide range of sources, including EHRs, clinical assessments, diagnostic testing, patient monitoring devices, smart technologies, mobile health applications, and social media. Firican (2017) estimates that mobile traffic generates 6.2 billion gigabytes of data per month, 300 hours of video is uploaded to YouTube every minute, and Google processes 40,000 search queries every second. This huge volume of information presents opportunities to generate new insights about health and disease management, effectiveness of interventions, and health system use. The sheer volume alone means that we cannot continue using the same techniques we always have. We must adopt new perspectives, new methods and tools, and new ways of conceptualizing health information management.

The concept of "big data" emerged around 2001. This term describes enormous data sets that exceed current capabilities of traditional database management approaches and methodologies to derive meaning from analysis (Brennan & Bakken, 2015; Gu, Li, Li, & Liang, 2017). Although the exact definition of "big data" continues to evolve and the number of Vs increases, the 5 Vs of big data are widely recognized and accepted (Westra, Sylvia, Weinfurter et al., 2017; Table 10.6). Firican (2017) suggested adding an additional 5Vs:

- Variability—inconsistencies in data or inconsistent speed of generation;
- Validity—data accuracy and correctness;
- Vulnerability—whether the data introduce any security issues;
- Volatility—the length of time data should be kept before becoming historic or irrelevant; and
- Visualization—finding a meaningful way to visually display the vast new data.

Harrington (2011, 2012) has advocated for the recognition of and a strategic approach to identifying and managing the **practice-based evidence** that is available in clinical environments and clinical information systems. This recognition of the full spectrum of information that reflects **clinical intelligence** about care delivery and outcomes of care, and acknowledgment of the value and potential impact of gaining insights from the data generated in practice, is aligned with the spirit of big data. Nurses spend a significant amount of time documenting in and managing digital health solutions in the course of their day, but are seldom provided with real-time feedback to inform or refine their practice (Jeffrey, 2019; Westra, Clancy, Sensmeier et al., 2015). Westra, Clancy, Sensmeier et al. (2015) refer to this phenomenon as being "data rich and information poor" (DRIP) and advocate for a more proactive approach to using the clinical intelligence that can be generated through big data analytics and **nursing data science**.

TABLE 10.6 The 5 Vs of Big Data

Characteristic	Description
Volume	The scale of data generated by a variety of sources, considered by many to be the hallmark of big data (Gu, Li, Li, & Liang, 2017; Westra, Sylvia, Weinfurter et al., 2017). Researchers projected that health care data will grow faster than data from all other sectors through to 2025 (Kent, 2018)
Velocity	The unparalleled speed of proliferation of data (Westra, Sylvia, Weinfurter et al., 2017)
Variety	Data are generated by a range of different data sources (Westra, Sylvia, Weinfurter et al., 2017)
Veracity	The degree of uncertainty of data elements and whether the data are fit for secondary analysis (Westra, Sylvia, Weinfurter et al., 2017; Topaz & Pruinelli, 2017)
Value	The perceived contribution that the data are able to provide to support the organizational mission and objectives

Sources: Gu, D., Li, J., Li, X., et al. (2017). Visualizing the knowledge structure and evolution of big data research in healthcare informatics, *International Journal of Medical Informatics 9*, 22–32. https://doi.org/10.1016/j.ijmedinf.2016.11.006; Kent, J. (2018, January). *Big data analytics, information governance, and informatics will be among the eight top issues of 2018, AHIMA predicts.* Retrieved from https://healthitanalytics.com/news/ahima-focus-on-healthcare-big-data-analytics-informatics-in-2018; Topaz, M., & Pruinelli, L. (2017). Big data and nursing: Implications for the future. In J. Murphy, W. Goossen, & P. Weber (Eds.), *Forecasting informatics competencies for nurses in the future of connected health* (pp. 165–171). Amsterdam, Netherlands: IMIA and IOS Press. https://doi.org/10.3233/978-1-61499-738-2-165; Westra, B. L., Sylvia, M., Weinfurter, E. F., et al. (2017). Big data science: A literature review of nursing research exemplars. *Nursing Outlook, 65*, 549–561. https://doi.org/10.1016/j.outlook.2016.11.021.

Early steps in understanding big data's magnitude prompted consideration of how best to systematically analyze and leverage the vast data holdings to improve outcomes and health care delivery. Brennan & Bakken (2015) recommended a principled, scientific approach to big data to complement the popular mainstream discussions—"data science," blending math, computer science, statistics, modelling, predictive analytics, and others, offering greater philosophical and methodological rigour to all phases of the data management cycle. Topaz and Pruinelli (2017) also defined data science as a multidisciplinary scholarship approach and noted that a variety of researchers are required to manage how "messy" health care data are and applying appropriate analytic methods, such as data mining, artificial intelligence, natural language processing, and visualization. Jeffrey (2019) has suggested that data science lies at the convergence of "domain knowledge, computer science, statistics, and data visualization/presentation" (p. 1).

With the increasing need to manage big data and analytics, many health care organizations are heavily investing by establishing dedicated institutes to study this domain and stimulate both innovation and collaboration. For example, Canada Health Infoway is investing in digital health data platforms for Canada's research hospitals and academic health sciences centres. HealthCareCAN (2019) will consult with Infoway, given its expertise in the development, adoption, and effective use of digital health solutions across the country. Numerous universities and teaching networks are also creating big data research programs and

CASE STUDY

Canadian Health Outcomes for Better Information and Care Project

The Canadian Health Outcomes for Better Information and Care (C-HOBIC) project represents a key Canadian initiative that links nursing practice and decades of research on standardized nursing data. C-HOBIC is a jointly funded initiative in partnership with the CNA, Canada Health Infoway, and three Canadian provinces to include nursing-sensitive patient information in EHRs. Ontario, Prince Edward Island, and Saskatchewan were the initial provincial participants, and in May 2008, Manitoba joined the initiative. Most recently, the C-HOBIC initiative completed a pilot project contributing data to CIHI's Discharge Abstract Database. Results of that pilot are currently being evaluated.

C-HOBIC uses ICNP, SNOMED CT, and interRAI (a comprehensive assessment tool) to enable collection and extraction of nursing data in secure jurisdictional EHRs, data repositories, or databases. C-HOBIC targets data on functional status, pain, fatigue, dyspnea, nausea, falls, and pressure ulcers and makes these data available to nurses for use in patient care across four sectors: acute care, complex continuing care, long-term care, and home care.

As a result of the work implemented in the C-HOBIC project, Canada has contributed to the development of the ICNP catalogue of terms by identifying new terms and recommending precoordination of terms to effectively capture the intent of the nursing item. The ICN has welcomed the C-HOBIC project as a leading example of standardized nursing data, and the C-HOBIC terms are being used by other countries, including Ireland.

The C-HOBIC project promotes widespread, systematic use in Canada of standardized patient assessments

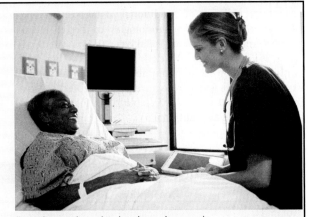

(istock.com/monkeybusinessimages)

and standardized related documentation. Based on the data captured by the C-HOBIC project, nurses are able to retrieve feedback about patient outcomes by comparing patient assessments at different times.

This groundbreaking initiative offers numerous benefits, including:

1. Relevant information to support clinical practice;
2. Improvements to patient care by fostering information access across care sectors; and
3. Opportunity to collect aggregated data that accurately reflect nursing activity.

Updates on the C-HOBIC project may be obtained through the CNA website.

collaborations, such as Dalhousie University in Halifax. Nine universities across Canada now offer master's programs focused on big data.

Brennan & Bakken (2015) have suggested that a key focus of the nursing profession should be ensuring that future nurse researchers and leaders are being adequately and appropriately prepared in data science and analytics—a priority echoed by Jeffrey (2019), Topaz and Pruinelli (2017), Westra, Clancy, Sensmeier et al. (2017), and Broome (2016), among others. Competency in advanced statistics, data modelling, visualization, data mining, and other advanced data management techniques will be required to position nursing to continue advancing knowledge using emerging vast data sets. The University of Victoria is innovating to meet this need by offering a dual master's degree in nursing and computer science and building skills to manage both advanced nursing scholarship and data/systems management. Many universities offer a Master of Health Informatics program, such as the University of Toronto, University of Waterloo, and Dalhousie University.

 APPLYING CONTENT KNOWLEDGE

Consider the CASN entry-to-practice competencies for registered nurses:
1. Do you think the recommended informatics competencies align with contemporary needs in clinical practice?
2. What additional factors might influence the development of competencies to support these outcomes?
3. Are there additional foundational technical skills that students should bring to their nursing programs?
4. What essential supports are required in the practice setting to enable the development of the nursing informatics competencies?

CANADIAN INFORMATICS AND DIGITAL HEALTH SHOWCASE

As digital health initiatives in Canada continue to mature, nurses serve as critical team members in projects that demonstrate innovations using technology to support practice and patient outcomes. Aside from the obvious clinical expertise nurses provide, Millard (2019) has noted that nurses are ideally positioned to function as leaders in transformation projects and expects their involvement to increase as nurses leverage their unique skills around technology, clinical practice and workflow management, and patient advocacy.

Figure 10.7 illustrates the seven-step model of health information technology adoption developed by the Healthcare Information and Management Systems Society (HIMSS). The Electronic Medical Record Adoption Model (EMRAM) is a maturity model of technology adoption that reflects increasing sophistication in the adoption of digital health technologies, with increasingly demanding requirements for the recognition of each stage. Health care organizations across Canada are generally at the lower stages of development, but an increasing number of facilities recognize the value of progression and are investing with their teams to improve health outcomes, strengthen their use of digital solutions, and earn higher EMRAM designations. Invariably, nurses are key leaders and team members in these examples.

Clinical and Systems Transformation Project, British Columbia

In British Columbia, health care is being transformed by the Clinical and Systems Transformation Project (CST), a major initiative involving Vancouver Coastal Health, the Provincial Health Services Authority, and Providence Health Care. Commencing in 2016, the CST Project started establishing common practices, assessments, and a clinical information system to support safety, quality, consistent care, and optimized health outcomes. Impacting everything from pharmacy and medication administration to radiology, labs, and clinical documentation, this initiative is transforming how data are collected, managed, and shared between partner organizations. Clinicians will see many changes, including real-time electronic charting, clinical decision-support tools, common clinical practices, and closed-loop medication systems. Patients will avoid duplicate testing and delays, minimize the need to repeat information to health care professionals, and have access to safer care. The concept of "collect once, use many times" is a key value in this initiative.

Since 2016, many sites have gone live with the new clinical information system and have reported positive responses from staff and patients. Nurses have played a critical role in the success of this massive and complex initiative. Sixteen clinicians from a variety of nursing practice settings, including maternal and child health, acute medicine, oncology, and others, were seconded to provide key clinical guidance on consolidating clinical practices and clinical contributions to configuration activities, training support, go-live support, and more (Clinical and Systems Transformation, 2014).

More information about the CST Project is available on the website.

HIMSS Analytics EMRAM

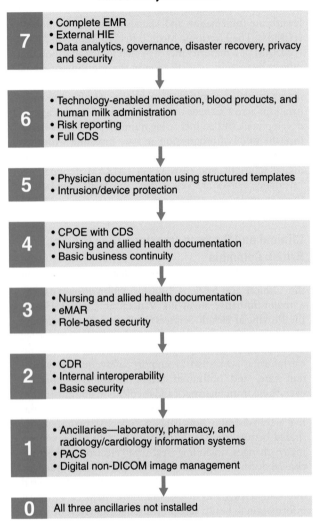

7
- Complete EMR
- External HIE
- Data analytics, governance, disaster recovery, privacy and security

6
- Technology-enabled medication, blood products, and human milk administration
- Risk reporting
- Full CDS

5
- Physician documentation using structured templates
- Intrusion/device protection

4
- CPOE with CDS
- Nursing and allied health documentation
- Basic business continuity

3
- Nursing and allied health documentation
- eMAR
- Role-based security

2
- CDR
- Internal interoperability
- Basic security

1
- Ancillaries—laboratory, pharmacy, and radiology/cardiology information systems
- PACS
- Digital non-DICOM image management

0   All three ancillaries not installed

Fig. 10.7 HIMSS Electronic Medical Record Adoption Model (EMRAM). CDR, Clinical data repository; CDS, clinical decision support; CPOE, computerized provider order entry; DICOM, Digital Imaging and Communications in Medicine; eMAR, electronic medication administration record; EMR, electronic medical record; HIE, health information exchange; PACS, picture archiving and communication system. (**Source:** HIMSS Analytics. (2019). *A strategic roadmap for effective EMR adoption and maturity.* Retrieved from https://www.himssanalytics.org/sites/himssanalytics/files/North_America_EMRAM_Information_2018.pdf.)

CASE STUDY

Digital Health Maturity Model and Mackenzie Health

HIMSS is a leader in digital health and health information management regulation and standards. With a head office located in the United States, HIMSS has branches located internationally to provide a network of leadership and informatics education and advocacy. HIMSS has also developed a maturity model that describes the hallmarks of progressive digital health adoption, known as the Electronic Medical Record Adoption Model (EMRAM). As the organization gains maturity and progresses through levels 0 to 7, various digital health components are added to generate increasing benefits and support for health care.

Mackenzie Health in Ontario planned to implement the full suite of Epic EMR systems in all departments to achieve improved health outcomes for patients and enhanced performance. Their goal was to achieve EMRAM level 6 within 2 years and level 7 within 3 years (Zeidenberg, 2016). Theirs was an aggressive goal, as most other hospitals in Canada have implemented only ambulatory or other selected Epic modules.

As Mackenzie built out their smart hospital, they successfully leveraged an enthusiastic clinical workforce. McKenzie is the first hospital in Canada to achieve level 7 (Zeidenberg, 2019). The effort and clinical engagement required to achieve this very rigorous milestone was significant, requiring nurses to be actively involved from the beginning. With working groups and nursing staff from across the organization actively collaborating and innovating practice improvements, developing standard operating policies, providing critical feedback on workflows and clinical practice requirements for documentation, providing training to end users, and providing go-live support, nurses were essential to the project's success. More information on this initiative is available on the Mackenzie Health website.

Sources: Zeidenberg, J. (2016. February 3). *Mackenzie Health moves ahead with Epic HIS.* Retrieved from https://www.canhealth.com/2016/02/03/mackenzie-health-moves-ahead-with-epic-his/; Zeidenberg, J. (2019, January 31). *Mackenzie Health makes the leap to EMRAM 7.* Retrieved from https://www.canhealth.com/2019/01/31/mackenzie-health-makes-the-leap-to-emram-7/.

The Hospital for Sick Children's Epic Implementation Project

In 2015, leaders of The Hospital for Sick Children in Toronto (SickKids) started planning for a major clinical information system implementation on what would be a 3-year journey (Greenwood, 2018). On January 1, 2016, SickKids commenced its enterprise-wide Epic implementation. With an aggressive time frame in which to implement the system and a commitment to using a "big bang" approach, in which the new solution goes live across the hospital for everyone at the same time, SickKids successfully went live in a completely digital environment in December 2018. Helen Edwards, Chief Nursing Informatics Officer, noted that SickKids' success was thanks to (1) having the full participation of clinical governance and clinical leaders who had shared accountability in their dedicated project roles and were passionate about supporting nurses during the transition; (2) supporting the working groups that provided leadership on design, configuration, and practice requirements; and (3) actively leading the Nursing Council where decisions were made (H. Edwards, personal communication, May 27, 2019). The next phases will include optimization of processes and developing analytics on the data being generated by the new clinical information system—activities in which nurses will again be actively involved. More information is available on the SickKids website.

North York General Hospital Wins HIMSS Davies Enterprise Award

HIMSS is a leading international organization focused on health information and innovation. The Davies Enterprise Award is presented annually to an organization that successfully applies health information and technology to significantly improve clinical care, health care outcomes, and population health (Canadian Healthcare Technology, 2017). North York General Hospital began a project in 2016 to raise their EMRAM status from level 2 to level 6 and improve their overall care delivery in the following four domains (HIMSS, 2019):

- Improving the prevention of nosocomial venous thromboembolism (VTE);
- Reducing preventable inpatient death;
- Reducing medication errors with a closed loop medication administration system; and
- Implementing a medication reconciliation system that reduces the risk of unintended medication discrepancies.

In early 2017, HIMSS presented the 2016 Davies Enterprise Award to North York General Hospital for their outstanding accomplishments related to leveraging technology to improve care. The hospital reduced their VTE rates by almost 40%, increased appropriate prophylaxis to 97%, and reduced mortality rates for inpatients from pneumonia and COPD exacerbations. They also implemented a closed-loop medication system to improve drug management and medication reconciliation, thereby minimizing the risk of preventable medication errors.

PRIVACY AND CONFIDENTIALITY IN A DIGITAL PRACTICE DOMAIN

A significant issue in nursing, regardless of the presence or absence of technology, relates to patient privacy and the security of patient information. Where computerized records are shared across jurisdictions, the protection of privacy and confidentiality becomes an even greater concern. The provincial standards of practice and the national *Code of Ethics for Registered Nurses* (CNA, 2017b) govern nurses' actions in regard to the protection of patient information. Privacy legislation varies among provinces, and nurses should have a working knowledge of the relevant legislation, both provincially and nationally.

There are two separate pieces of legislation that govern the privacy of personal information at the federal level. These are the *Privacy Act* and the *Personal Information Protection and Electronic Documents Act* (PIPEDA) (Government of Canada, 2018a). Each Act sets forth specific regulatory parameters with regard to personal information. In the *Privacy Act*, the regulation states that "Personal information under the control of a government institution shall not, without the consent of the individual to whom it relates, be disclosed by the institution" (Government of Canada, 2018b, s. 8.1). PIPEDA takes the *Privacy Act* one step further by addressing the specific risks associated with electronic data collection, storage, retrieval, and communication (Government of Canada, 2019). PIPEDA addresses personal health information specifically and notes that the personal health information of an individual, whether living or deceased, means

(a) information concerning the physical or mental health of the individual;

(b) information concerning any health service provided to the individual;

(c) information concerning the donation by the individual of any body part or any bodily substance of the individual or information derived from the testing or examination of a body part or bodily substance of the individual;

(d) information that is collected in the course of providing health services to the individual; or

(e) information that is collected incidentally to the provision of health services to the individual. (Government of Canada, 2019, s. 1.2)

PIPEDA further stipulates that the disclosure of personal information may be permitted only under the most stringent of conditions, such as when required by law enforcement (Government of Canada, 2019, s. 7.3).

Many provinces have enacted provincial privacy laws whose key tenets align with those of federal privacy legislation. The provinces have also included guidance on addressing privacy needs specific to their jurisdiction. In cases where the provincial laws are deemed to be "substantially similar" to PIPEDA, the provincial laws take precedence. Alberta, British Columbia, and Quebec have enacted provincial privacy laws governing the private sector that supersede PIPEDA owing to their close alignment in focus, while Nova Scotia, New Brunswick, Newfoundland, and Ontario have enacted privacy laws with a substantially similar focus, specifically on health information (Government of Canada, 2018a). PIPEDA applies to all other provinces and territories in Canada.

Regardless of the practice setting or mode, nurses are professionally and ethically obliged to protect the personal information of all patients in their care. Knowledge of these two pieces of federal privacy legislation, in addition to provincial privacy legislation, can support nurses as they uphold the standards of practice and *Code of Ethics*.

NURSING INFORMATICS COMMUNITIES AND RESOURCES

Internet access to nursing and health-related resources is immensely helpful to nurse clinicians, administrators, educators, and researchers. Websites have been launched by respected organizations, special interest groups, and individuals to provide information and assistance in relation to their mission or principal interests. Thus, information that previously might have taken nurses days or weeks to obtain can be accessed within minutes. Websites may also contain information about the principal staff and divisions of an organization as well as the names and telephone numbers of contacts for particular kinds of assistance, thereby providing valuable networking opportunities.

The plethora of health information available online is also reflective of the demand by patients and consumers to be involved in decision making about their health care. However, without the benefit of health care education, consumers are vulnerable to misinformation, and nurses must therefore be prepared to help guide health research activities and evaluate the quality and veracity of information discovered in consumer searches. Tools to evaluate the quality of information on websites exist for such a purpose. Perhaps the best recognized is the HONCode tool, which provide an eight-item assessment covering such topics as authority, attribution, privacy, and transparency

to determine the trustworthiness of the information (Health on the Net, 2017). Other similar tools include the DISCERN tool (DISCERN, n.d.), the Dalhousie University tool (Dalhousie University, 2019), the Delphi method (Boulkedid, Abdoul, Loustau et al., 2011), and a tool developed by Leite, Gonçalves, Teixeira et al. (2011).

Nurses routinely use the Web for accessing up-to-date health information or to network with professional colleagues. The success of electronic discussion groups is perhaps one of the most exciting professional developments for nurses. There are hundreds of online public discussion lists, newsgroups, chat rooms, and blogs that connect nurses around the globe. Feedspot is one such site that provides links to most other nursing blogs and provides opportunities for nurses to informally discuss professional information as well as pursue discussions that have a more educational flavour. Tools like LinkedIn, Twitter, Facebook, and other emerging social media platforms also offer channels for connecting with other nurses and interprofessional colleagues, networking and collegial support, nursing education, research and other scholarly activity, and political action.

Nurses interested in joining a network or nursing informatics community will find several groups readily accessible online. Although not every province has a nursing informatics special-interest group, the CNIA has a website offering access to a variety of educational resources, informatics events, and networking opportunities. Links to existing provincial nursing informatics groups are available on the CNIA website. IMIA-NI is an international organization of significant value to nurses interested in nursing informatics. This group has multiple working groups and represents the interests of nurses internationally.

Digital Health Canada (DHC; formerly known as COACH, Canada's Health Informatics Association), formed in 1975 by several health professionals and vendors in the medical industry, is another group of interest to nurses. DHC's more than 900 members include health care executives, physicians, nurses and allied health professionals, researchers and educators, chief information officers, information managers, technical experts, consultants, and information technology vendors. Organizational members include health care service delivery organizations, government and nongovernment agencies, consulting firms, commercial providers of information and telecommunications technologies, and educational institutions.

Today, there are a multitude of online resources for nurses. The library catalogues of most universities and major university health centres are for the most part fully online and provide access to full-text journal articles. Online lectures with leading experts are offered by many groups. The MyCNA site also incorporates many of these features to support nursing education and professional practice.

GLIMPSES INTO THE FUTURE

The CNA released its vision for future nursing practice in its landmark document *Toward 2020: Visions for Nursing* (CNA, 2006b). This document highlighted areas that would change between the document's publication and 2020. Changes predicted in the report included the use of robots to perform mundane or repetitive tasks, changes in human resource management, and an education revolution in how nursing programs are structured. These are all changes that have emerged or are emerging in Canada, and while not yet evident in every hospital or practice setting, these milestones are shaping nursing practice. Personalized medicine has enabled customized treatments that offer greater potential for successful outcomes, while artificial intelligence applications are providing more rapid diagnosis and treatment support. Care is being documented using mobile devices such as tablets and phones, and smart devices (glucometers, heart and blood pressure monitors, scales, spirometers, and more comprehensive solutions such as smart homes) are sending patient data directly to clinicians to enable remote monitoring. The boundaries of care settings are blurring, and visionary leaders are needed who can proactively manage how accountabilities and nursing practice evolve (Kennedy & Moen, 2017; Remus, 2016; Hussey & Kennedy, 2016).

CONCLUSION

Although the nursing practice environment has evolved significantly with the integration of technology, the philosophy and goals of nursing have remained constant. The patient-centred focus of the profession is as important now as ever. It may have assumed even more importance, with patients requiring more support and reassurance as they undergo new and potentially frightening diagnostic and treatment procedures.

The vast array of informational resources that have been made accessible by technological innovations will continue to benefit nurses and their patients. Enhancements to communication resources are occurring on an almost daily basis. Nurses will continue to advocate for patients in the midst of a health care environment that is laden with technology and continue to support the central goals of competent and caring nursing practice.

SUMMARY OF LEARNING OBJECTIVES

- Digital health and nursing informatics have evolved significantly since the 1960s and 1970s, with the term "nursing informatics" coined in the 1980s. Since the 1980s, definitions of both nursing informatics and digital health have progressed to reflect both the platforms (or technology) and the nature of how professional disciplines use technology to deliver services. Existing and emerging innovations continue to progress the concept of digital health and expand the scope of practice.
- While technology is increasingly ubiquitous, nursing informatics is recognized as a distinct practice. The CASN approved core competencies as necessary to practice in contemporary digital health environments, as well as additional foundational skills. Additionally, technology is also referenced in the CNA *Code of Ethics*, making competent use of technology both a regulatory and ethical requirement.
- Understanding the key federal health information agencies and their respective mandates is a necessity. Organizations such as the CIHI and Canada Health Infoway provide key leadership in defining health standards, funding and collaborating on innovation, and maintaining key data holdings for national use. Other key organizations include the CNIA and Digital Health Canada, both of which provide communities of practice and uniquely support and advance digital health in the Canadian health care system.
- Standardized languages such as ICNP and SNOMED CT are essential in digital health information systems and effectively represent nursing practice in the health care system in a systematic manner. Standardized nursing data enable comparison, analysis, and interpretation across practice domains, geography, and time. Nursing data standards prescribe how nursing data should be capture, stored, presented, and exchanged to enable nursing data to be consistently managed and compared. C-HOBIC is an example of a standardized outcomes tool that enables consistent analysis of nursing-sensitive outcomes across four domains of practice, and which can be easily integrated into health information systems for ease of use.
- Nursing data science is an emerging field of study, arising from the formalization of big data, and offers innovative philosophies, approaches, and analytical methods to understand past, current, and future health information; drive new insights and interpretations; and support future health care and nursing practice.
- Canada's health care organizations are benefitting from the adoption of digital health. SickKids, Mackenzie Health, and North York General Hospital have all

successfully applied digital solutions to improve the delivery of patient care and outcomes. EMRAM, a model of digital maturity, demonstrates how nurses' roles are evolving across care boundaries to include new ways of communicating with clients and how nurses are offering services using new modalities.

- First Nations communities in Atlantic Canada have experienced successes and challenges with implementing and using digital health technologies. Including Indigenous ways of knowing and being in clinical information systems better serves the needs of Indigenous peoples and is an important step toward reconciliation.

- In Canada, we are guided by both federal and provincial legislation that determines the provision of privacy and protection of personal health information. The *Privacy Act* and PIPEDA are two important pieces of federal legislation. Where provincial legislation is similar to PIPEDA, the provincial legislation takes precedence.

- Nurses can participate in digital health and informatics communities in many different ways. The CNIA, Digital Health Canada, and Infoway all offer communities of practice, while formal and informal communities also exist on the Web and through social media. Provincial nursing informatics groups exist in many provinces, and these can be accessed through the CNIA.

CRITICAL THINKING QUESTIONS

1. You are part of a multidisciplinary team that is planning for a new health information system at your local hospital or community centre. The members of what other disciplines are important to have as team members? Why? What specific competencies would you need to be an effective nursing representative? How will these competencies contribute to your participation?

2. You and your nursing team are examining ways to examine the outcomes of nursing care on your unit. The manager has required that a standardized nursing language must be used to perform the analysis. What are some of the issues you may confront with colleagues unfamiliar with such languages? How would you explain the necessity and value of standardized languages in nursing?

REFERENCES

Ball, M. J., & Hannah, K. J. (1984). *Using computers in nursing.* Reston, VA: Reston Publishing.

Branswell, H. (2013, March 6). Ten years later, SARS still haunts survivors and health-care workers. *The Globe and Mail.* Retrieved from https://www.theglobeandmail.com.

Brennan, P. F., & Bakken, S. (2015). Nursing needs big data and big data needs nursing. *Journal of Nursing Scholarship, 47*(5), 477–484. https://doi.org/10.1111/jnu.12159.

Broome, M. E. (2016). Big data, data science, and big contributions. *Nursing Outlook, 64*(2), 113–114. https://doi.org/10.1016/j.outlook.2016.02.001.

Boulkedid, R., Abdoul, H., Loustau, M., et al. (2011). Using and reporting the Delphi method for selecting healthcare quality indicators: A systematic review. *PLoS ONE, 6*(6), 1–9. https://doi.org/10.1371/journal.pone.0020476.

Canada Health Infoway. (2018). *Infoway 2018 annual report.* Retrieved from https://www.infoway-inforoute.ca/en/component/edocman/resources/i-infoway-i-corporate/annual-reports/3556-annual-report-2017-2018.

Canadian Association of Schools of Nursing. (2015). *Nursing informatics: Entry-to-practice competencies for registered nurses.* Ottawa, ON: Author.

Canadian Health Outcomes for Better Information and Care. (n.d.). *About C-HOBIC.* Retrieved from https://c-hobic.cna-aiic.ca/about/default_e.aspx.

Canadian Healthcare Technology. (2017 February, 1). *NYGH to receive prestigious HIMSS award.* Retrieved from https://www.canhealth.com/2017/02/01/nygh-to-receive-prestigious-himss-award/.

Canadian Institute for Health Information. (2018). *National health expenditure trends, 1975 to 2018.* Ottawa, ON: Author. Retrieved from https://www.cihi.ca/sites/default/files/document/nhex-trends-narrative-report-2018-en-web.pdf.

Canadian Institute for Health Information. (2019a). *About CIHI.* Retrieved from https://www.cihi.ca/en/about-cihi.

Canadian Nurses Association. (1993). *Papers from the Nursing Minimum Data Set Conference.* Ottawa, ON: Author.

Canadian Nurses Association. (2000). *Collecting data to reflect nursing impact: Discussion paper.* Ottawa, ON: Author.

Canadian Nurses Association. (2006a). *E-Nursing strategy for Canada.* Ottawa, ON: Author. Retrieved from https://www.cna-aiic.ca/~/media/cna/page-content/pdf-en/e-nursing-strategy-for-canada.pdf.

Canadian Nurses Association. (2006b). *Toward 2020: Visions for nursing.* Ottawa, ON: Author.

Canadian Nurses Association. (2017a). *Nursing informatics: Joint position statement.* Retrieved from https://www.cna-aiic.ca/-/media/cna/page-content/pdf-en/nursing-informatics-joint-position-statement.pdf.

Canadian Nurses Association. (2017b). *Code of ethics for registered nurses.* Ottawa, ON: Author. https://www.cna-aiic.ca/~/media/cna/page-content/pdf-en/code-of-ethics-2017-edition-secure-interactive.

Canadian Nurses Association. (2019). *Nursing informatics.* Retrieved from https://www.cna-aiic.ca/en/nursing-practice/the-practice-of-nursing/nursing-informatics.

Clark, J., & Lang, N. M. (1992). Nursing's next advance: An international classification system for nursing practice. *International Nursing Review, 39*(4), 109–112. 128.

Clinical and Systems Transformation. (2014). *About CST.* Retrieved from http://cstproject.ca/about-cst.

Dalhousie University. (2019). *Evaluation of health information on the web.* Retrieved from http://dal.ca.libguides.com/c.php?g=257155.

DISCERN. (n.d.). *Welcome to DISCERN.* Retrieved from http://www.discern.org.uk.

Firican, G. (2017, February 8). *The 10 V's of big data.* Retrieved from https://tdwi.org/articles/2017/02/08/10-vs-of-big-data.aspx.

Government of Canada. (2018a). *Summary of privacy laws in Canada.* Retrieved from https://www.priv.gc.ca/en/privacy-topics/privacy-laws-in-canada/02_05_d_15/.

Government of Canada. (2018b). *The Privacy Act. Bill C-21.* Retrieved from https://www.priv.gc.ca/en/privacy-topics/privacy-laws-in-canada/the-privacy-act/.

Government of Canada. (2019). *Personal Information Protection and Electronic Documents Act (PIPEDA).* Retrieved from https://www.priv.gc.ca/en/privacy-topics/privacy-laws-in-canada/the-personal-information-protection-and-electronic-documents-act-pipeda/.

Graves, J. R., & Corcoran, S. (1989). The study of nursing informatics. *Image: Journal of Nursing Scholarship, 21,* 227–231. https://doi.org/10.1111/j.1547-5069.1989.tb00148.x.

Greenwood, M. (2018 June 1). *This is how SickKids Hospital is going completely digital overnight.* Retrieved from https://techvibes.com/2018/06/01/sickkids-hospital-is-going-completely-digital.

Gu, D., Li, J., Li, X., & Liang, C. (2017). Visualizing the knowledge structure and evolution of big data research in healthcare informatics. *International Journal of Medical Informatics, 9,* 22–32. https://doi.org/10.1016/j.ijmedinf.2016.11.006.

Hannah, K. J. (2005). Health informatics and nursing in Canada. *Healthcare Information Management and Communications, 19*(3), 45–51.

Hannah, K. J., Ball, M., & Edwards, M. (2006). *Introduction to nursing informatics* (3rd ed.). New York, NY: Springer-Verlag.

Hannah, K. J., White, P., Nagle, L., et al. (2009). Standardizing nursing information in Canada for inclusion in electronic health records: C-HOBIC. *Journal of the American Medical Informatics Association, 16,* 524–530. https://doi.org/10.1197/jamia.M2974.

Harrington, L. (2011). Clinical intelligence. *Journal of Nursing Administration, 41*(12), 507–509. https://doi.org/10.1097/NNA.0b013e318237cca0.

Harrington L. (2012). The role of nurse informaticists in the emerging field of clinical intelligence. *Proceedings NI2012: 11th International Congress on Nursing Informatics,* Montreal, QC, Canada (2012). pp. 162–165.

HealthCareCAN. (2019). *Digital health and data platforms: An opportunity for Canadian excellence in evidence-based health research.* Retrieved from http://www.healthcarecan.ca/2019/01/25/digital-health-and-data-platforms-an-opportunity-for-canadian-excellence-in-evidence-based-health-research/.

Health on the Net. (2017). *HONCode.* Retrieved from https://www.healthonnet.org/HONcode/Conduct.html.

HIMSS. (2019). *North York General Hospital — Davies enterprise award.* Retrieved from https://www.himss.org/library/north-york-general-hospital-davies-enterprise-award.

Hussey, P., & Kennedy, M. A. (2016). Instantiating informatics within nursing practice for integrated patient centered holistic models of care: A discussion paper. *Journal of Advanced Nursing, 75*(5), 1030–1041. https://doi.org/10.1111/jan.12927.

International Council of Nurses. (2019a). *eHealth & ICNP.* Retrieved from https://www.icn.ch/what-we-do/projects/ehealth-icnp.

International Council of Nurses. (2019b). *ICNP browser.* Retrieved from https://www.icn.ch/what-we-do/projects/ehealth/icnp-browser.

International Council of Nurses. (2019c). *ICNP catalogues.* Retrieved from https://www.icn.ch/what-we-do/projects/ehealth-icnp/about-icnp/icnp-catalogues.

International Medical Informatics Association Special Interest Group – Nursing Informatics (IMIA-NI). (2009). *Definition of nursing informatics.* Retrieved from https://imianews.wordpress.com/2009/08/24/imia-ni-definition-of-nursing-informatics-updated/.

International Organization for Standardization. (2014). *ISO 18104: Health informatics—Categorial structures for representation of nursing diagnoses and nursing actions in terminological systems.* Retrieved from https://www.iso.org/standard/59431.html.

Jeffrey, A. (2019). ANI emerging leader project: Identifying challenges and opportunities in nursing data science. *Computers in Nursing, 37*(11), 1–3. https://doi.org/10.1097/CIN.0000000000000504.

Kennedy, M. A., & Moen, A. (2017). Nurse leadership and informatics competencies: Shaping transformation of professional practice. In J. Murphy, W. Goosen, & P. Weber (Eds.), *Forecasting informatics competencies for nurses in the future of connected health* (pp. 197–206). Amsterdam, Netherlands: IAMA and IOS Press.

Leite, P., Gonçalves, J., Teixeira, P., et al. (2011). A model for the evaluation of data quality in health unit websites. *Health Informatics Journal, 22,* 479–495. https://doi.org/1460458214567003.

Millard, M. (2019, May 6). *Nurses are well-positioned to lead innovation and digital transformation.* Retrieved from https://www.healthcareitnews.com/news/nurses-are-well-positioned-lead-innovation-and-digital-transformation.

Nagle, L., & White, P. (Eds.) (2018). *Proceedings of the 2018 national nursing data standards symposium.* Retrieved from https://www.cihi.ca/sites/default/files/document/nnds_2018_proceedings.pdf.

Naylor, D., Girard, F., Mintz, J., et al. (2015). *Unleashing innovation: Excellent healthcare for Canada. Report of the advisory panel on healthcare innovation.* (Health Canada catalogue no. H22-4/9-2015E-PDF). Retrieved from https://www.canada.ca/en/health-canada/services/publications/health-system-services/report-advisory-panel-healthcare-innovation.html.

Remus, S. (2016). The big data revolution: Opportunities for chief nurse executives. *Canadian Journal of Nursing Leadership, 28*(4), 18–28. https://doi.org/10.12927/cjnl.2016.24557.

SNOMED International. (2020). *5-step briefing.* Retrieved from https://www.snomed.org/snomed-ct/five-step-briefing.

Statistics Canada. (2016). *Population trends by age and sex.* Retrieved from https://www150.statcan.gc.ca/n1/pub/11-627-m/11-627-m2017016-eng.htm.

Statistics Canada. (2017). *The internet and digital technology.* Retrieved from https://www150.statcan.gc.ca/n1/pub/11-627-m/11-627-m2017032-eng.htm.

Topaz, M., & Pruinelli, L. (2017). Big data and nursing: Implications for the future. In J. Murphy, W. Goossen, & P. Weber (Eds.), *Forecasting informatics competencies for nurses in the future of connected health* (pp. 165–171). Amsterdam, Netherlands: IMIA and IOS Press. https://doi.org/10.3233/978-1-61499-738-2-165.

United Nations. (2019). *Ageing.* Retrieved from https://www.un.org/en/sections/issues-depth/ageing/.

Werley, H. H. (1988). Introduction to the nursing minimum data set and its development. In H. H. Werley, & N. M. Lang (Eds.), *Identification of the nursing minimum data set* (pp. 1–15). New York, NY: Springer.

Westra, B. L., Clancy, T. R., Sensmeier, J., et al. (2015). Nursing knowledge: Big data science—implications for nurse leaders.

Journal of Nursing Administration., 39, 304–310. https://doi.org/10.1097/NAQ. 0000000000000130.

Westra, B. L., Sylvia, M., Weinfurter, E. F., et al. (2017). Big data science: A literature review of nursing research exemplars. *Nursing Outlook, 65*, 549–561. https://doi.org//10.1016/j.outlook.2016.11.021.

White, P., Nagle, L., & Hannah, K. (2017). Adopting national nursing data standards in Canada. *Canadian Nurse, 113*(3), 18–23. Retrieved from https://www.canadian-nurse.com/en/articles/issues/2017/may-june-2017/adopting-national-nursing-data-standards-in-canada.

World Health Organization. (2015). *WHO global strategy on people centered and integrated health services interim report.* Retrieved from http://www.who.int/servicedeliverysafety/areas/people-centred-care/global-strategy/en/.

World Health Organization. (2017). *eHealth.* Retrieved from http://www.who.int/topics/ehealth/en/.

World Health Organization. (2019a). *10 facts on the state of global health.* Retrieved from https://www.who.int/features/factfiles/global_burden/en/.

World Health Organization. (2019b). *Noncommunicable diseases.* Retrieved from https://www.who.int/news-room/fact-sheets/detail/noncommunicable-diseases.

World Population Review. (2019). *Canada population.* Retrieved from http://worldpopulationreview.com/countries/canada-population/.

PART III

Nursing Care Delivery

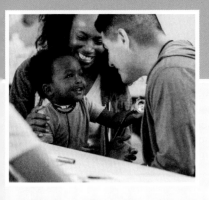

Primary Health Care: Challenges and Opportunities for the Nursing Profession

Lynn Anne Rempel

e http://evolve.elsevier.com/Canada/Ross-Kerr/nursing

LEARNING OBJECTIVES

After reading this chapter, you will be able to:
- Explain and provide examples of the five interrelated principles of primary health care.
- Describe the international and historical evolution of primary health care.
- Identify examples of primary health care initiatives in Canada.
- Explain the role of primary health care in addressing both physical and social determinants of health.

- Describe nursing's involvement and the potential leadership role of nursing in the evolution of primary health care in Canada.
- Identify how every nurse can practice using primary health care principles.
- Explain the challenges and complexities of providing health care that meets primary health care goals.

OUTLINE

KEY TERMS

accessibility	interdisciplinary collaboration	public administration
appropriate technology	intersectoral collaboration	public participation
comprehensiveness	LGBTQ2	social determinants of health
health equity	multilateral agencies	social justice
health promotion	population health	universality
illness prevention	portability	upstream

PERSONAL PERSPECTIVES

As a public health nurse in the 1980s, I promoted health in a variety of ways for people across the lifespan. I taught prenatal classes, visited new mothers, served as the neighbourhood school nurse, developed long-term supportive relationships with families experiencing parenting challenges, helped seniors manage their chronic conditions at home or at clinics where I also provided regular foot care, and assisted people with psychiatric problems to manage their medications and to develop supportive relationships. As district nurses, we were a first point of connection to the health care system.

Public health priorities changed, and nursing practice became more specialized. My own practice became more focused on prenatal and postpartum nursing and breastfeeding promotion. I valued breastfeeding as a healthy behaviour that provided the best start for baby. I observed that successful breastfeeding was often empowering for women, but noted that most women, especially those who were young or socioeconomically disadvantaged, stopped breastfeeding early. This started me on a journey of breastfeeding promotion research that prompted another public health nurse to organize a region-wide breastfeeding forum with health professionals and community members to consider ways to strengthen breastfeeding support. The result was Breastfeeding Buddies, a mom-to-mom breastfeeding support program. An intersectoral group of nurses, community partners, and breastfeeding mothers formed the steering committee that developed the program. It was determined that the appropriate way to deliver the program (the appropriate technology, in principles of primary health terminology) would be mothers with breastfeeding experience, trained with the 18-hour breastfeeding course, who would be matched with new mothers to provide telephone breastfeeding support or meet mothers at breastfeeding drop-in sites in shopping malls. Buddies connected mothers to nurses whenever there was a breastfeeding or other challenge that was beyond their scope as a volunteer. A breastfeeding mother was hired to coordinate the program from an office at the Downtown Community Health

Centre. In order to connect with mothers before birth, we developed *Me? Breastfeed?*, a prenatal breastfeeding workshop led by trained Buddies. My evaluation showed that this innovative technology was as effective as a traditional nurse-led breastfeeding class and that mothers found it more helpful to learn from the peer breastfeeding experiences (Rempel & Moore, 2012).

Over the 16 years since its inception, the program has grown and thrived. Accessibility is a high priority. There are Breastfeeding Buddies who have experience as teen mothers who join the coordinator at *Me? Breastfeed?* sessions at a community agency for teen mothers. There are Buddies for nontraditional families, including lesbian and transgender mothers. Support is provided in multiple languages. Arabic-speaking Buddies hold sessions in a mosque. *Me? Breastfeed?* workshops and drop-ins are offered in low-income neighbourhoods. A local hospital has invited Buddies to meet with mothers on the postpartum unit as a way of reducing nonmedical formula supplementation.

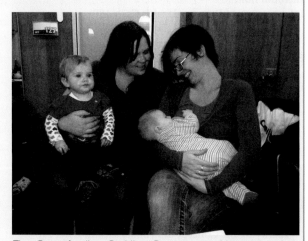

The Breastfeeding Buddies Program provides appropriate, accessible, participatory peer breastfeeding support. (Breastfeeding Buddies Program of Waterloo Region.)

As nurses, we successfully engaged in a participatory, intersectoral collaboration to develop and provide ongoing support for an accessible, appropriate technology for health promotion that meets community needs. Developing the Breastfeeding Buddies Program has been one of my best experiences in providing primary health care.

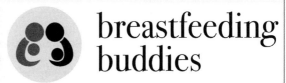

breastfeeding
buddies

Funded by Kitchener Downtown CHC and Region of Waterloo Public Health and Emergency Services

(Breastfeeding Buddies Program of Waterloo Region)

INTRODUCTION

With the Declaration of Alma-Ata in 1978, primary health care (PHC) was introduced as "the key to attaining . . . a level of health that will permit . . . all peoples of the world by the year 2000 . . . to lead a socially and economically productive life . . . as part of development in the spirit of social justice" (World Health Organization [WHO], 1978, p. 3). The goal of this international meeting was captured in the slogan "Health for All by the Year 2000." PHC was defined as

> *essential health care based on practical, scientifically sound and socially acceptable methods and technology made universally accessible to individuals and families in the community through their full participation and at a cost that the community and country can afford to maintain at every stage of their development in the spirit of self-reliance and self-determination. It forms an integral part both of the country's health system, of which it is the central function and main focus, and of the overall social and economic development of the community. It is the first level of contact of individuals, the family and community with the national health system bringing health care as close as possible to where people live and work, and constitutes the first element of a continuing health care process.* (WHO, 1978, pp. 3–4)

From the beginning, PHC was conceptualized as a **social justice** model. The nursing profession was envisioned as being key to attaining health for all (Mahler, 1985). Nurses around the world, including in Canada, embraced PHC as fundamental to nursing's role in enhancing health, and nurses have been actively involved in efforts to bring about PHC reform.

DECONSTRUCTING PRIMARY HEALTH CARE

Principles of Primary Health Care

Although the PHC concept is somewhat ambiguous, there is general agreement that PHC is based on five principles (see Figure 11.1).

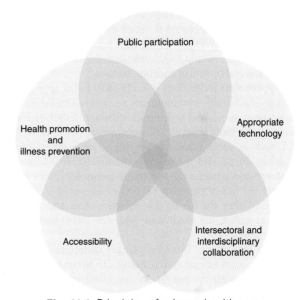

Fig. 11.1 Principles of primary health care.

Accessibility implies promotive, preventive, curative, rehabilitative, and palliative health care that is universally available to all people without unreasonable geographic or financial barriers (Canadian Nurses Association [CNA], 2015). Factors such as hours of service, physical features, or cultural safety also determine accessibility of health care services (CNA, 2005). In the spirit of the Health for All philosophy of reducing health inequities, the concept of accessibility can be expanded beyond its conventional meaning of access to health care services to access to the social, economic, environmental, and behavioural determinants of health (WHO, 2011), which often lie outside traditional health care services.

Public participation refers to individual and community involvement in the planning and operation of their health care and the health of their communities (CNA, 2005). Health committees and self-help, advocacy, community protection, or other civil society organizations can be directly involved in planning and implementing health care and can hold health care providers and government accountable for their policies and actions (WHO, 2003). Collaborative partnerships include partnerships at all levels—governmental, nongovernmental, corporate, and community.

The principle of **health promotion** and **illness prevention** stresses the importance of a strong focus on these aspects of health care in contrast to the generally greater emphasis on cure and treatment of illness (Lankshear, 2012). The Ottawa Charter (WHO, 1986) introduced the broad view of health promotion as enabling control over determinants of health, most of which are outside the direct control of the health care sector. Thus, health promotion requires public participation and intersectoral collaboration to achieve equity in health. Illness prevention is central to six of the eight essential elements of PHC (WHO, 1978): health education, nutrition, sanitation, maternal and child health care, immunization, and prevention and control of endemic diseases.

Appropriate technology refers broadly to the appropriate use of all health care resources, such as funds, facilities, equipment, tools, and techniques (Stewart, 2000). It also includes the most effective and appropriate use of personnel, such as using nurses to provide chronic illness care (Ritchie, 2012), and the use of evidence-informed interventions and strategies. Appropriate technology does not assume the use of the most current or advanced technology, but rather the use of cost-effective tools and methods that match the needs and values of individuals and communities.

Intersectoral and **interdisciplinary collaboration** is a crucial principle to achieving health for all and is highly interrelated with the previously described principles. As one of the key elements relevant to action on determinants of health (Canadian Council on Social Determinants of Health [CCSDH], 2015), collaboration is required with government and with nongovernmental and private sectors involved in national and community development (WHO, 2014), such as education, agriculture, industry, social services, housing, and public works (WHO, 1978). Addressing determinants of health also requires collaboration among many health care and other disciplines.

The Declaration of Alma-Ata, when examined closely, was a radical document when it was published in 1978. It implied a need for structural changes in how health services were delivered and changes in the health care skill mix needed to promote and maintain health. The changes involved a shift from a predominantly medical model of health care, delivered primarily via hospitals dominated by professionals, to health care provided in the community by a spectrum of health care workers that may include community health workers without professional training (Gillam, 2008). Such changes were difficult, and

geopolitical and economic challenges dashed aspirations to achieve health for all by the year 2000 (Birn, 2018). On the fortieth anniversary of the Declaration of Alma Ata, Birn (2018) reflected on the reasons for those dashed aspirations. These reasons included conservative shifts in political ideology, the debt crisis in developing countries in the 1980s, and reductions in spending on social welfare and reduced commitments to **multilateral agencies**. The 2008 WHO report *Primary Health Care—Now More Than Ever* suggested that people were healthier than in 1978, but the progress in health had been unequal, with growing health inequities within and between countries.

Health Equity—A Key Component of Health for All

Health equity (National Collaborating Centre for Determinants of Health [NCCDH], 2013b) remains a key factor impacting health for all. At a global summit in 2000, the United Nations adopted the following Millennium Development Goals, which were focused on reducing inequity by 2015: eradicating extreme poverty; universal primary education; gender equality and empowerment of women; reducing child mortality; improving maternal health; combating HIV/AIDS, malaria, and other diseases; environmental sustainability and access to safe drinking water and sanitation; and global partnerships for development (United Nations, 2015b). Recommendations for PHC reform (WHO, 2008) renewed a call for health equity. Trends noted as undermining equity included health systems focused on specialized curative care; disease control systems focused on short-term results; and increasing commercialization of health. To address such trends, the WHO report recommended the promotion of equity and social justice through universal coverage; people-centred health service delivery; an enhanced focus on the health of communities through public policy reforms across sectors; and promotion of inclusive, participatory health system leadership.

One important aspect of the WHO (2008) recommendations was the focus on the importance of intersectoral action toward public policy that would address the **social determinants of health**. The WHO Commission on the Social Determinants of Health was established in 2005 to examine evidence regarding models and practices that could promote health equity. The social determinants of health are the unequal distribution of power and resources and consequent unfair access to adequate education, living, and working conditions (Commission on Social Determinants of Health, 2008). The Toronto Charter for a Healthy Canada, developed following a conference of Canadian health and social policy experts, articulated the social determinants of health (Raphael, Bryant, & Curry-Stevens, 2004). A list of the social determinants of health can be found in the box Cultural Considerations: Determinants of Health. The commission also noted that women, especially women of colour, Indigenous women, and new Canadians, are especially vulnerable to the effects of poor social conditions. To support action on the social determinants of health, the WHO (2014) Helsinki statement encouraged governments to adopt principles of Health in All Policies in order to achieve health for all.

The goal of reducing inequity is challenging and, despite notable progress, the ambitious Millennium Development Goals were not met. In 2015, the 17 Sustainable Development Goals were developed to further the Millennium Development Goals agenda and work in global partnerships to end poverty and hunger, protect the planet, ensure economic, social, and technological progress in harmony with nature, and foster peaceful, just, and inclusive societies (United Nations, 2015a; see Figure 1.2 in Chapter 1). The Shanghai Declaration (WHO, 2016) focused on promoting health in the context of sustainable development and called for governments to enable decisions that will benefit the poorest and most vulnerable through policy orientation, fostering healthy cities, increasing health literacy, and social mobilization (WHO, 2017).

PRIMARY HEALTH CARE IN THE CANADIAN CONTEXT

Historical Perspectives

Prior to the 1978 Declaration of Alma Ata, the federal and provincial governments in Canada had moved in a direction congruent with some of the main tenets of PHC. Universal health care insurance was introduced in 1966 and the *Lalonde Report* (Lalonde, 1974) articulated the difference between health and health care and the need for intersectoral collaboration if the health status of the Canadian population was to improve in a significant way. In 1984, the *Canada Health Act* entrenched the principles of **accessibility, universality, portability, comprehensiveness,** and **public administration** of hospital and medical services (Government of Canada, 2020). The groundwork for building an accessible health care system oriented to prevention, health promotion, and intersectoral collaboration had been put in place. See Chapter 1 for details about the historic development of health care in Canada.

Canada is known globally in health promotion circles as the site of the first WHO international conference on health promotion and the resulting influential Ottawa Charter (WHO, 1986). The charter articulates the fundamental prerequisites of health—peace, shelter, education, food, income, a stable ecosystem, sustainable resources, social justice, and equity. The Ottawa Charter stressed the importance of not just promoting healthy lifestyles, but also coordinating the efforts of individuals, governments, and other sectors to promote the conditions that foster the prerequisites for health.

The same year, the *Epp Report* (Epp, 1986) outlined Canada's blueprint for achieving health for all. The *Epp Report* identified the major challenges to health as reducing inequities, increasing prevention, and enhancing coping. Self-care, mutual aid, and healthy environments were viewed as the relevant health promotion mechanisms. Fostering public participation, strengthening community services, and coordinating healthy public policy were suggested as implementation strategies. Together, the Ottawa Charter and the *Epp Report* reinforced four of the five principles of PHC.

The **population health** paradigm, articulated by the Canadian Institute of Advanced Research (CIAR) in the 1990s, significantly influenced the direction of government health initiatives and was adopted to guide federal policy in 1997 (Pederson, Rootman, Frohlich et al., 2017). This approach is characterized by a strong epidemiological research base requiring definition and measurement indicators of health status and determinants of health at a population level in order to develop multiple coordinated intervention strategies based on the best evidence available (Health Canada, 2001). Strategies should include **upstream** investments (NCCDH, 2014) that involve coordination of activities across sectors to address determinants of health, including income, income distribution, and social status; social support networks; education; employment and working conditions; social and physical environments; healthy child development; personal health practices, individual capacity, and coping skills; biology and genetic endowment; and health services.

Although there are clear similarities between population health and health promotion, there has been debate regarding the importance of the differences. It was argued that population health involved a top-down, research-driven approach to health as compared with the more bottom-up approach in which communities influence and advocate for their own healthy environments (Coburn, Denny, Mykhalovskiy et al., 2003). Health Canada integrated these two approaches in the Population Health Promotion Model (Hamilton & Bhatti, 1996), which clearly identified the contributions of each approach: the determinants of health that need to be addressed (population health) using the five broad action strategies from the Ottawa Charter (health promotion). Operational definitions of the population health approach continue to differ, but core elements identified by health system leaders using population health are consistent with PHC, including a focus on prevention, working together with communities to determine and address needs, addressing health disparities and multiple determinants of health, and embracing intersectoral action (Cohen, Huynh, Sebold et al., 2014).

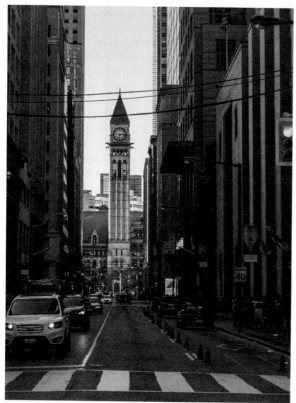

Intersectoral action requires participation with government, economic, educational, environment and other sectors to address determinants of health. (istock.com/Steven_Kriemadis)

Calls for health care reform in Canada have included principles of PHC in recommendations for a sustainable health care system. In 1997, the federal government established the 3-year Health Transition Fund to support projects across Canada to test and evaluate innovative ways to deliver health care, including 65 primary care/PHC projects that addressed one or more principles of PHC (Mable & Marriott, 2002). Many projects focused on improving the administration of primary care, some focused on cross-sectoral integration of care, and some focused on programs for people with chronic diseases or other issues among populations at risk. Numerous projects focused on the shift from solo physician practices to the development

of multidisciplinary teams, with some using nurses as the first line of care in rural and remote settings.

In September 2000, the First Ministers identified PHC reform as a priority for the renewal of Canada's health care system. Accordingly, the Government of Canada established the Primary Health Care Transition Fund to support the provinces and territories to improve the delivery of PHC over the next 4 years (Weatherill, 2007). The goals for the Primary Health Care Transition Fund were as follows: increase the number of people who have access to first-contact PHC organizations that are accountable for a clearly defined set of comprehensive health services to a defined population; increase health promotion, disease and injury prevention, and the management of chronic diseases; expand 24/7 access to essential health services; establish interdisciplinary PHC teams to ensure the most appropriate health care was provided by the most appropriate professional; and ensure that people's health care is coordinated and integrated with other health services. Some key learnings from those initiatives included the importance of educating health care providers to be ready to collaborate in PHC teams and the value of patients being at the centre of their care as active members of the interprofessional team engaged in the management of their own health. It was also noted that a strong health information infrastructure facilitates PHC change. Most of the projects ended when the funding ran out, although according to the CMA (2010), projects in Alberta and Ontario had lasting effects on primary care delivery.

The Romanow Commission (2002) supported PHC as a key element of health system reform. However, the commission argued that ideal approaches to PHC require too many changes at once. Thus, their focus was to support a model of PHC that included interdisciplinary teams providing 24-hour comprehensive care to a certain population with an increased emphasis on prevention, health promotion, and management of chronic diseases. There was a limited focus on improving accessibility to health care through a proposed rural and remote access fund, a home care access fund, and a new approach to Indigenous health. However, there was no clear call for action on the social determinants of health.

The *Romanow Report* and the Primary Health Care Transition Fund initiatives set the stage for the directions proposed in the First Ministers' 2003 health accord and the 2004 *10-Year Plan to Strengthen Health Care* (Health Council of Canada, 2013). There was a focus on health care quality, accessibility, sustainability. Federal funding was provided to implement reforms in PHC, home care, and catastrophic drug coverage. The Health Council of

Canada, created to report on these reforms, noted in its final report that despite these commitments, Canada's allocation of health dollars changed very little and that expenditures directed to hospitals, drugs, and physicians remained the largest areas of health care spending. There were more interdisciplinary teams and models for chronic disease management and care coordination, and greater use of electronic health records to provide health care information to members of the PHC team, but health disparities and inequities in health care persisted across Canada.

Negotiations for a renewed health accord following the end of the 2014 accord were challenging. In 2017, the First Ministers agreed on a common set of principles that would be used to determine bilateral agreements with the provinces for the next 10 years. These principles included improving access to mental health and addiction services and supports; improving access to home and community palliative and end-of-life care; and working with First Nations, Inuit, and Métis leadership to improve access to health services and health outcomes of Indigenous peoples (Government of Canada, 2017). There was no mention of the ongoing PHC reform that was advised by the Health Council of Canada or the ongoing health reforms recommended by the Standing Senate Committee on Social Affairs, Science, and Technology (2012).

LINKING NURSING, PRIMARY HEALTH CARE, AND THE CANADIAN CONTEXT

Given the congruence of the PHC principles with the key concepts underlying nursing practice, it should be no surprise that nurses quickly embraced the concept. The International Council of Nurses (ICN) pledged support for PHC, encouraging nurses worldwide to become involved in the planning and implementation of PHC in their own countries (Glass & Hicks, 2000). The ICN reiterated support for PHC following the Astana Global Conference on Primary Health Care (ICN, 2018).

MacPhail (1991, 1996) and Ogilvie and Reutter (2003), in past editions of this book, tracked the response of Canadian nurses to the challenge of PHC. In the 1970s, postgraduate nurse practitioner (NP) diploma programs, focusing on primary care and nurses as substitutes for physicians, developed in Canada primarily to increase access to essential first-contact PHC services in underserved areas (Kaasalainen, Martin-Misener, Kilpatrick et al., 2010). The skills needed for PHC were emphasized in such programs. Graduates were employed primarily in Northern health centres where consultation with physicians was available using telephone or other technology, and in urban centres, often in clinics serving marginalized populations.

However, these roles were challenging to sustain because provincial ministries of health did not fund NP positions. All the NP educational programs, except that at Dalhousie University, were phased out by the late 1980s, partly in recognition of the difficulty of adequately educating nurses through relatively short courses for the complexity of implementing PHC (MacPhail, 1996). Integrating knowledge, skills, and attitudes into baccalaureate nursing education was perceived as more appropriate. Since the 1990s, the thrust has been toward master's-level programs to prepare advanced practice nurses whose scope of practice encompasses extended clinical responsibilities and autonomy (Kaasalainen, Martin-Misener, Kilpatrick et al., 2010). Several nursing education programs, including a consortium of nine Ontario universities, focus on PHC.

Nursing Association Support for Primary Health Care

The Canadian Nurses Association (CNA), along with provincial and territorial nursing associations, has provided leadership for nursing contributions to PHC in Canada. Rodger and Gallagher (2000) have described the history of CNA action in Canada from 1985 to 1998. The CNA developed position statements on health care reform, implementation strategies for specific issues such as an aging population, Indigenous peoples, mental health, and comprehensive school health and wrote policy statements regarding the role of nurses in PHC and health care delivery. Briefs on the need for health care reform congruent with PHC principles were submitted to the Standing Committee of the House of Commons on Health and Welfare, Social Affairs, Seniors, and the Status of Women and to the National Forum on Health.

From 2001 to 2006, the CNA partnered on five projects funded under the government's Primary Health Care Transition Fund (Elliott, Rutty, & Villeneuve, 2008): a project led by the Arthritis Society that focused on chronic disease management in a multidisciplinary community health setting; a project led by the Canadian Psychological Association to support effective collaboration among health care providers; a project led by the College of Family Physicians of Canada aimed at improving collaboration between providers of mental health services; a project led by the Society of Obstetricians and Gynaecologists of Canada to develop collaborative primary maternity care models, and a major project led by the CNA on facilitating the integration of NPs in the health system (CNA, 2005; Elliott, Rutty, & Villeneuve, 2008). The CNA strongly endorsed PHC in presentations to the Commission on the Future of Health Care in Canada (the Romanow Commission) and the Standing Senate Committee on Social Affairs, Science, and Technology (Kirby Commission) (CNA, 2005). The CNA also developed documents and fact sheets in support of a public health system based on PHC principles (e.g., CNA, 2002, 2003, 2004). They advocated federally for Indigenous peoples' health at the 2006 meeting of First Ministers and Indigenous leaders and for mental health (Elliott, Rutty, & Villeneuve, 2008) and for health care reform (CNA, 2011).

The CNA further articulated its vision for PHC and the role of nurses in *Toward 2020: Visions for Nursing* (Villeneuve & MacDonald, 2006). Nurses were envisioned as providing health services in interprofessional collaborative teams with clients who shared responsibility for their own health (Elliott, Rutty, & Villeneuve, 2008). As managers, coordinators, and teachers, nurses would work with individuals, families, and communities and become "resources for everyday living." The shift to prevention would lead to a healthier population and would reduce the need for nurses in acute care areas, where they would take on more care team leadership. Nurses' use of increasingly sophisticated health-care technologies would facilitate these changes.

At the same time as the CNA was envisioning a PHC future, it also developed a primary care toolkit—an online set of evidence-based resources for nurses and NPs working in primary care teams (Elliott, Rutty, & Villeneuve, 2008). It continued to focus on primary care with a scoping review of ways to optimize the nursing role in primary care, noting the strong potential for nurses in chronic disease management and care (Martin-Misener & Bryant-Lukosius, 2014). The CNA noted that the vision of nurses practicing in collaborative teams to their full scope of practice requires knowledgeable, confident nurses who have clear roles that are understood by all members of the team and health system governance structures that create opportunity for nurses. The CNA's revised PHC position statement clarified the difference between primary care and PHC and reiterated the importance of effective interdisciplinary collaboration in multiple settings for optimal health outcomes (CNA, 2015; Ashley, 2015).

The CNA's advocacy for the role of NPs in a reformed PHC system led to the formation of the Canadian Nurse Practitioner Initiative (CNPI). Funded by the Primary Health Care Transition Fund, the goal of the CNPI was to facilitate sustained integration of the NP role in the health system. Following the launch of this initiative, the CNPI made recommendations regarding legislation, regulation, education, and remuneration mechanisms (CNA, 2006). The CNA's (2016a) revised position statement on the role of the NP summarized the key role of NPs in community and organizational development, interprofessional work and teamwork, capacity building,

and health policy development. The CNPI suggested that graduate education in nursing is essential and positions NPs to function independently and collaboratively, providing high-quality, cost-effective care in a variety of settings across the continuum of care. A summary of progress on the integration of NPs 10 years after the end of the NP initiative (CNA, 2016b) reported a 300% increase in the number of NPs in Canada, with three out of four NPs working in the family all-ages primary care stream. The report called for the education of more NPs and a focus on providing primary care in the community to vulnerable populations such as seniors, high users, refugees, Indigenous peoples, and people living in rural and remote settings.

In addition to the leadership provided at CNA, provincial and territorial nursing associations have encouraged nursing involvement in PHC. By the mid 1990s, all associations had developed a position statement on PHC and were involved in provincial or territorial government task forces for health system reform (Rodger & Gallagher, 2000). Advocacy for PHC is ongoing. For example, the Association of Registered Nurses of British Columbia issued a brief calling for increased provision of PHC through community health centres (Association of Registered Nurses of British Columbia, 2016). The Association of Registered Nurses of Newfoundland and Labrador (2012, 2013) issued an updated position statement regarding PHC and a briefing note advocating for full implementation of PHC in the health system. A nursing practice consultant from the Nurses Association of New Brunswick (2012) participated on the advisory committee for the development of the Primary Health Care Framework for New Brunswick. The College and Association of Registered Nurses of Alberta (2008) issued guidelines for the implementation of PHC and led the development of Alberta's Primary Health

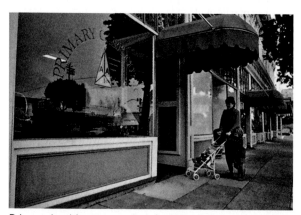

Primary health care requires facilities that are accessible and inviting for all.

Strategy (College and Association of Registered Nurses of Alberta, 2014).

The Registered Nurses' Association of Ontario (RNAO) has moved more explicitly in the direction of activity related to root causes and determinants of health than have other nursing associations. The RNAO was one of 11 Ontario member organizations of the Coalition for Primary Health Care, formed in 2000. Their PHC focus has been championing the role of NPs in PHC, calling for funding for more NP-led clinics and NP PHC positions, and calling for the removal of legislative and regulatory barriers to enable NPs with extended-care qualifications to practise to their full scope (RNAO, 2008). The RNAO also advocates for system reforms such as client-centred care and nursing and governmental action to address social and environmental determinants of health.

Canadian Nursing Contributions to Primary Health Care

Examples of early Canadian nursing contributions to PHC were identified by Rodger and Gallagher (2000). Much of the nursing activity was related to health promotion and disease and injury prevention, with nurses participating in projects related to bicycle helmets, tobacco use, and other health-related issues. Telephone health information systems staffed by nurses (e.g., Health Link in Alberta) were examples of health systems using nurses as the first point of contact for individuals seeking information for specific health concerns.

The Health Council of Canada (2014a, 2014b, 2014c, 2014d) reported on the diversity of PHC innovations that were implemented in Canada from 2004 to 2013, during the period of the health accord. Many initiatives included nurses as members of interdisciplinary PHC teams. Examples of innovations involving nurses included oncology nurse navigators; telehomecare for chronic obstructive pulmonary disease and congestive heart failure; a hospital interprofessional model of care; integrated care mental health care teams; and caregiver support programs. Innovations frequently focused on chronic care management and secondary illness prevention, with some adding a specific health promotion focus, such as one that integrated community strategies such as treks and biking. Several innovations increased the accessibility of health care for low-income or precariously housed or homeless people, including primary care outreach services, a health bus, a short-term cancer care unit, and the Insite safe injection site. Other initiatives were specifically developed with and for Indigenous communities, such as home and community care services on- and off-reserve; culturally based services to reduce chronic diseases; and an outreach project to increase tuberculosis screening and treatment. One

CASE STUDY

A Primary Health Care Nurse

Patti Melanson was one of the nurses highlighted in the CNA (2013) *Leadership in Primary Health Care* series. As a PHC nurse, Melanson developed the Halifax North End Community Health Centre's Mobile Outreach Street Health (MOSH) program. The MOSH team originally consisted of team lead Patti Melanson, three nurses, and an occupational therapist supported by physicians; the MOSH team now also includes an outreach NP. The mobile team brings health care to the streets, community agencies, and shelters. While working as a nurse coordinator at a youth centre, Patti identified the need for PHC for homeless, addicted, and at-risk adults and brought together a group of people from shelters, addictions counselling, needle exchange programs, and other stakeholders to identify gaps in services. MOSH was developed to provide access to primary care, such as wound care or physical assessments, as well as to assist people to address issues of importance to their health and quality of life, such as managing chronic diseases and medications, obtaining financial assistance, or learning to shop for food. They provide housing assistance and support using a housing-first model. MOSH is an outreach service of the North End Community Health Centre, which also offers primary care, including social work, mental health, foot care, nutrition, and dental services (North End Community Health Centre, n.d.; CNA, 2013). Patti Melanson's actions resulted in her being awarded the Order of Nova Scotia just before her death from cancer in 2018 ("Halifax nurse Patti Melanson," 2018).

Sources: Canadian Nurses Association. (2013). *Leadership in primary health care series*. Ottawa, ON: Author. Retrieved from https://www.cna-aiic.ca/en/policy-advocacy/primary-health-care/leadership-in-primary-health-care-series; North End Community Health Centre. (n.d.). *Programs and services*. Retrieved from https://nechc.com/; *Halifax nurse Patti Melanson was a champion of the vulnerable* (2018, December 17), *The Chronicle Herald*. Retrieved from https://www.thechronicleherald.ca/news/local/halifax-nurse-patti-melanson-was-a-champion-of-the-vulnerable-268977/.

initiative involved the use of trained community health aides working with nurses as culturally appropriate health care providers in Inuit communities experiencing difficulties retaining nurses. PHC principles most commonly exemplified in these interdisciplinary collaborations were improved accessibility and appropriate use of human and communication technologies. Innovations were client-focused, but few were described as explicitly including partnerships with community members in the development or implementation of the programs, and no programs involved sectors external to health-related organizations to address the root causes of health disparities.

In the CNA (2013) *Leadership in Primary Health Care* series, nurses shared personal stories about providing PHC in a variety of settings. These stories included a community health nurse in the Northwest Territories providing the full spectrum of health promotion, preventive, and acute illness treatment and emergency care (often via telemedicine) to a fly-in Dené community; a Quebec nursing consultant who worked on developing a program to reduce emergency admissions of older people living in long-term care; a New Brunswick community health centre nurse trained to recognize and treat common mental health disorders; an Ontario NP providing care at an NP primary care clinic and another in a family health team; a public health nurse working with high-risk new mothers in a nurse–family partnership program; an Indigenous NP providing care in an Ontario First Nations community; and the chronic pain management program at the Comox Valley Nursing Centre in British Columbia.

Nurse Practitioners and Primary Health Care

On August 30, 2007, the first NP-led clinic opened in Sudbury, Ontario, with funding from the provincial government. In 2015, there were 5.5 full-time equivalent NPs, an RN, a registered practical nurse, administrative staff, four part-time physicians, a dietitian, and a social worker. In addition to the main clinic, there were two satellite sites in smaller communities. The clinic reported high patient satisfaction, fewer emergency department visits, and medical outcomes comparable to those of physician practices at comparable or lower cost (Miedema, 2015). The number of clinics has increased, and as of 2019, there were 25 NP-led clinics in Ontario. NP-led clinics have also opened in other provinces. For example, the Collaborative Community Care project is a NP-led PHC project that began in 2018 (O'Rourke, Summach, & McDonald, 2018). Exam rooms are located in an Edmonton seniors' centre that collaborated on the development and implementation of the project. The centrally located centre provides social services, counselling, and a café in addition to health services.

The Role of Nurses in Primary Health Care

Nursing's main contribution within an interdisciplinary, intersectoral team is performing assessments that identify the effects of social determinants of health and integration of health promotion principles in a PHC system (Besner, 2006). The domain of nursing in which PHC is most integrated is community health nursing. Stewart (2000) proposed an influential framework for community health nurses based on PHC principles. This orientation has continued, as exemplified in the explicit inclusion of PHC principles in the Community Health Nurses of Canada (2019) *Standards of Practice*. According to the standards, community health nurses provide health promotion and protection wherever people live, work, and play. They engage in public participation through capacity building and community development focused on client strengths.

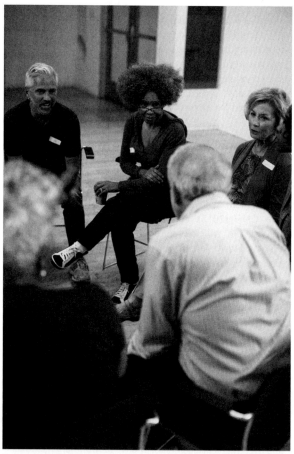

Meaningful client and public participation is required for effective primary health care. (istock.com/monkeybusinessimages)

Appropriate technology is reflected in the requirement to engage in evidence-informed decision making. Health promotion is expected to address the determinants of health within social, environmental, and political contexts and incorporate inclusiveness, equity, and social justice. CHNs are also expected to promote health through political action and by promoting healthy public policy.

Although the role of health promotion is clearly recognized in community health nursing, Dupéré, Perrault, Hills et al. (2012) posited that health promotion should also be central to nursing care in acute care settings. For example, nurses can develop care plans that include consideration of patients' access to community supports, or their ability to obtain and pay for medications, and advocate for needed resources. Other ways to engage in PHC might be working with members of the community on a hospital ward modernization committee, determining hospital room design, considering how to use technology effectively, and recommending ways to make care more accessible (Ashley, 2015). Innovative ideas for addressing health equity can be fostered by nurses' participation on boards in leadership positions at the centre of organizations; in these roles, nurses can foster the recalibration of health and nonhealth systems to act early and comprehensively, using a life-course approach that recognizes optimal points at which to promote individual and population health (Butterfield, 2017).

Nurses educated from a health promotion stance are more likely to focus on the primacy of people and provide empowering care in partnership with clients in all contexts (Dupéré, Perrault, Hills et al., 2012). It is becoming an expectation that all nurses be educated to promote health, and current Canadian entry-to-practice competencies for RNs explicitly contain PHC competencies (e.g., College of Nurses of Ontario, 2018; College and Association of Registered Nurses of Alberta, 2019). PHC can be a general framework guiding the nursing curriculum (Munro, Gallant, MacKinnon et al., 2000) and can be used by students to guide assessment and determine appropriate interventions in partnership with clients in an acute care setting (Blanchard & Murnaghan, 2010). A PHC curriculum framework can also be used to understand the nursing role in chronic care. A PHC focus can foster understanding of the nursing profession as **appropriate technology** for providing chronic care and stresses the client's right to self-determination as foundational to their participation in care. Concepts such as stigma and social isolation can be framed as issues limiting accessibility to chronic care. The importance of intersectoral collaboration with community services that meet the needs of people experiencing chronic illness is also highlighted when PHC is used to learn about chronic care (Ritchie, 2012).

Thus, when applied broadly, PHC principles can be used to guide all nursing care. Box 11.1 contains questions associated with each of the five principles that nurses can ask a when providing care in any setting.

BOX 11.1 How Can You Practice Using Primary Health Care Principles?

Nurses in all settings, not only in primary care, need to understand and take action on PHC principles. From the intensive care unit to long-term care, the principles are relevant and critical to comprehensive, client-centred practice. Nurses can strengthen their practice by considering the following questions:

- Accessibility. What issues affect the ability of your clients to access your services (e.g., hours, transportation, disability, cultural and economic factors)? How can your services be made more accessible?
- Health promotion. What are the effects of social, economic, and environmental factors on the health of your clients? Do you take these factors into account when you develop your interventions?
- Interdisciplinary collaboration. Do you work as a team with health professionals from other disciplines? What could be done to make this relationship more effective?
- Use of appropriate skills and technology. Are the skills of different health care and social service providers used in the most effective way to support your clients?
- Public participation. Does the community you work with have input into the kinds of programs you do or the way in which they are delivered?

The public respects nurses and considers them credible when they speak about health issues. Nurses can use this position to advocate for a better health system in the following ways:

- Educate decision makers, community leaders, and other health care providers about PHC and the role that nurses can play.
- Invite politicians and other decision makers to your workplace so they can see first-hand what you do and the issues that affect your work.
- Write a letter to the editor of your local newspaper—tell your story.
- Participate on planning committees at your workplace or in your community that are looking at PHC issues. Ensure that the nursing perspective is heard.

Source: Canadian Nurses Association. (2015) *Primary health care: A summary of the issues* (p. 4). Retrieved from https://www.cna-aiic.ca/-/media/cna/page-content/pdf-en/primary-health-care-position-statement.pdf. © Canadian Nurses Association. Reprinted with permission. Further reproduction prohibited.

APPLYING CONTENT KNOWLEDGE

Choose a nursing practice setting. How have you observed the five principles of PHC reflected in that setting? What is your vision for what it would look like if PHC was fully implemented there? What changes would you recommend in order to improve PHC practice in your chosen setting?

IMPLEMENTATION OF PRIMARY HEALTH CARE: ISSUES AND CHALLENGES

In Box 11.2, we present a summary of the challenges and issues discussed in this section.

Clarifying the Concept of Primary Health Care

Although there appears to be considerable movement toward PHC in Canada, several issues limit the full application of PHC. An overriding issue is that ambiguity remains about what is meant by PHC, which may limit its potential. PHC is often considered synonymous with primary medical care. For example, the Health Canada (2015) website articulates that PHC includes all services that contribute to health (e.g., income, housing, education, and environment) and that primary care, one element of PHC, focuses on health care services, including health promotion, illness and injury prevention, and the diagnosis and treatment of illness and injury. However, the website also notes that PHC serves a dual function within the health care system of direct provision of first-contact services and of the coordination of movement across the system. This traditional understanding of PHC as essentially provider-driven primary care has resulted in an overriding focus on addressing the accessibility principle, with the emphasis on 24/7 access and the availability of sufficient health human resources. Moreover, this emphasis inadvertently may have been "facilitated" by legislation permitting nurses to engage in extended services that were previously the purview of physicians. Although such activities may indeed enhance nursing's complementary role within an interdisciplinary team, they also have the potential to erode nursing's prominent emphasis on health promotion. Politically, extending nursing roles in primary care through legislation may be much easier than integrating health promotion into all facets of the health care system, into other relevant sectors, and into policy. Economic arguments oriented to short-term gains, under the guise of maintaining accessibility to illness care, may subvert real efforts at reform.

Nevertheless, it should be noted that there is room for greater accessibility to the whole range of health care services. As the Canadian Institute for Health Information

---

BOX 11.2   Issues and Challenges in the Implementation of Primary Health Care

- Clarifying the concept of PHC
- Equity-oriented PHC
- Effective interprofessional collaboration
- Insufficient PHC research and evaluation
- Need to strengthen government accountability for ongoing PHC reform
- Balancing accessibility to health determinants and health care
- Ensuring individual and community participation
- Removing legislative barriers for health care providers
- Implementing appropriate models of care

GENDER CONSIDERATIONS

One population that experiences challenges in access to safe, affirming health care is LGBTQ2 persons. Many health care providers lack sufficient knowledge about sexual orientation, nonheterosexual activity, and gender identity and expression and are therefore uncertain of the health care needs of LGBTQ2 individuals (Gahagan & Subirana-Malamet, 2018). A study of nonbinary youth documented their challenges in seeking gender-affirming care (Clark, Veale, Townsend et al., 2018). Nonbinary youth were less likely to have a family doctor than were binary youth, and they tended to feel uncomfortable speaking to doctors about their trans-specific health care needs (Clark, Veale, Townsend et al., 2018). Family-centered or youth-centered spaces, such as school or youth clinics, can be important places for promoting physical and mental health for this population. Quest Community Health Centre in St. Catharines, Ontario is an example of a queer-friendly PHC organization. One of their priority populations is sexually and gender-diverse communities. Quest provides health services, supports, and resources to individuals, families, and communities. They also organize health promotion initiatives such as the annual Pride Prom, which was developed by a nursing student in partnership with community members and community organizations (Quest Community Health Centre, n.d.).

Sources: Gahagan, J., & Subirana-Malamet, M. (2018). Improving pathways to primary health care among LGBTQ populations and health care providers: Key findings from Nova Scotia, Canada. *International Journal for Equity in Health, 17,* 76. https://doi.org/10.1186/s12939-018-0786-0; Quest Community Health Centre. (n.d.). *About Quest CHC.* Retrieved from https://questchc.ca/#; Clark, B. A., Veale, J. F., Townsend, M., et al. (2018). Non-binary youth: Access to gender-affirming primary health care. *International Journal of Transgenderism, 19,* 158–169. https://doi.org/10.1080/15532739.2017.1394954.

(CIHI, 2016) results suggest, timely access to primary care services is a concern for many Canadians. Vulnerable populations, such as those living in poverty, cultural minorities, people in rural communities, and Indigenous peoples, are particularly challenged in terms of health care accessibility. Immigrant and Indigenous populations may encounter linguistically inaccessible, culturally inappropriate, and culturally incomprehensible services. **LGBTQ2** persons also experience challenges in access to safe, affirming health care (Gahagan & Subirana-Malamet, 2018). See the Gender Considerations box.

Equity-Oriented Primary Health Care in Primary Care

Within primary care settings, it is argued that PHC is not actually the model of care that is being used unless equity and social determinants of health are a primary focus of care. The implementation of PHC requires an upstream approach that is people and community centred, embodying a "patients-first" perspective (Rayner, Muldoon, Bayoumi et al., 2018). Care should be provided by integrated interprofessional teams and should address the full spectrum of determinants of health. This can be accomplished through advocacy to address the impact of poverty, as well as through practical initiatives such as providing food boxes, organizing childcare, and establishing community gardens. PHC organizations should determine population needs and, using a community development approach, address them through partnerships with local organizations such as libraries, shelters, or programs for specific subgroups such as youth. Care needs to be accessible, culturally safe, anti-oppressive, and nonjudgmental, both in terms of relationships with care providers and in terms of physical space (Rayner, Muldoon, Bayoumi et al., 2018). Equity oriented health care means that providers make clients feel comfortable; talk openly about issues such as grief, mental health, and substance use and abuse; ask clients about their access to basic resources and help them reduce barriers to accessing health care. As a result, patients are more confident in their own ability to manage and prevent health problems and experience improvements in depression and symptoms of post-traumatic stress and improved quality of life (Ford-Gilboe, Wathen, Varcoe et al., 2018).

An aspect of accessibility and social justice that is often overlooked is religion and spirituality, particularly for some racialized and immigrant communities. Shared religious identity can be an important form of social capital, including bonding and support as well as engagement in social justice activities within their own faith communities and beyond (Reimer-Kirkham, 2014). However, religious identity can also lead to stigma and marginalization.

Reimer-Kirkham described Sikh and Muslim individuals who experienced inadequate care and situations in which religious observances were not honoured.

The crisis of increasing opioid overdoses demonstrates a failure of PHC to address social determinants of health and do effective health promotion and prevention. Deaths involve both users of prescription and illegal opioids, with the rise in deaths being related to the increasing toxicity of substances on the illegal market. Indigenous women and homeless or precariously housed people have been at higher risk of death (Belzak & Halverson, 2018). Modeled after Vancouver's Insite facility, supervised injection facilities received approval from the Canadian government to open in selected cities across Canada. These sites provide harm reduction services and a point of entry into health care and rehabilitation, but obtaining buy-in from law enforcement, policymakers, and community stakeholders can be challenging (Young & Fairburn, 2018). Ongoing advocacy is required to provide a full range of harm reduction services, prevention, and treatment accessible to all who need it and to address the social determinants that underlie the opioid crisis.

Equity-Oriented Community Health Nursing

Public health nurses carry out PHC through home visits, as school nurses, in clinics, and in other community settings with individuals and groups. Services are often universally available, but many programs such as prenatal classes or parenting programs are accessed more by people who are socially advantaged. Programs such as home visits for new families frequently target vulnerable families but tend to engage in "lifestyle drift" by addressing the consequences of inequities and focusing on behaviour change, rather than addressing the causes of inequities (NCCDH, 2013a).

In 2012, as a way to strengthen the equity focus of public health units, the Ontario Ministry of Health and Long-Term Care funded the development of an initiative in which 36 public health units could create two Social Determinants of Health (SDH) Public Health Nurse positions (NCCDH, 2015). These nurses focus on enhancing programs and services to meet the needs of priority populations most affected by inequity by using a combination of upstream health promotion strategies and the application of health equity approaches to direct client care.

Some of the SDH nurses are placed within a specific program area, where they provide direct service as outreach nurses to vulnerable populations in clients' homes or through community partner agencies, whereas other SDH nurses have cross-organizational positions where they are able to build equity capacity across departments (NCCDH, 2015). The Breastfeeding Outreach Nurse is an example of a program-specific nurse who offers lactation

◢◣ RESEARCH FOCUS

Using a mixed-methods ethnographic design, Browne and colleagues identified key dimensions of equity-oriented PHC services. Data were collected at two PHC centres located in low-income urban neighbourhoods in Western Canada through interviews with 62 patients, three focus groups with 11 patients, interviews with 33 staff members and a focus group with 8 staff members, over 900 hours of participant observation, and an analysis of key organizational documents. Purposive sampling was used to obtain a range of positive and negative experiences with the clinic. The four key dimensions of equity-oriented PCH services that arose were (1) inequity-responsive care, which addresses the social determinants of health as legitimate, routine, and priority aspects of care; (2) trauma- and violence-informed care, which recognizes the past and ongoing structural violence affecting people; (3) contextually tailored care, which addresses local population demographics and social issues; and (4) culturally competent care, which accounts for the cultural meaning of health and illness as well as the ways in which discrimination affects health and quality of life. Analyses also identified 10 strategies for enhancing capacity in equity-oriented services (Figure 11.2): articulate a commitment to equity in organizational vision, mission, and policy; develop supportive structures, policies, and processes; revise time-use expectations to meet clients' needs; address power differentials within the organization; tailor care and programs to the context of people's lives; implement strategies to counter oppression and barriers to health and access to care; foster community and participatory client engagement; tailor care to individual and group histories; engage in advocacy and intersectoral collaborations to enhance access to resources that address social determinants of health; and optimize clinic space and resources to create therapeutic, relational environments. These dimensions and strategies have been used to develop indicators that can be used to measure how this process can lead to improved health outcomes.

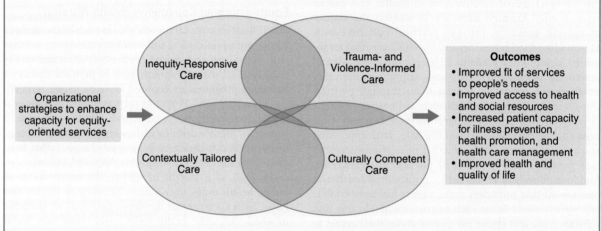

Fig. 11.2 Enhancing equity-oriented health care delivery. (**Source:** Adapted from Brown, Varcoe, Wong et al., 2012)

Source: Browne, A. J., Varcoe, C. M., Wong, S. T., et al. (2012). Closing the health equity gap: Evidence-based strategies for primary health care organizations. *International Journal for Equity in Health*, *11*, 59. https://doi.org/10.1186/1475-9276-11-59.

consultation, parenting, and mental health support to clients unable to access traditional programs and services. Nurses with cross-organizational positions use upstream strategies such as advocating for living wages, affordable housing, and universal drug and dental coverage. Some nurses collaborate with community stakeholders to complete health impact assessments to determine the potential effects that programs and policies may have on the health of a population and the distribution of those effects within the population. Others have coordinated training for colleagues and community partners on Indigenous cultural safety, LGBTQ2 issues, healthy equity, and other determinants of health. A study of the integration of SDH nurses into public health departments indicated that the extension of the knowledge and expertise of SDH nurses was effective in shifting some health units away from a previously entrenched biomedical focus and enhanced the focus on social determinants of health in organizations that had already embraced an equity orientation (NCCDH, 2015).

Public health nurses sometimes experience barriers to being able to engage in upstream health promotion that can involve challenging current public policy. Public health employers who depend on government funding may constrain challenges to the status quo, and nurses may fear for the security of their jobs if they speak out (Falk-Rafael & Betker, 2012). Another challenge is frequent restructuring, reorganization, and reassignment of roles (Falk-Rafael & Betker, 2012). For example, the Government of Ontario recently announced that 35 health units will be combined to form 10 regional entities, a plan that is feared to seriously disrupt frontline services, including those provided by public health nurses (Ontario Association of Public Health Nursing Leaders, 2019). School nursing is a specific example of PHC that has experienced many shifts due to budget cuts and reorientation of public health priorities. Using a comprehensive school health approach, nurses can provide physical and mental health care and engage in school-wide health promotion activities in collaboration with school and community partners. However, the changing focus of public health programs has often prevented nurses from working to their full scope of practice within schools and sometimes has resulted in a total elimination of nurses in schools (Community Health Nurses Initiatives' Group, 2015).

Primary Health Care Issues for Indigenous Peoples

Equity-oriented and culturally safe care is paramount for Indigenous PHC. Historical and ongoing colonialism and the associated reservation system are considered to be fundamental determinants of Indigenous health (de Leeuw, Lindsay, & Greenwood, 2018). One significant effect of colonization is suicide, which is a leading cause of death in Indigenous communities (Pollock, Healey, Jong et al. 2018; Ansloos, 2018). Another notable ongoing effect of colonization is the unacceptable quality of drinking water in many Indigenous communities, with the water system of up to 30% of communities being at high risk of bacterial or chemical contamination (Bharadwaj & Bradford, 2018). Water is considered an important spiritual lifeforce for many Indigenous peoples, yet their water frequently causes gastrointestinal infections, skin conditions, and other health concerns (Bradford, Bharadwaj, Okpalauwaekwe et al., 2016). Many Indigenous communities do not have access to adequate water treatment infrastructure or the experts to construct or repair treatment facilities when they fail (Bharadwaj & Bradford, 2018).

Counteracting colonization requires Indigenous voices, rooted in Indigenous knowledge, to have primacy in conversations about their own health and health care (de Leeuw, Lindsay, & Greenwood et al., 2018). Indigenous community development leaders have suggested that common models of determinants of health insufficiently reflect an Indigenous worldview (Nesdole, Voigts, Lepnurm, & Roberts, 2014). When compared with the Public Health of Agency key determinants of health, the missing determinants identified by Indigenous leaders included spirituality, and a sense of purpose; life-sustaining values, morals and ethics; adequate power; social justice and equity; cultural integrity and identity; healthy eco-system and a sustainable relationship between human beings and the natural world; and meaningful work and service to others (Nesdole, Voigts, Lepnurm, & Roberts, 2014, p. 211).

For more information, see the Cultural Considerations box, which provides three conceptions of determinants of health for comparison.

Counteracting colonization also requires public policy that enshrines Indigenous human rights and provides Indigenous sovereignty over resources and services (Pollock, Healey, Jong et al., 2018). Such actions are foundational to health equity, health promotion, and suicide prevention. Most Indigenous communities have some responsibility for the planning and delivery of community-based services; however, further reform is required in order to address the Truth and Reconciliation Commission Calls to Action to reorient services for Indigenous populations (Henderson, Montesanti, Crowshoe et al., 2018; Tompkins, Mequaint, Barre et al., 2018). Suggestions for innovation identified by Indigenous leaders, provincial health system leaders, and PHC physicians and nurses in Alberta include having a coherent model for community engagement and outreach; learning from the success of other sectors, such as the reduction in violence through the involvement of Elders; and the use of technology such as telehealth to link Indigenous patients to Elders for support on their healing journeys (Henderson, Montesanti, Crowshoe et al., 2018).

Stable funding models for innovative programs and for clinical services in Indigenous communities has been identified as an important issue. Most Indigenous communities receive federal funding for health care, with the remaining funds obtained from a variety of sources,

⊕ CULTURAL CONSIDERATIONS

Determinants of Health: Non-Indigenous and Indigenous Perspectives

Perspectives on determinants of health have evolved over time and with a growing understanding of the significant role of social factors in determining the health of individuals and communities. Indigenous knowledge, worldviews, and history have provided another perspective in the form of the Four Worlds First Nations–derived determinants of health. This table compares a list of determinants from this Indigenous perspective with determinants listed in two non-Indigenous perspectives on determinants of health.

Public Health Agency of Canada Key Determinants of Health	Social Determinants of Health	Four Worlds First Nations–Derived Determinants of Health
• Income and social status • Employment and working conditions • Education and literacy • Childhood experiences • Physical environments • Social supports and coping skills • Healthy behaviours • Access to health services • Biology and genetic endowment • Gender • Culture • Race/racism (Public Health Agency of Canada, 2019)	• Indigenous ancestry • Disability • Early life • Education • Employment and working conditions • Food security • Gender • Geography • Health care services • Housing • Immigrant status • Income and its distribution • Race • Social safety net • Social exclusion • Unemployment and employment security (Raphael, 2016)	• Physical needs • Spirituality and a sense of purpose • Life-sustaining values, morals, and ethics • Safety and security • Adequate income and sustainable economies • Social justice and equity • Cultural integrity and identity • Community solidarity and social support • Strong families and healthy child development • Healthy ecosystems and a sustainable relationship between human beings and the natural world • Critical learning opportunities • Adequate human services and social safety net • Meaningful work and service to others (Nesdole, Voigts, Lepnurm, & Roberts, 2014)

Sources: Public Health Agency of Canada. (2019, July 25). *Social determinants of health and health inequalities*. Retrieved from https://www.canada.ca/en/public-health/services/health-promotion/population-health/what-determines-health.html; Raphael, D. (2016). *Social determinants of health: Canadian perspectives* (3rd ed., p. 11). Toronto, ON: Canadian Scholars' Press; Nesdole, R., Voigts, D., Lepnurm, L., & Roberts, R. (2014). Reconceptualizing determinants of health: Barriers to improving the health status of First Nations peoples (p. e210). *Canadian Journal of Public Health, 105*, e209–e213. https://doi.org/10.17269/cjph.105.4308.

including the province, the tribal council, and other sources (Tompkins, Mequaint, Barre et al., 2018). There are also notable regional variations in funding for innovative programs, such as community-based diabetes care strategies (Tompkins, Mequaint, Barre et al., 2018). System-wide funding and health system innovations have been implemented in Ontario and British Columbia, but gaps remain (RNAO, 2018). Community health nurses and home care nurses form the majority of PHC professionals in Indigenous communities (Tompkins, Mequaint, Barre et al., 2018). Insufficient resources perpetuate the inequitable access to the important PHC work that nurses do alongside their Indigenous partners.

Interprofessional Collaboration and Primary Health Care

Interprofessional collaboration is foundational to effective PHC and has been demonstrated to improve health outcomes (CNA, 2019). Team-based care can improve patient-centredness and coordination of care and can increase prevention and health promotion activities (Jesmin, Thind, & Sarma, 2012). Nurses and NPs are important members of collaborative interprofessional teams. They possess a diverse set of psychomotor clinical skills, and their holistic orientation to patient care facilitates the development of relationships with patients that foster cost-effective health promotion and continuity of care, especially for high-needs patients (Kennedy, 2014; Roots & MacDonald, 2014). For example, an NP with a geriatric focus provided care at a family health team site, retirement homes, and through home visits and collaborated with multiple community agencies, which led to decreased lengths of stay in hospital and more older clients discharged to home (Prasad, Dunn, Hillier et al., 2014).

Expansion of a team to include additional roles such as dental care, while considered valuable, can be met with organizational and funding constraints and concerns about role ambiguity by nurses and other team members (Harnagea, Lamothe, Couturier et al., 2018). The integration of social workers is also challenged by limited understanding of social workers' roles and scope of practice (Ashcroft, MacMillan, Ambrose-Miller et al., 2018). Traditional health professional hierarchies can undermine authentic collaboration. Undergraduate and postgraduate professional education programs need to facilitate changing attitudes away from those that perpetuate hierarchical systems (CNA, 2019). Effective interprofessional teams must communicate regularly and well to maximize the value that each member can have in promoting health.

A question that arises when considering nurse-led clinics is whether NPs should be replacing physicians as the first point of care. A Cochrane review of studies in which nurses were substituted for doctors in primary care found that NPs and trained RNs provided equal and sometimes better quality of care than physicians, which probably resulted in equal or better outcomes for patients (Laurant, van der Biezen, Wijers et al., 2018). Many family doctors fear that they could be replaced by NPs (Owens, 2019). Although it could be argued that independent NP clinics have done so, the CNA website states that NPs do not replace doctors, but rather work collaboratively with other health care providers.

Another issue related to the role of NPs in the health care system is the addition of physician assistants (PAs) to the team mix. PAs are unregulated care providers who are currently licenced to practice in Manitoba, Ontario, New Brunswick, and Alberta, extending physician services under the supervision of physicians (Canadian Association of Physician Assistants, n.d.). The RNAO (2012), in their response to an application for regulation of PAs in Ontario, argued that NPs, who are more highly educated than PAs, provide more effective care. Furthermore, the RNAO contended that RNs, clinical nurse specialists, pharmacists, and midwives, if practicing to their full scope, can independently provide all aspects of care as currently regulated health care providers. It is likely that the preference of some physicians to hire PAs is related to the ability to maintain professional hierarchy and control in a manner that is not appropriate when working in collaboration with an independent regulated health care provider, such as an NP.

Primary Health Care Research and Evaluation

Researchers have argued that strong, coordinated implementation of PHC in Canada has been hampered by the paucity of research and evaluation of PHC (Montesanti, Robinson-Vollman, & Green, 2018). An example of the type of research that has been conducted is that reported by the Canadian Institute for Health Information using data collected on selected PHC indicators from various data sets developed in the decade prior to 2014 (CIHI, 2016). PHC was simply defined as care provided by family doctors and nurses at the first point of contact, resulting in indicators that were all associated with primary care rather than full PHC. For example, the report noted that the number of RNs in PHC settings had remained consistent, but that the number of physicians and their use of information and communication technology and electronic medical records had increased. About 85% of participants had access to a family doctor, but more than 50% reported difficulty obtaining care after hours or on weekends. Social determinants of health indicators were focused on individual health-promoting behaviours. Smoking had declined and obesity had increased, while fruit and vegetable consumption had decreased and physical activity had increased slightly. Health output indicators focused on preventive activities such as smoking cessation advice, eye exams for people with diabetes, influenza immunization, and colorectal and cervical cancer screening. Paré-Plante, Boivin, Berbiche et al. (2018) similarly conducted a PHC study that was focused on what improved accessibility, narrowly defined as the ability to get an appointment with a doctor as quickly as a patient wanted. They found that, even in clinics that included a nurse, it was only the ability to walk in or book same-day appointments that increased accessibility.

Montesanti, Robinson-Vollman, & Green (2018) suggested that research is needed to determine appropriate structures and delivery of PHC services that are focused on health equity and the full range of determinants of health. To facilitate coordinated research, a group of 12 community-based PHC research teams identified core dimensions for PHC indicators, namely access, comprehensiveness, team and system coordination, effectiveness in terms of patient management of chronic diseases and hospitalizations for select diseases, and equity in terms of access to care (Canadian Institutes of Health Research, n.d.). Developing common indicators is laudable, but it should be noted that the chosen dimensions indicate the ongoing focus on access to primary care rather than a full understanding of equity and social determinants of health. Given the complexity of PHC, deciding on common-health related outcomes that should be used to determine the effectiveness of care and other important aspects such as patient engagement is challenging (Santaguida, Dolovich, Oliver et al., 2018). Yet, a robust set of recommended measures is vital to research that would inform governments of the value of funding an expansion of PHC in Canada.

A valid measure of PHC engagement is also important for robust future PHC research. Kosteniuk, Stewart, Karunanayake et al. (2017) developed a measure with subscales measuring accessibility of clinical services, community participation, interdisciplinary and intersectoral collaboration, and population orientation and equity. These subscales can be used as independent variables to determine what components of a PHC system are responsible for optimal health outcomes.

An example of a research study that examined the effect of true PHC compared it with primary medical care in terms of the care provided to immigrant populations in Canada (Batista, Pottie, Bouchard, et al., 2018). Primary care was more oriented to improving the organization and quality of clinical care, whereas PHC implemented more strategies aimed at health promotion and socioeconomic or political contexts and structures that affect migrants' health, including developing partnerships with organizations such as legal services, food distribution, and transportation. PHC organizations also were more likely to use community health workers or health promotors to connect the community and health services.

Government Accountability for Ongoing Primary Health Care Reform

The accountability of governments to focus on PHC is an issue in terms of ongoing system reform. In its final letter to the First Ministers and Ministers of Health after removal of its funding, the Health Council of Canada (2014e) indicated that the results of the government funding over the previous 10 years had been less than optimal. They suggested that government efforts should be concentrated on PHC, seniors' care, mental health, and Indigenous health. The Health Council stressed their concern that accountability for the quality of the health system would be lost with the cessation of their mandate, and they called for the creation of a new mechanism to continue to hold the government accountable. Such a mechanism has not been developed.

A symptom of health system challenges is crowding and long stays in Canadian emergency departments, which has been noted as a significant, ongoing healthcare issue (CIHI, 2018a; Morley, Unwin, Peterson et al., 2018).

Insufficient access to primary care, inadequate staffing, and the high number of patients with complex, chronic conditions are drivers of crowding. Mandated limits on wait times and extended primary care opening hours have been shown to reduce crowding, but the primary solutions lie beyond the emergency department (Morley, Unwin, Peterson et al., 2018). To address this issue, the Ontario Premier's Council on Improving Healthcare and Ending Hallway Medicine (2019) identified three areas for health care improvement: considering technology solutions such as email contacts and virtual appointments; integrated timely care across the continuum of health, including proactive interventions and considering the social determinants of health; and evidence-based short- and long-term strategies such as prevention and early intervention to improve health outcomes. Nurses can be important drivers of these solutions.

Technology solutions and appropriate technology are often equated with using ever-improving information technology. It is important for nurses to be knowledgeable about evolving technology that can enhance health care. Appropriate use of the Internet, social media, and communication applications can facilitate effective health assessment, health promotion, and illness management by improving collaboration with clients and members of the health team. When using these resources with clients, however, it is important to be aware that lower education and literacy levels can reduce accessibility to information from these sources (Hardman & Ho, 2015).

One method to improve integration of care across the system is to use electronic medical records. Electronic medical records that can be accessed by all providers associated with the care of an individual can significantly improve the coordination and effectiveness of health care and increase patient safety. Yet only 75% of Canadian physicians used electronic medical records in 2015 (CIHI, 2016), and fewer than half used them to support quality of care decisions, such as to alert physicians to potential drug interactions or prompt guideline-based interventions. Challenges that have limited the widespread adoption of this important technology include cost, multiple incompatible platforms, and limited computer literacy of staff (Chang & Gupta, 2015).

Balancing Accessibility to Health Determinants and Accessibility to Health Care

A continuing challenge with the full implementation of PHC is the need to balance the focus on accessibility to health care services with a greater emphasis on those determinants of health that lie outside the health care system. Accessibility must include access to the prerequisites and determinants of health, which can be achieved only through intersectoral collaboration. Given that the underlying impetus for the PHC movement in 1978 was the observed health inequities brought about by social inequality, it is indeed noteworthy that social determinants, social inequality, and access to health (over and above access to health care) have received less attention from both nursing associations and government health departments. Advocacy, intersectoral collaboration, and political action become important nursing roles. The CIHI (2016) PHC health outcome indicators demonstrate a continued focus on individual behaviours, such as healthy eating, physical activity, and healthy weights, and do not address inequities in health or the social determinants of health.

Many frameworks have been developed to explain the impacts of the determinants of health on individuals, communities, and populations and the relationships between determinants; a review of these frameworks was conducted by the Canadian Council on Social Determinants of Health (2015). Consistent among the 36 frameworks they reviewed were holistic and intersectoral approaches, the recognition of social exclusion, and the importance of upstream action. Upstream action requires political action and effective messaging to effectively advocate for Health in All Policies. Private-sector leaders can be engaged by focusing on the value of investment in employee health and the positive image associated with corporate social responsibility actions; public-sector leaders need to be reminded that health is a consistent priority for Canadians, ill health and chronic disease are costly, and that focusing on prevention is valuable (CCSDH, 2012). It must be stressed that PHC benefits all members of society (van Weel, Turnbull, Bazemore et al., 2018).

The Pan-Canadian Public Health Network (2018) documented the extent of health disparities and the factors leading to disparities. Significant inequalities in health outcomes were found for Indigenous peoples, people with lower socioeconomic status, sexual and racial minorities, and people living with functional limitations. Recommendations included adopting a human rights approach to upstream and downstream interventions across the lifespan. Actions should also address living, working, and environmental conditions, power, privilege, and exclusion. To accomplish these actions requires a Health in All Policies approach, because the most significant influences on health lie outside the health care sector.

Nurses and nursing associations at the provincial and federal levels also need to expand their efforts to address the social determinants of health. The CNA (2018) position paper advocated for the Health in All Policies orientation. It encouraged all nurses to include social determinants of health in their assessments and interventions and to strive to reduce inequity. Nurses can engage in policy advocacy regarding social determinants of health within their organization, educate patients and others about determinants of health, become involved in collaborations with partners such as housing or food chain managers, learn the policy agendas of local agencies and legislators, be aware of issues, join their professional organization and work on policy statements, ask legislators for their position on issues, and vote in elections (Williams, Phillips, & Koyama, 2018). Climate change is a more recently recognized determinant of health inequity that most affects those that experience other social and physical vulnerabilities. Nurses have a professional responsibility to find ways to mitigate climate change in their workplaces and educate and advocate for climate justice (Travers, Shenck, Rosa et al., 2019). Of all the provincial associations, the RNAO appears to be a leader in advocacy efforts directed to determinants of health such as poverty reduction, housing, and the environment.

Ensuring Individual and Community Participation

Another challenge in implementing PHC relates to the principle of ensuring individual and community participation. Overall, there has been increasing emphasis on citizen participation in program and policy development (Lenihan, 2012), as citizen participation is important in ensuring that programs and policies are relevant and effective. The concept of empowerment, which requires participation in defining problems and determining solutions, is the essence of health promotion. It is important, however, to consider the types of participation and the degree to which this participation is empowering. If participation is to be truly meaningful, people should be able to influence the configuration of services available and not just the ways in which already mandated services are to be delivered. In recognition of the need to empower clients, as of 2016, Accreditation Canada standards require patient engagement in their own care as well as on planning and advisory committees (Ontario Hospital Association, 2015; Health PEI, 2016). Participation in the political process, through elections and public forums, provides civil society with a voice in decisions related to health and health care. As well, there is a need to ensure inclusivity for disadvantaged groups who have traditionally had little voice in decision making by providing the supports needed to enable their participation and ensuring that they have meaningful participation (O'Mara-Eves, Brunton, McDaid et al., 2013). Thus, although public participation is challenging, the expectation that patients and community members will be engaged in planning health care is growing.

Removing Legislative Barriers for Health Care Providers

Legislative barriers that constrain access to appropriate health care providers (Lankshear, 2012) is another challenge related to the principle of appropriate technology. The *Canada Health Act, 1984* privileges hospital-based and physician services. In hospitals, physicians currently are the gatekeepers to most nonphysician services. In the community, the public has always had direct access to public health nurses and increasingly has access to NPs and midwives, but this is not the case with other health care providers. Without changes in how physician services are funded, it will be difficult to shift rules for entry into the system. It has been argued that the fee-for-service system also has limited the economic contribution of PHC (van Weel, Turnbull, Bazemore et al., 2018) and that new models of team-based remuneration are needed (Lankshear, 2012).

Changes to health professions Acts, enacted in some jurisdictions and underway in others, allow increases in the scope of practice for health care providers. For example, Ontario changed the *Nursing Act* in 2017 to allow nurse prescribing (College of Nurses of Ontario, 2019), and the 2019 Ontario budget promises further expansions to scope of practice for other health professions such as NPs, pharmacists, and optometrists (Ontario Minister of Finance, 2019). These legislative changes open possibilities for nurses to take on multiple roles and be part of more effective collaborative teams. The boundaries among health care provider scopes of practice are more flexible. For example, pharmacists in most provinces can already renew prescriptions or prescribe some medications for patients, provided that a diagnosis has been established, and prescribe for minor ailments (Canadian Pharmacists Association, 2019). Telehealth, through Internet health databases and information, computer transmission of images, and conversations and assessments across long distances, is revolutionizing the need for specialist services to be located near the patient. What services need to be where, with what provider, is a question that should be addressed.

The shortage of health care providers, particularly family physicians and nurses, is a key challenge for health care systems, making health human resource planning of interest worldwide. Canada has fewer doctors per capita than most other high-income countries, with greater general practitioner shortages in rural areas (Globerman, Barua, & Hasan, 2018). The number of nurses in Canada grew gradually since 2008, with 2018 showing the slowest growth rate in the decade because of the aging workforce and low numbers of new nursing graduates

(CIHI, 2018b). But this growth has not been sufficient to mitigate the ongoing shortage of nurses (CNA, 2008). The situation is compounded by the concern that nurses often are not working to their scope of practice (Martin-Misener & Bryant-Lukosius, 2014). The labour shortage may be an incentive for working in intradisciplinary and multidisciplinary teams, with each professional group working to its scope of practice. See Chapter 17 for a detailed discussion of the Canadian nursing workforce. Caution must be exercised, however, to ensure that nurses use their health promotion expertise and do not merely take on a medical role.

Implementing Appropriate Models of Care: Community Health Centres

What service model of health care delivery will best serve the health needs of Canadians? The answer, of course, is that nobody knows for sure. Community health centres—with their salaried multidisciplinary teams; integration of curative, preventative, and health-promotion programs; accessibility to the population being served; facilitation of public participation; and creation of intersectoral links—are viewed by many as the best options for a health care system truly oriented to PHC. Community health centres in Canada generally offer both PHC and social programs and services, thereby addressing many social determinants of health (Hay, Varga-Toth, & Hines, 2006). For example, the Calgary Urban Project Society offers a variety of services in inner-city Calgary, including multidisciplinary health clinics (e.g., prenatal and maternal–child clinics, chiropractic care, dentistry, shared-care mental health, eye care); counselling and advocacy; family resource centre (e.g., life skills and parenting programs; breakfast and hot lunch; basic needs services, referrals, socialization); community outreach (e.g., home visits, referrals, emergency transportation); educational and early intervention programs; and a housing registry (Calgary Urban Project Society, 2019). The promise of community health centres is reflected in the number of centres represented by the Canadian Association of Community Health Centres (n.d.), the federal voice of people-centred, community-based PHC organizations across Canada.

THE WAY FORWARD

There are promising developments to move the PHC agenda forward. Nursing associations have served nurses well in setting the guidelines for their potential involvement in a PHC system. At the political level, there seems to be openness to trying to do things differently. Funding for innovative projects and research is available. The Institute of Population and Public Health, one of the Canadian Institutes of Health Research (n.d.), has a priority area for community-based PHC that funded 12 teams in 2016 to research a variety of PHC initiatives. There is also at least one Canada Research Chair focused on PHC.

Substantial scholarly work in nursing exists to provide guidance, in Canada and elsewhere. Nursing textbooks and curricula emphasize PHC. The international journal *Primary Health Care Research and Development* is devoted to disseminating PHC research and practice. Nurses need to embrace the challenge and, perhaps most importantly, contribute to the research evidence that a system truly based on PHC principles can enhance the health of Canadians.

To meet the challenge of reforming the health system such that it operates according to PHC principles, nursing education will need to concentrate on several key areas. First, nurses must be educated to work in community settings. Currently, many nursing programs concentrate students' clinical practice in hospital settings. As first-contact providers in PHC teams, nurses will require advanced assessment skills. Curricula should include basic physical assessment skills and assessment of the influence of the social context on health situations to strengthen nurses' unique holistic contributions to the PHC team. To better prepare nurses to work in multidisciplinary teams, interdisciplinary education will need to be strengthened (CNA, 2019).

Finally, to realize the health promotion contribution of nursing, nurses will need a comprehensive understanding of the whole range of health determinants that influence individual health; moreover, they will require skills to work collaboratively with other sectors and disciplines to influence these determinants through strategies such as policy advocacy and community development. Nursing curricula must therefore provide a strong foundation in health promotion principles and strategies at the individual, community, and societal levels in the spirit of social justice. Such a health promotion focus is crucial to implementing a PHC model.

CONCLUSION

As a set of five interrelated principles, PHC requires a fundamental change in values, priorities, funding structures, and organization of health services if potential health gains for populations are to be achieved. Health reform for health equity—not merely increased accessibility to existing services provided in new ways—is required in order to achieve health for all. Nurses, with a strong focus on health promotion and public participation, need to continue to advocate for the inclusion of all the principles of PHC.

Nurse academics, educators, administrators, and practitioners need to join forces with nursing associations, other health professionals, consumers, and other public sectors if a system based on PHC principles is to become a viable alternative to Canada's current health system. Or, perhaps more alarmingly, to prevent a move to a more privatized system with greater inequities than currently exist. Meeting the challenges addressed in this chapter will require risk and innovation by nurses and nursing associations as they work collaboratively with others to create a health care system that will meet the needs of Canadians.

SUMMARY OF LEARNING OBJECTIVES

- PHC is a social justice model that includes five interrelated principles that are foundational to achieving health for all: accessibility to the full range of health care; public participation in the planning and management of health and health care; a focus on health promotion and illness prevention to achieve health equity; use of appropriate technology; and intersectoral and interdisciplinary collaboration.
- PHC was first articulated in 1978, in the Declaration of Alma Ata. As the site of the Ottawa Charter, Canada is perceived as world leader in PHC. There continue to be challenges worldwide with accomplishing full implementation of PHC.
- There are many examples of a variety of PHC initiatives in Canada.
- To effectively implement PHC, health care needs to be equity oriented and address both physical and social determinants of health.

- Nursing has been deeply involved in promoting PHC and in engaging in ways of caring that demonstrate the evolution of PHC in Canada. Nurses must continue to provide leadership to strengthen PHC implementation.
- Every nurse can practice in any setting using PHC principles.
- Providing health care that meets PHC goals is challenging and complex. It requires a broad understanding of PHC and the foundational concept of health equity, effective interprofessional collaboration and collaboration with government and non–health care sectors, prioritizing individual and community participation in care, and conducting research to evaluate the effectiveness of PHC models of health promotion and care.

CRITICAL THINKING QUESTIONS

1. How can the use of multidisciplinary teams facilitate a PHC approach to care?
2. What might it look like if an RN was the first point of care in a fully implemented PHC system?
3. What attitudes, knowledge, and skills do you think are most fundamental to nurses working within a PHC system?
4. What are some priorities issues in your community that challenge the achievement of health equity?
5. How do the challenges associated with global PHC differ from the challenges in Canada?

REFERENCES

Ansloos, J. (2018). Rethinking Indigenous suicide. *International Journal of Indigenous Health, 13*, 8–28. https://doi.org/10.18357/ijih.v13i2.32061.

Ashcroft, R., MacMillan, C., Ambrose-Miller, W., et al. (2018). The emerging role of social work in primary health care: A survey of social workers in Ontario family health teams. *Health and Social Work, 43*, 1110–1117. https://doi.org/10.1093/hsw/hly003.

Ashley, L. (2015). Primary health care in practice. *Canadian Nurse, 111*, 7.

Association of Registered Nurses of British Columbia. (2016). *Community health centres*. Retrieved from https://www.arnbc.ca/pdfs/policies-and-advocacy/issues-briefs/community-health/ARNBC-IB-Community-Health-Centres.pdf.

Association of Registered Nurses of Newfoundland and Labrador. (2012). *Position statement: Primary health care*. Retrieved from https://www.arnnl.ca/primary-health-care-2012.

Association of Registered Nurses of Newfoundland and Labrador. (2013). *Brief. Supporting health system sustainability through investments in primary health care*. Retrieved from https://www.arnnl.ca/supporting-health-system-sustainability-through-investments-primary-health-care-2013.

Batista, R., Pottie, K., Bouchard, L., et al. (2018). Primary health care models addressing health equity for immigrants: A systematic scoping review. *Journal of Immigrant and Minority Health, 20*, 214–230. https://doi.org/10.1007/s10903-016-0531-y.

Bharadwaj, L., & Bradford, L. (2018). Indigenous water poverty: Impacts beyond physical health. In H. Exner-Pirot, B. Norbye, & L. Butler (Eds.), *Northern and Indigenous health and health care* (Chapter 4). Saskatoon, SK: University of Saskatchewan. Retrieved from https://openpress.usask.ca/northernhealthcare/chapter/chapter-4-indigenous-water-poverty-impacts-beyond-physical-health/.

Bradford, L. E. A., Bharadwaj, L. A., Okpalauwaekwe, U., et al. (2016). Drinking water quality in Indigenous communities in Canada and health outcomes: A scoping review. *International Journal of Circumpolar Health, 75*(1), 32336. https://doi.org/10.3402/ijch.v75.32336.

Belzak, L., & Halverson, J. (2018). Evidence synthesis—The opioid crisis in Canada: A national perspective. *Health Promotion and Chronic Disease Prevention in Canada, 38*, 6. https://doi.org/10.24095/hpcdp.38.6.02.

Besner, J. (2006). Optimizing nursing scope of practice within a primary health care context: Linking role accountabilities to health outcomes. *Primary Health Care Research and Development, 7*, 284–290. https://doi.org/10.1017/S1463423606000387.

Birn, A. (2018). Back to Alma-Ata, from 1978 to 2018 and beyond. *AJPH, 108*, 1153–1155. https://doi.org/10.2105/AJPH.2018.304625.

Blanchard, J. F., & Murnaghan, D. A. (2010). Nursing patients with chest pain: Practice guided by the Prince Edward Island conceptual model for nursing. *Nurse Education in Practice, 10*, 48–51. https://doi.org/10.1016/j.nepr.2009.03.010.

Butterfield, P. G. (2017). Thinking upstream: A 25-year retrospective and conceptual model aimed at reducing health inequities. *Advances in Nursing Science, 40*, 2–11. https://doi.org/10.1097/ANS.0000000000000161.

Calgary Urban Project Society. (2019). *Programs*. Retrieved from https://www.cupscalgary.com.

Canadian Association of Community Health Centres. (n.d.). *About us*. Retrieved from https://www.cachc.ca/about/.

Canadian Association of Physician Assistants. (n.d.). *About PAs*. Retrieved from https://capa-acam.ca/about-pas.

Canadian Council on Social Determinants of Health. (2012). *Communicating the social determinants of health: Guidelines for common messaging*. Retrieved from http://ccsdh.ca/images/uploads/Communicating_the_Social_Determinants_of_Health.pdf.

Canadian Council on Social Determinants of Health. (2015). *A review of frameworks on the determinants of health*. Retrieved from http://ccsdh.ca/images/uploads/Frameworks_Report_English.pdf.

Canadian Institute for Health Information. (2016). *Primary health care in Canada: A chartbook of selected indicator results, 2016*. Ottawa, ON: Author. https://secure.cihi.ca/free_products/Primary%20Health%20Care%20in%20Canada%20-%20Selected%20Pan-Canadian%20Indicators_2016_EN.pdf.

Canadian Institute for Health Information. (2018a). *Emergency department wait times in Canada continuing to rise*. Ottawa, ON: Author. Retrieved from https://www.longwoods.com/newsdetail/11387.

Canadian Institute for Health Information. (2018b). *Canada's nursing workforce experiences slowest growth in a decade*. Ottawa, ON: Author. Retrieved from https://markets.businessinsider.com/news/stocks/canada-snursing-workforce-experiences-slowest-growth-in-adecade-1027010894.

Canadian Institutes of Health Research. (n.d.). *Community-based primary health care*. Retrieved from http://www.cihr-irsc.gc.ca/e/43626.html.

Canadian Medical Association. (2010). *Health care transformation in Canada: Change that works, care that lasts*. Retrieved from https://www.cma.ca/health-care-transformation-canada-change-works-care-lasts.

Canadian Nurses Association. (2002). *Effective health care equals Primary Health Care. Fact Sheet*. Retrieved from https://www.cna-aiic.ca/~/media/cna/page-content/pdf-fr/fs17_effective_health_care_equals_primary_health_care_nov_2002_e.pdf.

Canadian Nurses Association. (2003). Primary health care: The time has come. *Nursing Now*, 16, 1–4.

Canadian Nurses Association. (2004). *Building a strong, viable, publicly funded, not-for-profit health system*. Ottawa, ON: Author. Retrieved from https://cna-aiic.ca/~/media/cna/page-content/pdf-fr/cna_platform_e.pdf.

Canadian Nurses Association. (2005). *Primary health care: A summary of the issues*. Ottawa, ON: Author. Retrieved from https://www.cna-aiic.ca/-/media/cna/page-content/pdf-en/bg7_primary_health_care_e.pdf.

Canadian Nurses Association. (2006). *Practice framework for nurse practitioners in Canada*. Ottawa, ON: Author. Retrieved from https://www.cna-aiic.ca/-/media/cna/page-content/pdf-en/04_practice-framework.pdf.

Canadian Nurses Association. (2008). *Tested solutions for eliminating Canada's registered nursing shortage*. Ottawa, ON: Author. Retrieved from https://cna-aiic.ca/~/media/cna/page-content/pdf-en/rn_highlights_e.pdf.

Canadian Nurses Association. (2011). *Review of the 10-year plan to strengthen health care*. Ottawa, ON: Author. Retrieved from https://www.cna-aiic.ca/-/media/cna/page-content/pdf-en/brief_10_year_plan_e.pdf.

Canadian Nurses Association. (2013). *Leadership in primary health care series*. Ottawa, ON: Author. Retrieved from https://www.cna-aiic.ca/en/policy-advocacy/primary-health-care/leadership-in-primary-health-care-series.

Canadian Nurses Association. (2015). *Primary health care position statement*. Ottawa, ON: Author. Retrieved from https://www.cna-aiic.ca/~/media/cna/page-content/pdf-en/primary-health-care-position-statement.pdf.

Canadian Nurses Association. (2016a). *The nurse practitioner position statement*. Ottawa, ON: Author. Retrieved from https://www.cna-aiic.ca/-/media/cna/page-content/pdf-en/the-nurse-practitioner-position-statement_2016.pdf.

Canadian Nurses Association. (2016b). *The Canadian Nurse Practitioner Initiative: A 10-year retrospective*. Ottawa, ON: Author. Retrieved from https://www.cna-aiic.ca/-/media/cna/page-content/pdf-en/canadian-nurse-practitioner-initiative-a-10-year-retrospective.pdf.

Canadian Nurses Association. (2018). *Social determinants of health position statement*. Ottawa, ON: Author. Retrieved from https://www.cna-aiic.ca/-/media/cna/page-content/pdf-en/social-determinants-of-health-position-statement_dec-2018.pdf.

Canadian Nurses Association. (2019). *Interprofessional collaboration position statement*. Ottawa, ON: Author. Retrieved from https://www.cna-aiic.ca/-/media/cna/page-content/pdf-en/interprofessional-collaboration-ps-2019.pdf.

Canadian Pharmacists Association. (2019). *Pharmacists' scope of practice in Canada*. Ottawa, ON: Author. Retrieved from https://www.pharmacists.ca/cpha-ca/assets/File/cpha-on-the-issues/Scope%20of%20Practice%20in%20Canada_April2019.pdf.

Chang, F., & Gupta, N. (2015). Progress in electronic medical record adoption in Canada. *Canadian Family Physician*, 61, 1076–1084.

Coburn, D., Denny, K., Mykhalovskiy, E., et al. (2003). Population health in Canada: A brief critique. *American Journal of Public Health*, 93, 393–396. https://doi.org/10.2105/AJPH.93.3.392.

Cohen, D., Huynh, T., Sebold, A., et al. (2014). The population health approach: A qualitative study of conceptual and operational definitions for leaders in Canadian healthcare. *Sage Open Medicine*, 2. https://doi.org/10.1177/2050312114522618.

College and Association of Registered Nurses of Alberta. (2008). *Primary health care*. Edmonton, AB: Author. Retrieved from https://docplayer.net/31448189-Guidelines-primary-health-care.html.

College and Association of Registered Nurses of Alberta. (2014). *Annual report 2013–2014*. Edmonton, AB: Author. Retrieved from https://nurses.ab.ca/docs/default-source/annual-andfinancial-reports/annual-report-2014-2015.pdf.

College and Association of Registered Nurses of Alberta. (2019). *Entry level competencies for the practice of registered nurses*. Edmonton, AB: Author. Retrieved from https://www.nurses.ab.ca/docs/default-source/document-library/standards/entry-to-practice-competencies-for-the-registered-nurses-profession.pdf.

College of Nurses of Ontario. (2018). *Entry-to-practice competencies for registered nurses*. Toronto, ON: Author. CNO Publication No. 41037. Retrieved from http://www.cno.org/globalassets/docs/reg/41037-entry-to-practice-competencies-2020.pdf.

College of Nurses of Ontario. (2019). *Journey to nurse prescribing*. Toronto, ON: Author. Retrieved from http://www.cno.org/en/trending-topics/journey-to-rn-prescribing/.

Commission on Social Determinants of Health. (2008). *Closing the gap in a generation: health equity through action on the social determinants of health. Final Report of the Commission on Social Determinants of Health*. Geneva, Switzerland: World Health Organization. Retrieved from https://www.who.int/social_determinants/thecommission/finalreport/en/.

Community Health Nurses Initiatives' Group. (2015). *Healthy schools, healthy children: Maximizing the contribution of public health nursing in school settings (Version 2.0)*. Toronto, ON: Author. Retrieved from http://www.ontariohealthyschools.com/uploads/2/1/7/6/21766954/school-nursing-paper-2.pdf.

Community Health Nurses of Canada. (2019). *2019 Canadian community health nursing professional practice model & standards of practice*. Retrieved from https://www.chnc.ca/standards-of-practice.

de Leeuw, S., Lindsay, N. M., & Greenwood, M. (2018). Introduction to the second edition: Rethinking (once again) determinants of Indigenous peoples' health. In

M. Greenwood, S. de Leeuw, & M. N. Lindsay (Eds.), *Determinants of Indigenous peoples' health: Beyond the social* (2nd ed.). Toronto, ON: Canadian Scholars' Press.

Dupéré, S., Perreault, R., Hills, M., et al. (2012). Perspectives on health promotion from different areas of practice. In I. Rootman, M. S. Dupéré, A. Pederson et al. (Eds.), *Health promotion in Canada* (3rd ed., pp. 3–19). Toronto, ON: Canadian Scholars' Press.

Elliott, J., Rutty, C., & Villeneuve, M. (2008). *Canadian Nurses Association: One hundred years of service.* Ottawa, ON: Canadian Nurses Association. Retrieved from https://www.cna-aiic.ca/html/en/CNA-ONE-HUNDRED-YEARS-OF-SERVICE-e/files/assets/basic-html/page-1.html.

Epp, J. (1986). *Achieving health for all: A framework for health promotion.* Ottawa, ON: Health and Welfare Canada. Retrieved from https://www.canada.ca/en/health-canada/services/health-care-system/reports-publications/health-care-system/achieving-health-framework-health-promotion.html.

Falk-Rafael, A., & Betker, C. (2012). Witnessing social injustice downstream and advocating for health equity upstream: "The trombone slide" of nursing. *Advances in Nursing Science, 35,* 92–112. https://doi.org/10.1097/ANS.0b013e31824fe70f.

Ford-Gilboe, M., Wathen, C. N., Varcoe, C., et al. (2018). How equity-oriented health care affects health: Key mechanisms and implications for primary health care practice and policy. *The Millbank Quarterly, 96,* 636–671. https://doi.org/10.1111/1468-0009.12349.

Globerman, S., Barua, B., & Hasan, S. (2018). *The supply of physicians in Canada: Projections and assessment.* Vancouver, BC: Fraser Institute. Retrieved from https://www.fraserinstitute.org/sites/default/files/supply-of-physicians-in-canada.pdf.

Gillam, S. (2008). Is the declaration of Alma Ata still relevant to primary health care? *BMJ, 336,* 536–538. https://doi.org/10.1136/bmj.39469.432118.AD.

Glass, H., & Hicks, S. (2000). Health public policy in health system reform. In M. J. Stewart (Ed.), *Community nursing: Promoting Canadians' health* (2nd ed., pp. 156–170). Toronto, ON: W.B. Saunders.

Government of Canada (2017). *A common statement of principles on shared health priorities.* Retrieved from https://www.canada.ca/en/health-canada/corporate/transparency/health-agreements/principles-shared-health-priorities.html.

Government of Canada. (2020). *Canada Health Act.* Retrieved from https://www.canada.ca/en/public-health/services/publications/science-research-data/canada-health-act-infographic.html.

Hamilton, N., & Bhatti, T. (1996). *Population health promotion: An integrated model of population health and health promotion.* Ottawa, ON: Health Promotion Development Division, Health Canada. Retrieved from https://www.canada.ca/en/public-health/services/health-promotion/population-health/population-health-promotion-integrated-model-population-health-health-promotion.html.

Hardman, S., & Ho, K. (2015). The effect of educational attainment levels on use of nontraditional health information resources: Findings from the Canadian survey of experiences with primary health care. *Knowledge Management &*

E-Learning, 7(4), 677–687. https://doi.org/10.34105/j.kmel.2015.07.044.

Harnagea, H., Lamothe, L., Couturier, Y., et al. (2018). How primary health care teams perceive the integration of oral health care into their practice: A qualitative study. *PLoS ONE, 13*(10), e0205465. https://doi.org/10.1371/journal.pone.0205465.

Hay, D., Varga-Toth, J., & Hines, E. (2006). *Frontline health care in Canada: Innovations in delivering services to vulnerable populations. Research Report F/63.* Family Network (CPRN). Toronto, ON: Canadian Policy Research Networks.

Health Canada. (2001). *The population health template: Key elements and actions that define a population health approach.* Retrieved from https://www.canada.ca/en/public-health/services/health-promotion/population-health/population-health-approach.html.

Health Canada. (2015). *About primary health care.* Retrieved from https://www.canada.ca/en/health-canada/services/primary-health-care/about-primary-health-care.html.

Health Council of Canada. (2013). *Better health, better care, better value for all: Refocusing health care reform in Canada.* Retrieved from https://healthcouncilcanada.ca/773/.

Health Council of Canada. (2014a). *Health innovation portal: Archive of innovative practices theme: Patient-centered care* (Vol. 1). Retrieved from https://healthcouncilcanada.ca/files/access_and_wait_times_1.pdf.

Health Council of Canada. (2014b). *Health innovation portal: Archive of innovative practices theme: patient centered care* (Vol. 2). Retrieved from https://healthcouncilcanada.ca/files/Access_and_Wait_Times_2.pdf.

Health Council of Canada. (2014c). *Health innovation portal: Archive of innovative practices theme: Health promotion and disease prevention* (Vol. 1). Retrieved from https://healthcouncilcanada.ca/files/Access_and_Wait_Times_1.pdf.

Health Council of Canada. (2014d). *Health innovation portal: Archive of innovative practices theme: Health promotion and disease prevention* (Vol. 2). Retrieved from https://healthcouncilcanada.ca/files/Access_and_Wait_Times_2.pdf.

Health Council of Canada. (2014e). *The Health Council of Canada's departing message in support of future health care reform.* Retrieved from https://healthcouncilcanada.ca/834/.

Health PEI. (2016). *Engagement toolkit.* Retrieved from http://www.gov.pe.ca/photos/original/hpei_engagetool.pdf.

Henderson, R., Montesanti, S., Crowshoe, L., et al. (2018). Advancing Indigenous primary health care policy in Alberta. *Canada. Health Policy, 122,* 638–644. https://doi.org/10.1016/j.healthpol.2018.04.014.

International Council of Nurses. (2018). *International Council of Nurses and Nursing Now statement. Astana Declaration on primary health care: From Alma-Ata towards universal health coverage and the Sustainable Development Goals.* Geneva, Switzerland: Author. Retrieved from https://www.icn.ch/nursing-policy/endorsements-joint-statements.

Jesmin, S., Thind, A., & Sarma, S. (2012). Does team-based primary health care improve patients' perception of outcomes? Evidence from the 2007-08 Canadian Survey of Experiences with Primary Health. *Health Policy, 105,* 71–83. https://doi.org/10.1016/j.healthpol.2012.01.008.

Kaasalainen, S., Martin-Misener, R., Kilpatrick, K., et al. (2010). A historical overview of the development of advanced practice nursing roles in Canada. *Nursing Leadership, 23*(Special Issue), 35–60. https://doi.org/10.12927/cjnl.2010.22268.

Kennedy, V. (2014). The value of registered nurses in collaborative family practice: Enhancing primary healthcare in Canada. *Nursing Leadership, 27*, 32–61.

Kosteniuk, J. G., Stewart, N. J., Karunanayake, C. P., et al. (2017). Exploratory factor analysis and reliability of the Primary Health Care Engagement (PHCE) Scale in rural and remote nurses: Findings from a national survey. *Primary Health Care Research and Development, 18*. 692-622. https://doi.org/10.1017/S146342361700038X.

Lalonde, M. (1974). *A new perspective on the health of Canadians: A working paper*. Ottawa, ON: Government of Canada.

Lankshear, S. (2012). *Primary Health Care Summit summary report. Report prepared for Canadian Nurses Association and Canadian Medical Association*. Tiny, ON: Relevé Consulting Services. Retrieved from https://www.cna-aiic.ca/-/media/cna/page-content/pdf-en/primary_health_care_report_e.pdf.

Laurant, M., van der Biezen, M., Wijers, N., et al. (2018). Nurses as substitutes for doctors in primary care. *Cochrane Database of Systematic Reviews, 7*. https://doi.org/10.1002/14651858.CD001271.pub3.

Lenihan, D. (2012). *Rescuing public policy: The case for public engagement*. Ottawa, ON: Public Policy Forum.

Mable, A., & Marriott, J. (2002). *Sharing the learning: Health Transition Fund: Synthesis Series: Primary Health Care*. Ottawa, ON: Health Canada.

MacPhail, J. (1991). Primary health care: The means for reaching nursing's potential in achieving Health for All. In J. Kerr, & J. MacPhail (Eds.), *Canadian nursing: Issues and perspectives* (2nd ed., pp. 321–335). Toronto, ON: Mosby.

MacPhail, J. (1996). Primary health care: The means for reaching nursing's potential in achieving Health for All. In J. Ross-Kerr, & J. MacPhail (Eds.), *Canadian nursing: Issues and perspectives* (3rd ed., pp. 390–406). Toronto, ON: Mosby.

Mahler, H. (1985). *Nurses lead the way. WHO Features (No. 97)*. Geneva, Switzerland: World Health Organization.

Martin-Misener, R., & Bryant-Lukosius, D. (2014). *Optimizing the role of nurses in primary care in Canada. Final report*. Ottawa, ON: Canadian Nurses Association. Retrieved from https://www.cna-aiic.ca/~/media/cna/page-content/pdf-en/optimizing-the-role-of-nurses-in-primary-care-in-canada.pdf.

Morley, C., Unwin, M., Peterson, G. M., et al. (2018). Emergency department crowding: A systematic review of causes, consequences and solutions. *PLoS ONE, 13*(8), e0203316. https://doi.org/10.1371/journal.pone.0203316.

Montesanti, S., Robinson-Vollman, A., & Green, L. A. (2018). Designing a framework for primary health care research in Canada: A scoping literature review. *BMC Family Practice, 19*, 44. https://doi.org/10.1186/s12875-018-0839-x.

Miedema, B. (2015). Thinking outside the primary health care box. Alternative models of primary health care for New Brunswickers. *Info Nursing, 46*, 31–33.

Munro, M., Gallant, M., MacKinnon, M., et al. (2000). The Prince Edward conceptual model for nursing: A nursing perspective of primary health care. *Canadian Journal of Nursing Research, 32*, 39–55.

National Collaborating Centre for the Determinants of Health. (2013a). *Let's talk: Universal and targeted approaches to health equity*. Antigonish, NS: National Collaborating Centre for Determinants of Health, St. Francis Xavier University. Retrieved from http://nccdh.ca/resources/entry/lets-talk-universal-and-targeted-approaches.

National Collaborating Centre for the Determinants of Health. (2013b). *Let's Talk: Health equity*. Antigonish, NS: National Collaborating Centre for Determinants of Health, St. Francis Xavier University. Retrieved from http://nccdh.ca/images/uploads/Lets_Talk_Health_Equity_English.pdf.

National Collaborating Centre for the Determinants of Health. (2014). *Let's talk: Moving upstream*. Antigonish, NS: Author. Retrieved from http://nccdh.ca/images/uploads/Moving_Upstream_Final_En.pdf.

National Collaborating Centre for the Determinants of Health. (2015). *Learning to work differently: Implementing Ontario's Social Determinants of Health Public Health Nurse Initiative*. Antigonish, NS: Author. Retrieved from http://nccdh.ca/resources/entry/learning-to-work-differently-implementing-ontarios-sdoh-public-health-nurse.

Nesdole, R., Voigts, D., Lepnurm, L., & Roberts, R. (2014). Reconceptualizing determinants of health: Barriers to improving the health status of First Nations peoples. *Canadian Journal of Public Health, 105*, e209–e213. https://doi.org/10.17269/cjph.105.4308.

North End Community Health Centre. (n.d.). *Programs and services*. Retrieved from http://nechc.com.

Nurses Association of New Brunswick. (2012). *Primary health care framework: An investment in patients*. Retrieved from http://www.nanb.nb.ca/media/resource/NANB-PR-PHCAnnouncement-2012-E.pdf.

Ogilvie, L., & Reutter, L. (2003). Primary health care: Complexities and possibilities from a nursing perspective. In J. Ross-Kerr, & M. Wood (Eds.), *Canadian nursing: Issues and perspectives* (4th ed., pp. 441–465). Toronto, ON: Elsevier.

O'Mara-Eves, A., Brunton, G., McDaid, D., et al. (2013). Community engagement to reduce inequalities in health: a systematic review, meta-analysis and economic analysis. *Public Health Research, 1*(4), https://doi.org/10.3310/phr01040.

Ontario Association of Public Health Nursing Leaders. (2019, May 2). *Open letter re: Modernizing Ontario's Public Health Units*. Retrieved from https://cdn.ymaws.com/www.alphaweb.org/resource/resmgr/OAPHNL_PHR_020519.pdf.

Ontario Hospital Association. (2015). *Patient and family engagement requirements for accreditation: A guidance document*. Retrieved from https://www.oha.com/Documents/Patient%20and%20Family%20Engagement%20Requirements%20for%20Accreditation%20with%20Appendix.pdf.

Ontario Minister of Finance. (2019). 2019 *Ontario budget: Protecting what matters most*. Retrieved from http://budget.ontario.ca/2019/bg-matters.html.

Ontario Premier's Council on Improving Healthcare and Ending Hallway Medicine. (2019). *Hallway health care: A system under strain: First interim report from the Premier's Council on Improving Healthcare and Ending Hallway Medicine.* Retrieved from http://www.health.gov.on.ca/en/public/publications/premiers_council/default.aspx.

O'Rourke, T., Summach, A., & McDonald, K. (2018). Reshaping primary health care for older adults. *Alberta RN, 74*(2), 30–31. Retrieved from https://nurses.ab.ca/docs/default-source/alberta-rn/abrn_summer18.pdf.

Owens, S. (2019, January 30). Roles of nurse practitioners and physician assistants in medicine still under debate. *CMAJ News.* Retrieved from https://cmajnews.com/2019/01/30/roles-of-nurse-practitioners-and-physician-assistants-in-medicine-still-under-debate-cmaj-109-5708/.

Pan-Canadian Public Health Network. (2018). *Key health inequalities in Canada: A national portrait.* Ottawa, ON: Minister of Health. Retrieved from https://www.canada.ca/content/dam/phac-aspc/documents/services/publications/science-research/key-health-inequalities-canada-national-portrait-executive-summary/hir-full-report-eng.pdf.

Paré-Plante, A., Boivin, A., Berbiche, D., et al. (2018). Primary health care organizational characteristics associated with better accessibility: Data from the QUALICO-PC survey in Quebec. *BMC Family Practice, 19,* 188. https://doi.org/10.1186/s12875-018-0871-x.

Pederson, A., Rootman, I., Frohlich, K. L., et al. (2017). The continuing evolution of health promotion in Canada. In M. O'Neill, I. Rootman, A. Pederson, et al. (Eds.), *Health promotion in Canada* (4th ed., pp. 3–19). Toronto, ON: Canadian Scholars' Press.

Pollock, N. J., Healey, G. K., Jong, M., et al. (2018). Tracking progress in suicide prevention in Indigenous communities: a challenge for public health surveillance in Canada. *BMC Public Health, 18,* 1320. https://doi.org/10.1186/s12889-018-6224-9.

Prasad, S., Dunn, W., Hillier, L. M., et al. (2014). Rural geriatric glue: A nurse practitioner–led model of care for enhancing primary care for frail older adults within an ecosystem approach. *Journal of the American Geriatrics Society, 62*(9), 1772–1780. https://doi.org/10.1111/jgs.12982.

Raphael, D., Bryant, T., & Curry-Stevens, A. (2004). Toronto charter outlines future health policy directions for Canada and elsewhere. *Health Promotion International, 19,* 269–273. https://doi.org/10.1093/heapro/dah214.

Rayner, J., Muldoon, L., Bayoumi, I., et al. (2018). Delivering primary health care as envisioned: A model of health and well-being guiding community-governed primary care organizations. *Journal of Integrated Care, 26,* 231–241. https://doi.org/10.1108/JICA-02-2018-0014.

Registered Nurses' Association of Ontario. (2008). *Briefing note: Primary health care - increasing access.* Retrieved from https://rnao.ca/policy/briefing-notes/primary-health-care-increasing-access.

Registered Nurses' Association of Ontario. (2012). *Proposal feedback: Regulation of physician assistants under the Regulated Health Professions Act.* Retrieved from https://rnao.ca/sites/rnao-ca/files/RNAO_submission_to_HPRAC_re-PAs_April_2_2012.pdf.

Registered Nurses' Association of Ontario. (2018). *Indigenous health backgrounder.* Retrieved from https://rnao.ca/sites/rnao-ca/files/Indigenous_health_backgrounder.pdf.

Reimer-Kirkham, S. (2014). Nursing research on religion and spirituality through a social justice lens. *Advances in Nursing Science, 37.* 249-237. https://doi.org/10.1097/ANS.0000000000000036.

Rempel, L. A., & Moore, K. (2012). Peer-led prenatal breastfeeding education: A viable alternative to nurse-led education. *Midwifery, 28,* 72–79. https://doi.org/10.1016/j.midw.2010.11.005.

Ritchie, L. (2012). Integration of chronic illness care into a primary healthcare focused nursing curriculum. *Nurse Educator, 37,* 23–24. https://doi.org/10.1097/NNE.0b013e3182383717.

Rodger, G. L., & Gallagher, S. M. (2000). The move toward primary health care in Canada: Community health nursing from 1985 to 2000. In M. J. Stewart (Ed.), *Community nursing: Promoting Canadians' health* (2nd ed., pp. 33–55). Toronto, ON: W.B. Saunders.

Roots, A., & McDonald, M. (2014). Outcomes associated with nurse practitioners in collaborative practice with general practitioners in rural settings in Canada: A mixed methods study. *Human Resources for Health, 12,* 69. https://doi.org/10.1186/1478-4491-12-69.

Romanow, R. (2002). *Building on values. The future of health care in Canada—final report.* Commission on the Future of Health Care in Canada. Retrieved from http://publications.gc.ca/collections/Collection/CP32-85-2002E.pdf.

Santaguida, P., Dolovich, L., Oliver, D., et al. (2018). Protocol for a Delphi consensus exercise to identify a core set of criteria for selecting health related outcome measures (HROM) to be used in primary health care. *BMC Family Practice, 19,* 152. https://doi.org/10.1186/s12875-018-0831-5.

Standing Senate Committee on Social Affairs, Science, and Technology. (2012). *Time for transformative change: A review of the 2004 Health Accord.* Retrieved from https://sencanada.ca/content/sen/Committee/411/soci/rep/rep07mar12-e.pdf.

Stewart, M. J. (2000). Framework based on primary health care principles. In M. J. Stewart (Ed.), *Community nursing: Promoting Canadians' health* (2nd ed., pp. 58–82). Toronto, ON: W.B. Saunders.

Tompkins, J. W., Mequaint, S., Barre, D. E., et al. (2018). National Survey of Indigenous primary healthcare capacity and delivery models in Canada: The TransFORmation of IndiGEnous PrimAry HEAlthcare delivery (FORGE AHEAD) community profile survey. *BMC Health Services Research, 18,* 828. https://doi.org/10.1186/s12913-018-3578-8.

Travers, J. L., Shenck, E. C., Rosa, W. E., et al. (2019). Climate change, climate justice, and a call for action. *Nursing Economics, 37,* 9–12.

United Nations. (2015a). *Transforming our world: The 2030 Agenda for Sustainable Development.* New York, NY: Author.

United Nations. (2015b). *The Millennium Development Goals report, 2015.* New York, NY: Author.

van Weel, C., Turnbull, D., Bazemore, A., et al. (2018). Implementing primary health care policy under changing global political conditions: Lessons learned from 4 national settings. *Annals of Family Medicine, 16*, 179–180. https://doi.org/10.1370/afm.2214.

Villeneuve, M., & MacDonald, J. (2006). *Toward 2020: Visions for nursing.* Ottawa, ON: Canadian Nurses Association.

Weatherill, S. (2007). *Laying the groundwork for culture change: The legacy of the Primary Health Care Transition Fund.* Ottawa, ON: Health Canada. Retrieved from https://www.canada.ca/content/dam/hc-sc/migration/hc-sc/hcs-sss/alt_formats/hpb-dgps/pdf/prim/2006-synth-legacy-fondements-eng.pdf.

Williams, S. D., Phillips, J. M., & Koyama, K. (2018). Nurse advocacy: Adopting a health in all policies approach. *Online Journal of Issues in Nursing, 23*(3). https://doi.org/10.3912/OJIN.Vol23No03Man01.

World Health Organization. (1978). *Primary health care: Report of the International Conference on Primary Health Care: Alma-Ata, USSR.* Geneva, Switzerland: Author.

World Health Organization. (1986). *Ottawa Charter for Health Promotion.* Retrieved from https://www.who.int/healthpromotion/conferences/previous/ottawa/en/.

World Health Organization. (2003). *World Health Report 2003: Shaping the future.* Retrieved from https://www.who.int/whr/2003/en/whr03_en.pdf?ua=1.

World Health Organization. (2008). *World Health Report 2008: Primary health care—Now more than ever.* Retrieved from https://www.who.int/whr/2008/whr08_en.pdf.

World Health Organization. (2011). *Rio Political Declaration on social determinants of health.* Retrieved from https://www.who.int/sdhconference/declaration/Rio_political_declaration.pdf.

World Health Organization. (2014). *Health in all policies: Helsinki statement. Framework for country action.* Retrieved from https://apps.who.int/iris/handle/10665/112636.

World Health Organization. (2016). *Shanghai Declaration on promoting health in the 2030 Agenda for Sustainable Development.* Retrieved from https://www.who.int/healthpromotion/conferences/9gchp/shanghai-declaration.pdf.

World Health Organization. (2017). *Promoting health: Guide to national implementation of the Shanghai Declaration.* Geneva, Switzerland: Author. Retrieved from https://www.who.int/healthpromotion/publications/guide-national-implementation-shanghai-declaration/en/.

Young, S., & Fairburn, N. (2018). Expanding supervised injection facilities across Canada: lessons from the Vancouver experience. *Canadian Journal of Public Health, 109*, 227–230. https://doi.org/10.17269/s41997-018-0089-7.

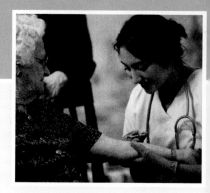

12

Quality of Care: From Quality Assurance and Improvement to Cultures of Patient Safety

Sharon M. Goodwin

 http://evolve.elsevier.com/Canada/Ross-Kerr/nursing

LEARNING OBJECTIVES

After reading this chapter, you will be able to:

- Define the concept of quality assurance in health care.
- Review the historical development of quality assurance and quality improvement.
- Outline the limitations of quality assurance.
- Describe the key concepts of continuous quality improvement.
- Review the steps of continuous quality improvement processes.
- Outline the applicable tools used when examining and assessing outcomes related to quality improvement and assurance.

- Discuss the role of patient safety, nursing-sensitive outcomes, and best practice guidelines in current quality improvement initiatives.
- Situate quality improvement and quality assurance in the current health care context.
- Describe possible future directions of quality improvement and quality assurance in Canadian nursing.

OUTLINE

KEY TERMS

best practice guidelines

change management

continuous quality improvement

nursing-sensitive outcomes

outcomes standards or criteria

patient safety

patient–family engagement

process standards or criteria

quality assurance

quality improvement

structural standards or criteria

total quality management

PERSONAL PERSPECTIVES

When gaps are identified in a system or process, getting involved to influence change can pay dividends. A good example is when VON Canada participated in the revision and updating of the Canadian national guidelines for treating patients with intravenous therapies. Nan Cleator, VON's National Practice Consultant, worked with the Canadian Vascular Access Association (CVAA) to shape the best practice guidelines to reflect practice in the home and community sector. Community is an emerging area of care delivery as the health system shifts care delivery into the community. However, the CVAA's 1999 guidelines did not reflect the home and community sector. VON was able to influence practice changes by participating with the national association in their review and revision process (VON Canada, 2019).

In 2012, VON undertook a major improvement initiative. Lean quality management and change management methods were used to create a whole system change in the service delivery chain. The lean way focuses on the flow of work versus simply standards. The team started by mapping the current process. They discovered that there were 170 steps from client referral to service! That explained the frustration and delays that were occurring. The team then identified waste, rework, and steps that added no value, reducing the process to 50 steps. This resulted in better and faster access to care, happier staff, and better financial outcomes (Goodwin & Miller, 2014).

Sources: Goodwin, S., & Miller, L. (2014). System overhaul. *The HIROC Connection, 33* (Summer 2015), 2731; VON Canada. (2019, May 21). *Shaping guidelines for IVs and infusions.* Retrieved from https://www.von.ca/en/story/may-2019.

INTRODUCTION

Health care organizations in Ontario are required by the Ministry of Health to have quality improvement plans in place. Sunnybrook Hospital in Toronto uses their plan to drive organizational improvement each year, and they proudly share the plan on their public website. The plan consists of five categories where improvements can be made: **patient–family engagement**, timeliness of care, effective care, safe care, and efficient care. An example of a **quality improvement** initiative that they undertook to improve safety was to increase the percentage of patients screened for risk of suicide in the emergency department (Sunnybrook Health Sciences Centre, 2019).

Increasing diversification and sophistication in the health care field have accompanied steady increases in national expenditures on health care. Meanwhile, public attitudes reflect parallel changes in social values about health, and better-informed health consumers are demanding increased accountability in health care. The activities of consumers' rights groups have attracted media attention and raised public awareness; health lobbyists have argued for environmental protection, health promotion, and provision of health care services that are accessible, effective, and appropriate. As a result, North American attitudes toward health care and health care providers have undergone a significant transition. This change is reflected in the perception that health care is a right rather than a privilege and the expectation that health care providers deliver not just care, but quality care.

Historically, **quality assurance** (QA) in health care was defined as the self-regulating activities of various professions. In 2009, quality improvement in health care included actions designed to improve both processes and outcomes of care, specifically actions aimed at increasing the value of services, improving responsiveness to those receiving care, and enhancing overall outcomes of care (Alexander & Hearld, 2009). Donabedian (2003) describes quality assurance as "all actions taken to establish, protect, promote, and improve the quality of health care" (p. xxiii). Continuous quality improvement has been evolving in health care, and **lean quality improvement** methods borrowed from manufacturing are being used to augment quality approaches in health care (Spear, 2004).

The traditional view that only relevant health care providers could describe the nature of competent practice meant that physicians, nurses, and other professionals were not challenged about how they dealt with matters of professional misconduct. Today, the situation is very different. Although professional groups still have the privilege of autonomously conducting regulatory functions, there is more public scrutiny of the process. In many provinces, lay members of professional governing boards and their disciplinary committees are appointed by the government to represent the public interest in professional deliberations. The professional conduct of physicians, nurses, and other health care providers is a subject for public discussion and debate, something that was unheard of in the past. The media have constantly pressured professional groups for full and open disclosure of the results of disciplinary operations. In the past decade, several provincial governments have introduced omnibus legislation for the regulation of health care providers that includes mandatory quality assurance and continuing competence programs as well as professional conduct hearings that are open to the public.

HISTORICAL DEVELOPMENTS IN QUALITY ASSURANCE

The assessment of nursing care quality has been an important and essential strategy for monitoring and stimulating excellence in nursing practice, administration, education, and research. The first documented study in health care and nursing, based on the use of standards, is attributed to Florence Nightingale, who in 1858 investigated the quality of care provided to military personnel (Nightingale, 1858). The development of standards for health care was formalized in the United States in 1918. The US standards were subsequently adopted in Canadian hospitals and applied to all disciplines and services. In 1952, the Joint Committee on Accreditation of Hospitals was formed, assuming responsibility for accrediting Canadian hospitals until 1958 (Joint Commission, 2019). At that time, the Canadian Council on Hospital Services Accreditation (CCHSA) was established to accredit health care agencies in Canada. Since then, the CCHSA has provided the external stimulus for quality assurance programs in nursing. Accreditation standards and requirements have been revised regularly and reflect increasingly strenuous monitoring. Beginning in the 1970s, the CCHSA standards required the presence of a quality assurance program in hospitals across Canada (Accreditation Canada, 2019).

Although quality assurance activities were visible in all disciplines, the primary focus was directed toward developing quality-monitoring programs in nursing, undoubtedly because nursing was the largest and most critically important service in health care agencies. Provincial professional associations in nursing also instituted quality assurance activities by developing guidelines for implementing quality assurance programs and nursing practice standards. Nursing consultants with quality assurance expertise were retained by professional associations to assist nursing service departments in provincial health care agencies with developing programs or ongoing quality assurance activities. Many hospitals established a quality assurance department within the division of nursing with responsibility for implementing and monitoring quality-related activities. Nursing expertise has also been important in developing standards at the past CCHSA Board of Directors, where the Canadian Nurses Association (CNA) was also represented.

In 2008, the CCHSA launched the Qmentum Accreditation Program and changed its name to Accreditation Canada. Accreditation Canada led the way by establishing standards and required organizational practices related to **patient safety**. In 1999 the Institute of Medicine conducted a study which "estimated that about 98,000 Americans die in hospitals each year from preventable medical errors" (Land & Stefl, 2007, p. 90). This study developed a new sense of urgency within health care to solve safety and quality problems. Baker, Norton, Flintoff et al. (2004) completed the "Canadian Adverse Events Study: The Incidence of Adverse Events Among Hospital Patients in Canada," with findings similar to those of the American study. The authors of this study and pioneers in patient safety made recommendations to establish what is now the Canadian Patient Safety Institute (CPSI) to foster a safer health care system for Canadians. Since its establishment in 2003, the CPSI has worked in collaboration with Accreditation Canada and the provincial health councils to further efforts to make health care safer for patients.

The common denominator of quality assurance programs has been standards. Standards set a level of expected functioning in health care systems to allow assessment against the standard. Standards in accreditation assess topics such as leadership, infection practices, and medication management, all of which affect the quality of care that people receive (Health Standards Organization, 2019). Donabedian (1980, 2003) proposed three levels for assessing quality: structure, process, and outcome. **Structural standards or criteria** focus on relationships among available human and material resources within a health care setting. Examples include the philosophy of the institution, resources and supplies, staffing patterns, and environmental characteristics. **Process standards or criteria** focus on nursing roles and activities to meet patient care goals. Examples of process standards are the nursing process, communication between nurses and patients, and nursing activities. Process and structure indicators dominated health care quality measurement until the 1990s (Doran & Pringle, 2011). **Outcomes standards or criteria** are mainly patient oriented and describe anticipated results of the care process. Outcomes generally refer to the results of health care delivery. It has been difficult to attribute outcomes to any one health care profession because a team effort is necessary to achieve results. Outcome measurement has also been slower to develop in health care because of the relatively slow uptake of clinical computerization (Doran & Pringle, 2011). With increasing use of electronic health information, systems outcome measurement is becoming more feasible.

The major effort in quality assurance programs was directed at process levels of care because health care provider activities could be assessed and measured directly at this level. This assessment was concurrent or, more frequently, retrospective. If concurrent, nursing care was reviewed or measured as it was delivered; if retrospective, the review took place after care was provided. Concurrent methods have the potential for collecting more and better information and direct information from patients. Because information was gathered sooner, any necessary changes could be made quickly. Disadvantages included increased costs and possible disruption to nursing unit activities. Retrospective reviews were attractive because costs tended to be lower, with less disruption to the nursing unit because the review usually focused on the patient's record. However, it was not usually possible to collect information directly from the patient, and nurses responsible for chart data were not available to elaborate or answer questions that arose. Because both concurrent and retrospective reviews provided valuable and unique information about the process of care, many agencies implemented both types in their quality assurance programs.

The literature on quality assurance has been plentiful (Trussel & Strand, 1978; Ventura, Hageman, Slakter, & Fox, 1980; Giovannetti, Kerr, Bay, & Buchan, 1986), with descriptive publications covering the nature of quality; components of a quality assurance model or framework; categorizations of quality; rationale for developing quality assurance techniques and programs; and establishing, maintaining, and improving quality assurance programs. The research literature dealing with quality assessment has been limited, focusing primarily on instrument development with little attention to the type of testing that should be integral to the process. Most instruments demonstrated little more than face validity, raising questions about the value of results in quality assessment programs using inadequately tested instruments. This has also posed problems for the interpretation of research based on instruments purporting to measure the quality of nursing care.

LIMITATIONS OF QUALITY ASSURANCE PROGRAMS

As a result of the previously noted issues, quality assurance programs have shown some significant limitations. A constant and major challenge facing executive officers of agencies is the cost effectiveness of all programs, including quality assurance programs. As the number of professionals required for successful operation of quality-monitoring programs increased, so did costs that were associated with programs implemented by external consultants. Funds expended were considerable and, some suggest, disproportionate to the results achieved.

Another area of concern was whether those responsible for design and implementation were knowledgeable in research and quality assessment. Knowledge about the research literature was important, as was the ability to assess strengths and weaknesses of various approaches to quality that maximize the former and minimize the latter in programs selected for implementation. Many nurses responsible for in-service education were also given responsibility for managing quality assurance activities in health care agencies. Although this was an expedient way for agencies to implement quality monitoring, it assumed that those responsible had the time, interest, background, and expertise to function effectively in both spheres. Limited testing of instrument reliability and validity for monitoring quality was a major concern for nursing departments. Many instruments did not measure dimensions of quality consistently and therefore provided little value for judging performance within the institution based on the results obtained. Ventura, Hageman, Slakter, and Fox (1980) and Giovannetti, Kerr, Bay, and Buchan (1986) noted that measurements must be made carefully so that quality-monitoring processes yield reliable findings. Controlled conditions required that raters be carefully trained and monitored. This meant that certain nurses were designated as quality auditors and seconded to the program for a specific period of time. Although this system supported principles of good data collection, the process was seen as delegating the responsibility for quality care to a few individuals whose role was primarily inspection. Another limitation of many quality assurance programs was the retrospective focus on achievement of standards. Considerable emphasis on quality-monitoring activities occurred after the fact, when it was least possible to make necessary changes. Also, minimum standards of achievement were acceptable in determining whether criteria were met.

One of the greatest limitations was the largely department-specific focus of quality assurance programs. This limited the resolution of interdisciplinary issues such as admission, transfer, discharge, consultation, and materials distribution, which have been resistant to change despite a variety of quality-monitoring techniques. The other major limitation of quality assurance programs was the "blame culture" associated with them. Traditional approaches to quality assurance tended to focus on the quality of clinical practice as well as assigning blame to individuals when something went wrong. This negative approach set up a cycle of blame and fear, resulting in a decrease of both discussion and focus on solving problems (Canadian Patient Safety Institute, 2017; Darr, 1999).

Finally, the foundation of quality assurance programs—achieving predetermined standards in the clinical setting—became seen as somewhat arbitrary. Administrators and program directors established the level to which each standard was to be achieved. Critical standards were expected to be achieved 100% of the time, while less critical standards, perhaps 80% to 90% of the time. For example, within nursing, random chart reviews were completed to determine how often nurses recorded their assessment of medication efficacy when analgesia was given as needed in the postoperative period. Eighty percent achievement was considered acceptable but the target was an arbitrary number. Where was the evidence that achieving 80% on a particular standard was an appropriate goal? Was the goal even reasonable? In the world of quality assurance, a standard could be achieved to the desired level without any discussion as to its appropriateness or to evidence to support the goal. For example, anesthetic and surgical procedures could be performed to standard 100% of the time, yet the particular surgical procedure might be performed too often or not often enough. In quality assurance chart reviews, questions of timing, frequency, or indication for the procedure were rarely asked. Perhaps the provider performing a procedure was not the most appropriate; could it have been completed more cost effectively by a health care provider from another discipline?

Although quality assurance had for several decades provided the focus for improving the care given to patients, a new approach to quality—using processes of continuous improvement rather than achieving predetermined standards—began to stir the corporate health care environment in the early 1990s. This approach to quality was initially known as **total quality management** (TQM); however, the lasting moniker is **continuous quality improvement** (CQI).

THE TRANSITION TO TOTAL QUALITY MANAGEMENT AND CONTINUOUS QUALITY IMPROVEMENT

The first wave of change in the quality movement in health care was TQM, described as a "structured, systematic process for creating organization-wide participation in planning and implementing continuous improvement in quality" (Whetsell, 1990, p. 16). Its origins date back to the 1930s, when Dr. W. Edwards Deming, a graduate from Yale University and consultant in statistical studies, put forward his theory of continuous improvement to Western Electric Laboratories (later AT&T Bell Laboratories) and other US industries. Deming became the "father of quality improvement" because he believed that problems with, and therefore opportunities to improve, quality were built into complex production processes and that defects in quality could rarely be attributed to the people involved with the process. Problems were generally caused not by poor motivation or effort but rather by job design. In his theory of continuous improvement, Deming (1986) advocated for a strong, long-term commitment by management, including the need for clearly defined mission and vision statements. He believed quality should be the central focus of the organization and that emphasis needed to shift from inspection to prevention. Preventing defects and improving processes so that defects do not occur are the goals toward which all organizations should strive. Establishing long-term relationships with suppliers was more important than accepting the lowest bid. Deming believed that training and retraining employees was critical to organizational success and that management's role was to coach employees. Finally, he believed that reducing variability in processes would ultimately lead to sustained process improvements.

Dr. Deming's nomenclature of CQI continues today. His work with improving processes and the Japanese acceptance of the plan–do–check–act plan (also known as the Deming cycle) was a major success for manufacturing processes in Japan (Johnson, 2002). Lean quality improvement is the adoption of the Toyota Production System that has demonstrated success in manufacturing and increasingly in health care settings (Miller, 2016; Moraros, Lemstra & Nwankwo, 2016; Toussaint & Berry, 2013).

In the 1980s, both Canadian and American health care agencies began to face significant pressures, previously experienced in industry, to improve the quality of services while reducing steadily increasing costs. Quality assurance programs in hospitals were not providing the foundation on which to make the significant changes thought to be necessary. Further, the culture of quality, so much a part of the fabric of successful industries, was not identifiable in the health care industry. The successes that industries made in improving quality and reducing costs caught the attention of hospital managers. Could the quality improvement principles proven to be successful in industry have application in hospitals? Many were skeptical that any relationships could be found between manufacturing products and the highly complex, people-focused hospital milieu.

Donald Berwick (Berwick, Godfrey, & Roessner, 1990), professor of pediatrics at Harvard Medical School and pediatrician with the Harvard Community Health Plan, and colleagues disagreed with this view. In 1987, he launched the National Demonstration Project on Quality Improvement in Health Care, an exploratory study designed to answer the question, "Can the tools of modern quality improvement, with which industries have achieved breakthroughs in performance, improve health care?" This landmark study, described in the book *Curing Health Care* (Berwick, Godfrey, & Roessner, 1990), documented the efforts of 21 health care organizations—paired with an equal number of industrial quality management experts—that used quality management principles to implement hospital-based pilot projects.

During the 8-month demonstration study, 17 hospitals completed projects that improved processes such as transport of critically ill neonates, use of portable X-ray machines, appointment waiting times, patient discharge, and hiring of nurses. At least 15 projects were considered successful, leading to several discoveries. These pioneer teams found that quality improvement methods and tools were applicable to health care; cross-functional teams were valuable in improving health care processes; data useful for quality improvement abounded; and poor quality correlated with high cost.

Involving physicians in the quality improvement process was difficult but essential, and quality transformation was dependent on leadership. This work was the first documented evidence that quality management principles initially implemented in industry could be applied to hospital processes. Many hospitals have continued to make profound changes, providing a model for successful implementation of a quality improvement philosophy in Canadian hospitals.

In Canada and the United States, lean quality improvement spread through health care systems starting in the late 1990s and today is widely used as a quality improvement methodology. The Saskatchewan Health Authority was the largest implementation of lean quality improvement in Canada (Saskatchewan Health Quality Council, 2013). The Health Authority initiative was promoted to improve health care by reducing errors, to improve patient satisfaction, and to trim costs while improving outcomes of care. The difference with using a lean quality improvement approach is the focus on the flow of the work, the involvement of the people who do the work to design change, and the focus on objective data to quantify the problem and the results. Although results from projects are promising, research is required to study quality improvement projects and evaluate the outcomes achieved (Moraros, Lemstra, & Nwankwo, 2016).

EVOLUTION OF NURSING-SENSITIVE INDICATORS

Nursing classification systems and computerization have influenced the evolution of nursing measurement and indicator development. Nursing as a profession has struggled to describe its unique contribution to care in comparison to other health professions. One of the major challenges in nursing was the absence of a common nursing language to classify and quantify nursing work.

Nursing classification systems are a precursor to indicator development because a common language is needed to describe observations and action. Effective measurement of outcomes is dependent on standard definitions and data collection practices (Doran, Mildon, & Clarke, 2011). Once a common language is available, indicators of quality can be determined through common methods of defining the indicators, collecting the data, and reporting the data. Nursing diagnoses provide a standard way to describe and document the diagnoses that registered nurses make. Two widely known classification systems are the North American Nursing Diagnosis Association (NANDA) system and the National Information Classification (NIC) system. NANDA has 13 domains, 476 classes, and 172 diagnoses, while NIC has 7 domains, 30 classes, and 514 interventions (Popoola, Wahl, Dupont et al., 2008). The research team that developed NIC was from the University of Iowa. NIC and NANDA were developed in the United States because the country was promoting university education and also because of how the United States finances health care.

A plethora of nursing-sensitive indicators were developed from the late 1970s onward as interest in nursing indicators increased. A knowledge synthesis was undertaken in Canada to understand what was known within Canada and internationally. This synthesis included the development of a set of nursing-sensitive indicators that could help the profession measure the outcomes of the care nurses provide (Doran, Mildon, & Clarke, 2011). The CNA began to work on a nursing minimum data set, and by 1997 consensus was achieved on five care elements: patient/client status, nursing care interventions, patient/client outcomes, primary nurse identifier, and nursing care intensity (Hannah & White, 2012). Promising work on quality measurement specific to nursing is occurring in terms of comparative data, benchmarking, and measurement across the continuum of care. Work on establishing scorecards in nursing and nursing-specific indicators is emerging and will help the nursing field to quantify the quality of care and the unique contribution of nursing (Jeffs, Doran, VanDeVelde-Coke et al., 2015).

Research has demonstrated the importance of evidenced-informed practice on the outcomes of clinical care. Numerous studies on the Registered Nurses' Association of Ontario (RNAO) **best practice guidelines** (BPGs) have demonstrated improvement in outcomes. Examples include a 20% reduction in fall rates in an Ontario hospital study using the prevention of falls BPG, and improved wound outcomes in Ontario and Saskatchewan when a wound care BPG was implemented (VanDeVelde-Coke, Doran, Grinspun et al., 2012). To ensure that outcome measurement of BPG usage occurs, the RNAO developed the NQuIRE database to collect appropriate data and work within the International Classification of Nursing Practice systems to design methods to collect the data systematically.

Although progress is being made, measurement and indicator use in nursing is still lagging in many health care organizations. Three major initiatives in Canada are providing leadership to advance effective measurement for nursing practice to enable better patient outcomes. The Canadian National Nursing Quality Report (NNQR(C)) team, Canadian Health Outcomes for Better Information and Care (C-HOBIC), and Nursing Quality Indicators for Reporting and Evaluation (NQuIRE) are working together and leading the way to ensure effective outcome measurement of the quality of care. These three initiatives are informing nursing how to continuously improve quality using standard nursing-sensitive indicators for outcome evaluation (VanDeVelde-Coke, Doran, Grinspun et al. 2012).

CASE STUDY

Engaging Patients and Families in Quality Improvement

An example of patient–family engagement is the Ontario home and community care system run through the Local Health Integration Networks (LHIN). The LHIN arranges care coordination services and contracts out nursing and home support services to providers. The LHIN contacts a third-party agency to conduct a survey of a sample of patients and their families, and they use a valid and reliable patient experience instrument. These results are posted annually on the public Health Quality Ontario website.

Source: Health Quality Ontario. (n.d.). *Home care performance in Ontario.* Retrieved from https://www.hqontario.ca/System-Performance/Home-Care-Performance.

Patient Satisfaction and Patient Experience Indicators

Patient satisfaction is a simple concept that is difficult to define and measure. The development and use of valid and reliable instruments is an ongoing process in the nursing profession. Patient satisfaction is an important quality indicator that is being used more widely in nursing management. Researchers are developing common instruments to measure patient satisfaction, and the research is finding valid instruments to measure nursing care satisfaction (Laschinger, Gilbert, & Smith, 2011).

A surgical medical centre in a Midwestern hospital in the United States instituted a relationship-based care model to improve the quality of nursing care and care outcomes. The centre first conducted a thorough literature review and based their care model on previous studies where intentional actions to improve the relationship with patients had improved care outcomes (Woolley, Perkins, Laird et al., 2012). The intervention involved the education of all staff, whiteboard communication, and hourly rounding with patients as well as team meetings to review indicators (Woolley, Perkins, Laird et al., 2012). Rounding on patient units was found to increase patient satisfaction and improve pain control. The study was evaluated using the Hospital Consumer Assessment of Healthcare Providers and Systems, and all indicators were progressing in a positive direction after the intervention.

The American Nurses Association (1995), as cited in Laschinger, Gilbert, and Smith (2011), identified patient satisfaction with care as a nurse-sensitive indicator of importance. With the emergence of public reporting and the inclusion of patient satisfaction data in all reporting, it is clear that nursing must pay particular attention to this indicator. Although the definition of patient satisfaction varies, the concept is that the patient is satisfied with the care experience they received. It can be argued that patients do not have adequate knowledge to accurately assess the quality of the care they received, so any rating has more to do with their perceptions of the quality of care and with the interpersonal approaches used in the delivery of the care. Laschinger, Gilbert, and Smith (2011) found that the key components of patient satisfaction with nursing care involve effective support from nursing staff, access to health information, control over decisions, and competence of the professionals caring for the patient.

The concept of patient experience as more robust than patient satisfaction is emerging. Patient satisfaction is increasingly seen as an inadequate way to assess the quality of service. Often satisfaction simply indicates that the patient is not dissatisfied, but it does not provide information on what the experience of the patient was. A recent study questions the lagging nature of patient satisfaction surveys and the usefulness of the data for that reason. Immediate feedback from patients may be more useful in changing nursing practice than the annual results that are the current norm (Thornton et al., 2017). Patient experience surveys are meant to help organizations understand whether the patient felt safe, whether the patient felt involved as a partner in their care planning, and whether they felt they were treated with dignity and compassion. More specific questions can allow organizations to take actions to improve the experience of the patient (Shale, 2013).

KEY CONCEPTS OF CONTINUOUS QUALITY IMPROVEMENT

A number of key concepts are central to the CQI approach and reflect a significant shift in thinking away from quality assurance. Successful implementation in industry and health care have guided the development of these concepts (Walton, 1986; McLaughlin & Kaluzny, 1990; Thompson, 1991; Harrigan, 2000; Moraros, Lemstra, & Nwankwo, 2016).

Processes of Health Care and Health Care Delivery

CQI focuses on key processes rather than individual people. This approach is based on the premise that 85% of problems encountered in organizations result from cumbersome or poorly defined processes. Problems are attributable to staff performance only 15% of the time. Health care processes are complex and cross traditional departmental and disciplinary boundaries (Miller, 2016).

Most processes flow across the organization and between departments rather than up and down the hierarchy. Therefore, quality teams are made up of people who are most knowledgeable about the process. The team leader could be anyone in the organization who is knowledgeable about the process under review and who has demonstrated group leadership skills, knowledge of the quality improvement process, and skill in using quality tools. Only after a process is carefully analyzed to determine what it entails can changes be made to improve it. Staff are dedicated to providing high-quality care; it is the process itself that requires improvement.

Customer Focus

A customer is anyone who receives or is affected by a product or a process. Therefore, patients, families, hospital visitors, hospital employees, physicians, volunteers, and suppliers are all viewed as customers of particular processes. In fact, service providers often have other service providers as their customers, and internal providers may also serve groups that are external to the organization (Toussaint & Berry, 2013). In this way, everyone within the organization is serving a customer and often is a customer.

Continuous Monitoring of Quality

Meeting and exceeding the needs of patients and staff is a priority goal and involves not only an evaluation of current services but expectations and ideas for improvement. These expectations and requirements are data driven. Decisions are made based on facts and data, not opinions. Quality improvement tools and techniques are used by teams to create a systematic approach to problem analysis, resolution, and evaluation. The process of improvement adapted by the organization provides a consistent proactive approach to problem solving that is used by all teams. Approximately 50% to 70% of the time spent on a quality improvement process is focused on collecting and analyzing data (Miller, 2016). Team members frequently report that data analysis revealed information about root causes that differed from commonly held opinion.

Quality improvement is a continuous cycle of improving processes before errors are made or complaints are received. Doing the right thing right the first time and all the time is considered much more cost effective than redoing work. Responsibility for improving processes rests with those directly involved in the process. CQI involves more than improving one process at a time or in one moment in time. It is an ongoing initiative for continuous improvement of all care processes and services within the organization. There is no point at which a final solution is achieved. The central tenet of CQI is that there is always room for further improvement.

Education and Learning

Everyone in the organization is involved in CQI. Working within the guidelines and boundaries established by managers, staff are empowered by receiving information, resources, and authority to improve work processes that will benefit patients and themselves. Problem resolution occurs as close to the work or point-of-care delivery as possible in the organization, where staff has the greatest knowledge about potential causes and solutions. Staff education and training at all organizational levels is central to a motivated and contributing workforce. Education programs include an awareness of CQI principles, steps in quality improvement, use of quality improvement tools, just-in-time training, and teamwork skills. Staff are expected to embrace quality improvement as part of their everyday work rather than viewing it as an added responsibility. It is a way of individual as well as corporate thinking and managing, rather than a task to be completed and checked off a list.

Long-Term Commitment

The process of cultural transformation is a long-term commitment that may take 5 to 10 years in most hospitals or health care organizations. Even with a 5-year implementation plan, results will depend on a variety of factors, including resources, dedication, organizational stability, organizational priority setting, and commitment by staff and physicians. Knowledge translation is the spread of new research knowledge and is based on a paradigm of organization as machines. Research has found that knowledge translation alone is insufficient to transform organizational culture and that coupling knowledge translation with stakeholder engagement, **change management** approaches, and expert facilitation creates greater uptake of new knowledge (Kitson, 2008).

THE PROCESS OF CONTINUOUS QUALITY IMPROVEMENT

The following steps in the quality improvement process are generic and reflect a basic scientific approach:
1. Select and define a problem.
2. Organize a knowledgeable team.
3. Gather data to identify the root causes of the problem.
4. Implement a plan of action based on the data analysis.
5. Continuously monitor results.

Two more formalized methods are now being widely used to standardize the process of improvement. The first shows the sequence of steps designed by Juran (1989), a student of Deming. This model conceptualizes the process as a journey having four phases: project definition and organization, a diagnostic journey, a remedial journey, and holding the gains.

A second commonly used model involves a nine-step method called FOCUS-PDCA (James, 1989; Figure 12.1):
- *Find a process to improve.*
- *Organize a team familiar with the process.*
- *Clarify current knowledge of the process.*
- *Understand sources of variation.*
- *Select the process improvement.*
- *Plan a change.*
- *Do—carry out the change.*
- *Check and observe the effects of the change. (Also referred to as the "study" step.)*
- *Act, adapt, or modify the plan* (p. 33).

These two methods, and others less commonly used, are cyclical. As a process is improved, the cycle begins again, either to achieve a new level of performance or to address a new quality improvement opportunity. The goal

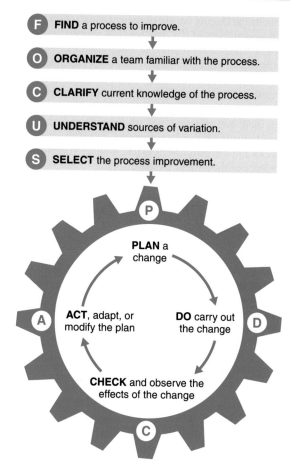

Fig. 12.1 FOCUS-PDCA is a management method used to improve processes in health care.

is prevention, not detection, of errors through continuous improvement.

RESEARCH FOCUS

A recent study using the FOCUS-PDSA cycle and lean continuous improvement was successful in improving team-based rounding in a hospital. The team developed, executed, and evaluated an interprofessional teamwork model. The team evaluation reported increased communication and time savings and reduced 30-day readmissions to hospital. There was no effect on emergency department same-day visits.

Source: Li, J., Talari, P., Kelly, A., et al. (2018). Interprofessional Teamwork Innovation Model (ITIM) to promote communication and patient-centred, coordinated care. *BMJ Quality & Safety, 27*(9), 700–709. https://doi.org/10.1136/bmjqs-2017-007369.

THE TOOLS OF QUALITY IMPROVEMENT

Several tools can be used to identify and analyze work processes and data pertinent to the problem a team is working on (Plsek, 1990; Miller, 2016). These quality tools and other techniques have gradually replaced routine auditing associated with quality assurance programs (Figure 12.2). Some examples include:

- A process map (also known as a flow chart or value stream map) provides a pictorial representation of the steps in a process, how they relate to each other, and where there are opportunities to reduce steps, increase flow, and so on. For example, mapping the process of patient admission provides common understanding for team members and is usually enlightening. This creates awareness in the whole team of the current state to enable mapping a future state that improves patient flow.
- A check sheet is a form that shows the frequency of events and is particularly useful in showing patterns and translating opinions into facts. Recording the number of times equipment is unavailable or broken provides factual data.
- A Pareto chart uses data derived from a check sheet that shows the frequency of occurrence. Using data, the Pareto (or 20/80) rule is applied, which states that 20% of issues account for 80% of occurrences. If a team is studying reasons for delays in patient transport to radiology, a check sheet will identify the factors contributing to delays, and a Pareto chart will determine the specific factors that cause delays 80% of the time.
- A cause-and-effect (or fish-bone) diagram is used to record contributing causes of a problem—for example, methods, materials, people, or equipment. A check sheet and Pareto chart are then used to determine the "vital few" that require improvement.
- A histogram is a bar graph that displays the distribution of data within a category. If a team were studying the response time of the hospital's pharmacy to a narcotic order, this instrument would show the frequency with which the response time fell within a time interval.
- A run chart is used to display data over time, such as the length of time a nonemergent patient waits to see a triage or other nurse in an emergency department.
- A scatter diagram is used to plot two variables to determine whether a correlation exists. For example, the number of patient days per month could be plotted with the number of nursing hours to see whether staffing is efficient.
- A plan–do–study–act (PDSA) chart (also known as the Deming cycle) is appropriate for simpler projects that are within one department. The "plan" section describes the problem and what data were used to identify it; the "do" section sets out a plan of action; the "study" (or "check") section outlines how to evaluate the data; and the "act" section discusses what modifications should be made and plans for the next test.
- A-3 is for improvement projects that cross departments and require coordination. The A-3 (so named because it was originally printed on large 14 × 17 paper) describes the project in summary so that everyone can understand what problem is being solved, what the goals are, how the team will measure success, who the team members are, and what the milestones are.

QUALITY IMPROVEMENT INDICATORS

Accreditation Canada's Qmentum program has updated standards that measure patient safety and patient–family engagement as a priority. The Qmentum program also evaluates the organization as a whole in terms of the systems and processes necessary to achieve CQI. Accreditation Canada has online survey measurement tools for patient safety culture, worklife pulse, and board governance for organizations to have staff complete before their accreditation (Accreditation Canada, 2019). Health care agencies are now monitoring quality indicators such as wait times for emergency care, cancer surgery, preoperative deaths, readmissions, and others.

The quality improvement movement originated in times of recession and reform that necessitated deep cuts in health and social service spending with resultant major shifts in roles and functions of all health team members. The move of care from the acute setting to the community was also a factor influencing the continuing development of quality improvement programs. With regionalization of health care authorities from many independent hospital boards, the quality indicators being measured shifted from health care delivery indicators to include more general population health indicators. Accreditation Canada's Qmentum Program evaluates the three main categories of standards: system-wide areas, population-based aspects, and service excellence components of health care organizations (Accreditation Canada 2019). Overall, the Qmentum accreditation program "emphasizes health system performance, risk prevention planning, patient safety, performance measurement, and governance" (Accreditation Canada, 2019).

HEALTH REFORM

Health reform and the restructuring of health care delivery systems have had a significant impact on the ability of health care agencies to provide quality care in a consistent

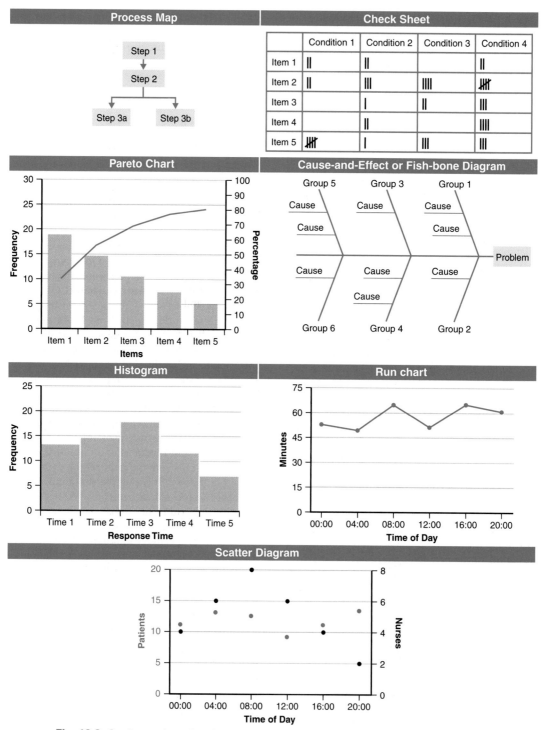

Fig. 12.2 Quality tools and techniques associated with quality assurance programs.

and seamless fashion (Cummings & Estabrooks, 2003; Hetherington, 1998). The 1990s were times of rapid and unprecedented change in health care. All structures, functions, roles, and expectations that defined delivery and consumption of health care services were challenged. Traditional hierarchical models were reconfigured, and functions historically organized by department (such as nursing, medicine, pharmacy, and laboratory) were redefined to flatter structures with less hierarchy and to interdisciplinary models of organization.

Management literature is clear that structural changes alone will not lead to lasting organizational quality changes. Structural changes must be supported by modifications in roles, relationships, attitudes, and resource allocation. Concepts such as cross-functional teams, seamless organizations, clinical treatment teams, functional work groups, empowerment, coaching, and CQI are central to the paradigm shift from traditional management processes to a system-wide quality improvement philosophy. Transformational leadership within health care can mitigate the external forces of change, leading to opportunities to improve organizations and services, as well as improve outcomes for patients (Cummings, Hayduk, & Estabrooks, 2005; Foubert, 2014; Goodwin & Miller, 2014; Wong & Cummings, 2007).

In 1998, the International Study of Hospital Organization and Staffing on Patient Outcomes was launched in Canada, the United Kingdom, Scotland, Germany, and the United States to analyze the impact of the restructuring of health care on quality of care, availability of professional nurse staffing, and patient outcomes, including complication rates and mortality. Numerous reports have shown relationships between lower patient mortality and more hours of nurse staffing, a richer nurse skill mix, nurse education, and physician–nurse relationships (Aiken, Clarke, Sloane et al., 2002; Estabrooks, Midodzi, Cummings et al., 2005; Manojlovich & Laschinger, 2007).

Since the mid-2000s, one movement in health reform has focused on the patient and their family in their health care journey, known as patient-centered care. Health care was traditionally a model where the expert practitioner provides advice and care to the patient. As societal expectations began to change, so did health care begin to accept change. As a result of this societal and health cultural shift, people are now able to find health information online, newer generations are less deferential to authority and want control over health care decisions, and a customer-service orientation is an expectation. The addition of standards for accreditation that assess the involvement of patients and families in care delivery and design of systems is targeting that change in societal expectations (Accreditation Canada, 2019).

Patient Safety Movement

Another recent phenomenon in the international media is the focus on the epidemic of patient injury caused by health care (Wilson, 2001). The Canadian Adverse Events Study (Baker, Norton, Flintoff et al., 2004) followed on the heels of the US Institute of Medicine's (IOM) seminal report *To Err Is Human: Building a Safer Health System* (Institute of Medicine [IOM], 2000) and the *Quality in Australian Health Care Study* (Wilson, 1995). In Canada, 1 in 13 adult patients admitted to acute-care hospitals in fiscal year 2000 experienced adverse events, sparking renewed interest in patient safety (Baker, Norton, Flintoff et al., 2004). A 7.5% incidence rate for adverse events, of which 36.9% were highly preventable, accounted for 1.1 million additional hospital days. Patient safety continues to be a major concern for health care consumers and providers while, at the same time, hospitals struggle with declining revenues and climbing costs.

In a follow-up to the *To Err Is Human* report, the IOM pointed to the critical role nursing plays in providing safe care and identified health care management practices necessary to create a positive patient safety culture (IOM, 2004). Identified practices included creating and maintaining trust throughout the organization, deploying health care workers in adequate numbers, creating a culture of openness regarding reporting and prevention of errors, involving workers in decision making pertaining to work design and work flow, and actively managing the process of change (IOM, 2004). The report specifically targeted the salient role of strong nursing leadership to implement effective management practices that create "cultures of safety" (IOM, 2004, p. 253) and improve patient outcomes. The Canadian safety report also profiled the need for safer patient care environments and echoed the call for leadership to make the required changes (Baker, Norton, Flintoff et al., 2004). The IOM emphasized that quality of patient care is directly affected by the degree to which hospital nurses are active and empowered participants in decisions about their patients' plans of care and by the degree to which they have an active and central role in organizational decision making (IOM, 2004).

In 2002, the National Steering Committee on Patient Safety reported 19 recommendations for a comprehensive and integrated national strategy to make patient safety a national priority for the Canadian health care system (National Steering Committee on Patient Safety [NSCPS], 2002). One recommendation included the establishment of the CPSI in 2005 with a mission to provide leadership on patient safety issues by advising governments, stakeholders, and the public on effective strategies; fostering information sharing; influencing culture change; supporting systems change; and collaborating with stakeholders in an ongoing dialogue on patient safety (NSCPS, 2002). In addition to producing original resources, the CPSI provides peer-reviewed and annotated links to externally developed tools, articles, and other resources, and they link with key health care organizations and other groups involved in patient safety. The CPSI played a critical role working with Accreditation Canada to embed patient safety standards into the Canadian accreditation process. Accreditation Canada now ensures patient safety standards are being followed by health care organizations. The nursing profession plays a role in advocating for safe care systems for patients. The CNA (2019) describes advocacy as working with others to mobilize change in policy and practice and to speak out against inequality and inequity.

NURSING-SENSITIVE OUTCOMES AND BEST PRACTICE GUIDELINES

The majority of care to patients in most health sectors is delivered by nurses, but insufficient information about the influence of nursing care is documented in administrative databases (Pringle & Doran, 2003). With the increasing imperative for professional and financial accountability in health care, we need health databases and electronic health record systems to be more pertinent to nursing practice so that better information about the contributions of nurses is collected at the point of care.

Recent efforts by professional and regulatory groups in both the United States and Canada have recommended that health databases be expanded beyond mortality and morbidity (clinical complications) to include nurse-sensitive outcomes to measure the quality of nursing care. The American Nurses Association (2000) included patient satisfaction with pain management and patient education in the *Nursing Care Report Card for Acute Care*. The Ministry of Health and Long-Term Care of Ontario and its Expert Panel on Nursing and Health Outcomes recommended including functional status, symptom control, therapeutic self-care, pressure ulcers, and falls in Ontario administrative databases (Pringle & White, 2002). **Nursing-sensitive outcomes** are those that are relevant, based on nurses' domain and scope of practice, and linked to nursing inputs and interventions by empirical evidence (Doran, 2003).

In a feasibility study conducted with 890 patients from acute-care hospitals and long-term care facilities, Doran, Harrison, Laschinger et al. (2006) demonstrated that the outcomes tools, functional status, symptom (pain, nausea, dyspnea, fatigue) severity and frequency, and therapeutic self-care used were sensitive to change in patient condition and that select nursing interventions were related to these outcomes. These findings suggest that it is possible to collect data on nursing-sensitive patient outcomes in a reliable and valid way and to integrate these data collection into routine and daily nursing assessment and documentation.

Inclusion of nursing-sensitive outcomes in health system monitoring is still in its early stages but much progress has been made in the last 10 years. The Canadian National Nursing Quality Report (NNQR(C)) team established an initial set of process, structure, and outcomes indicators for nursing through a modified Delphi study of nursing experts. The group then selected standardized definitions for the indicators chosen through a collaboration between NNQR(C), C-HOBIC, and NQuIRE. The indicators were pilot tested by eight health care organizations from the acute, long-term care and mental health sectors. A subsequent phase of additional testing is currently underway, and the group is working with the Canadian Institute for Health Information (CIHI) to ensure that these indicators become part of the pan-Canadian database that CIHI manages (VanDeVelde-Coke, Doran, & Jeffs, 2015).

An associated domain of outcomes measurement is the use of evidence-informed BPGs as support to nurse decision making in the delivery of quality nursing care. BPGs are systematically developed statements based on the best available evidence to assist clinician and patient decision making about appropriate health care for specific clinical circumstances (Field & Lohr, 1990; Siering, Eikermann, Hausner et al., 2013). The implementation of evidence-informed BPGs contributes to improved care outcomes. In Ontario, the RNAO has developed, piloted, evaluated, disseminated, and supported the uptake of nursing BPGs since 1999 (Virani & Grinspun, 2007). The BPG program is funded by Ontario's Ministry of Health and Long-Term Care. There are now more than 55 BPGs grouped into streams such as foundational, clinical, mental health, and healthy workplace environments. There are also individual BPGs on topics such as asthma; breastfeeding; diabetic foot complications; delirium, dementia, and depression; smoking cessation; venous leg ulcers; and substance misuse.

The RNAO attributes the success of the BPG program to four key factors: intense grassroots engagement in BPG guideline development, dissemination, and uptake; comprehensive recommendations; government funding support; and strong staff leadership and expertise (Virani & Grinspun, 2007). The rationale behind the BPG project is that nurses are knowledge professionals whose practice must be based on the most valid and reliable evidence. This is essential to achieve best health and clinical outcomes for patients and positive organizational results. See the Canadian Research Focus box for an example of research that has evolved from the RNAO's work on BPGs and how BPGs can be examined to inform quality improvement processes. A number of studies on the RNAO BPGs have demonstrated improvement in outcomes (VanDeVelde-Coke, Doran, Grinspun et al., 2012). The combined leadership of the NNQR(C), HOBIC, and NQuIRE to standardize the indicators used in nursing will increase comparability within organizations and across the health care continuum. In addition, these advances will enable better planning for improved health outcomes when the unique contribution of nursing is quantified for decision makers.

APPLYING CONTENT KNOWLEDGE

1. How is quality improvement and assurance actualized in your setting and how can you participate in ensuring the care provided to patients and their families fosters positive outcomes?
2. How do individual-level actions for improving patient care enhance the overall efforts of CQI?

RESEARCH FOCUS

A National Nursing Data Standards symposium was held in April 2016 in Toronto, Ontario, with 60 nurse leaders (by invitation), student scribes and vendor representatives. "Symposium participants focused on developing the beginnings of a national strategy to promote the adoption of a core set of nursing data standards" (Nagle & White, 2016, p. 6). This work builds on the efforts described earlier in the chapter; the CNA facilitated consensus on a nursing minimum data set on five care elements: patient/client status, nursing care interventions, patient/client outcomes, primary nurse identifier; and nursing care intensity (Hannah & White, 2012). Because nursing is the largest health profession, they are major users and contributors of clinical data. With the movement toward the usage of electronic health records in Canada, the time is right for the nursing profession to unite in promoting a coherent and comprehensive data strategy in support of the measurement of nursing-sensitive outcomes. This adoption of a core set of nursing data standards will inform further research and improvement in nursing care, contribute to health policy, strengthen patient safety, and improve outcomes of care.

Sources: Nagle, L., & White, P. (Eds.). (2016). *Proceedings from the National Nursing Data Standards Symposium*. Toronto, ON: Canadian Nurses Association. Retrieved from https://www.cna-aiic.ca/en/~/media/cna/page-content/pdf-en/national-nursing-data-standards-symposium-proceedings-report; Hannah, K., & White, P. (2012). C-HOBIC: Standardized clinical outcomes to support evidence-informed nursing care. *Canadian Journal of Nursing Leadership, 25*(1), 43–46.

FUTURE DIRECTIONS TO ENSURE QUALITY OF CARE

Accreditation Canada and the Qmentum accreditation program are currently committed to playing a major role in improving patient safety through accreditation. The accreditation process is a way of identifying conditions of unsafe practice and supporting health care organizations to promote safe care. When Qmentum standards are met, the potential for adverse events occurring within health care and service organizations is reduced. Consequently, the Qmentum accreditation program has made patient safety an essential element, reinforcing that health service cannot be of high quality unless it is safe. Accreditation Canada added client- and family-centered care (CFCC) in 2017 as a major focus of accreditation. The new standards associated with CFCC set the expectation that clients and families should be involved in mutually planning their care and that all health care organizations should include patient representatives to make major changes, to set strategy, and to participate at many levels in organizations (Accreditation Canada, 2019).

Nursing has directed and will continue to direct quality monitoring of nursing care, thus ensuring that professional standards are maintained for individual nurses. Quality-monitoring instruments, which have underpinned nursing quality assurance programs, continue to be used to monitor standards of nursing practice; however, the audit process is being replaced by new methodologies associated with a CQI philosophy, the ongoing measurement of nursing-sensitive outcomes, and the implementation of nursing BPGs. As more consistent data standards are implemented and electronic health records become the norm for patient records, the outcomes of care will become more evident. CQI and lean methods will provide the tools for nurses to evaluate and improve practice. By using BPGs that become embedded in our electronic systems, best practice information will be available at clinicians' fingertips.

Many factors determine successful CQI, all of which must be addressed by leaders in the organization. The way forward through all the significant quality issues addressed in this chapter is to place patients or clients and their needs at the centre. Then, by using the best available evidence to determine required care processes, measurement to inform and direct the processes, an organizational rather than an individualized approach, and the application of process-change management, a culture of CQI will result in improved outcomes. These improvements are based on a true cultural transformation; a well-developed quality strategy; ongoing educational programs available to all staff regardless of level in the organization; well-prepared team leaders; empowerment of frontline staff; and a quality improvement council charged with prioritizing quality issues, developing policy, and identifying a process for the identification of projects and teams.

The shift from quality assurance programs to a system-wide quality improvement philosophy has shown promising results in the pursuit of cost-effective quality care. Nurses have been at the forefront in developing and monitoring standards of practice that have provided the foundation for the future. Efforts by the nursing profession to improve patient care and public accountability by refining and enhancing quality processes will continue to be instrumental in the ongoing redesign of health care. Quality improvement and patient safety cultures are interdisciplinary, interdependent approaches to managing our health care system, for which comprehensive and integrated data

need to be a driver. These data and commitment at all levels of the health care system will ensure a cyclical and continual improvement to quality of care regardless of internal and external challenges.

> ### 👤 APPLYING CONTENT KNOWLEDGE
>
> 1. What might quality improvement within nursing look like in the future?
> 2. What working groups are in place to study and/or investigate issues related to quality improvement in Canada?
> 3. How do you envision using best practice guidelines in your nursing practice?

SUMMARY OF LEARNING OBJECTIVES

- The development of quality assurance started in the 1950s in response to the need to ensure quality of care. Over time, the health system evolved, and it became obvious that quality assurance had deficiencies.
- CQI approaches have evolved over the last 20 or more years into systematic, organization-wide approaches to embed improvement into the daily work of all health care providers and are demonstrating positive results.
- Lean quality management is an emerging, systematic approach to CQI with a focus on using process maps, PDSA cycles, and A3s, for example.
- Patient safety issues were discovered in two sentinel studies (one in Canada and one in the United States),

and the patient safety movement emerged. Accreditation standards now have standards that contribute to safer patient care, and health care organizations are required to be compliant.
- Evidence-informed practice has been recognized as the basis for excellent outcomes in care delivery, and much effort has been expended to develop BPGs that ensure this evidence is available in a format clinicians can easily access and use.
- In the last 10 to 15 years, patient and family engagement has been recognized as another important way to improve care. This approach is being embraced by health care organizations and promoted by Accreditation Canada.

CRITICAL THINKING QUESTIONS

1. A nurse has been appointed to participate on a committee to reduce the number of families without access to adequate respite care in the community. What tools or processes should the nurse suggest to help explore and improve the issue?
2. How does the concept of CQI differ from quality assurance?
3. Why is it important for health care databases to include information about nursing interventions and nursing-sensitive outcomes?

4. What are some ways in which a nurse in any clinical setting can make patient safety improvement and error reduction not just an organizational priority but a personal one in their everyday practice?
5. How can nurses demonstrate effective leadership related to quality improvement?

REFERENCES

Accreditation Canada. (2019). *Qmentum accreditation program.* Retrieved from https://accreditation.ca/accreditation/qmentum/.

Accreditation Canada. (2019). *Our history.* Retrieved from https://accreditation.ca/intl-en/about/our-history/.

Aiken, L. H., Clarke, S. P., Sloane, D. M., et al. (2002). Hospital nurse staffing and patient mortality, nurse burnout, and job dissatisfaction. *Journal of the American Medical Association, 288*(16), 1987–1993.

Alexander, J. A., & Hearld, L. R. (2009). Review: What can we learn from quality improvement research? A critical review of research methods. *Medical Care Research and Review, 66*, 235.

American Nurses Association. (2000). *Nurse staffing and patient outcomes in the inpatient hospital setting: Report*. Washington, D.C.: Author.

Baker, G. R., Norton, P. G., Flintoff, V., et al. (2004). The Canadian Adverse Events Study: The incidence of adverse events among hospital patients in Canada. *Canadian Medical Association Journal, 170*(10), 1678–1686.

Berwick, D., Godfrey, A. B., & Roessner, J. (1990). *Curing health care: New strategies for quality improvement*. San Francisco, CA: Jossey-Bass.

Canadian Nurses Association. (2019). *Policy and advocacy*. Retrieved from https://www.cna-aiic.ca/en/policy-advocacy.

Canadian Patient Safety Institute. (2017). *Module 1: Systems thinking: Moving beyond blame to safety*. Retrieved from https://www.patientsafetyinstitute.ca/en/education/PatientSafetyEducationProgram/PatientSafetyEducationCurriculum/Pages/Module-1-Systems-Thinking.aspx.

Cummings, G., & Estabrooks, C. A. (2003). The effects of hospital restructuring that included layoffs on individual nurses who remained employed: A systematic review of impact. *International Journal of Sociology and Social Policy, 8–9*, 8–53.

Cummings, G. G., Hayduk, L., & Estabrooks, C. A. (2005). Mitigating the impact of hospital restructuring on nurses: The responsibility of emotionally intelligent leadership. *Nursing Research, 54*(1), 2–12. Retrieved from https://www.ncbi.nlm.nih.gov/pubmed/15695934.

Darr, K. (1999). Nexus: Risk management and quality improvement: Together at last—Part 1. *Hospital Topics, 77*(1), 27–32. https://doi.org/10.1080/00185869909596516.

Deming, W. E. (1986). *Out of crisis*. Cambridge, MA: MIT Press.

Donabedian, A. (1980). *Explorations in quality assessment and monitoring* (Vol. 1). Ann Arbor, MI: Health Administration Press.

Donabedian, A. (2003). *An introduction to quality assurance in health care*. New York, NY: Oxford University Press.

Doran, D. (Ed.). (2003). *Nursing sensitive outcomes: The state of the science*. Boston, MA: Jones and Bartlett Publishers.

Doran, D. M., & Pringle, D. (2011). Patient outcomes as an accountability. In D. M. Doran (Ed.), *Nursing outcomes: The state of the science* (2nd ed., pp. 1–28). Sudbury, MA: Jones and Bartlett.

Doran, D. M., Harrison, M. B., Laschinger, H. S., et al. (2006). Nursing-sensitive outcomes data collection in acute care and long-term care settings. *Nursing Research, 55*(2S), S75–S81.

Doran, D., Mildon, B., & Clarke, S. (2011). *Toward a national report card in nursing: A7 knowledge synthesis*. Toronto, ON: Nursing Health Services Research Unit.

Estabrooks, C. A., Midodzi, W. K., Cummings, G. G., et al. (2005). Determining the impact of hospital nursing characteristics on 30-day mortality among patients in Alberta acute care hospitals. *Nursing Research, 54*(2), 74–84.

Field, M. J., & Lohr, K. N. (Eds.). (1990). *Guidelines for clinical practice: Directions for a new program*. Washington, D.C.: Institute of Medicine, National Academies Press.

Foubert, T. (2014). Lean reform. *The HIROC Connection, 33* (Summer 2015), 12–15.

Giovannetti, P., Kerr, J. C., Bay, K., & Buchan, J. (1986). *Measuring quality of nursing care: Analysis of reliability and validity of selected instruments*. Edmonton, AB: University of Alberta Faculty of Nursing.

Goodwin, S., & Miller, L. (2014). System overhaul. *The HIROC Connection, 33*(Summer 2015), 27–31.

Hannah, K., & White, P. (2012). C-HOBIC: Standardized clinical outcomes to support evidence informed nursing care. *Canadian Journal of Nursing Leadership, 25*(1), 43–46.

Harrigan, M. L. (2000). *Quest for quality in Canadian health care: Continuous quality improvement* (2nd ed.). Ottawa, ON: Health Canada.

Health Quality Ontario. (n.d.). *Home care performance in Ontario*. Retrieved from https://www.hqontario.ca/System-Performance/Home-Care-Performance.

Health Standards Organization. (2019). *Why standards matter*. Retrieved from https://healthstandards.org/standards/why-standards-matter/.

Hetherington, L. T. (1998). Evaluating quality management systems. *Journal of Nursing Care Quality, 13*(2), 56–66.

Institute of Medicine. (2000). *To err is human: Building a safer health system*. Washington, D.C.: National Academies Press.

Institute of Medicine. (2004). *Keeping patients safe: Transforming the work environment of nurses*. Washington, D.C.: National Academies Press.

James, B. C. (1989). *Quality management of health care delivery*. Chicago, IL: American Hospital Association.

Jeffs, L., Doran, D., VanDeVelde-Coke, S., et al. (2015). Implementation of the National Nursing Quality Report Initiative in Canada: Insights from pilot participants. *Journal of Nursing Care Quality, 30*(4), E9–E16. https://doi.org/10.1097/NCQ.0000000000000122.

Joint Commission. (2019). *History of the Joint Commission*. Retrieved from https://www.jointcommission.org/about_us/history.aspx.

Johnson, C. N. (2002). The benefits of PDCA. *Back to Basics. Quality Progress, 35*. (5), 120–121.

Juran, J. M. (1989). *Juran on planning for quality*. New York, NY: Free Press.

Kitson, A. L. (2008). The need for systems change: reflections on knowledge translation and organizational change. *Journal of Advanced Nursing, 65*(1), 217–228. Retrieved from https://doi.org/10.1111/j.1365-2648.2008.04864.x.

Laschinger, H. K., Gilbert, S., & Smith, L. (2011). Patient satisfaction as a nurse-sensitive outcome. In D. Doran (Ed.), *Nursing outcomes: The state of the science* (2nd ed., pp. 359–400). Mississauga, ON: Jones & Bartlett Learning.

Land, T., & Stefl, M. E. (2007). Health care we must get it right: To make real progress in healthcare reform, healthcare organization leaders need to make quality and safety a priority. *Healthcare Financial Management, 61*(7), 90–95.

Manojlovich, M., & Laschinger, H. (2007). The Nursing Worklife Model: Extending and refining a new theory. *Journal of Nursing Management, 15,* 256–263.

McLaughlin, C., & Kaluzny, A. (1990). Total quality management in health: Making it work. *Health Care Management Review, 15*(3), 7–14.

Miller, L. (2016). *The lean coach: Developing the habits of continuous improvement.* Potomac, MD: Author.

Moraros, J., Lemstra, M., & Nwankwo, C. (2016). Lean interventions in healthcare: Do they actually work? A systematic literature review. *International Journal for Quality in Health Care, 28*(2), 150–165. https://doi.org/10.1093/intqhc/mzv123.

National Steering Committee on Patient Safety. (2002). *Building a safer system: A national integrated strategy for improving patient safety in Canadian health care.* Ottawa, ON: Author.

Nightingale, F. (1858). *Notes on matters affecting the health, efficiency and hospital administration of the British army.* London, UK: Harrison & Sons.

Plsek, P. (1990). A primer on quality improvement tools. In D. Berwick, A. Godfrey, & J. Roessner (Eds.), *Curing health care* (pp. 177–220). San Francisco, CA: Jossey-Bass.

Popoola, M. M., Wahl, M., Dupont, J., et al. (2008). Nursing Information Classification system education. *West African Journal of Nursing, 19*(1), 42–45.

Pringle, D., & Doran, D. M. (2003). Patient outcomes as an accountability. In D. M. Doran (Ed.), *Nursing-sensitive outcomes: State of the science* (pp. 1–25). Sudbury, MA: Jones and Bartlett.

Pringle, D. M., & White, P. (2002). Nursing matters: The Nursing and Health Outcomes Project of the Ontario Ministry of Health and Long-Term Care. *Canadian Journal of Nursing Research, 33,* 115–121.

Saskatchewan Health Quality Council. (2013, August). FAQs about Lean and Healthcare in Saskatchewan. Saskatchewan Healthcare Management System. Retrieved from http://hqc.sk.ca/portals/0/documents/lean-faq.pdf.

Shale, S. (2013). Patient experience as an indicator of clinical quality in emergency care. *Governance: An International Journal, 18*(4), 285–292. https://doi.org/10.1108/CGIJ-03-2012-0008.

Siering, U., Eikermann, M., Hausner, E., et al. (2013). Appraisal tools for clinical practice guidelines: A systematic review. *PLoS ONE, 8*(12), e82915. https://doi.org/10.1371/journal.pone.0082915.

Spear, S. (2004, May). Learning to lead at Toyota. *Harvard Business Review.* Retrieved from https://hbr.org/2004/05/Learning-to-lead-at-toyota.

Sunnybrook Health Sciences Centre. (2019). *Quality Improvement Plan 2019/2020.* Retrieved from https://sunnybrook.ca/content/?page=quality-improvement-plan.

Thompson, R. (1991). The six faces of quality. *Health Care Executive, 6*(2), 26–27.

Thornton, R. D. Nurse, N., Snavely, L., Hackett-Zahler, S., Frank, K., & DiTomasso, R. A. (2017). Influences on patient satisfaction in healthcare centers: a semi-quantitative study over 5 years. *BMC Health Services Research, 17,* 361

Toussaint, J. S., & Berry, L. L. (2013, January). The promise of Lean in health care. *Mayo Clinic Proceeding, 88*(1), 74–82. https://doi.org/10.1016/j.mayocp.2012.07.025.

Trussel, P. M., & Strand, N. (1978). A comparison of concurrent and retrospective audits of the same clients. *Journal of Nursing Administration, 8*(5), 33–38.

VanDeVelde-Coke, S., Doran, D., Grinspun, D., et al. (2012). Measuring outcomes of nursing care, improving the health of Canadians: NNQR(C), C-HOBIC and NQuIRE. *Nursing Leadership, 25*(2), 26–37.

VanDeVelde-Coke, S., Doran, D., & Jeffs, L. (2015). Update on the NNQR(C) pilot project. *Canadian Nurse, 111*(2), 10–11. Retrieved from https://www.canadian-nurse.com/en/articles/issues/2015/march-2015/update-on-the-nnqr-c-pilot-project.

Ventura, M., Hageman, P. T., Slakter, M. J., & Fox, R. N. (1980). Inter-rater reliabilities for two measures of nursing care quality. *Research in Nursing and Health, 3*(1), 25–32.

Virani, T., & Grinspun, D. (2007). Best practice guidelines— RNAO's Best Practice Guidelines Program: Progress report on a phenomenal journey. *Advances in Skin & Wound Care, 20*(10), 528–535.

Walton, M. (1986). *The Deming management method.* New York, NY: Dodd, Mead.

Whetsell, G. (1990). Total quality management. *Health Progress, 71*(8), 16–19.

Wilson, R. (1995). The Quality in Australian Health Care Study. *Medical Journal of Australia, 163,* 458–471.

Wilson, R. (2001). Quality improvement will require a major commitment. *Hospital Quarterly, 4*(3), 20–24.

Wong, C., & Cummings, G. G. (2007). The relationship between nursing leadership and patient outcomes: A systematic review. *Journal of Nursing Management, 15,* 508–521.

Woolley, J., Perkins, R., Laird, P., et al. (2012). Relationship-based care: Implementing a caring, healing environment. *Medsurg Nursing, 21*(3), 179–184.

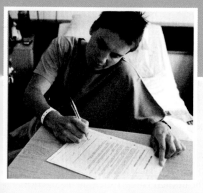

The Practising Nurse and the Law

Lyle G. Grant

🅔 http://evolve.elsevier.com/Canada/Ross-Kerr/nursing

LEARNING OBJECTIVES

After reading this chapter, you will be able to:
- Discuss some common legal issues that may involve nurses.
- Highlight the role of nurses as professionals and the obligations of self-regulation.
- Outline the elements of a nursing negligence action.
- Appreciate the complexities required for a valid consent to health care treatment, informed consent, and capacity to consent for minors and dependent adults.

- Identify the legal obligation of nurses to keep treatment records.
- Understand the legal obligation to maintain the privacy and confidentiality of patients.
- Understand that the legal aspects of nursing practice are not static and evolve with the development of nursing practice.

OUTLINE

KEY TERMS

capacity
confidentiality
consent
duty of care
electronic health record
electronic medical record

informed consent
negligence
privacy
scope of practice
tort

PERSONAL PERSPECTIVES

Jennifer is called into her manager's office. Upon arriving, she discovers that a union representative is also present. The manager shows Jennifer screenshots of her social media postings. Included in the materials are the following comments:

We had a heck of day saving lives in our ER today. A 3-year old who attends the same pre-school as my daughter had swallowed a "foreign body" that turned out to be illicit drugs. Social Services became involved and I think the parents were arrested. Poor young girl is now staying with strangers.

The manager suggests to Jennifer that there is sufficient information in her posting, given the small community in which she lives, for others to identify the child and the parents involved. Jennifer states that her Facebook page is by invitation only to nurses who also work at the same hospital, and that they are all bound by the hospital's confidentiality agreements, so there should not really be any problem. She is apologetic.

What factors might be considered in determining whether there has been a breach of confidentiality and its seriousness if there has? Are there other legal issues or implications to her practice that Jennifer should consider?

INTRODUCTION

On a daily basis, nurses confront a myriad of factors that directly affect their ability to make informed decisions about the quality of care they give. Legal challenges to nursing activities were once rare and posed little concern in the nursing profession. However, circumstances have changed. The extension of nurses' **scope of practice**, substantial improvements in salaries and working conditions, and a greater propensity for the public to seek damages for professional **negligence** are all reasons for nurses to be aware of the risks and responsibilities inherent in their practice (Grant, 2015). The potential benefit of understanding rights and responsibilities under the law, particularly as they apply to the health care field, is clear when one considers the close and continuing contact between patients and nurses in health care environments.

Nurses' responsibilities have evolved over time and often do not match traditional public notions of nursing. Legislative, institutional, and other social structures have fashioned higher degrees of independence in nursing practice than in the past. This includes an increasing latitude of nurse-initiated treatment procedures and interventions. Along with these structural changes in practice, nursing and nurses' roles are affected by the far-reaching impacts of an exponential increase in knowledge, an increased emphasis on understanding and applying best practice, and the increased use of technologies.

As the scope of practice expands, modern nursing, regardless of practice setting, sees nurses assuming increased responsibility for decision making and performing procedures that entail considerable risk. The primary types of legal proceedings that may affect nurses' professional practices throughout their careers include negligence actions, disciplinary proceedings, public inquiries, coroner's inquests, criminal charges, and employment arbitrations. Although each proceeding differs, they all require that nurses become not only knowledgeable and competent in the practice of their profession, but also aware and respectful of the legal rights of their patients. This chapter provides an overview of important areas of law related to nursing clinical practices and pertinent areas of nurses' involvement in the legal system. The information is not intended as a comprehensive treatment of the subject, but rather as a cursory review to introduce areas of concern, stimulate thinking about different issues, and encourage further research.

PROFESSIONAL STATUS OF NURSES

In all provinces and territories in Canada, nurses have professional status, which imparts autonomy of practice, the right of self-regulation, and the obligation to monitor and discipline its own members. Nurses are governed in some provinces and territories by individual health profession legislation. However, other jurisdictions have moved to umbrella legislation for all health care providers. A common principle among all jurisdictions, however, is the designation of a governing body whose role is to register, monitor, and discipline nurses within the province or territory.

Each jurisdiction's nursing governing bodies are charged by legislation to provide and enforce standards of practice and a code of conduct as well as to establish requirements for entry to practice. Even after nurses have met the qualifications and competencies required for registration, they have a continuing legal obligation to remain familiar with developments in the profession and to remain capable of performing tasks and making decisions that the public would expect a competent nurse to perform. In addition to their regulatory functions, most nursing associations or colleges take on voluntary functions in the interest of promoting the nursing profession, except for a few jurisdictions whose legislation requires that the regulatory body and the voluntary functions remain separate; for example, this includes the College of Nurses of Ontario and the Registered Nurses' Association of Ontario.

When incidents occur that involve complaints against a nurse for failure to meet the standards of practice, for incompetence, or for incapacity, the governing body protects the public by investigating such complaints about members' practice. Investigations performed by the registrar, employer through mandatory reporting, or regulated health care provider may arise as a result of complaints from patients, colleagues, or members of the public. Any professional conduct or discipline process must meet the requirements of the governing legislation. A hearing related to a complaint may be held when issues are of a serious nature and the allegations of professional misconduct or incompetence are supported by evidence. A hearing is similar to a court proceeding; each side has opening and closing statements, examinations and cross-examinations, and the testimony of expert witnesses. The board or committee hearing the complaint will be empowered by the governing legislation to issue a decision with the appropriate penalty, the most severe being revocation of registration.

Each regulatory body will set out the appeal process of decisions of the board or committee of the hearing. Following the appeal, a further appeal to the appropriate court may be available. Where available, the appeal court has the ability to confirm the decision, to substitute its own decision, or to send the issue back for a new hearing. Complaints of professional misconduct or incompetence may also result in a negligence lawsuit and criminal charges. As discussed below, negligence lawsuits are primarily about compensation for damages, whereas the complaints of professional misconduct or incompetence concern registration and practice permits. Using criminal charges as a means of protecting the public is a useful policy in legal considerations for nursing practice. However, criminal charges focus on punishment and deterrence to achieve the safety outcome and may be limited to one occurrence. Ensuring public safety is a broader endeavour of public policy, the law, regulatory bodies, and the nursing profession.

LAWSUITS AND HEALTH CARE PROVIDERS

The majority of lawsuits against health care providers arise in tort law. A **tort** is a wrongful act from which an individual has been harmed. Torts can be classed as either intentional or unintentional. As the names suggest, intent is something of a distinguishing feature. Examples of intentional torts include assault, battery, fraud, wrongful imprisonment, defamation, and trespass. Unintentional torts might look like accidents of carelessness, which can be viewed in law as negligent acts where there is a legal **duty of care** owed to another. Examples of unintentional torts include car accidents, slips and falls, product liability, medical malpractice, and other professional negligence in practice. Those injured can bring legal action as a plaintiff for a claim of damages to help remedy their situation to a position closer to one they would have been in but for the tort. Damages

can sometimes also be assessed as a deterrent against others committing a similar wrongful act. Actions for claims in monetary damages in tort are commonly referred to as suing for damages. The bulk of lawsuits against health care providers are unintentional torts based on complaints of negligence that have resulted in personal injury or suffering. These types of lawsuits will be the focus of this discussion.

Elements of Negligence

Patients place their trust in nurses on a daily basis and have a right to expect the best possible care based on a reasonable standard of skill and knowledge. There is a duty of nurses to exercise a degree of care in their actions that the public can reasonably expect. **Negligence** in this context is commonly defined as a nursing action falling below the standard of care that a reasonable and prudent nurse would follow in particular or similar health care circumstances. Professional practice standards are often looked at first in helping to define expected degrees of care for nursing actions. Through case commentary, the courts have provided an indication of the generally expected standards of care of health practitioners:

Every medical practitioner must bring to his task a reasonable degree of skill and knowledge and must exercise a reasonable degree of care. He is bound to exercise that degree of care and skill which could reasonably be expected of a normal, prudent practitioner of the same experience and standing. (Crits v. Sylvester, [1956], p. 601)

A claim of negligence will succeed if the essential elements can be demonstrated by a plaintiff. These elements include the following: (1) the defendant must owe the plaintiff a duty of care; (2) the duty of care was not met or was breached—that is, the nurse must have been careless or negligent; (3) there must be reasonable foreseeability in the consequences; (4) the breach must have caused the damages or injury; and (5) the damages or injury would not have occurred but for the negligence (Dickens, 2011, p. 117).

In order to establish that a duty of care is owed to a patient by a nurse, a relationship between the patient and nurse must be demonstrated. A duty of care is seldom disputed, as

the extreme vulnerability and dependency of patients upon their nurses and the obvious capacity of nurses to cause harm to their patients by substandard care combine to create in the eyes of the law an unquestionable duty owed to each patient to provide appropriate care and professional skill. (Irvine, 2013, p. 188)

Most often, this element will be satisfied by the reliance on records documenting the nurse's involvement with the patient's care.

The second element, breach of duty or standard of care, tends to provide the focus of debate when a nurse is sued.

The care need not be the best care, or even the optimum care, but the standard of care that a "reasonable and prudent nurse" would have provided in a particular situation. The evidence establishing the standard of a "reasonable and prudent nurse" is developed in a number of ways, including relevant statements in articles and books by nursing authors that document the acceptability of certain practices, nursing practice standards developed by federal and provincial/territorial professional nursing associations, curriculum content in schools of nursing, and testimony by expert witnesses who are nurses. As well, the individual nurse's practice, educational background, and experience are scrutinized by the court. In one important case (*Dowey v. Rothwell*, [1974]), a nurse who had worked in a physician's office in Alberta for 22 years was found negligent after the court learned that she had failed to take any continuing education courses since the year after her graduation, some 40 years before. Even if there is more than one recognized method of care, a nurse would not be negligent as long as the nurse provided care that was consistent with accepted practice.

The next element requires that the consequences of the event caused harm that was reasonably foreseeable (Grant, 2015, p.83). This helps to distinguish accidents or errors in judgement from actions or omissions (Dickens, 2011; Irvine, 2013). The distinction is important for determining liability.

The fourth element requires a plaintiff to establish that the breach of duty caused the patient's injury. Although health care providers, including nurses, tend to view actions involving negligence as negative to reputation and integrity, the purpose of the law pertaining to torts is to compensate the party who is injured through the actions of another. For example, in the case of *Strachan (Guardian ad litem of) v. Reynolds* [2004], a mother and child were entitled to recover damages against a nurse who had failed to recognize the signs and symptoms of developing uterine rupture, which caused the child's oxygen deprivation and subsequent brain injury. The issue here is not punishment, but rather to compensate the plaintiff for injury by moving responsibility for loss from the plaintiff to the defendant. If a patient is not able to demonstrate damages, then there

🔍 RESEARCH FOCUS

A public inquiry was conducted in the wake of a high-profile criminal case involving a Canadian nurse who deliberately used insulin to end the lives of eight people in long-term care. The commissioner focused on significant systemic vulnerabilities that permitted the offences and that would need to be addressed to improve the safety and operations of long-term care services. Collaboration, cooperation, and communication were viewed as key to identifying the necessary improvements.

One of the main recommendations concerned the need for heightened awareness of the potential deliberate harm that could be done to patients by health care providers, particularly by serial murderers. "A growing body of research and literature shows that healthcare serial killing is a phenomenon which, while rare, is long-standing and universal in its reach, with documented cases dating back to the 1800s" (Gillese, 2019, p. 4). Among the many recommendations made to bolster awareness of health care providers deliberately harming those in their care is Recommendation 40:

The College of Nurses of Ontario must educate its membership and staff on the possibility that a nurse or other healthcare provider might intentionally harm those for whom they provide care. (Gillese, 2019, p. 31)

Recommendations also included the need to increase awareness among those "who work, volunteer, or visit family and friends in long-term care homes about their reporting obligations under section 24(1) of the [Ontario] *Long-Term Care Homes Act, 2007* (LTCHA)" (Gillese, 2019, p. 26). Similar to reporting requirements in other Canadian provinces and territories, s. 24(1) of the LTCHA requires that any person who has reasonable grounds to suspect improper or incompetent treatment or care, or the abuse or neglect of residents (among other things), must report their suspicion and the information not just to facility management but also to the government ministry.

Systemic responses to the systemic issues explored by the commission included recommendations grouped into the themes of prevention, awareness, deterrence, and detection. It is likely that as the recommendations are more carefully considered for implementation, health care providers will have increased standards of care, heightened awareness, and increased legal responsibility to those for whom they care and to the systems in which they operate. The commission signalled that the significant systemic shortcomings of long-term care services have implications for health care providers in all health service areas.

Source: Gillese, E. E. (2019). *Public inquiry into the safety and security of residents in the long-term care homes system. Vol. 1— Executive summary and consolidated recommendations.* Retrieved from https://longtermcareinquiry.ca/en/final-report/.

would be no basis for a civil action, notwithstanding that a patient could still initiate discipline proceedings.

The fifth element requires that the injury or damages would not have occurred but for the nurse's negligence. It must be demonstrated on the balance of probabilities that if the nurse's actions or inactions caused the harm and if the nurse had not been negligent, then the injury would not have been suffered. Expert witnesses often help to determine whether this linkage exists. In *MacDonald v. York County Hospital* [1972], a patient treated for a fractured dislocation of the ankle developed gangrene and was forced to undergo an amputation of his leg below the knee. The trial judge found that the nurses had been aware that the patient's condition was deteriorating over an 18-hour period but had failed to advise a physician. The judge also found the hospital and nursing staff partially responsible for the injuries. On appeal, the nurses' negligence was found not to have caused any harm to the plaintiff, as the physician had provided evidence that he would not have acted even if the appropriate standard of care had been met by the nurses.

In some jurisdictions, there may be legislation that affords nurses protection from liability if the applicable legislation contains an appropriate statutory limitation of liability. This was the case in *Wowk v. Edmonton (Health Board)* (1994), in which the plaintiff suffered an injury as a result of an influenza shot given by the defendant, a community health nurse. The court found that the *Public Health Act* (Alberta) shielded the community health nurse from liability for any act done or omitted in good faith in performing the services, as negligence was not itself a lack of good faith.

APPLYING CONTENT KNOWLEDGE

What is the legal differentiation between an error and negligence of a nurse in nursing practice?

CONSENT TO NURSING CARE

A fundamental human right, historically respected in law, is the right to be free from interference. Except in the case of emergencies and other extraordinary circumstances, **consent** must be obtained from the individual prior to the provision of health care treatment. In 1993, the Supreme Court of Canada confirmed this right in stating that

> [e]veryone has the right to decide what is to be done to one's own body. This includes the right to be free from medical treatment to which the individual does not consent. This concept of individual autonomy is fundamental to the common law. (Ciarlariello v. Schacter, [1993], p. 135)

The tort of battery involves intentional touching of another person without consent (Peppin, 2011, p. 155). There need not be any injury for the tort to be established and upheld by the courts. Because nursing practice involves much touching of patients, patient consent must be obtained for any nursing procedures that involve touching. Thus, the aim here is to provide a cursory discussion of the fundamental requirements for legal consent. The present discussion represents a brief summary only. More specific references should be consulted to obtain a deeper understanding of the issues.

Age, health, and mental status of patients, and the circumstances surrounding the situation, often make it difficult for nurses to obtain **informed consent**. Nurses usually rely on the patient's verbal expression of consent to nursing-care activities. In the past, the majority of these activities have been considered low risk. However, with the steady expansion of the scope of nursing practice and the increase in independent nursing functions, many current nursing-care procedures are considered high risk. Thus, it is crucial that nurses understand all the fundamental requirements for a valid consent and their role in documenting it. Health care providers who rely on implied consent in the absence of an emergency or for high-risk procedures and without understanding the limitations of implied consent or what may imply that the consent is withdrawn may expose patients to unauthorized intrusion on their bodies and themselves to liability (Irvine, 2013). In *Canadian AIDS Society v. Ontario* (August 4, 1995), the court had to consider whether consent could have been implied by a blood donor to have his donated blood tested 10 years after the fact. Express consent is preferred even if implied consent may be valid.

Much of the law surrounding consent has been settled in case law or by the relevant legislation in the provinces. In an attempt to provide a degree of certainty, some provinces have enacted legislation that defines how and by whom consent can be given. For example, Ontario's *Health Care Consent Act, 1996* holds that valid consent relating to treatment must be informed and voluntary and must not be obtained by misrepresentation or fraud. In the absence of specific legislation within the nurse's jurisdiction, the law has recognized four basic requirements for consent to be valid: (1) it must relate to the treatment; (2) it must be informed; (3) it must be given voluntarily; and (4) the patient must have the **capacity** to consent to the proposed treatment. A brief explanation of each of these four elements will reveal the importance and complexity of this issue.

Treatment and the Provider of Treatment

Consent to care given must be specific to the proposed treatment or procedure. As noted in *Dixon v. Calgary Health*

Region [2006], a patient sued after being treated with multiple intramuscular injections of Demerol, which the patient claimed caused weakness in his right leg, causing him to fall and injure his back. The court ruled that informed consent had been provided and that separate written consents were not required for each injection. Additionally, consideration should be taken if a patient consented to the performance of a procedure by a particular health care provider; this requirement does not authorize substitution of another, less qualified, or different type of, health practitioner.

Informing Patients of the Nature and Risks of Treatment

Informed consent is foundational to obtaining a valid consent for treatment. In all provinces, for consent to be informed prior to commencing treatment, the patient must be provided with information concerning the nature of the treatment and its gravity, the expected benefits of the treatment, the material risks of the treatment and material side effects of the treatment, alternative courses of action, and potential consequences of not having the treatment. The patient should also have an opportunity to ask questions and receive responses to the questions. The courts have found that "material risk" is dependent on each situation. Not every conceivable risk or mere possibility needs to be disclosed, but normally just those risks that may result in serious consequences (Peppin, 2011). Through the *Health Care Consent Act* in s. 11(3), Ontario has set out the "reasonable person" as the standard used as a basis for determining how much information needs to be disclosed to a patient.

Voluntary Consent

To be considered voluntary, consent must be freely given and must be obtained without undue influence or misrepresentation about the nature of the treatment. Even though each case depends on its facts, fundamentally patients have the full right to control their own medical treatment. The court will examine any pressure brought on a patient and determine whether it was sufficient to affect the decision making of that individual. In *Re T* [1992], a minor who was 34 weeks pregnant refused to have a blood transfusion. Though the minor was no longer a Jehovah's Witness, her mother was a member of that faith. Upon the request of the minor's father, the court granted application to order the transfusion. On appeal, the court held that there was undue influence upon the minor by her mother and so upheld the decision to authorize the transfusion.

It is also important to remember that patients have a right to make their own health care decisions. A patient also has a right to withdraw consent to any procedure at any time before or during the procedure. The Supreme

Court of Canada confirmed that if there is any basis for the withdrawal of consent to a medical procedure even while it is underway, the procedure must be halted except if termination of the procedure either would be life threatening or would cause serious problems for the patient (*Ciarlariello v. Schacter*, [1993], p. 135).

Capacity to Consent

The patient must have the legal capacity to consent to treatment or substitute consent must be obtained from a person with legal standing to make the treatment decision. Capacity in this context refers to the individual's age and mental competence to understand the nature and ramifications of their decision making. Adults with disabilities, those with progressive diseases affecting the mind or ability to communicate, and children are groups for whom questions of consent in health matters may become complex. It can be difficult not only to identify the appropriate decision maker, but also to determine the basis on which the decision is to be made.

The limits on decision-making authority depend on a number of factors. For adults without capacity, most jurisdictions have enacted comprehensive legislation to deal with the substitute consent and the ability to create a legally valid personal or advance directive or to appoint a health care agent (Peppin, 2011). British Columbia, Ontario, Prince Edward Island, and Yukon provide examples of these types of Acts. Guardianship Acts also provide means of appointing substitute decision makers for those without legal capacity.

In addition to the legislation for adults without capacity, health care providers should be aware of relevant provincial or territorial legislation that addresses age of consent for minors. Although parents are routinely consulted in regard to treatment, their decisions are not absolute. The courts have the jurisdiction to challenge a parent's decision if it is not deemed to be in the best interests of the child. Some jurisdictions have enacted legislation that creates an independent tribunal to review decisions that are not in the best interests of the child. For example, in Ontario, the Consent and Capacity Board, an independent body created by the Government of Ontario under the *Health Care Consent Act*, considers whether the substitute decision maker followed the principles for making substitute decisions.

A common situation occurs when, for example, in the opinion of health care providers, a blood transfusion is required but is refused by parents for religious reasons. The courts will take into consideration age, intelligence, education, and previous experiences in determining whether a child can understand the nature and consequences of the proposed treatment and thus give consent. In the 1986 decision by the Alberta Court of Appeal, *C. (J.S.) v. Wren* [1986], a 16-year-old sought an abortion and obtained the consent of her doctor and the Therapeutic Abortion Committee, both of which were required at the time. Her parents attempted to stop the procedure, arguing that their daughter was a minor and therefore could not give consent to the abortion. Although the court confirmed parental rights, it held that the evidence established that the daughter was a normal 16-year-old who had sufficient intelligence and understanding to make up her own mind. Thus, the court upheld the committee's original order.

Along with physicians, nurses often face the issue of consent, as they are often involved in asking patients to sign consent-to-treatment documents. The case of *B.H. (Next friend of) v. Alberta (Director of Child Welfare)* [2002] illustrates the complexity of this issue. In February 2002, a 16-year-old minor was diagnosed with acute myeloid leukemia, and based on her religious beliefs, she refused to consent to blood transfusions or the administration of blood products. The Alberta Director of Child Welfare made an application to the Provincial Court for an apprehension order and a medical treatment order. The court granted the orders that made the minor a ward of the state, and the essential treatment was administered. The decision was upheld by the Alberta Court of Appeal, and leave to appeal to the Supreme Court of Canada was refused. Although this difficult issue has arisen before, it is worth revisiting, as it serves as a reminder of the complexities involved in obtaining a minor's consent.

Consent may also be importantly influenced by the known wishes of an adult expressed while they were competent (Grant, 2015). Many provinces and territories have legislation that addresses advance directives that acknowledge the individual's right to contemplate and direct or refuse consent to treatments and interventions in advance. An express wish not to be intubated or to deny cardiopulmonary resuscitation (CPR) are simple forms of possible advance directives. Acting against the known wishes of a patient who contemplated potential loss of decision-making capacity may disrespect nursing duties to the patient and may create legal liability.

Recent examples of the impact of loss of capacity to consent concern legislative provisions that acknowledge the right of Canadians to obtain and instruct medical assistance in dying (MAID) in certain circumstances. There are specific legislative requirements and safeguards for consent, including a 10-day waiting period and second acknowledgement of consent immediately prior to commencing MAID. Patients are often subject to deteriorating mental function or increasing analgesics as a result of their underlying medical condition, and some lose the capacity to provide the necessary second confirmation of consent, thus preventing MAID from taking place. Some of the specific requirements of consent are detailed in Bill C-14: An Act to Amend the

Criminal Code and to Make Related Amendments to Other Acts (Medical Assistance in Dying), 2016.

RESEARCH FOCUS

The case of *Starson v. Swayze* put the issue of capacity to consent to treatment front and centre in Canada (Sklar, 2007). The decision of the Supreme Court of Canada (SCC) focused on the interpretation of the "understanding" requirement for capacity in Ontario's *Health Care Consent Act.* The court looked at many factors, including the question of whether the patient's best interests are to be factored into the determination of a patient's capacity and subsequently the right of a capable patient to refuse treatment. In this 2007 article, the author discusses and analyses the SCC's decision, including its clinical and constitutional implications for Ontario and the rest of Canada.

Source: Sklar, R. (2007). *Starson v. Swayze*: The Supreme Court speaks out (not all that clearly) on the question of "capacity." *Canadian Journal of Psychiatry, 52*(6), 390–396.

NURSING DOCUMENTATION

Most health care providers are legally obligated to maintain an account of the care and treatment they give to the minimum standard set out by legislation as well as standards set by the health profession's governing body. The primary purpose of creating health records is to facilitate communication among health care providers in treating a patient. Health records reflect a contemporaneous account of the care and treatment of patients and are a vital part of communication among members of the health care team. Once created, the health record becomes a legal document. Documentation should be done in compliance with a number of legal requirements with respect to content, retention, and disclosure of the health record. Other sources that set out the frequency, quantity, and detail of documentation include provincial/territorial legislation, hospital bylaws, policies and procedures, standards of the professions, regulatory guidelines, and complexity and severity of the patient's health problems.

Courts have over time recognized that in many situations a written record may be more dependable than a witness's oral recollection of events. The leading case with respect to admissibility of hospital records into evidence, including nurses' notes, is the Supreme Court of Canada case *Ares v. Venner* [1970]:

Hospital records, including nurses' notes made contemporaneously by someone having a personal knowledge

of the matters then being recorded and under a duty to make the entry or record, should be received in evidence as prima facie proof of the facts stated therein. This should in no way preclude a party wishing to challenge the accuracy of the records or entries from doing so. (p. 626)

The decision changed the legal landscape on the importance of nursing notes, such that when a chart entry is made by a nurse contemporaneously with the events as part of their nursing duty, the contents shall be presumed true unless the party challenging their accuracy can persuade a Court otherwise (Irvine, 2013, p. 198).

In some cases, problems with nursing notes introduced as evidence in court have invited criticism from the court during legal proceedings. Court accounts of the deficiencies noted in nursing records present an opportunity for nurses to learn of the importance of their often routine work. Frequent court criticisms have included failure to record events contemporaneously, gaps in recording, and recording of care by someone other than the nurse who provided the care. As illustrated in the case of *Kolesar v. Jefferies* (1974), the case involved a patient who was found dead the morning after a spinal fusion operation. The chart was important in establishing liability, as no nursing entries were made from 2200 to 0500 hours, when the death was discovered. Where this is a positive duty for a nurse to make observations or take any action for the safety and health of a patient, a lack of nursing notes will be seen as a failure to take such required nursing actions. This case may be the basis for the nursing expression "not charted, not done."

However, the law is full of complexities. The *Kolesar v. Jefferies* case was distinguished from the case of *Ferguson v. Hamilton Civic Hospitals* (1983) to allow for inference that a patient's condition remained unchanged on each observation unless noted otherwise. This is perhaps akin to and commonly understood by nursing to be charting by exception. Mr. Justice Krever rejected the notion that the absence of nursing notes for a limited period of time was to infer a failure in the provision of care by attending nursing staff in a recovery room setting. Instead, he would infer that there was no observable change during the period that justified being recorded. In emphasizing the difference between this case and the *Kolesar v. Jefferies* case, he pointed to the positive duty required for a nurse to perform a physical act, rather than to simply make a routine observation. The former would require a nursing note and the latter not.

In general, it is difficult to verify that any care not recorded was actually provided. Cases often come to trial long after the events in question occurred. In these circumstances, it is difficult for those directly involved in the care to remember details of what happened. Thus, clear, accurate, and complete recording of events at the time of the event is essential, as the contemporaneous record will generally be accepted over anyone's recollection of the events. The court in *Chancey v. McKinstry* [2000] demonstrated this principle by its reliance on the medical record. The case involved a patient who assaulted his wife after he had stopped taking lithium after 20 years of treatment for a bipolar disorder. The patient at trial alleged that his psychiatrist had told him to stop taking the lithium. The court accepted the psychiatrist's notes as demonstration that it was his standard practice not to interfere with patients' prescriptions.

The desired documentation practices for nursing care consist of many essential elements. The recording of information should be done by the nurse who had firsthand knowledge of what was described in the record. It is considered poor practice to record the actions of another health care provider, as the recording nurse would not have personal knowledge of the event and would not be able to testify as to the truth of it. Therefore, nurses should record only what they performed, saw, and heard. It is important to record chronologically, frequently, and accurately in preparing a "factual, concise and totally objective" record of the events (Ross, 1973, pp. 102–103). These principles are exemplified in the case of *Meyer v. Gordon* [1981], which involved an infant who suffered a serious brain injury during birth. The trial was held 5 years after the incident, and the nurse's sole evidence was her chart. The chart was found to be insufficient to demonstrate that she provided adequate care to the patient and she was found to be negligent.

Nevertheless, many believe that nurses are required to do a good deal of unnecessary charting in which they spend too much time recording routine care. This is thought to be wasteful both in using the time of highly skilled nurses unnecessarily and the space and time required for storage and retrieval of the data. Thus, "charting by exception" is being used in many health care centres. This is a method by which routine care and normal procedures are documented in an abbreviated method and only unusual occurrences and exceptions are recorded by a narrative. Nevertheless, charting by exception should be used only when it is supported by standards and policies to ensure that consistency and commitment to documentation is maintained.

There may be failures or honest mistakes made in the documentation process. The best course of action is to strike out the incorrect information and fill in the correct information with the date and time corrected. Nurses may be considered negligent if information is erased, as the court must assume that important facts were hidden and the person or persons responsible for the act did so in self-interest. It is evident that dishonesty in matters pertaining to care will usually be discerned in court proceedings and will not reflect positively on the character, conduct, or professionalism of the nurse or nurses involved. Additionally, any falsification and destruction of nursing records by nurses will most likely result in criminal and disciplinary action initiated by the employer as well as the regulatory body.

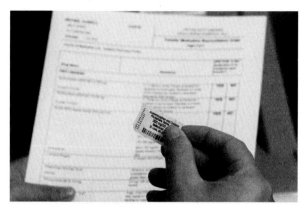

Nurse checking the label of a medication against the patient's medical administration record to ensure accuracy.

Electronic Health Records

All the principles with respect to nursing documentation apply whether the notes are in paper or electronic format. The obligation for documenting is the same regardless of the form of charting. The guidelines and professional standards created by the regulatory bodies support the notion that it is acceptable to maintain **electronic health records (EHRs)**. New discussions are occurring about the need for national nursing standards that support the goals for creating national EHRs (see Canada Health Infoway at https://infocentral.infoway-inforoute.ca/en/). There are four common considerations for electronic records: (1) they must be secure from interference or unauthorized access; (2) it is possible to display and print each patient's record separately; (3) the records have automatic backup and recovery; (4) and an audit trail is maintained.

Distinctions should be drawn between an EHR and an **electronic medical record (EMR)**. An EHR provides an integrated and comprehensive collection of a person's encounters with the health care system, including a patient's health history (Canada Health Infoway, 2019a). EMRs are the computer equivalent to the patient chart and are computer-based patient records specific to a single clinical practice or setting, such as a hospital, clinic, or doctor's office. The EMRs are sources of communication between various health care providers within a practice environment (Canada Health Infoway, 2019b).

EHRs promise improved ways to bring efficiency to maintaining, storing, and retrieving patient health files and improving the exchange of information between health care providers to deliver improved care to patients. Nevertheless, as EHRs contain the personal health information of patients, these records raise significant concerns regarding **privacy**, **confidentiality**, and security. Issues of patient confidentiality are important and are discussed below, and the parameters for maintaining confidentiality do not change with computerization.

PRIVACY AND CONFIDENTIALITY

The right to privacy and the duty of confidentiality are related. However, they may be differentiated in that the duty of confidentiality is owed by a health care provider to a patient (Gibson, 2011) to hold their personal information private. The right to privacy is vested in the patient (*R. v. Duarte*, 1990) and is the right of the individual to control their own personal information. Statutes of the provinces that include laws addressing the patient's right to confidentiality in health records are usually included in hospitals' and health agencies' specific privacy legislation; legislation that regulates nursing also contains provisions that reiterate the nurse's professional responsibility to maintain patient confidentiality. To fail in this responsibility is to be subject to allegations of professional misconduct.

This issue is illustrated in an unreported Ontario case (Sanchez-Sweatman, 1997) in which a charge nurse was found to have breached confidentiality by using her access card to call up information on her nurse manager, who had been admitted to the hospital the previous day. It was determined that the nurse had inadvertently called up the chart on the screen and was initially dismissed for these actions. Although the nurse was reinstated, the fact that it is possible for many people to access computerized records underscores the need to implement systems that allow only those with the right to access patient records to do so.

Privacy laws in Canada remain a bit of a patchwork in providing protection of personal health information while imposing obligations and responsibilities on health care institutions and their employees (Grant, 2015). The landscape of privacy laws continues changing and developing. Canadians take their rights to privacy seriously and find support in the *Canadian Charter of Rights and Freedoms, 1982*, s. 7 and 8. The Charter provides that "everyone has the right to life, liberty and security of the person and the right not to be deprived thereof except in accordance with the principles of fundamental justice and to freedom from unreasonable search and seizure" (*Canadian Charter of Rights and Freedoms, 1982*, s. 7). The Supreme Court has upheld the Charter's provisions as respecting individual's rights to privacy in both civil and criminal cases unless the infringement can be justified under section 1 of the Charter.

The modern health care system, with its rapid advances in technology, has created not only significant benefits to health, but also situations that have never before arisen in health and communications. Patients are in a vulnerable position. Concepts of autonomy require that patients retain control over their health records, including the ability to access those records and control their disclosure. Federal and provincial/territorial governments have attempted to respond to the public's concern by putting in place comprehensive legislation that provides a clear framework governing the rights of access and the collection, use, and disclosure of personal health information.

The privacy of personal health information remains an important priority of governments and health authorities across the country. Health authorities have taken an increasing number of actions to discipline employees who inappropriately access the health information of others as violations of confidentiality and the breaching of patient privacy rights. Processes to protect privacy are extremely important to safeguard personal and sensitive information from unauthorized access, collection, and disclosure. The difficulty in providing protection for personal information from access, collection, and disclosure must be balanced with the needs of health care providers who require the information to provide treatment to patients.

Currently, individual health records are protected through a variety of federal and provincial/territorial legislative acts, policies, and regulations. The federal government's initiative, the *Personal Information Protection and Electronic Documents Act, 2000* (PIPEDA) endeavours to control the collection, use, and disclosure of most forms of personal information. The provisions of PIPEDA, now well established in Canadian law, affect interprovincial and international flows of personal information as well as personal health information in any province without supplemental legislation acceptable to the federal government.

Most provinces have also enacted dedicated health privacy statutes aimed specifically at substantially transforming their practices and policies relating to protecting the privacy of health information. The aim of the legislation is to establish minimum standards for the collection, use, disclosure, and safeguarding of the information. Other objectives of the legislation include providing patients with access to their health records; the ability to correct erroneous information; the ability to request an independent review to resolve complaints relating to the handling of health information; and the ability to obtain remedies for contraventions of the legislation. Exceptions to the obligation to maintain individuals' privacy include (1) patient consent (implied or express, depending on the application legislation) for disclosure of health information to persons; (2) statutory provisions for reporting certain diseases and child abuse to appropriate health and social services personnel; and (3) court orders, which are often used to obtain health records for the use of plaintiffs or defendants in trials. With regard to privacy, these legislative initiatives are a welcome start to standardizing the health sectors dealing with patients' personal information.

New technology has revolutionized the advancement and adoption of information and telecommunications technologies in the delivery of health care. Applications such as remote presence, telehealth, and EHRs continue to transform health care delivery in the information age by improving the accessibility, quality, and efficiency of health care. With the advancement of nursing practice, new technologies for information sharing and new ways of seeking treatment across jurisdictions are adopted, giving rise to new legal issues. Some of the most prevalent issues are licensure, patient identification, privacy, and protection of personal and health information (Province of BC Health Authorities, 2014).

Policies and legislation are emerging to deal with these legal issues. For example, British Columbia enacted the *E-Health (Personal Health Information Access and Protection of Privacy) Act*, 2008. That legislation conceptualized an EHR for every individual in the province and governs the collection, use, and disclosure of personal health information in government databases. As most jurisdictions continue to build their capacity to use the new information and telecommunication technologies advance, only the passage of time will demonstrate whether the new legislation achieves the correct balance between access and protection for health care providers and patients.

CASE STUDY

Liam lives in Inuvik, Northwest Territories. Today, he will attend a consultation with a cardiac specialist who practices in and is based in Ottawa. They will discuss a relatively new surgical procedure that is only available at an Ottawa hospital. The consultation will occur across a computer connection via telehealth and use robotic remote presence technology to assist the surgeon in physically examining and interviewing Liam to screen his suitability for this new surgical intervention. Amongst other things, the surgeon will discuss the procedure, review the potential risks and benefits, and answer any of Liam's questions. What privacy and confidentiality matters might be important to consider with these types of remote interactions that also cross provincial and territorial boundaries? How might some of the issues be practically addressed?

UNDERSTANDING THE LEGAL ASPECTS OF NURSING

The professional nurse must have some knowledge of the law, legal processes, the judicial system, and patient rights. The increasing complexity of professional practice has been associated with increased risks in nursing procedures, and higher-risk procedures increase the potential for legal action. Nurses' roles have changed over time, and the pace of development has accelerated in recent years. The establishment of the baccalaureate standard for entry to practice for registered nurses is likely to result in even more change in the direction of augmented responsibility and increased risks for the registered nurse. There is no substitute for maintaining a high level of competence in nursing practice, excellent communication with patients, and an awareness of the risks involved in performing various procedures.

The Canadian Nurses Protective Society (CNPS) was established by the Canadian Nurses Association in 1988 at the request of the provincial and territorial professional nursing associations in response to the escalating cost of professional liability insurance. The CNPS is a nonprofit organization that offers liability insurance purchased by 10 of the 12 provincial and territorial associations on behalf of their members. It also offers advice about professional liability to nurses 24 hours a day all year round. Nurses may contact the CNPS if they have had personal involvement in or knowledge of any situation in which there are ethical or legal implications of concern. The CNPS offers the opportunity to speak with those who can provide immediate advice and assistance, including an indication of the steps to be taken in documenting an unusual occurrence, understanding legal processes that might be applicable, and referring nurses to experienced legal counsel.

Nurses have an obligation to respect their own professional and ethical guidelines and to follow the law. To meet these obligations, nurses require extensive knowledge and skills for legal, competent, ethically based practice. More than ever before, nurses engaged in practice need a fundamental understanding of the law and legal aspects of nursing. This chapter is not meant to be a comprehensive discussion of the issues nor should it be considered legal advice. It is meant to shed light on and raise awareness of some of the legal issues that nurses may face in their practice and encourage further thought and study on the topic.

SUMMARY OF LEARNING OBJECTIVES

- Understanding the common legal issues involving nursing practice is part of maintaining competencies in nursing, meeting professional standards of practice, and respecting or advocating for the rights of patients.
- Nurses, by virtue of their work, can expose themselves to risks from a legal perspective such as liability for negligence or battery.
- Negligence includes a duty of care owed to another that was breached and that caused damages or injury that could have been reasonably foreseen. Nurses can be held legally liable for negligence. Professional practice standards are important indicators of the expected level of care in determining relevant duties of care nurses owe to others.
- Consent is required for all nursing care. To be valid it must relate to the treatment, be informed, and be given freely by those with legal capacity to consent. Various legislative provisions may assist in establishing who has legal capacity to consent or who can consent on behalf of another, and these laws vary significantly between provinces and territories.
- Nursing documentation plays in important part in patient care delivery and communication. In any legal enquiry, this documentation often establishes the level and nature of nursing care provided. If this documentation is made contemporaneously to events, as part of routine practices and nursing duties, it creates a presumption in legal proceedings that the account is accurate and true. The care that nurses must take in this documentation follows its importance.
- Privacy and confidentiality are serious matters to Canadians. Nurses have clear obligations to protect the privacy and confidentiality of patients and their health and personal information. Amid some variation, all provinces and territories have laws that govern these protections. Breaches have serious consequences for nurses and for those they serve.

CRITICAL THINKING QUESTIONS

1. Identify the principles of informed consent to health care treatment.
2. What elements constitute negligence in nursing practice?
3. What would your advice be to a new nurse about being informed about one's legal obligations? How might they meet these obligations?

REFERENCES

Ares v. Venner, [1970] S.C.R. 608 at 626.

B.H. (Next friend of) v. Alberta (Director of Child Welfare) 2002 ABQB 371, 2002 ABCA 109, [2002] S.C.C.A. No. 196.

C. (J.S.) v. Wren, [1986] 76 A.R. 118 (Alta. C.A.).

Canada Health Infoway. (2019a). *Electronic health records.* Retrieved from https://www.infoway-inforoute.ca/en/solutions/digital-health-foundation/electronic-health-records.

Canada Health Infoway. (2019b). *Electronic medical records.* Retrieved from https://www.infoway-inforoute.ca/en/solutions/digital-health-foundation/electronic-medical-records.

Canadian AIDS Society v. Ontario, unreported August 4, 1995 (Ont. Gen. Div.).

Chancey v. McKinstry, [2000] B.C.J. No. 2008 (S.C.).

Ciarlariello v. Schacter, [1993] 2S.C.R. 119 at 135.

Crits v. Sylvester [1956] SCR 991, 5 D.L.R. (2d) 601.

Dickens, B. (2011). Medical negligence. In J. G. Downie, T. A. Caulfield, & C. M. Flood (Eds.), *Canadian health law and policy* (4th ed., pp. 115–151). Markham, ON: LexisNexis Canada.

Dixon v. Calgary Health Region, [2006] ABQB 235, 398 A.R. 199, 2006 Carswell Alta 378.

Dowey v. Rothwell, [1974] 5W.W.R. 311, 49 D.L.R. (3d) 82 (*Crits v. Sylvester* [1956] O.R. 132, 1 D.L.R. (2d) 502 (C.A.) affirmed 1956 Carswell Ont 84, Alta. S.C.).

Ferguson v. Hamilton Civic Hospitals (1983), 1983 Carswell Ont 705, 40 O.R. (2d) 577, 23.

Gibson, E. (2011). Health information: Confidentiality and access. In J. G. Downie, T. A. Caulfield, & C. M. Flood (Eds.), *Canadian health law and policy* (4th ed., pp. 253–294). Markham, ON: LexisNexis Canada.

Grant, L. G. (2015). Legal issues. In P. S. Yoder-Wise, L. G. Grant, & S. Regan (Eds.), *Leading and managing in Canadian nursing* (1st Canadian ed., pp. 69–89). Toronto, ON: Elsevier Canada.

Irvine, J. C. (2013). Nursing liability. In J. C. Irvine, P. H. Osborne, & M. Shariff (Eds.), *Canadian medical law: An introduction for physicians, nurses, and other health care professionals* (4th ed.). Scarborough, ON: Thomson Carswell.

Kolesar v. Jeffries (1974), 9 O.R. (2d) 41, 59 D.L.R. (3d) 367 (H.C.).

MacDonald v. York County Hospital, [1972] 3 O.R. 469, 28 D.L.R. (3d), [1976] 2S.C.R. 825.

Meyer v. Gordon, [1981] B.C.J. NO. 524 (S.C.)(QL).

Peppin, P. (2011). Informed consent. In J. G. Downie, T. A. Caulfield, & C. M. Flood (Eds.), *Canadian health law and policy* (4th ed., pp. 153–194). Markham, ON: LexisNexis Canada.

Re T, [1992] All. E.R. 649 (C.A.).

R. v. Duarte, [1990] 1 SCR 30.

Province of BC Health Authorities. (2014). *Telehealth clinical guidelines.* Retrieved from http://www.phsa.ca/Documents/Telehealth/TH_Clinical_Guidelines_Sept2015.pdf.

Ross, M. W. (1973). The nurse as an employee. In S. R. Good, & J. C. Kerr (Eds.), *Contemporary issues in Canadian law for nurses* (pp. 95–106). Toronto, ON: Holt, Rinehart & Winston.

Sanchez-Sweatman, L. (1997). Nurses, computers and confidentiality. *The Canadian Nurse, 93*(7), 47–48.

Strachan (Guardian ad litem of) v. Reynolds (2004), [2004] B.C.J. No. 1418.

Wowk v. Edmonton (Health Board), [1994] 19 Alta L.R. (3d) 232.

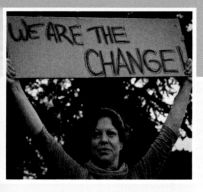

14

Decolonizing and Anti-Oppressive Nursing Practice: Awareness, Allyship, and Action

Sonya L. Jakubec and R. Lisa Bourque Bearskin

http://evolve.elsevier.com/Canada/Ross-Kerr/nursing

LEARNING OBJECTIVES

After reading this chapter, you will be able to:

- Understand allyship, anti-oppressive practice, diversity, culture, race, and ethnicity.
- Understand specific types of diversity in Canada: ethnic, linguistic, religious, sexual, and physical abilities.
- Describe key demographic groups for whom the nursing profession must take up anti-oppressive approaches.
- Describe how racism and discrimination are determinants of health.

- Explain awareness and cultural competence and their relevance to the nursing profession.
- Explain the concept of cultural safety and relevance to the nursing profession.
- Describe how relational practice and anti-oppressive practice are central to the nursing profession.
- Discuss some important skills and tools required for anti-oppressive practice, advocacy, and action at individual and organization levels.

OUTLINE

KEY TERMS

action	cultural skill	prejudice
allyship	cultural understanding	privilege
anti-oppressive practice	culture	race
awareness	decolonization	racializing
bias	diversity	racially visible
client	ethnicity	racism
colonization	ethnocentrism	refugee
cultural awareness	immigrant	relational practice
cultural blindness	intersectionality	sexual orientation
cultural competence	LGBTQ2	social justice
cultural knowledge	microaggressions	stereotyping
cultural pluralism	multiculturalism	trans
cultural safety	newcomer	visible minority
cultural sensitivity	oppression	white supremacy

PERSONAL PERSPECTIVES

"Start with Awareness"

LaRon E. Nelson is a Toronto-based public-health nurse practitioner and researcher who works with people who routinely face well-intended but racist or oppressive care. His experiences as a person of colour and a nurse who has made assumptions and errors around cultural safety have made him think critically about how to work with populations who are stigmatized and marginalized and the "innocent" ways that providers can cause harm. He describes the very failure to acknowledge racism and other forms of oppression in Canada as a significant health problem. He asserts that racism, not race, is the determinant of health. Of course, racism is not easy to own up to, especially in a profession that credits itself with caring and meeting the needs of all people. Many oppressive practices or behaviours are hidden, not intentional, but nonetheless harmful. Nelson explains how, without seeing the impact of white **privilege** as discriminating against Black and brown people and Indigenous peoples, nurses are complicit in systems of oppression—and this does not excuse him, a Black nurse with training and awareness to spare! While awareness is only the beginning, it is an essential starting place for anti-oppressive practice and much-needed change (Nelson, 2018).

Source: Nelson, L.E. (2018, January 14). It happened to me: Racism and health care. *The Globe and Mail.* Retrieved from https://www.theglobeandmail.com/news/national/what-its-like-to-deal-with-racism-in-canadas-health-caresystem/article37600473/.

INTRODUCTION

Nursing is organized within a context of complex, rapidly changing, and interconnected contemporary global political, social, and economic environments. In this context, the nursing profession is also embedded within multiple sites and forms of visible and invisible **oppression**, where one group or individual uses power to maintain privilege and dominance over another. Many of the concepts of **social justice** that have previously framed nursing knowledge and practice do not fully address the dimensions of power or sufficiently work to challenge such deep, and often taken for granted, structures of oppression (Tuck & Yang, 2012; Smith, 2019). This chapter sets out to identify key dimensions of oppression and **allyship** in nursing, where nurses coming from dominant or privileged groups take action to reject and dismantle conditions of oppression (Happell, Scholz, Gordon et al., 2018). This chapter focuses on a broad notion of **diversity**, **culture** including **ethnicity** and **race** as well as diversity with respect to gender identity, age, and ability diversity (among others). Awareness, allyship, and **action** are relevant to the profession in terms of nursing practice and the health of **clients** and communities, as well as the development of the profession as a relevant, responsive, and respectful institution. (Note that the term client is used in this chapter. It implies collaboration and partnership and is more consistent with allyship and anti-oppressive practice than other terms used to refer to the people and groups nurses work with.) This integrated understanding of diversity, disparities, and social determinants of health is increasingly recognized as central to the relevance of the profession and a framework for the future (Villarruel, Bigelow, & Alvarez, 2014).

Here, we particularly emphasize allyship in regard to Indigenous culture as well as strategies for providing nursing care that result in culturally competent and safe service to clients. A review of the history of health care and nursing in early settler Canada serves to illustrate how the profession can learn and grow from carefully analyzing the ways in which oppression and **colonization** have materialized and impacted health, knowledge, and the nursing profession.

In early settler Canada, Indigenous knowledge heavily influenced health care, as Westernized medicine drew upon Indigenous peoples' practices (Donahue, 2010; McCallum, 2014). However, the rapid influx of settlers, along with advances in Western medicine, fundamentally transformed the relationship between Indigenous peoples and early nursing leaders, creating and sustaining disparities in nursing knowledge development (McCallum, 2007, 2008). Historical suppression of Indigenous nursing and knowledge systems is associated with the marginalization of traditional practices and poorer health outcomes for Indigenous peoples (Goodman, Fleming, Markwick et al., 2017).

Core values, beliefs, and practices associated with Indigenous worldviews are evidence of an adaptive integrity that is as valid for today's generations as for generations past. Nonetheless, the values, beliefs, and practices of professional health knowledge continue to deny and obscure the complex and direct relationship of Indigenous knowledge practices to Indigenous wellness (Wood, Kamper & Swanson, 2018). The dominance of Western health knowledge and beliefs continues to overshadow Indigenous wellness perspectives, creating barriers for Indigenous peoples seeking health services that respect Indigenous ways of being, knowing, and doing. Health research is highlighting the role that health care providers and health policy play in supporting systemic discrimination against and mistreatment of Indigenous clients and communities.

To develop the profession in a way that supports care for all clients as well as professional and social change, diversity must be understood with a view toward developing **anti-oppressive practice** as a professional value. Awareness, allyship, and anti-oppressive practice involve not just accepting and valuing people of different cultures, ages, genders, sexual orientation, abilities, and all lifestyles, beliefs, and practices, but seeking to dismantle the forces and contexts of oppression and colonization (Gray, 2018). This chapter introduces **relational practice** and how it establishes a path toward **awareness** and action, as well as anti-oppressive practices from a minimalist approach, positive action, equality schemes, and mainstreaming equal opportunities.

AWARENESS: OPPRESSION AND COLONIZATION

Awareness is foundational to anti-oppressive practice and sets the stage for allyship and action. Nurses' personal awareness of the privilege afforded to the dominant biomedical model and the power afforded to their role as nurses is critical to building and strengthening trusted, helping relationships and getting beyond the conditions that sustain inequities (Smith, 2019; Van Herk, Smith, & Andrew, 2011). Through awareness, allies understand and name oppression, including how it is organized, held together, and sustained both formally and informally. Being an ally involves "taking responsibility for one's own learning, acknowledging unearned privilege, and being willing to be confronted, to consider change, and to commit to action" (Spencer, 2008, p. 101). As discussed in Chapter 5, Feminist theory and postcolonial theory seek to understand and provide ways of understanding oppression and colonization. An **intersectionality** paradigm has arisen from these feminist and postcolonial theories and attends to, and enables, a view into the range of experiences within shared experiences of oppression, something that is often obscured in dominant viewpoints in nursing and health care (Van Herk, Smith, & Andrew, 2011). Additionally, both feminist and postcolonial theory provide analyses of power relations, with a particular concern for the objectification, subordination, and commodification of people and land (Tuck & Yang, 2012).

Awareness in an intersectional paradigm calls for just such wider analyses, knowing that there is always more to be known. Awareness requires humility, self-evaluation, continual learning, and perseverance to illuminate the best path for action. In both anti-oppressive and decolonizing practices, particular attention is paid to relationships, justice, truth, and power (Tuck & Yang, 2012). Decolonizing practices require, in part, some of these same processes and attributes of relationship and justice through awareness and allyship. **Decolonization,** however, is specifically concerned with dismantling the systematic oppression of Indigenous peoples, Indigenous culture, and the sites of oppression from colonization. **Decolonizing practices** are hard and unsettling work with and by Indigenous communities concerning settler relations. This is work that requires a commitment to truth and reconciliation and a right relationship with people and place.

For the scope and purposes of this chapter, broad dimensions of oppression are explored. We exclude discussion about the diverse groups and individuals with whom nurses work, the people who face oppression every day and with whom the profession must ally to advocate for and provide safe and effective care. Nurses provide care for diverse clients, and nurses themselves are diverse. Diversity and diverse groups' concerns are highlighted with a specific emphasis on the concerns of Indigenous peoples. Health inequity among Indigenous populations continues to widen despite advances in Indigenous health research (Greenwood, De Leeuw, & Lindsay, 2018). Although Canada's universal health care system is considered one of the best in the world, Indigenous populations continue to experience much poorer health outcomes due to the legacies and intersections of colonialism and **racism** (Allan & Smylie, 2015). Calls for an immediate response to increasing the number of Indigenous health care providers and programs aimed at improving Indigenous health are priorities outlined in the Truth and Reconciliation Commission of Canada's (2015) Calls to Action.

While professional nursing codes and standards provide guidance, acknowledging, confronting, and transforming oppressive practices is the work of everyone within the profession (Lancellotti, 2008). All nurses, for example, are responsible for ensuring that nursing practice is culturally congruent with and culturally responsive to the beliefs of the individuals, families, groups, organizations, and communities that nurses serve. At times, the very codes and norms require scrutiny for their taken-for-granted assumptions that perpetuate oppression and racism (Smith, 2019).

AWARENESS: DIVERSITY, CULTURE, RACE, AND ETHNICITY

Nurses work with people from a variety of backgrounds and identities, and the profession as a whole must be informed by common and unique experiences of diversity, culture, race, and ethnicity in nursing practice. Diversity in a cultural context considers similarities, differences, and power relations across age, gender, race, religion, occupation, **sexual orientation**, and poverty (Campinha-Bacote, 2002; Lowe & Archibald, 2009; Racine & Petrucka, 2011; Spector, 2012). The two types of diversity are visible and invisible (Clair, Beatty, & MacLean, 2005). Visible diversity includes attributes such as age, physical appearance, and gender identification (Clair, Beatty, & MacLean, 2005). People who are visibly diverse have a greater risk of experiencing discrimination, **stereotyping**, and marginalization (Srivastava, 2007). Invisible diversity includes attributes that are not readily seen, such as religion, national origin, occupation, sexual orientation, and illness. Consideration must also be given to people who are invisibly diverse, such as people with disabilities and those who are neurodiverse, because their inconspicuous attributes may not be acknowledged (Srivastava, 2007).

Throughout this chapter, the two terms **visible minority** and **racially visible** will be used, as they are the terms used by Statistics Canada under the *Employment Equity Act*. According to Statistics Canada (2015c), the term visible minority is used to describe people of colour; that is, people who are neither Indigenous nor white. However, the term racially visible is more accurate in describing diverse aggregates and indicates visible diversity by way of colour. Srivastava (2007) and Nestel (2012) identify limitations that occur when the terms visible minority or people of colour are used: heterogeneous groups of people of colour are slotted into one category, which ignores class and ethnic differences. In health care, this practice, known as **racializing,** has many of the pitfalls of categorization, including

bias, discrimination, and limiting opportunities for diversity (Varcoe, Browne, Wong et al., 2009). Being able to identify the limitations of these terms and their implications for health care enables nurses to embrace their roles as allies and take action against the oppression and racism that deeply impact individual and community health as well as professional practice.

The concepts of culture, race, and ethnicity also influence our understanding of human beliefs, perceptions, and behaviour as well as actions in health care practice (Napier, Arcano, Butler et al., 2014). Culture provides direction on the appropriate behaviours for situations in everyday life (Allender & Spradley, 2005). It also provides cues to nurses on how individuals may interact—but not as a predictive or in any way essentialist frame. The terms "race" and "ethnicity" are used to identify distinguishable groups within cultures (Jarvis, 2004). However, the imprecise use of these terms is problematic and can cause misidentification of various populations and a limited scope of understanding (Bourque Bearskin, 2011; Nestel, 2012).

Although culture has many definitions, Srivastava (2007) defines it as "a term that applies to all groups of people where there are common values and ways of thinking and acting that differ from those of another group" (p. 15). Srivastava also describes culture using the acronym CULTURE, where C is commonly, U is understood, L is learned, T is traditions, U is unconscious, R is rules of, and E is engagement.

Culture has six distinguishing features:

1. Culture is learned. It is based on the events and experiences that we internalize as we grow and develop from infancy onward. We are not born with culture.
2. Culture is adaptive. It adjusts to environmental and technological changes that occur over time.
3. Culture is dynamic. It is not static. It responds to changes created by new situations and demands.
4. Culture is invisible. It is something one experiences. It is apparent through rituals, language, celebrations, and dress.
5. Culture is shared. Persons from the same culture identify with the same values, beliefs, and patterns of behaviour, yet maintain individuality. Everyone is unique.
6. Culture is selective. It differentiates between outsiders and insiders through boundaries for desirable, acceptable, or unacceptable behaviour. It also influences how people view and respond to situations and issues. (Srivastava, 2007, p. 15)

Race is primarily a social classification based on an imagined hierarchy of human value that relies on phenotypes, skin colour, and other expressions of group superiority and inferiority to identify group membership (Nestel, 2012). Individuals may be of the same race but of different ethnicities and cultures. For example, Black people—who may have been born in Africa, the Caribbean, North America, or elsewhere—are a heterogeneous group, but they are often (wrongly) viewed as culturally and racially homogeneous.

Racism and other forms of oppression (for example, through social exclusion, medicalizing social issues) operate to produce health inequities and limit professional knowledge and agency (McGibbon, 2012). McGibbon and Etowa (2009) promote antiracist frameworks to guide the profession and to prevent the many forms of racism that often become invisible to nurses. For example, individual racism, internalized racism, systemic racism, environmental racism, and cultural racism negatively affect health status. Awareness and understanding of the different varieties of racism enables nurses to be more culturally sensitive and to adopt aspects of cultural safety, a topic that will be discussed later in this chapter.

Ethnicity is the state of belonging to a social group that shares common cultural patterns (e.g., beliefs, values, customs, behaviours, and traditions). It is influenced by education, income level, geographic location, and association with individuals from ethnic groups other than one's own. Therefore, a reciprocal relationship exists between the individual and society. Some examples of ethnicity are Berbers, Chinese, Greek, Irish, Italian, Peruvian, Ukrainian, Tuareg, and Vietnamese. Ethnicity is used more often than race to identify and categorize individuals (Srivastava, 2007).

KEY DEMOGRAPHICS FOR NURSING IN CANADA

In Canada, key demographic groups that have implications for awareness, allyship, and action in nursing are the aging older adult population, people with disabilities, Indigenous peoples, and **immigrant** communities. Demographic trends are important for the nursing profession in many ways, as they can help to inform professional position statements and advocacy for city or municipal design as well as social, health, and community services planning. For example, the rapidly growing aging and immigrant populations will affect planning for translators/interpreters, adapted/accessible/universal design, and the location of health care services. Awareness of people's diverse needs can support allyship and action to obtain supports and resources that may be otherwise out of the dominant, privileged view.

For instance, awareness of the experiences of a demographic group in a particular region could alert decision makers to a community's inequitable access to transportation or the additional sexual health support services required in a community. Professional associations, which are both part of and unique to the national Canadian Nurses Association, play a role in this allyship and action.

An Aging Population

Demographic trends around age, such as an aging population, an increase in older adults living in suburban neighbourhoods, and the overall declining birth rate, highlight the diversity of health needs and concerns. A key contributor to the changing demographic landscape in Canada is the growing older adult population. This trend has emerged because people are living longer (Statistics Canada, 2018). About 1 in 6 Canadians is aged 65 years and older, and this proportion is steadily increasing (Statistics Canada, 2014). In 2011, more people were aged 55 to 64 than the number that were aged 15 to 24 (Statistics Canada, 2012b). In 2014, older adults represented 15.7% of the population, and this percentage is projected to rise to between 24% and 28% by 2063 (Statistics Canada, 2014).

The largest proportion of older adults live in the Atlantic provinces, while the Western provinces and Northern Territories have the youngest populations (Statistics Canada, 2014). The fastest-aging population is reported to be in Newfoundland and Labrador (Statistics Canada, 2014). A growing number of older adults are living in Canadian suburbs, which has important implications for older adult belonging, community connection, and health and well-being in those areas (Jakubec, Olfert, Choi et al., 2019; Statistics Canada, 2011a) (Figure 14.1). Age discrimination impacts people of all ages. It has implications for the practice of nursing and in the organization of an increasingly intergenerational workforce with diverse abilities and perspectives (Kydd & Fleming, 2015; Stanley, 2010).

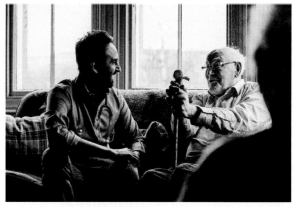

Fig. 14.1 Demographic trends of an aging population are highlighting discourses and discrimination related to both aging and disabilities within the nursing profession. (istock.com/Dean Mitchell)

Indigenous Peoples

Prior to European contact, an estimated 500,000 Indigenous peoples lived in what is now known as Canada. By 1871, this population was reduced to 102,000 because of Indigenous peoples' lack of immunity to influenza, small-pox, measles, and tuberculosis (Indian and Northern Affairs Canada, 1996). Early European immigrants forced First Nations, Inuit, and Métis communities to relocate and claimed the land and resources as their own. This displacement has caused First Nations, Inuit, and Métis communities to become resistant to the government's agenda to control and monopolize Canadian resources through its numerous assimilation policies (Indian and Northern Affairs Canada, 1996). Early colonization and assimilation policies—which led to residential schools, the Sixties Scoop, and other harmful child welfare practices—are today considered cultural genocide of Indigenous peoples. The influx of settler **newcomers** and government policies continues to perpetuate similarly oppressive and racist practices in contemporary health care systems, all of which have detrimental impacts on health, well-being, and professional practice.

The disastrous legacy of European colonization is captured in *Out of Sight*, a report about the death of Brian Sinclair, an Indigenous man who died in 2008 while waiting for care for 36 hours in a Winnipeg emergency room. The report states that Sinclair was killed by racism and that the subsequent inquest into his death did not address the real problem (Browne, Hill, Lavallee, et al., 2017). Though inquests, governmental apologies, and changes are issued, allyship and action at all levels of influence, including antiracist organizing and protest within the nursing profession, are still very much in early development in Canada. Advocacy for client safety and safe work environments (such as those in Nova Scotia; Figure 14.2) must consider racism and other oppressive practices that place clients and populations at risk.

White privilege and colonization are only beginning to be understood as part of professional nursing history, resulting in an unsettling of colonial assumptions and some tensions that have yet to be addressed (Smith, 2019). DiAngelo (2011) describes the unsettling and tensions with the concept of "white fragility," asserting that white people are protected from racial stress because of pervasive social environments. Individual claims that "I am not a racist" or defensiveness about the "good intentions of the nursing profession" at a broader level are mechanisms that reinforce white privilege and hinder **cultural safety**.

In Canada, Indigenous peoples are now the fastest-growing population in the country. At 1.4 million, they represent almost 4.3% of Canada's population. Of these, 61% self-identify as First Nations people, 32.3% as Métis, and 4.2%

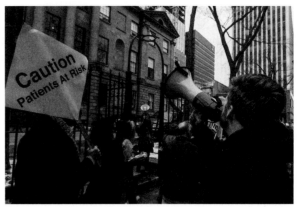

Fig. 14.2 A nursing protest in Nova Scotia to advocate for quality health care. (istock.com/shauni)

as Inuit (Statistics Canada, 2013b). The term Indigenous often refers to the original inhabitants of a country who identify with a particular heritage based on their home nation and/or linguistic family. The following brief introduction on the diversity of First Nations people, Inuit, and Métis living in Canada presents statistics for each group to provide a greater understanding of the differences among them.

First Nations People

Canada has more than 600 different First Nations communities (Statistics Canada, 2013b), each with its own unique history, language, traditions, art, and ceremonies. Some First Nations people identify with their linguistic group (e.g., Cree, Blackfoot, Dené, or Chipewyan), whereas others identify with their community of origin (e.g., Blood Tribe or Beaver Lake Cree Nation) or treaty area (e.g., Treaty 6 or Treaty 7). The most important means of Canadian control over First Nations communities was and still is the *Indian Act*, which consolidated the various laws relating to "Indians" (a now-outdated term) that was passed by the Canadian government in the years since Confederation and by the British colonial authorities before them.

Inuit

Three quarters of Inuit in Canada reside in 53 communities spread across the Northwest Territories, Yukon, Nunavut, Northern Quebec, and Labrador (Indigenous and Northern Affairs Canada, 2015). Over 90% of these communities are accessible by air only. Inuit communities are located in four land-claim regions: Nunatsiavut (Labrador), Nunavik (Northern Quebec), Nunavut Territory, and Inuvialuit Settlement Region (Northwest Territories and Yukon). Of the Inuit who live in southern Canada, about half live in cities. The largest populations are in Edmonton, Montreal, Ottawa, Yellowknife, and St. John's (Indigenous and Northern Affairs Canada, 2015).

Métis

The Métis National Council (n.d.) defines a Métis as "a person who self-identifies as Métis, is distinct from other Aboriginal peoples, is of historic Métis Nation Ancestry and who is accepted by the Métis Nation." The "historic Métis Nation" refers to the Indigenous people historically known as Métis, or mixed blood (with parents of Indigenous and European ancestry), who resided in the "historic Métis Nation Homeland," an area of land in west-central North America used and occupied as the traditional territory of the Métis. "Métis Nation" refers to the Indigenous people descended from the historic Métis Nation, which now comprises all Métis Nation citizens. Métis are members of the "Aboriginal peoples of Canada" per section 35 of the *Constitution Act, 1982*. Métis have their own distinct dialect (the Michif language) but are also diverse linguistically, with their language depending on ancestry (e.g., Cree, Dené, English, French).

Immigrant Communities

With the development and colonization of Canada came an influx of immigrants into the country. Historically, the patterns of immigration to Canada have changed over time, with a variety of places of origin represented. Many immigrants have come from Europe, Asia, the United States, Africa, and the Caribbean. Often, people's reasons for leaving their country of origin have included lack of economic prosperity, persecution, and war.

Citizenship and Immigration Canada (2016a) and the *Immigration and Refugee Protection Act* delineate permanent resident status categories such as economic classes (e.g., federal skilled trades class, live-in caregivers) and noneconomic classes (e.g., family members, people seeking humanitarian and compassionate consideration). This classification also defines the temporary status of residents as temporary workers, students, and visitors (Citizenship and Immigration Canada, 2016b).

Canada's ethnocultural composition has also changed over time. While in the past, immigrants came mainly from European countries, currently the largest source of immigrants is Asia, accounting for 61% of newcomers to Canada (Statistics Canada, 2017). The number of people immigrating from African countries is increasing and newcomers from Africa account for 13% of newcomers, outranking European newcomers for the first time (Statistics Canada, 2017). About 1 in 5 people in Canada are foreign born, representing about 21% of the overall population (Statistics Canada, 2017). About half of the foreign born population is from Asia and just under 10% are from Africa (Statistics Canada, 2017).

The majority of newcomers move to urban centres in Ontario, British Columbia, Quebec, and Alberta (Statistics Canada, 2017). However, an increasing number of newcomers are moving to urban centres in the Prairies. Toronto, Vancouver, and Montreal are the most racially and culturally diverse cities in Canada. Changes to the *Citizenship Act* in 2015 have required immigrants to prove that they have an attachment to Canada and are contributing to the economy. These changes are impacting where new immigrants choose to take up residence.

Canada has a history of admitting large numbers of immigrants of various ethnic origins. In 2015, Canada planned to welcome 260,000 to 285,000 new permanent residents, 65% of which were economic immigrants (Citizenship and Immigration Canada, 2015). In 2017, Canada admitted 321,035 permanent residents. This is the highest number of permanent residents admitted to Canada since 1913. Of this total, 45,758 people were admitted as refugees and protected persons (Immigration, Refugees and Citizenship Canada, 2018).

TYPES OF DIVERSITY

In Canada, diversity is expressed in many ways, including ethnic, religious, linguistic, sexual (also discussed in Chapter 5 Gender in Nursing), age, and physical abilities (which also relates to age). Understanding that diversity is expressed and experienced uniquely in the population, but with shared concerns and issues around social determinants of health (discussed further in Chapter 11), is essential to advocacy and supporting client strengths in an asset-based approach to nursing practice.

Ethnic Diversity

Over 200 ethnic groups live in Canada, with 13 of these groups having populations of over 1 million people. In 2011, visible minorities represented 19.1% of the total population, of which 30.9% were born in Canada and 65.1% were born outside of Canada. The median age of the visible minority population was about 7 years younger than that of the total population (Statistics Canada, 2013f). In all, 4% of the visible minority population consisted of nonpermanent residents (Statistics Canada, 2013f). Visible minorities are projected to represent an ever-increasing proportion of the population. For example, in 2031, it is estimated that 55% of the foreign-born population in Canada could be born in Asia and 20% in Europe (Statistics Canada 2010b). The nursing profession in Canada will need to consider training and development needs for direct care and both services and community development to address the realities of these changing demographics.

The ethnocultural population varies according to generations. The 2011 census indicated that 22% of the overall Canadian population was first-generation Canadian (born outside of Canada). Second-generation Canadians accounted for 17.4% of the overall population and are defined as individuals born in Canada but with one or both parents born outside of Canada. Third-generation Canadians accounted for 60.7% of the overall population and are defined as individuals born in Canada with parents who were also born in Canada. Three out of 10 second-generation Canadians were visible minorities. The median age of all second-generation visible minorities was 13.6 years, whereas the median age of the second generation who are not visible minorities was 43.4 years (Statistics Canada, 2013e).

Canada's ethnic mix is changing rapidly, particularly in urban areas, mainly because of increased rates of non-European immigration in recent decades. Immigrants make up an increasingly large proportion of the population. This means that a growing number of Canadians do not speak English or French as their mother tongue. Most, however, are able to at least carry out a conversation in one of the official languages. Furthermore, more and more Canadians identify with a religion other than Christianity. These changing demographics affect how health care is delivered to large segments of the community and the ability of newcomers to access health care.

Nurses' awareness of the context and circumstances of their clients is highly consequential to the quality of care and outcomes for the diversity of newcomers to Canada. A newcomer is a person who arrives in a new country to settle there for a variety of reasons and with a variety of backgrounds and experiences. Newcomers come from all parts of the world and bring with them unique cultural, health care, and religious backgrounds. Newcomers include immigrants, **refugees**, and persons in need of protection. An **immigrant** is a person who has chosen to live in Canada and has been accepted by the Government of Canada and who may apply for permanent residency. A **refugee** is a person who was forced to leave their home country because of a well-founded fear of persecution or because of war. By contrast, a person in need of protection is a person who cannot return to their country because of a risk of torture, a risk of cruel and unusual treatment or punishment, or a risk to their life; consequently, they have been given protection by the Government of Canada (Government of Canada, 2019b).

Newcomers may have limited access to health care if they lack health care benefits, financial and social resources, English or French language abilities, and transportation. Nurses need to consider the background of newcomer clients. Often, the community and the family (if available) must be relied on to provide information, support, and other aid. Nurses also need to know the major health concerns and risk factors for the cultural groups they work with, such as vulnerability to specific diseases, and consider related social determinants of health.

Nurses must consider the following dimensions of inequity and oppression that influence the health of individuals, families, groups, and the community (Beckmann Murray, Proctor Zentner, Pangman et al., 2009):

- *Language barriers;*
- *Low literacy levels;*
- *Poverty and economic constraints (higher for refugees than for immigrants);*
- *Discrimination by health care providers;*
- *Health care providers' lack of knowledge about high-risk diseases in the newcomer groups they care for;*
- *Reliance by many newcomers on traditional healing or folk health care practices that may be unfamiliar to their Canadian health care providers; and*

RESEARCH FOCUS

Making Access to Primary Health Care Services Easier

Immigrant and refugee families from Africa form a growing proportion of the population in Manitoba. This study examined African immigrant and refugee families' ($n = 83$) experiences of access to primary health care in Manitoba, including the barriers to accessing this care. Qualitative data were collected in open-ended interviews conducted in six different languages and analyzed for key themes. Challenges in the families' pursuits of primary health care were represented by three themes: (1) expectations not quite met, (2) facing a new life, and (3) let's buddy up to improve access. With "expectations not quite met," families struggled to understand a new health system while facing barriers that included lengthy wait times, shortages of health care providers, high cost of medication and nonbasic health care, and in some cases suboptimal care. With "facing a new life," immigrant and refugee families expressed challenges adjusting to their new and unfamiliar environments with social barriers (such as transportation, employment, language and cultural differences, and a lack of social support) that impacted access to health care services. Privately sponsored families and families with children experienced even less social support. With the theme of "let's buddy up to improve access," networking approaches were suggested by families as ways to engage and improve their access to primary health care services. To improve access, the authors recommended that decision makers develop culturally relevant programs, collaborative networking approaches, and policies that focus on addressing social determinants of health.

Source: Woodgate, R., Crockett, M., Dean, R., et al. (2017). A qualitative study on African immigrant and refugee families' experiences of accessing primary health care services in Manitoba, Canada: It's not easy! *International Journal for Equity in Health, 16*(1), 5. https://doi.org/10.1186/s12939-016-0510-x.

• *Physical and mental health problems, which are higher for refugees than immigrants.* (p. 210)

When working with newcomer populations, nurses need to recognize that their own background, beliefs, and knowledge may differ significantly from those of their clients. Moving beyond awareness as the starting place within the profession, nurses must next assess how both their privilege and lack of awareness may interfere with nursing care. Deeper orientation to the role of family and community and knowledge of strengths, resources, and talents are perspectives that can be taught to nurses and revisited continually as demographics change.

Population projections are estimates of how a population will grow and change in the future. Statistics Canada data indicate important trends in Canadian demographics by the year 2031:

• 3 in 10 Canadians (between 29% and 32%) could be a visible minority (i.e., South Asian, Chinese, Arab, West Asian, Black, Filipino, Latin American, Japanese, or Korean) (Statistics Canada, 2010b).
• The population that is not from a visible minority group is also projected to grow between 2001 and 2017, but at a slower rate of only 1% to 7% (Statistics Canada, 2010a).
• Visible minorities will continue to live in urban centres. Almost 96% of the racially visible population will live in census metropolitan areas, with more than 71% residing in Toronto, Vancouver, and Montreal (Statistics Canada, 2010b).

In 2011, South Asian, Chinese, and Black people formed the largest racially visible groups in Canada, representing 61.3% of the overall visible minority population, with Arabs and West Asians making up the fastest-growing segment of the population (Statistics Canada, 2013f). Projections for 2031 indicate that approximately 36% of visible minorities will be under 15 years of age and 18% will be over 65 years of age (Statistics Canada, 2010b). Nurses need to be aware of these changing demographic patterns to effectively advocate for services and uncover where existing programs may unintentionally limit access or oppress certain groups.

Table 14.1 presents population projections for 2031 on the median age of different groups in Canada. These statistical projections have implications for policy development and health care service delivery. For example, First Nations people, Inuit, and Métis and visible minorities will be, on average, much younger than the rest of the population (Statistics Canada, 2015c, 2015d). These age projections might be used to advocate for heath equity and social justice, to lend support for the continuation or expansion of existing programs or the development of new programs that better respond to age-based client health concerns.

TABLE 14.1 Projections for 2031 Median Age of Racially Visible and Indigenous Groups and the Rest of Canada

Group	2031 Projections (Median Age in Years)
Racially visible*	35.5
Canadian-born	16.6
Born outside of Canada	44.3
Rest of Canada[†]	43.3
Indigenous peoples	26.6
Rest of Canada[‡]	43.1

*Refers to Chinese, South Asian, Black, Filipino, Latin American, Southeast Asian, Arab, West Asian, Japanese, and Korean groups and excludes Indigenous peoples.
[†]Refers to all persons, including Indigenous peoples, but not persons included under "racially visible."
[‡]Refers to all persons, including racially visible, but not Indigenous peoples.
Sources: Statistics Canada. (2010). *Projections of the diversity of the Canadian population: 2006–2031.* Ottawa, ON: Minister of Industry. Retrieved from http://www.statcan.gc.ca/pub/91-551-x/91-551-x2010001-eng.pdf; Statistics Canada. (2015b). *Population projections by Aboriginal identity in Canada, 2006 to 2031.* Retrieved from http://www.statcan.gc.ca/pub/91-552-x/2011001/hl-fs-eng.htm.

Multiculturalism

In 1971, Canada was the first country to adopt **multiculturalism** as an official policy. Multiculturalism recognizes the diverse ancestry of citizens and supports the ideals of equality and mutual respect among the population's ethnic and cultural groups (Burnet & Driedger, 2011). In some cases, multiculturalism is seen as a protective wellness factor within diverse populations. School policies on multiculturalism were found to be a protective factor for students who experienced interpersonal violence in school environments (Le & Johansen, 2011).

Some critics of multiculturalism argue that it downplays the special status of Indigenous peoples and French Canadians (Citizenship and Immigration Canada, 2010). Others suggest that multiculturalism could be viewed as another form of assimilation and colonialism that further marginalizes diverse populations (Turner, 2006). Multiculturalism is less popular in Quebec than in other provinces because of the belief that the federal government's multicultural policy minimizes Quebec's nationalist aspirations (Citizenship and Immigration Canada, 2010). Quebec emphasizes a multiethnic policy—a form of interculturalism that aims to preserve historical identity and achieve sovereignty within the Canadian state (Parliament of Canada, 2018).

Linguistic Diversity

Language is the basis of culture and fundamental to how people make sense of their everyday lives. Language is a universal tool for translating information and knowledge within cultural groups, and each language has its own nuances, meanings, rules, and symbols (Hoffman-Goetz, Donelle, & Ahmed, 2014). The National Collaborating Centre for Indigenous Health considers language to be a social determinant of health that is essential to improving health outcomes for Indigenous peoples (Reading & Wien, 2013).

More than 200 languages are spoken in Canada. The proportion of the population that speaks English most often, with or without a language other than French, is 37.9%. The proportion of the population that speaks French most often, with or without a language other than English, is 4.2%. Between 2006 and 2011, the English–French bilingualism rate rose minimally, from 17.4% to 17.5%. The proportion of people that speaks a language other than English or French (Canada's two official languages) at home is 20%. At the same time, two-thirds of people who speak a nonofficial language at home also speak English or French (Statistics Canada, 2012d).

The proportion of Canadians who are **allophones,** or people whose first language is neither French nor English, is thought to be between 21% and 25% (Statistics Canada, 2011b). This means that one-fifth of the Canadian population speaks an immigrant language in their home on a regular basis (Statistics Canada, 2011b); 80% of this population lives in one of Canada's six largest cities. Chinese languages continue to be the most frequently used in the homes of the immigrant population. The number of people who speak Tagalog, a Philippine-based language, increased the most (+64%) between 2006 and 2011 (Statistics Canada, 2012d). The most common immigrant language is Punjabi (Statistics Canada, 2012c). The use of multiple languages at home increased from 9.1% in 2006 to 11.5% in 2011. Interestingly, of the 6.4 million people who speak a language other than English or French at home, 25,000 reported using sign language at home (Statistics Canada, 2012d).

Among the more than 60 Indigenous languages in Canada, the largest language family is Algonquian, which includes Cree, Ojibway, Innu/Montagnais, and Oji-Cree. Those whose first language is Algonquian live mainly in Saskatchewan, Manitoba, Alberta, Quebec, Nova Scotia, and New Brunswick (Statistics Canada, 2012a). Not all people who reported speaking an Indigenous language at home reported it as their mother tongue; that is, they reported another language (e.g., English or French) as their primary language, indicating that they may be learning an Indigenous language as another language at school. One in six Indigenous peoples reported being able to conduct a conversation in their mother tongue, with 22% of First Nations people, 2.5% of Métis, and 63% of Inuit able to do so (Statistics Canada, 2013a). In addition, 18.7% of First Nations people, 1.8% of Métis, and 58.7% of Inuit reported an Indigenous language as their primary language. This trend indicates that more people who self-identify as learning to speak Indigenous languages are reporting it as their primary language (Statistics Canada, 2012f). The highest proportion of people who reported having an Indigenous mother tongue live in Quebec (20%), Manitoba (17.7%), and Saskatchewan (16%) (Statistics Canada, 2012a).

Language is obviously an important part of the everyday expression of a profession's work. Language strongly impacts relationships with clients and other members of the health care team as well as the reputation of the profession. Respectful, relational nursing care requires a deep commitment to developing therapeutic communication, and attention to what is both spoken and unspoken.

Nurses must be aware of language that enacts disrespect, racism, and discrimination, including **microaggressions**—the subtle, often automatic, and unconscious verbal and nonverbal slights, insults, and disparaging messages directed toward people in relation to their gender, age, disability, and cultural or racial group membership (Sue, 2010). These expressions are perceived as racist by racialized targets, and while they rarely reflect vindictive intent, inadvertently inflict insult and create unsafe environments for work, services, or care; when unchecked in our institutions and professions, microaggressions contribute to and reinforce systemic racism (Fleras, 2016).

Particularly well hidden in professional nursing discourse are these unchecked patterns of microaggressions—manifested in the terminology used, the subtle comments, the hidden normalization, and the practices of oppression—upheld by a long history of racism within the nursing profession. The extent to which white privilege and colonialism are embedded in the language of science, medicine, nursing, and health have contributed to the subtle and not-so-subtle forms of racism in the nursing profession (Smith, 2019).

Religious Diversity

According to the 2011 National Household Survey, 67.3% of Canadians reported that they were affiliated with Christianity. In addition, 7.2% of Canadians reported affiliation with Islam, Hinduism, Sikhism, or Buddhism. The proportion of the population that reported having no religious affiliation was 23.9% (an increase of about 7% from 10 years earlier). Roman Catholics comprise the largest Christian denomination in Canada, with the largest number living in Quebec and Ontario. In all, 4.5% of the Indigenous population reported an affiliation to traditional Indigenous spirituality, representing 0.2% of the overall Canadian population (Statistics Canada, 2013f). Census data projections suggest that the number of non-Christians will more than double by 2031 (Statistics Canada, 2010b).

Sexual Diversity

Canadians have become much more accepting of—and open to celebrating—sexual diversity. In 2005, after a long series of court battles over same-sex marriage, Canada became the fourth country in the world to legalize same-sex marriage through the *Civil Marriage Act, 2005.* Ten years later, in 2015, a landmark ruling in the United States made same-sex marriage a nationwide legal right there. According to the 2011 census, the number of same-sex couple families in Canada was up by 42% from 2006, and same-sex marriages tripled during the same time period (Statistics Canada, 2012e).

Practice and policy in community health has begun to consider the sexual diversity of clients, including different sexual orientations and gender identities, same-sex families, and gender transitions from female to male and male to female. Nurses should understand sexual diversity to be able to support their **LGBTQ2** clients in a nondiscriminatory manner—and to ally with clients to address discrimination and oppression. As discussed at length in Chapter 5, the acronym LGBTQ2 stands for lesbian, gay, bisexual, transgender, and two-spirit. Sexual orientation refers to how people think of themselves in terms of their sexual attraction to people, whereas gender identity indicates one's personal sense of gender. Within an Indigenous context, individuals who feel that their body has both a masculine and feminine spirit may refer to themselves as two-spirited (Wilson, 1996). Understanding the language of sexual diversity is important for building knowledge and sensitivity that informs community health practices and policies.

Scientific and medical sources vary considerably in their conception of sexual diversity because insufficient data have been collected on this topic and because sexual orientation and gender identity are generally underreported information. People do not always feel safe publicly reporting their gender identity or sexual orientation because they fear discrimination, **prejudice**, physical harm, or other expressions of hatred and intolerance (Hurley, 2010). Within the LGBTQ2 community itself, there is also a lack of information on sexual diversity (Scheim & Bauer, 2015). Recent statistics suggest that perhaps 0.5% of the adult population identifies as a **trans** person, broadly defined. In Ontario, an estimated 23% of trans people had completed social and medical gender transition. Like any group, the trans population is heterogeneous: some trans people will live in their felt gender full time and others part-time.

Nurses who understand sexual diversity will be better positioned to expose intolerance and oppression, which is apparent in the increased rates of hate crimes toward the LBGTQ2 community (Statistics Canada, 2015b). Consider that 28% of lesbian, gay, and bisexual youth are at higher risk for suicide versus 4% of heterosexual youth (Centre for Suicide Prevention, n.d.). In Ontario alone, 1 in 10 youth identify as LGBTQ2. Nurses who are open to discussing gender and sexuality in relation to health care can reduce these risk factors for LGBTQ2 clients.

Nurses must face health concerns regarding gender and sexuality with awareness and sensitivity. Most home health care providers have not felt comfortable asking specific questions about sexuality and gender because of a lack of knowledge regarding the appropriate terminology to use (Daley & MacDonnell, 2015). The Registered Nurses' Association of Ontario (Registered Nurses' Association of Ontario [RNAO], 2007) recommends that nurses receive education and training on human rights and health equity that address LGBTQ2 health issues. Cultivating an atmosphere of acceptance and understanding of LGBTQ2 identities requires people to change the belief that sexual identity is a private matter, when in fact it is a community health concern that requires public attention (Canadian Centre for Diversity and Inclusion, n.d.). These practices are only one aspect of allyship, however. Again, nurses must work at the systemic level to dismantle discrimination with the hallmarks of humility and continuous education. There is always more to be learned.

Disability and Diverse Abilities

Disability is a narrow term used to describe any impairment that restricts daily activities and participation. Almost 14% of Canadians aged 15 and over have a disability, over 42% of those with a disability are 75 years of age or older, and slightly more women than men have reported having a disability (Statistics Canada, 2013c). The most common types of disability are pain, flexibility, and mobility; these disability types are prevalent in 25% of adults with a disability aged 15 years and over (Statistics Canada, 2015a). Over 25% of people living with a disability report having a severe disability, and more than 8 out of 10 people use aids or assistive devices (Statistics Canada, 2013d).

The stereotypical view that people with a disability live with a specific injury or genetic predisposition such as deafness or blindness does not capture the full meaning of the concept. A nurse may encounter people with chronic or progressive mobility disorders; visual, hearing, or other sensory impairment; chronic illness; mental illness or problematic substance use; or cognitive or intellectual disabilities. Often a disability is an underlying reality, but serious consideration must be given to access to care or adaptive services when a person is seeking other health and support (e.g., immunization, postpartum care, trauma-informed care, or sexual health support). Access to social care and supports (e.g., housing, education, employment, and recreation and socialization activities) must also be considered for the health and well-being of people who experience the diversity of disabilities.

According to the World Health Organization (World Health Organization [WHO], 2015), disability rates are increasing because of an aging population and a rise in chronic health conditions. Chronic diseases are the largest cause of death worldwide (WHO, 2020). In Canada, 67% of deaths every year are caused by four major chronic conditions: cancer, diabetes, cardiovascular disease, or chronic respiratory disease (Public Health Agency of Canada, 2013). Chronic diseases cost the Canadian economy $190 billion per year, with $68 billion going to treatment and the rest to lost productivity (Elmslie, 2012).

Patterns of disability involve a range of personal factors (e.g., self-confidence, self-efficacy, and social supports), environmental factors (e.g., accessible housing, transit and walkways, and supported employment programs), and health conditions (e.g., psychological health, and physical injuries or illnesses). Individuals, families, and communities living with disabilities continue to have poorer health outcomes, lower educational achievement, and higher rates of poverty and social isolation. Historically, people with disabilities have been provided services that have led to segregation in institutions or hospital-type settings. However, many individuals have not allowed their disability to define who they are and lead productive and fulfilling lives. Understanding disability through a human rights lens requires nurses to think differently and become aware of issues that prevent people with disabilities from reaching their full potential when addressing activities of daily living.

In 2010, Canada ratified the UN Convention on the Rights of Persons with Disabilities. Included in the convention's articles are strategies that promote inclusion, awareness, collaboration, and engagement with all stakeholders from a human rights perspective. In its first report on the convention, the Government of Canada recognized that although progress had been made in increasing the inclusion and participation of people with disabilities, "there continues to be challenges, including barriers to language and communication, learning and training, and safety and security" (Government of Canada, 2014, p. 2). See Figure 14.3 for an example of an accessible ramp.

Awareness of the demographics and statistics around disability is just one area of concern for nurse allies. Awareness of the structural inequities and systemic

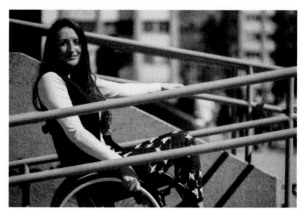

Fig. 14.3 Ramps and railings can provide access for people who use wheelchairs and other mobility aids as part of universal design. (istock.com/Constantinis)

oppression of people with disabilities is essential to supporting the health and well-being of all people. These inequities are discussed later in this chapter, including an elaboration on strategies for allyship.

DIVERSITY, DISCRIMINATION, AND THE DETERMINANTS OF HEALTH

The circumstances in our daily lives are shaped by the distribution of money, power, and resources globally, nationally, and locally as well as by public policy decisions. "The social determinants of health are mostly responsible for health inequities—the unfair and avoidable differences in health status seen within and between countries" (WHO, n.d.). Box 14.1 presents data that indicate how diversity—including race, immigrant or refugee status, access to health care, sexual diversity, ethnicity, gender, and disability—impacts the health of Canadians. From an equity perspective, the WHO (2008) recommends that actions on the social determinants of health focus on (1) improving living conditions; (2) tackling the inequitable distribution of power, money, and resources; and (3) measuring and understanding the problem and assessing the impact of action (p. 2). But for nurses, these are not simply recommendations or guidelines to consider. To act as allies in these crucial social transformations, nurses need to examine the underlying conditions that shape even seemingly unquestioned medical and nursing diagnoses, as well as how the social determinants of health and various challenges are organized and upheld— including through nursing's own privilege (Van Herk, Smith, & Andrew, 2011). For instance, nurses must ask why the experiences of racism, poverty, discrimination, access challenges, and so on, as described in Box 14.1, exist in Canada at this time?

BOX 14.1 Determinants of Health and Diversity

- 1 in 6 Canadian adults has experienced racism.*
- Racism is a form of social exclusion and a social determinant of health,†‡ and it contributes to lower income and social status, another social determinant of health.
- Racism not only has a direct effect on a person's health but also influences how health practitioners provide care.§
- People who have immigrant or refugee status are more likely to be refused health care and therefore are less likely to use preventive health care services.‖
- The use of health care services among visible minorities varies. For example, Japanese and Korean people tend to visit family physicians less often than South Asians.#
- Over 34% of lesbian, gay, or bisexual individuals self-reported living with extreme levels of stress, whereas almost 23% of the general Canadian population lives with high levels of stress.**
- Indigenous workers earn between 30% and 40% less than non-Indigenous workers with the same level of education.††
- In 2005, recent-immigrant men earned 63 cents for every dollar earned by Canadian-born men, and recent-immigrant women earned 56 cents for every dollar earned by Canadian-born women,‡‡ thereby contributing to lower socioeconomic status.

- Full-time working women make 20% less on average than full-time working men, which represents less than a 2% reduction in the gender gap over the last 20 years.††
- Visible minority workers with a high school diploma working full-time in the private sector earn 27% less than their nonvisible minority counterparts. This gap decreases by about 12% in the public sector.††
- Almost 66% of Indigenous children take part in sports regularly (about the same as non-Indigenous children), with Métis and Inuit children being the most involved in sports. First Nations children living off reserve have higher rates of sports participation than those living on reserve, and parents of Indigenous children participating in sports generally have higher levels of education and income than the parents of nonparticipating children.§§
- In 2006, 7.3% of the visible minority population in Canada was over 65 years of age compared with 13% of the total population,‡‡ indicating that, as a whole, the visible minority population is younger than the overall population in Canada.
- In 2012, 13.7% of the adult population in Canada reported limited daily activities due to a disability.‖

Sources:

* Ipsos-Reid. (2005). *March 21st, International Day for the Elimination of Racial Discrimination: One in six Canadians say they have been the victim of racism.* Retrieved from http://www.dominion.ca/Downloads/IRracismSurvey.pdf.

† Allan, B., & Smylie, J. (2015). *First peoples, second class treatment: The role of racism in the health and well-being of Indigenous peoples in Canada.* Toronto, ON: Wellesley Institute; Cameron, B., Carmargo Plazas, P., Santos Salas, A., et al. (2014). Understanding inequalities in access to healthcare services for Aboriginal people: A call for nursing action. *Advance Nursing Sciences, 37*(3), E1–E16. https://doi.org/10.1097/ans.0000000000000039.

‡ Mikkonen, J., & Raphael, D. (2010). *Social determinants of health: The Canadian facts.* Toronto, ON: York University School of Health Policy and Management. Retrieved from http://www.thecanadianfacts.org

§ Williams, D. R., & Mohammed, S. A. (2013). Racism and health I: Pathways and scientific evidence. *The American Behavioral Scientist, 57*(8), 1152–1173. https://doi.org/10.1177/0002764213487340.

‖ Pollock, G., Newbold, K. B., Lafranière, G., et al. (2012). Discrimination in the doctor's office: Immigrants and refugee experiences. *Critical Social Work, 13*(2), 60–79.

Quan, H., Fong, A., DeCoster, C., et al. (2006). Variation in health services utilization among ethnic populations. *Canadian Medical Association Journal, 174*(6), 787–791. https://doi.org/10.1503/cmaj.050674.

** Mental Health Commission of Canada. (2015). *Informing the future: Mental health indicators for Canada.* Retrieved from http://www.mentalhealthcommission.ca/English/document/68796/informing-future-mental-health-indicators-canada.

†† McInturrff, K., & Tulloch, P. (2014). *Narrowing the gap: The difference that public sector wages make.* Retrieved from https://www.policyalternatives.ca/publications/reports/narrowing-gap.

‡‡ Statistics Canada. (2009). *Earnings and incomes of Canadians over the past quarter century, 2006 census: Findings* (Cat. No. 97-563-XIE2006001). Ottawa, ON: Author. Retrieved from http://www12.statcan.ca/census-recensement/2006/as-sa/97-563/index-eng.cfm.

§§ Statistics Canada. (2007). *Study: Sports participation among Aboriginal children.* Retrieved from http://www.statcan.gc.ca/daily-quotidien/070710/dq070710b-eng.htm.

‖ Statistics Canada. (2013d). *Disability in Canada: Initial findings from the Canadian Survey on Disability.* Ottawa, ON: Minister of Industry. Retrieved from http://www.statcan.gc.ca/pub/89-654-x/89-654-x2013002-eng.pdf.

ANTI-OPPRESSIVE ACTION AND APPROACHES FOR THE NURSING PROFESSION

The nursing profession in Canada is taking a wide-ranging approach to addressing the oppressive practices and policies that operate to produce (and reproduce) health inequities (see Box 14.1) (Arya & Piggott, 2018). Numerous approaches, models, strategies, and skills exist to guide nurses in working with diverse populations and to act as allies. **Cultural competence**, anti-racist approaches, cultural safety, trauma-informed care, and relational practice are all approaches that frame current discourse aimed at action and allyship in the nursing profession. To be effective, all these actions must be strategic and occur within a framework of accountability within the profession. Moreover, it is crucial that nursing reframe what have long been referred to as individual vulnerabilities—or the deficiencies of individuals or groups—as inequities caused by oppression, against which members of health professions hold a moral responsibility to act (McGibbon, 2012).

Nursing has an obligation to contribute to people's health and well-being and to respond to diverse communities and their needs. The Canadian Nurses Association (Canadian Nurses Association, 2010) issued a position statement on promoting cultural competence in nursing, stating that nurses require "knowledge, skills, attitudes or personal attributes to maximize respectful relationships with diverse populations" (p. 1) (see the Canadian Nurses Association links on the Evolve website). Action is not simply a matter of individual behaviour; organizational awareness of and action on racism and oppression involves values, principles, and policies that will establish the context and resources whereby nurses and other health care providers can work effectively in diverse contexts (Andrews, Boyle, & Collins, 2019).

CULTURAL COMPETENCE

In response to Canada's diverse cultural landscape, the demand has grown for nurses to provide high-quality, effective, and culturally competent care. Many different definitions of cultural competence exist, with some being contested for their essentialist views of culture. Cultural essentialism suggests that there are "natural" and unchanging characteristics of people within cultural groups that fit defined categories (Curtis, Jones, Tipene-Leach et al., 2019; Wesp, Scheer, Ruiz et al., 2018).

The definition of cultural competence adopted here views it as an ongoing process rather than an outcome. A culturally competent health care provider is aware of their own cultural identity and views on different cultures and is sensitive to and accepting of clients' differing views (Srivastava, 2007). In order to address unique individuals in their specific contexts and environments, nurses need to move beyond essentialist perspectives of cultural competence that provide a checklist of attributes (Gray & Thomas, 2006; Gregory, Harrowing, Lee et al., 2010). A more emancipatory view of cultural competence draws on the intersectional, feminist, postcolonial,

---

⚡ RESEARCH FOCUS

An Intersectional Lens on Harm Reduction and Methadone Maintenance Treatment in Canada

Smye and colleagues (2011) conducted a study of harm reduction and methadone maintenance treatment (MMT) using an intersectional lens to better understand how harm reduction and MMT are experienced by people who are marginalized. The authors refined the notion of harm reduction using an intersectional lens by specifying the conditions in which both harm and benefit arise and how experiences of harm are continuous with wider experiences of domination and oppression. This ethnographic study, which involved individual interviews, focus groups, and observations, was conducted in a large city in Canada. Participants included Indigenous peoples accessing mainstream mental health, addictions, and primary health care as well as health care providers. All participants had extensive histories of abuse and violence, most often connected to colonialism (e.g., residential schooling) and experienced racism on a daily basis. Participants lived with co-occurring illnesses such as HIV/AIDS, hepatitis C, diabetes, mental illness, and substance use, and most lived in poverty. Participants expressed mistrust of the health care system owing to their everyday experiences within and outside a system that further marginalized them. Issues that impacted access to MMT were found to be stigma and prejudice, social and structural constraints influencing enactment of people's agency, and homelessness. Based on the study's intersectional approach, the authors concluded that harm reduction must move beyond harms related directly to drugs and drug use to addressing the harms associated with systemic oppression and the determinants of drug use and drug and health policy.

Source: Smye, V., Browne, A., Varcoe, C., & Josewski, V. (2011). Harm reduction, methadone maintenance treatment and the root causes of health and social inequities: An intersectional lens in the Canadian context. *Harm Reduction Journal, 8*(1), 17. https://doi.org/10.1186/1477-7517-8-17.

BOX 14.2 Eight Steps to Developing Cultural Competence

1. Know yourself by analyzing your values, behaviours, views, and assumptions.
2. Be aware of racism and the systems or behaviours that foster racism.
3. Reframe your thinking by engaging in activities that encourage others' views and perspectives.
4. Become familiar with the core cultural aspects of your community.
5. Partner with clients to facilitate a comparison of their perceptions and your findings of the core cultural aspects of the community.
6. Familiarize yourself with different cultures and their perceptions and practices for health and illness, and explore with clients their cultural uniqueness (diversity) regarding health and illness.
7. Establish rapport, respect, and trust with clients and coworkers by being open, understanding, and willing to accept varying perceptions.
8. Establish an environment that is welcoming for the diverse cultures within your community.

Source: Nova Scotia Department of Health. (2005). *A cultural competence guide for primary health care professionals in Nova Scotia* (p. 13). Retrieved from https://www.mycna.ca/~/media/nurseone/page-content/pdf-en/cultural_competence_guide_for_primary_health_care_professionals.pdf.

and critical race theories explored earlier in this chapter (Wesp, Scheer, Ruiz et al., 2018).

Cultural competence is also not a standalone quality assurance marker but a process. The cultural competence process helps nurses to understand culture as socially constructed within an historical context that reflects the values and assumptions of the society at a particular time (Campinha-Bacote, 1999; Narayanasamy, 2002). According to this view, culture is not to be thought of in terms of race or bloodline, but rather as "everyday experiences of marginalization" (Kirkham & Anderson, 2002, p. 2).

Cultural competence begins by acknowledging the fundamental variations in the ways that clients respond to health care challenges. A nurse can begin by asking clients questions about health inequities, poverty, and policies and practices that may include or exclude access to appropriate services (Rowan, Rukholm, Bourque Bearskin et al., 2013). At the same time, the nurse would seek to understand the client's health promotion activities; social connections; ability to cope with pain; grieving practices; and culturally specific beliefs, values, and practices (e.g., modesty, eye contact, closeness, and how one touches others).

The Nova Scotia Department of Health produced a *Cultural Competence Guide for Primary Health Care Professionals in Nova Scotia.* The guide consists of tools and resources that can assist health care providers in administering culturally competent health care (see the link on the Evolve website). This document addresses key concepts that impact the health status of Nova Scotia's diverse communities, such as power, privilege, equity, racism, and oppression (Nova Scotia Department of Health, 2005). It also includes a discussion on the eight steps to developing cultural competence (Box 14.2) as well as consideration of the social determinants of health, such as equity and access, and inequitable access to primary health care.

CASE STUDY

Building Culturally Safe Services Through Respect, Trust, and Collaboration

In this community-based project, a coalition was forged between two Saskatchewan Indigenous communities, a health region, and three tertiary educational institutions to improve cultural competence. The objective was to determine which cultural elements would ensure respect in the delivery of direct health care and ways to deliver health education programs for Indigenous peoples that were respectful of their cultural diversity. The resulting coalition led to an enhanced mutual understanding of Indigenous culture, specifically Indigenous healing and ways of knowing. The approach used by these communities demonstrated cultural competence because they worked in a collaborative way that was respectful and promoted trust.

Sources: Health Council of Canada. (2012). Empathy, dignity, and respect Creating cultural safety for Aboriginal people. Retrieved from https://healthcouncilcanada.ca/files/Aboriginal_Report_EN_web_final.pdf; Petrucka, P., Bassendowski, S., & Bourassa, C. (2007). Seeking paths to culturally competent health care: Lessons from two Saskatchewan Aboriginal communities. *Canadian Journal of Nursing Research, 39*(2), 166–182. Retrieved from https://cjnr.archive.mcgill.ca/article/viewFile/2059/2053.

Anti-oppressive practice requires that nurses build on the strengths of individuals and communities without imposing their own biases. As a starting place toward anti-oppressive practice, nurses need to be aware of their own traditions, values, beliefs, and biases toward healing and health care practices. Nurses also need to cut through "the rhetoric of caring" to acknowledge the history of discrimination, white privilege, Western scientific dominance, and oppression within the profession (Smith, 2019). Honouring

Indigenous nursing knowledge (see Research Focus) requires this awareness along with a desire to understand Indigenous approaches at a personal and systemic level.

RESEARCH FOCUS

Indigenous Nursing Knowledge for Personal and Systemic Awareness and Action

Mâmawoh kamâtowin is a Cree term used to describe the meaning of Indigenous community development. Drawing from the experiences of four Indigenous nurse scholars, this research explored how Indigenous knowledge is employed by Indigenous nurses and how it can better serve individuals, families, and communities. Indigeneity as a "way of being" framed the research approach and analysis that established how Indigenous knowledge has always been fundamental to the ways Indigenous nursing is practiced, regardless of the systemic and historical barriers endured over time. Identifying as Indigenous was found to be integral to the nurses' identities and practices. The multiple levels of intervention and integrated practice cutting across health care systems were viewed as essential to Indigenous nursing practice, in that such an approach could reduce health disparities for Indigenous peoples and all others experiencing the harmful effects of inequities. Indigenous nursing practice, in this way, was integrated with community development.

Source: Bourque Bearskin, R., Cameron, B., King, M., & Weber Pillwax, C. (2016). Mâmawoh kamâtowin, "Coming together to help each other in wellness": Honouring Indigenous nursing knowledge. *International Journal of Indigenous Health, 11*(1), 18–33. https://doi.org/10.18357/ijih111201615024.

Developing Culturally Responsive Care

The values of inclusivity, respect, celebrating differences, equity, and commitment underlie culturally competent care for individuals, families, groups, and communities. These values should be embedded in all processes, policies, and practices of nurses and health care organizations (RNAO, 2007). Culturally competent care is provided not only to individuals of racial or ethnic groups but also to individuals belonging to groups that differ based on age, religion, sexual orientation, and socioeconomic status. Nurses need to be culturally competent to provide nursing care that meets everyone's needs and reframes the profession to become a relevant and responsive ally. Cultural nursing assessment is discussed later in this chapter.

Developing cultural competence is a lifelong process that involves every aspect of professional and organizational development. It is challenging and at times painful as nurses and institutions confront historic practices and struggle to adopt new ways of thinking and being (Smith, 2019). Leininger (2002) suggests that the following two principles are useful for developing cultural competence:

1. Maintain a broad, objective, and open attitude toward individuals and their cultures; and
2. Avoid seeing all individuals as alike.

Nurses and organizations develop cultural competence in different ways, but the key elements are having direct experience with clients of other cultures, reflecting on this experience, and promoting mutual respect for differences. Burchum (2002) identified five attributes of cultural competence:

1. **Cultural awareness;**
2. Cultural knowledge;
3. **Cultural understanding;**
4. Cultural sensitivity; and
5. **Cultural skill.**

Two other attributes of cultural competence are cultural interaction and cultural proficiency.

Through listening and awareness, nurses can support the individual health and well-being of diverse clients and groups as well as participate in dismantling the structures of oppression and colonialism. Educational or self-help groups facilitated by nurses or other professionals can help community members learn new adaptation strategies and ways to relate to individuals, families, communities, schools, and workplaces.

An important nursing role as an ally with diverse populations is that of an advocate who speaks out against inequities alongside people from marginalized groups. Nurses have an obligation to support access to health care for diverse groups who may not have that access. Nurses also advocate at the local, provincial, and federal levels for policies that support adaptation of diverse groups, such as by assisting newcomers in their new or unfamiliar environment. For example, a policy change that was initiated by a municipality to assist a culturally diverse group of wheelchair users involved the requirement that all local public buildings have ramps to accommodate wheelchairs. As a result of this change, all public buildings in the community now have wheelchair access. Nurses can use tools such as environmental scans to ensure that inequities that disproportionately affect certain groups are addressed.

To provide culturally competent care, nurses need to appreciate and understand the issues experienced by and the cultural backgrounds of their clients. Although research has identified certain health beliefs and practices within Indigenous, Francophone, Black, Chinese, and other cultures, nurses need to remember that beliefs and practices differ regionally, within communities, and among individuals. One person from a cultural group, in the LGBTQ2 community, or experiencing a disability does not represent "all" such individuals. Specialized and intentional integrated practices are organizational strategies to both enhance nursing practice and support a diverse nursing workforce (Pearce, 2015). Indigenous Health Nursing is an approach and specialization that concentrates on **cultural knowledge** and nurses' participation. It empowers nurses to enhance clients' access to traditional Indigenous wellness practices within culturally safe and secure health care environments.

Inhibitors to Culturally Responsive Care

There are a number of challenges to building culturally responsive and diversity-conscious capacities for nurses and within organizations. Some of the all-too-commonplace inhibitors may result from a limited understanding of relational practice; institutional pressures to improve productivity, efficiency, or expanded organizational reporting needs; or pressures from colleagues who do not yet possess the same awareness and commitment to allyship. These and similar forces that inhibit cultural safety are indeed commonplace (Racine, 2014), as they compromise on the delivery of culturally responsive care and may result in some of the following behaviours:

- Ethnocentrism. **Ethnocentrism** is a type of cultural prejudice wherein one believes that their "own cultural values, beliefs, and behaviours are the best, preferred, and the most superior ways" (Srivastava, 2007, p. 5). For example, nurses who assume that their way of providing nursing care is the only right way are ethnocentric.
- Cultural blindness. **Cultural blindness** is a denial of diversity and the inability to recognize the uniqueness of individual clients. For example, a nurse, attempting to be culturally unbiased, treats all clients the same, conducts nursing assessments with the same questions, and consequently fails to gain an understanding of each client's culture and diversity.
- Bias. Bias is "the negative evaluation of one group and its members relative to another" (Blair, Steiner, & Havranek, 2011). Bias may be intentional or unconscious. For example, a nurse who is biased implements nursing care based on personal attitudes, cognitive errors, prejudices, and stereotypes.
- Culture shock. Culture shock is a condition that involves feelings of anxiety because of exposure to unfamiliar environments and culture. The person feels threatened and helpless while trying to adapt to the unfamiliar culture with its different practices, values, and beliefs. For example, a newcomer from Somalia who arrives in Canada and finds the unfamiliar environment and culture overwhelming is experiencing culture shock.
- Stereotyping. Stereotyping occurs when generalizations are applied to an individual without exploring their individual values, beliefs, and behaviours. For example, a nurse decides that an Italian client with diabetes eats too much pasta and therefore cannot control blood sugar levels. As a result, the nurse does not ask the client about the kinds of foods they eat on a regular basis.
- Prejudice. Prejudice is a negative attitude about a person or group without factual data (Srivastava, 2007). For example, "older adults do not have sex."
- Racism. Racism is a form of prejudice in which members of one cultural group perceive themselves to be superior to another cultural group (Ontario Human Rights Commission, 2008). For example, "the white race in Canada is superior to all newcomers."

Awareness and commitment to allyship may help nurses to be less judgmental, more accepting of cultural variations, and less likely to engage in the behaviours that inhibit cultural competence.

Anti-Racist Approaches

Racism is most frequently thought of as a hateful response to skin colour, ethnic origin, or religion; however, it can be directed at other aspects of culture such as cultural celebrations, traditional dress, and traditional food. The most common types of racism cited in the literature are overt and systemic. Overt racism is an open demonstration by attitudes, actions, policies, and practices of a feeling of superiority over individuals or groups with the intent of harming or damaging (Government of Canada, 2019a). Hate crimes, for example, are considered one example of overt racism.

Systemic racism, also known as institutional racism, means the unequal application of policies within organizations, corporations, and institutions (Bourque Bearskin, 2011; RNAO, 2007). Broader structural racism can be defined as "The macrolevel systems, social forces, institutions, ideologies and processes that interact with one another to generate and reinforce inequalities among racial and ethnic groups" (Gee & Ford, 2011). Systemic, or structural, racism is founded on the ideology of **white supremacy**, an "historically based, institutionally perpetuated system of exploitation and oppression of continents, nations, and peoples of color by white peoples and nations of the European continent, for the purpose of maintaining and defending a system of wealth, power, and privilege" (Challenging White Supremacy Workshop, 2000, p. 16).

Racism may be encountered within the nursing profession at all levels (RNAO, 2007). A nurse may experience racism in client interactions, collegial nursing interactions, workplace organizational systems, and community systems. Racism in nursing practice (whether toward a client or toward the nurse) needs to be labelled and addressed when it occurs, otherwise it can lead to oppression. Structural racism shapes client health and access to health care services as well as the development of the profession:

> *Achieving one's full potential is difficult when basic needs are not satisfied, resources are inadequate and do not promote sustainable wellness, and chronic life stressors persist* (Benoit, Cotnam, O'Brien-Teengs et al., 2019, p. 1)

Health disparities are an effect of racism, not of race, and the profession of nursing is beginning to bring awareness to this distinction. A study on the racism experienced by Indigenous women in two major urban centres in Ontario, for example, identified that the women's experiences spanned individual, collective and institutional, and cultural racism (Benoit, Cotnam, O'Brien-Teengs et al., 2019). As allies, nurses must consider the broad and individual impacts of racism, and the way that race privileges some while disadvantaging others, in terms of each nurse–client interaction. Commitment to allyship and anti-oppressive practice is supported by cultural safety practice and professional standards, which demand commitment and ongoing action at individual, institutional, and structural spheres of influence (Aurilio, 2013). Allyship as a feature of the profession of nursing must become more than a slogan and brought into action.

CULTURAL SAFETY

Cultural safety is defined by the client in nurse–client interactions (De & Richardson, 2008). **Cultural safety** refers to gaining an understanding of others' health beliefs and practices so that health care actions work toward equity and avoid discrimination. There is recognition of and respect for cultural identity so that power balance exists between the health care provider and the client (Anderson, Perry, Blue et al., 2003; Ramsden, 2002; Srivastava, 2007).

The term cultural safety was first coined by Irihapeti Ramsden, a Māori nurse in New Zealand who worked to improve health outcomes for Māori people. She identified the need to address cultural issues in relation to health care interactions between Māori clients and non-Māori health care providers. Ramsden asserted that cultural safety extends beyond the concept of cultural competence and that nurses need to be self-aware, be conscious of their own culture, and understand theories of power relations. In this context, cultural safety is an outcome of nursing care that enables those receiving the service to define safe service. Ramsden's research offers insight into the historical and political issues surrounding the delivery of health care services to the Māori population (Ramsden, 2002). Recently, Curtis, Jones, Tipene-Leach et al. (2019) proposed a definition of cultural

safety that addresses and works to transform key factors responsible for ethnic inequities in health care.

The National Aboriginal Health Organization asserted that cultural safety is built on the principle of biculturalism, which differs from transcultural nursing concepts in that transcultural nursing care develops from the dominant culture Yeung (2016). Gray and Thomas (2006) have supported the view of culture as relational, and as a sociopolitical construct it involves power relationships in nurse–client interactions. Therefore, when nurses use a cultural safety lens, they involve the client in addressing health inequities and striving for social justice. Cultural safety is about fostering an understanding of the relationship between minority status and health status so that practices and systems of health care that do not support the health of minority groups are identified and addressed (Arieli, Friedman, & Hirschfeld, 2012).

According to De and Richardson (2008), cultural safety is based on the following elements:

- The health care provider's analysis of their cultural self and its influence on client interactions;
- Acknowledgement of the power imbalance between the health care provider and the client; and
- The health care provider learning and applying basic skills.

For the nurse to work effectively with clients from various cultural backgrounds and to provide culturally responsive health care, cultural safety and cultural competence need to be addressed and implemented in client interactions (Bourque Bearskin, 2011; De & Richardson, 2008; Dion Stout & Downey, 2006).

The concept of cultural safety has become widely applied by organizations working with First Nations people, Inuit, and Métis. The Canadian Indigenous Nurses Association, Indigenous Physicians Association of Canada, NAHO (2008), and the National Collaborating Centre for Indigenous Health identified Indigenous peoples as a key group requiring culturally safe practice.

According to the Truth and Reconciliation Commission of Canada (2015), colonization continues to affect the traditional values and social structures of Indigenous peoples in Canada. It also contributes to inequities in the health status of Indigenous peoples in Canada. Colonialism encouraged the development of dominant systems of care that resulted in discrimination against and disempowerment of Indigenous peoples. Some of these influences have carried over to postcolonial times, sparking a desire for improved cultural competence and safety and a renaissance of honouring Indigenous knowledge (Bourque Bearskin, Cameron, King et al., 2016; NAHO, 2008).

Cultural safety requires a set of basic skills that can be learned through **cultural sensitivity** and cultural competence training (Kurtz, Janke, Vinek et al., 2018). A culturally safe nurse–client relationship requires that nurses understand the need for the following: Indigenous peoples' access to traditional health care practices and ceremonies; engagement, dialogue, and consultations with health care administrators and providers; health administrators' and providers' respect for the rights of diverse knowledge; and the enactment of ethical commitments, culturally safe practices, and collective thinking. All these elements can lead to a holistic understanding of culture and a sense of humility to raise nurses' consciousness of cultural safety.

The Canadian Indigenous Nurses Association website provides further information on its cultural competence and cultural safety initiative (see the link on the Evolve website).

Cultural Humility

The concept of cultural humility is relatively new for health care providers. It is a process that requires nurses to continually engage in self-reflection and self-critique as life-long learners and reflective practitioners. Cultural humility also brings into check the power imbalances that exist in the dynamics of a health care setting (Tervalon & Murray-Garcia, 1998). Nurses will be better prepared for culturally safe practice by learning cultural humility (Levi, 2009). Approaching health care with cultural humility goes beyond the concept of cultural safety; it means encouraging individuals to identify and acknowledge their own biases. Cultural humility acknowledges that it is impossible to be adequately knowledgeable about cultures other than one's own and requires that we take responsibility for our interactions with others beyond acknowledging or being sensitive to our differences (Juarez, Marvel, Brezinski, et al., 2006). Having a sense of humility is being comfortable with a position of not knowing and not being the expert.

Cultural humility is not an end in itself but rather a commitment to a way of being and an active process of relating to one another (Hoskins, 1999; Racher & Annis, 2007). Hoskins (1999) outlined five major processes that can help people work toward cultural humility:
1. Acknowledging the pain of oppression;
2. Engaging in acts of humility;
3. Acting with reverence;
4. Engaging in mutuality; and
5. Maintaining a position of not knowing.

Relational Practice: Gaining Awareness and Connecting as Allies for Action

Relational practice "is guided by conscious participation with clients using a number of relational skills including listening, questioning, empathy, mutuality, reciprocity,

self-observation, reflection and a sensitivity to emotional contexts" (College of Nurses of Ontario, 2014, p. 13). It places nursing care within the context of relationships (Bergum & Dossetor, 2005; Pollard, 2015; Spadoni, Hartrick Doane, Sevean, & Poole, 2015). Such an approach has been shown to improve health outcomes for clients and the job satisfaction of nurses (Andersen & Havaei, 2015; Johannessen, Werner, & Steihaug, 2013).

A framework of relational practice has been endorsed by professional associations and nursing bodies across Canada over the past decade. Relational practice—an approach that is increasingly being integrated into nursing education and practice guidelines—builds professional awareness and action for the concerns address in this chapter (e.g., oppression and diversity of gender identities, sexual orientation, abilities, spirituality, culture and race, income, language, and geographic locations) (RNAO, 2006). Canadian nursing scholars have led the profession to look beyond the restrictive labels of ethnicity, visible minority, age, and so on to see clients as individuals with their own history and identity (Hartrick Doane & Varcoe, 2015).

In relational practice, nurses engage with individuals, families, groups, and communities that have varying degrees of "differences." Nurses must listen to and care for all clients, regardless of their personal views on those differences. It is in these "hard spots" of nursing where holistic relational views can provide a basis for understanding culture and diversity and help nurses to ensure they are providing safe, competent, and ethical nursing care (Hartrick Doane & Varcoe, 2006). Relational practice requires a commitment to respect, which means different things to different people. At the heart of relational practice is the recognition that individuals are diverse in their personal characteristics as well as how they perceive the world and react to others. Nurses who seek to understand diversity through a cultural safety lens become more aware of their personal views on ethnicity and recognize that ethnicity is intersected by other markers that are socially and culturally constructed—these are often difficult conversations to have in nursing (Arieli, Friedman, & Hirschfeld, 2012; Greenwood, Wright, & Nielsen, 2006). Nursing is not yet as culturally and socially diverse as the general Canadian population or the people and communities that nurses work with at this time (Lowe & Archibald, 2009).

The hallmark of professional nursing practice is safe, client-focused care founded on trusting therapeutic relationships. There are many examples of how trusting therapeutic relationships have been severed in clinical practice. For example, cultural safety studies have noted the prevalence of stereotyping, perceived discrimination, and derogatory comments by health care providers (Allan & Smylie, 2015; Martin & Kipling, 2006). Hartrick Doane &

BOX 14.3 The Process of Relational Practice in Action

1. Enter into relation.
   - Participate consciously and intentionally.
   - Stop to look and listen.
   - Show unconditional positive regard for the client.
   - Get "in sync" with the client.
   - Walk alongside the client.
2. Be in collaborative relation.
   - Understand that the client collaborates with the nurse.
   - Understand that the client and nurse work together to assess and intervene.
3. Inquire into the health and healing experience.
   - Ask the client what is meaningful and significant with regard to their circumstances.
   - Keep the client (individual, family, group, or community) as the central focus.
4. Follow the lead of the client.
   - Take cues from the client.
   - Take a stance of unknowing and uncertainty.
   - Use theoretical knowledge to enhance sensitivity to client experience.
   - Scrutinize theoretical knowledge against client experience.
5. Listen.
   - Listen through phenomenological, critical, and spiritual lenses.
   - Listen through a socioenvironmental health promotion lens.
6. Engage in self-observation.
   - Be self-aware.

7. Practice letting be and support change.
   - Get to know who clients are and what is happening without imposing your views.
   - Create the opportunity for clients to learn more about their own experience, patterns, capacities, challenges, and contextual constraints.
8. Engage in collaborative knowledge development.
   - Draw on client knowledge (experiential, historical, sociocultural) to build understanding and plan interventions (scientific, theoretical, biomedical, political, practical).
9. Recognize patterns.
   - Identify underlying patterns of experience.
   - Identify client responses.
   - Identify patterns of capacity.
   - Identify capacity–adversity patterns.
10. Name and support client capacity.
    - Recognize the client's capacity.
    - Look beyond the surface.
    - Honour the client's version of the story.
    - Work with the client (at an individual and community level) to enhance capacity and address adversity.
11. Engage in emancipatory action.
    - Recognize and name inequities.
    - Recognize and name structural conditions.
    - Draw on and share contextual knowledge.
    - Introduce alternative discourses.
    - Devote energy to remedying structural inequities.
    - Create coalitions.

Source: Hartrick Doane, G., & Varcoe, C. (2004). *Family nursing as relational inquiry: Developing health-promoting practice.* Philadelphia, PA: Lippincott, Williams & Wilkins.

Varcoe (2005) have explained that relational practice builds on the strengths of individuals and recognizes differences without bias, keeping in mind the power dynamics involved in delivering health care services to clients. Relational practice helps nurses work with differences, thereby neutralizing the power dynamic.

Key concepts in relational practice are a heightened sense of self-awareness, self-reflexivity in relation to others, a holistic perspective of the context and culture, and relational capacities. Relational capacities are ways of being in a relationship; that is, being able and willing to understand others and express or share your own personal meaning. Nurses who engage in relational practice are fully present with clients and demonstrate mindfulness, mutuality, intentionality, genuineness, warmth, respect, care,

knowledge of boundaries, the ability to provide and receive constructive feedback, assertiveness, conflict-resolution skills, and a willingness to share information in meaningful ways (Hartrick Doane & Varcoe, 2005).

Relational practice requires good communication skills. Active listening skills, nonverbal communication skills, awareness, and compassion increase nurses' ability to develop effective therapeutic relationships with clients. They also provide nurses with greater self-awareness and awareness of clients' cues that can reveal the root causes of pain, suffering, or challenging behaviours (Hartrick Doane & Varcoe, 2005). This expanded awareness of context and emancipatory action is necessary to motivate anti-oppressive action at multiple levels (e.g., individual, group, policy). Box 14.3 highlights the process of relational practice in action.

Organizational Action and Anti-Oppressive Practices

A model of positive action for anti-oppressive practice at an organizational level incorporates activities that can shape the profession of nursing and the role of nurses within the health care system. Dismantling the systemic language, practices, and activities that uphold oppression requires action in many spheres of influence—at the interpersonal and relational levels, certainly, but also right at the heart of the technologies and mechanisms of our organizations.

Organizational action can include meeting minimal legal requirements for diversity and antidiscrimination, specific positive action measures, equality schemes, and mainstreaming equal opportunities (Nzira & Williams, 2009). For example, women in the nursing profession continue to be affected by persistent, systemic barriers around gender, such as a lack of respect for part-time workers, inflexible working hours, sexual harassment and bullying, intangible cultural factors, and few visible role models in leadership. Professional association standards and codes as well as bargaining and collective agreements allow for collective action around the minimal requirements to address the rights of nurses facing these barriers.

Moving beyond minimum legal requirements could involve taking proactive steps within the parameters of the law, engaging in positive action to challenge the discrimination that has produced the dominance of one group. For instance, white, nondisabled men dominate significant positions of power within health care institutions to the exclusion of women, visible minorities, and people with disabilities. Positive action means providing typically disadvantaged people and groups with special training and focused encouragement. Positive action does not put in place reverse discrimination quotas or preferential treatment, but rather applies an approach to diversifying a professional group in all roles to support better representation; this strategy counteracts the effects of past discrimination and helps to eliminate gender and racial stereotyping.

Additional far-reaching equality schemes and the mainstreaming of integrated organizational approaches (such as specific equity measures or new policies within an organization) can extend the reach of positive action to begin to shift institutionalized discrimination, inequity, and racism (Nzira & Williams, 2009). Mainstreaming positive action and anti-oppressive practices requires organizational policy and activities at multiple levels, including preservice and in-service training and education and hiring practices to enhance diversity (Phillips & Malone, 2014; Smith, 2019). Decolonizing practices focus on the unsettling of dominant approaches through Indigenous leadership and knowledge. Nursing education is increasingly including curricular and experiential engagement on this crucial awareness, allyship, and action. The diversity of the profession and nursing work requires this understanding and multi-level action at this time—it is a moral responsibility to face the historical legacy of racism and discrimination from within and beyond the profession.

SUMMARY OF LEARNING OBJECTIVES

- Diversity is an element of Canadian society and all aspects of nursing practice. Culture, race, and ethnicity are aspects of diversity that influence health and health care. Key demographic groups for nursing in Canada are older adults, Indigenous peoples, and immigrants.
- Canada's multicultural society is diverse in terms of ethnicity, language, religion, sexuality, and abilities. As a multicultural society that recognizes the diverse ancestry of the population and values **cultural pluralism**, Canada is in a process of addressing the Calls to Action for Truth and Reconciliation with Indigenous peoples.
- Practices of oppression operate to produce health inequities in relation to race, gender, culture, age, ability, and other domains of social inclusion.
- Cultural competence is an ongoing process rather than an outcome. In order to bring cultural competence to nursing practice and the organization of the profession, nurses apply cultural knowledge and skills appropriate to client interactions without personal biases.
- A cultural safety lens provides an understanding of others' health beliefs and practices so that health care actions work toward equity and avoid discrimination. Cultural safety incorporates self-awareness and awareness of the client's beliefs, values, attitudes, and behaviours. Cultural safety is an all-encompassing approach that brings sensitivity toward history and context into action (individual or policy level).
- Relational practice is an approach to awareness, allyship, and action and supports critical, emancipatory professional transformation. At the heart of relational practice is the recognition of diversity and how each individual perceives the world they live in and how they react to others.

CRITICAL THINKING QUESTIONS

1. What barriers do individual nurses and the profession face to becoming allies to racialized and marginalized people and groups?

2. What tools and skills do individual nurses and the profession need to become allies to racialized and marginalized people and groups?

3. What roles do individuals and professional organizations play in awareness, allyship, and action?

4. What is distinct about decolonization as part of anti-oppressive practice for the profession of nursing?

REFERENCES

Allan, B., & Smylie, J. (2015). *First peoples, second class treatment: The role of racism in the health and well-being of Indigenous peoples in Canada*. Toronto, ON: Wellesley Institute.

Allender, J. A., & Spradley, B. W. (2005). *Community health nursing: Promoting and protecting the public's health* (6th ed.). Philadelphia, PA: Lippincott, Williams & Wilkins.

Andersen, E., & Havaei, F. (2015). Measuring relational care in nursing homes: Psychometric evaluation of the relational care scale. *Journal of Nursing Measurement, 23*, 82–92. https://doi.org/10.1891/1061-3749.23.1.82.

Anderson, J., Perry, J., Blue, C., et al. (2003). Rewriting cultural safety within the postcolonial and postnational feminist project: Towards new epistemologies of healing. *Advances in Nursing Science, 26*(3), 196–214. https://doi.org/10.1097/00012272-200307000-00005.

Andrews, M. M., Boyle, J. S., & Collins, J. W. (2019). *Transcultural concepts in nursing care* (8th ed.). Philadelphia, PA: Wolters Kluwer, Lippincott, Williams & Wilkins.

Arieli, D., Friedman, V. J., & Hirschfeld, M. J. (2012). Challenges on the path to cultural safety in nursing education. *International Nursing Review, 59*(2), 187–193. https://doi.org/10.1111/j.1466-7657.2012.00982.x.

Arya, A., & Piggott, T. (2018). *Under-served: Health determinants of Indigenous, inner-city, and migrant populations in Canada*. Toronto, ON: Canadian Scholars' Press.

Aurilio, D. M. (2013). *Characteristics of and path to become an anti-racist direct-entry midwife*. (Publication No. 1551720) [Master's thesis, Bastyr University]. ProQuest Dissertations Publishing. Retrieved from http://search.proquest.com/docview/1499837437/.

Beckmann Murray, R., Proctor Zentner, J., Pangman, V., et al. (2009). *Health promotion strategies through the life span* (2nd ed.). Toronto, ON: Pearson Prentice Hall.

Bergum, V., & Dossetor, J. (2005). *Creating environment. Relational ethics: The full meaning of respect*. Hagerstown, MD: University Publishing Group.

Benoit, A., Cotnam, J., O'Brien-Teengs, et al. (2019). Racism experiences of urban Indigenous women in Ontario, Canada: "We all have that story that will break your heart." *International Indigenous Policy Journal, 10*(2). https://doi.org/10.18584/iipj.2019.10.2.1.

Blair, I., Steiner, J. L., & Havranek, E. L. (2011). Unconscious (implicit) bias and health disparities: Where do we go from here? *The Permanente Journal, 15*(2), 71–78.

Bourque Bearskin, R. L., Cameron, B. L., King, M., et al. (2016). Mâmawoh Kamâtowin, "Coming together to help each other in wellness": Honouring Indigenous nursing knowledge. *International Journal of Indigenous Health, 11*(1), 5–19.

Browne, A. J., Hill, E., Lavallee, B., et al. (2017). *Out of Sight*. Winnipeg, MB: Brian Sinclair Working Group. Retrieved from http://ignoredtodeathmanitoba.ca/index.php/2017/09/15/out-of-sight-interim-report-of-the-sinclair-working-group/.

Burchum, J. L. (2002). Cultural competence: An evolutionary perspective. *Nursing Forum, 37*(4), 5–15. https://doi.org/10.1111/j.1744-6198.2002.tb01287.x.

Burnet, J., & Driedger, L. (2011). Multiculturalism. *The Canadian Encyclopedia*. Retrieved from http://www.thecanadianencyclopedia.ca/en/article/multiculturalism/.

Campinha-Bacote, J. (1999). A model and instrument for addressing cultural competence in health care. *Journal of Nursing Education, 38*(5), 204–207. https://doi.org/10.3928/0148-4834-19990501-06.

Campinha-Bacote, J. (2002). The process of cultural competence in the delivery of healthcare services: A model of care. *Journal of Transcultural Nursing, 13*(3), 181–184. https://doi.org/10.1177/10459602013003003.

Canadian Centre for Diversity and Inclusion. (n.d.). *Research and tool kits*. Retrieved from http://www.ccdi.ca/what-we-do/research-toolkits/.

Canadian Nurses Association. (2010). *Position statement: Promoting cultural competence in nursing*. Retrieved from https://www.cna-aiic.ca/~/media/cna/page-content/pdf-en/ps114_cultural_competence_2010_e.pdf.

Centre for Suicide Prevention. (n.d.). *Sexual minorities and suicide prevention. A suicide prevention toolkit*. Retrieved from https://www.suicideinfo.ca/resource/sexual-minorities-suicide-prevention/.

Challenging White Supremacy Workshop. (2000). *A glossary of some terms used in CWS workshops*. Retrieved from http://www.cwsworkshop.org/about/6Glossary_of_Terms.PDF.

Citizenship and Immigration Canada. (2010). *The current state of multiculturalism in Canada and research themes on Canadian multiculturalism 2008-2010*. Retrieved from http://www.cic.gc.ca/english/pdf/pub/multi-state.pdf.

Citizenship and Immigration Canada. (2015). *Report on plans and priorities 2015-2016*. Retrieved from http://www.cic.gc.ca/english/resources/publications/rpp/2015-2016/.

Citizenship and Immigration Canada. (2016a). *Permanent resident program*. Retrieved from http://www.cic.gc.ca/english/resources/tools/perm/index.asp.

Citizenship and Immigration Canada. (2016b). *Temporary residents.* Retrieved from http://www.cic.gc.ca/english/resources/tools/temp/index.asp.

Clair, J., Beatty, J., & MacLean, T. (2005). Out of sight but not out of mind: Managing invisible social identities in the workplace. *Academy of Management Review, 30*(1), 78–95. https://doi.org/10.5465/amr.2005.15281431.

College of Nurses of Ontario. (2014). *Competencies for entry-level registered nurse practice.* Toronto, ON: Author.

Curtis, E., Jones, R., Tipene-Leach, D., et al. (2019). Why cultural safety rather than cultural competency is required to achieve health equity: A literature review and recommended definition. *International Journal for Equity in Health, 18*(1), 1–17. https://doi.org/10.1186/s12939-019-1082-3.

Daley, A. E., & MacDonnell, J. A. (2015). That would have been beneficial": LGBTQ education for home-care service providers. *Health and Social Care in the Community, 23*(3), 282–291. https://doi.org/10.1111/hsc.12141.

De, D., & Richardson, J. (2008). Cultural safety: An introduction. *Pediatric Nursing, 20*(2), 39–43. https://doi.org/10.7748/paed2008.03.20.2.39.c6529.

DiAngelo, R. (2011). White fragility. *International Journal of Critical Pedagogy, 3*(3), 54–70.

Dion Stout, M., & Downey, B. (2006). Nursing, Indigenous peoples and cultural safety: So what? Now what? *Contemporary Nurse, 22*, 327–332. https://doi.org/10.5172/conu.2006.22.2.327.

Donahue, M. P. (2010). *Nursing the finest art: An illustrated history* (3rd ed.). Philadelphia, PA: Mosby/Elsevier.

Elmslie, K. (2012). *Against the growing burden of disease* [PowerPoint]. Ottawa, ON: Public Health Agency of Canada. Retrieved from http://www.csih.org/sites/default/files/resources/2016/10/elmslie.pdf.

Fleras, A. (2016). Theorizing micro-aggressions as racism 3.0: Shifting the discourse. *Canadian Ethnic Studies Journal, 48*(2), 1–19. https://doi.org/10.1353/ces.2016.0011.

Gee, G. C., & Ford, C. L. (2011). Structural racism and health inequities: Old issues, new directions. *Du Bois Review: Social Science Research on Race, 8*(1), 115–132. https://doi.org/10.1017/S1742058X11000130.

Goodman, A., Fleming, K., Markwick, N., et al. (2017). "They treated me like crap and I know it was because I was Native": The healthcare experiences of Aboriginal peoples living in Vancouver's inner city. *Social Science & Medicine, 178*, 87–94. https://doi.org/10.1016/j.socscimed.2017.01.053.

Government of Canada. (2019a). *Canada's Anti-racism Strategy.* Retrieved from https://www.canada.ca/en/canadian-heritage/campaigns/anti-racism-engagement/anti-racism-strategy.html.

Government of Canada. (2019b). How Canada's Refugee System Works. Retrieved from https://www.canada.ca/en/immigration-refugees-citizenship/services/refugees/canada-role.html.

Government of Canada. (2014). *Convention on the Rights of Persons with Disabilities: First report of Canada.* Ottawa, ON: Her Majesty the Queen in Right of Canada. Retrieved from http://www.ccdonline.ca/en/international/un/canada/crpd-first-report.

Gray, P. D., & Thomas, D. J. (2006). Critical reflections on culture in nursing. *Journal of Cultural Diversity, 13*(2), 76–82.

Greenwood, M., de Leeuw, S., & Lindsay, N. M. (Eds.). (2018). *Determinants of Indigenous peoples' health in Canada: Beyond the social.* Toronto, ON: Canadian Scholars' Press.

Greenwood, S., Wright, T., & Nielsen, H. (2006). Conversations in context: Cultural safety and reflexivity in child and family health nursing. *Journal of Family Nursing, 12*(2), 201–224. https://doi.org/10.1177/1074840706287405.

Gregory, D., Harrowing, J., Lee, B., et al. (2010). Pedagogy as influencing nursing students' essentialized understanding of culture. *International Journal of Nursing Education Scholarship, 7*(1), 1–17. https://doi.org/10.2202/1548-923x.2025.

Gray, A. (2018). *Doing the right something: A grounded theory approach to understanding advocacy and allyship among college students* (Publication No. 11007102) [Doctoral dissertation, North Carolina State University]. ProQuest Dissertations Publishing. Retrieved from http://search.proquest.com/docview/2133044607/.

Hartrick Doane, G., & Varcoe, C. (2005). *Family nursing as relational inquiry: Developing health-promoting practice.* Philadelphia, PA: Lippincott, Williams & Wilkins.

Hartrick Doane, F., & Varcoe, C. (2006). The "hard spots" of family nursing: Connecting across difference and diversity. *Journal of Family Nursing, 12*(1), 7–21. https://doi.org/10.1177/1074840705284210.

Hartrick Doane, G., & Varcoe, C. (2015). *How to nurse? Relational inquiry with individuals and families in changing health and healthcare contexts.* Philadelphia, PA: Lippincott, Williams & Wilkins.

Happell, B., Scholz, B., Gordon, S., et al. (2018). "I don't think we've quite got there yet": The experience of allyship for mental health consumer researchers. *Journal of Psychiatric and Mental Health Nursing, 25*(8), 453–462. https://doi.org/10.1111/jpm.12476.

Hoffman-Goetz, L., Donelle, L., & Ahmed, R. (2014). *Health literacy in Canada: A primer for students.* Toronto, ON: Canadian Scholars' Press.

Hoskins, M. L. (1999). Worlds apart and lives together: Developing cultural attunement. *Child and Youth Care Forum, 28*(2), 73–85. https://doi.org/10.1023/A:1021937105025.

Hurley, M. (2010). *Sexual orientation and legal rights.* Ottawa, ON: Library of Parliament.

Immigration, Refugees and Citizenship Canada. (2018). *Table 1: Permanent residents admitted in 2017, by top 10 source countries.* Retrieved from https://www.canada.ca/en/immigration-refugees-citizenship/corporate/publications-manuals/annual-report-parliament-immigration-2018/permanent-residents-admitted.html.

Indian and Northern Affairs Canada. (1996). *Report of the Royal Commission on Aboriginal Peoples (RCAP).* Retrieved from http://www.collectionscanada.gc.ca/webarchives/20071115053257/ http://www.ainc-inac.gc.ca/ch/rcap/sg/sgmm_e.html.

Indigenous and Northern Affairs Canada. (2015). *Inuit.* Retrieved from https://www.aadnc-aandc.gc.ca/eng/1100100014187/1100100014191.

Jakubec, S. L., Olfert., M., Choi., L., et al. (2019). Understanding belonging and community connection for seniors living in the suburbs. *Urban Planning, 4*(2), 43–52. https://doi.org/10.17645/up.v4i2.1896.

Jarvis, C. (2004). *Physical examination and health assessment* (4th ed.). St. Louis, MO: Elsevier Science.

Johannessen, A. -K., Werner, A., & Steihaug, S. (2013). Work in an intermediate unit: Balancing between relational, practical and more care. *Journal of Clinical Nursing, 23*, 586–595. https://doi.org/10.1111/jocn.12213.

Juarez, J. A., Marvel, K., Brezinski, K. L., et al. (2006). Bridging the gap: A curriculum to teach residents cultural humility. *Family Medicine, 38*, 97–102. https://doi.org/10.1016/s0197-4572(86)80164-1.

Kirkham, S., & Anderson, J. M. (2002). Postcolonial nursing scholarship: From epistemology to method. *Advances in Nursing Science, 25*(1), 1–17. https://doi.org/10.1097/00012272-200209000-00004.

Kurtz, D., Janke, R., Vinek, J., et al. (2018). Health sciences cultural safety education in Australia, Canada, New Zealand, and the United States: A literature review. *International Journal of Medical Education, 9*, 271–285. https://doi.org/10.5116/ijme.5bc7.21e2.

Kydd, A., & Fleming, A. (2015). Ageism and age discrimination in health care: Fact or fiction? A narrative review of the literature. *Maturitas, 81*(4), 432–438. https://doi.org/10.1016/j.maturitas.2015.05.002.

Lancellotti, K. (2008). Culture care theory: A framework for expanding awareness of diversity and racism in nursing education. *Journal of Professional Nursing, 24*(3), 179–183. https://doi.org/10.1016/j.profnurs.2007.10.007.

Le, T. N., & Johansen, S. (2011). The relationship between perceived school multiculturalism and interpersonal violence: An exploratory study. *Journal of School Health, 81*(11), 688–695. https://doi.org/10.1111/j.1746-1561.2011.00645.x.

Leininger, M. (2002). Essential transcultural nursing care concepts, principles, examples, and policy statements. In M. Leininger, & M. R. McFarland (Eds.), *Transcultural nursing: Concepts, theories, research, and practices* (3rd ed., pp. 45–69). New York, NY: McGraw-Hill.

Levi, A. (2009). The ethics of nursing student international clinical experiences. *Journal of Obstetric, Gynecologic, and Neonatal Nursing, 28*(1), 94–99. https://doi.org/10.1111/j.1552-6909.2008.00314.x.

Lowe, J., & Archibald, C. (2009). Cultural diversity: The intention of nursing. *Nursing Forum, 44*(1), 11–18. https://doi.org/10.1111/j.1744-6198.2009.00122.x.

Martin, D., & Kipling, A. (2006). Factors shaping Aboriginal nursing students' experiences. *Nurse Education Today, 26*(8), 688–696. https://doi.org/10.1016/j.nedt.2006.07.013.

McCallum, M. J. L. (2007). *Twice as good: A history of Aboriginal nurses.* Ottawa, ON: Aboriginal Nurses Association of Canada.

McCallum, M. J. L. (2008). *Labour, modernity and the Canadian state: A history of Aboriginal women and work in the mid-twentieth century* [Unpublished doctoral thesis]. University of Manitoba.

McCallum, M. J. L. (2014). *Indigenous women, work, and history.* Winnipeg, MB: University of Manitoba Press.

McGibbon, E. A. (Ed.). (2012). *Oppression: A social determinant of health.* Blackpoint, NS: Fernwood Publishing.

McGibbon, E., & Etowa, J. (2009). *Anti-racist health care practice.* Toronto, ON: Canadian Scholars' Press.

Métis National Council. (n.d.). *Métis Nation citizenship.* Retrieved from http://www.metisnation.ca/index.php/who-are-the-metis/citizenship.

Napier, A. D., Arcano, C., Butler, B., et al. (2014). Culture and health. *The Lancet, 384*(9954), 1607–1639. https://doi.org/10.1016/S0140-6736(14)61603-2.

Narayanasamy, A. (2002). The ACCESS model: A transcultural nursing practice framework. *British Journal of Nursing, 11*(9), 643–655. https://doi.org/10.12968/bjon.2002.11.9.10178.

National Aboriginal Health Organization. (2008). *Cultural competency and safety: A guide for health administrators, providers, and educators.* Ottawa, ON: Author. Retrieved from https://en.unesco.org/interculturaldialogue/resources/249.

Nelson, L. E. (2018, January 14). It happened to me: Racism and health care. *The Globe and Mail.* Retrieved from https://www.theglobeandmail.com/news/national/what-its-like-to-deal-with-racism-in-canadas-health-caresystem/article37600473/.

Nestel, S. (2012). *Colour coded health care: The impact of race and racism on Canadians' health.* Toronto, ON: Wellesley Institute.

Nova Scotia Department of Health. (2005). *A cultural competence guide for primary health care professionals in Nova Scotia.* Retrieved from http://www.healthteamnovascotia.ca/cultural_competence/Cultural_Competence_guide_for_Primary_Health_Care_Professionals.pdf.

Nzira, V., & Williams, P. (2009). *Anti-oppressive practice in health and social care.* Los Angeles, CA: SAGE Publications.

Ontario Human Rights Commission. (2008). *Racism and racial discrimination: Your rights and responsibilities.* Retrieved from http://www.ohrc.on.ca.

Parliament of Canada. (2018). *Canadian Multiculturalism.* Retrieved from https://lop.parl.ca/sites/PublicWebsite/default/en_CA/ResearchPublications/200920E#a1.

Pearce, L. (2015). The workforce with strength in diversity. *Nursing Standard, 30*(7), 18–20. https://doi.org/10.7748/ns.30.7.18.s21.

Phillips, J., & Malone, B. (2014). Increasing racial/ethnic diversity in nursing to reduce health disparities and achieve health equity. *Public Health Reports (1974–), 129*, 45–50. https://doi.org/10.1177/00333549141291S209.

Pollard, C. L. (2015). What is the right thing to do: Use of a relational ethic framework to guide clinical decision-making. *International Journal of Caring Sciences, 8*(2), 362–368.

Public Health Agency of Canada. (2013). *Preventing chronic disease strategic plan 2013-2016.* Ottawa, ON: Her Majesty the Queen in Right of Canada. Retrieved from http://publications.gc.ca/collections/collection_2014/aspc-phac/HP35-39-2013-eng.pdf.

Racher, F. E., & Annis, R. C. (2007). Respecting culture and honoring diversity in community practice. *Research and Theory for Nursing Practice, 21*(4), 255–270. https://doi.org/10.1891/088971807782427985.

Racine, L. (2014). The enduring challenge of cultural safety in nursing. *Canadian Journal of Nursing Research, 46*(2), 6–9. https://doi.org/10.1177/084456211404600202.

Racine, L., & Petrucka, P. (2011). Enhancing decolonization and knowledge transfer in nursing research with non-Western populations: Examining the congruence between primary healthcare and postcolonial feminist approaches. *Nursing Inquiry, 18*(1), 12–20. https://doi.org/10.1111/j.1440-1800.2010.00504.x.

Ramsden, I. (2002). *Cultural safety and nursing education in Aotearoa and Te Waipounamu.* Wellington, New Zealand: Victoria University.

Reading, C. L., & Wien, F. (2013). *Health inequalities and social determinants of Aboriginal peoples' health.* Prince George, BC: National Collaborating Centre for Aboriginal Health. Retrieved from http://www.nccah-ccnsa.ca/Publications/Lists/Publications/Attachments/46/health_inequalities_EN_web.pdf.

Registered Nurses' Association of Ontario. (2006). *Establishing therapeutic relationships—Best practice guideline.* Retrieved from http://rnao.ca/bpg/guidelines/establishing-therapeutic-relationships.

Registered Nurses' Association of Ontario. (2007). *Embracing cultural diversity in health care: Developing cultural competence.* Retrieved from http://rnao.ca/bpg/guidelines/embracing-cultural-diversity-health-care-developing-cultural-competence.

Rowan, M. S., Rukholm, E., Bourque-Bearskin, R. L., et al. (2013). Cultural competence and cultural safety in Canadian schools of nursing: A mixed methods study. *International Journal of Nursing Education Scholarship, 10*(1), 1–10. https://doi.org/10.1515/ijnes-2012-0043.

Scheim, A. E., & Bauer, G. R. (2015). Sex and gender diversity among transgender persons in Ontario, Canada: Results from a respondent-driven sampling survey. *Journal of Sex Research, 52*(1), 1–14. https://doi.org/10.1080/00224499.2014.893553.

Smith, K. (2020). Facing history for the future of nursing. *Journal of Clinical Nursing, 29*(9–10), 1429–1431. https://doi.org/10.1111/jocn.15065.

Spadoni, M., Hartrick Doane, G., Sevean, P., & Poole, K. (2015). First-year nursing students—Developing relational caring practice through inquiry. *Journal of Nursing Education, 54*(5), 270–275. https://doi.org/10.3928/01484834-20150417-04.

Spector, R. (2012). *Cultural diversity in health and illness* (8th ed.). Upper Saddle River, NJ: Pearson Prentice Hall.

Spencer, M. S. (2008). A social worker's reflections on power, privilege, and oppression. *Social Work, 53*(2), 99–101. https://doi.org/10.1093/sw/53.2.99.

Srivastava, R. H. (2007). *The health care professional's guide to clinical cultural competence.* Toronto, ON: Elsevier Canada.

Stanley, D. (2010). Multigenerational workforce issues and their implications for leadership in nursing. *Journal of Nursing Management, 18*(7), 846–852. https://doi.org/10.1111/j.1365-2834.2 010.01158.x.

Statistics Canada. (2010a). *Canada's ethnocultural mosaic, 2006 census: National picture.* Retrieved from http://www12.statcan.ca/census-recensement/2006/as-sa/97-562/p2-eng.cfm.

Statistics Canada. (2010b). *Projections of the diversity of the Canadian population: 2006-2031.* Ottawa, ON: Minister of Industry. Retrieved from http://www.statcan.gc.ca/pub/91-551-x/91-551-x2010001-eng.pdf.

Statistics Canada. (2011a). *2011 National Household Survey.* Ottawa, ON: Author.

Statistics Canada. (2011b). *The Canadian population in 2011: Population counts and growth.* Retrieved from https://www12.statcan.gc.ca/census-recensement/2011/as-sa/98-310-x/98-310-x2011001-eng.cfm.

Statistics Canada. (2012a). *Aboriginal languages in Canada.* Ottawa, ON: Minister of Industry. Retrieved from http://www12.statcan.gc.ca/census-recensement/2011/as-sa/98-314-x/98-314-x2011003_3-eng.pdf.

Statistics Canada. (2012b). *The Canadian population in 2011: Age and sex.* Ottawa, ON: Minister of Industry. Retrieved from https://www12.statcan.gc.ca/census-recensement/2011/as-sa/98-311-x/98-311-x2011001-eng.pdf.

Statistics Canada. (2012c). *Immigrant languages in Canada.* Ottawa, ON: Minister of Industry. Retrieved from http://www12.statcan.gc.ca/census-recensement/2011/as-sa/98-314-x/98-314-x2011003_2-eng.pdf.

Statistics Canada. (2012d). *Linguistic characteristics of Canadians.* Ottawa, ON: Minister of Industry. Retrieved from http://www12.statcan.gc.ca/census-recensement/2011/as-sa/98-314-x/98-314-x2011001-eng.pdf.

Statistics Canada. (2012e). *Portrait of families and living arrangements in Canada.* Ottawa, ON: Minister of Industry. Retrieved from http://www12.statcan.gc.ca/census-recensement/2011/as-sa/98-312-x/98-312-x2011001-eng.pdf.

Statistics Canada. (2012f). *Visual census—Language, Canada.* Retrieved from https://www12.statcan.gc.ca/census-recensement/2011/dp-pd/vc-rv/index.cfm?Lang=eng&TOPIC_ID=4.

Statistics Canada. (2013a). *Aboriginal peoples and language.* Ottawa, ON: Minister of Industry. Retrieved from http://www12.statcan.gc.ca/nhs-enm/2011/as-sa/99 011 x/99 011 x2011003_1-eng.pdf.

Statistics Canada. (2013b). *Aboriginal peoples in Canada: First Nations people, Métis and Inuit.* Ottawa, ON: Minister of Industry. Retrieved from http://www12.statcan.gc.ca/nhs-enm/2011/as-sa/99-011-x/99-011-x2011001-eng.pdf.

Statistics Canada. (2013c). *Canadian survey on disability: Data tables (Catalogue no. 89-654-X).* Ottawa, ON: Minister of Industry. Retrieved from http://www.statcan.gc.ca/pub/89-654-x/89-654-x2013001-eng.pdf

Statistics Canada. (2013d). *Disability in Canada: Initial findings from the Canadian Survey on Disability.* Ottawa, ON: Minister of Industry. Retrieved from http://www.statcan.gc.ca/pub/89-654-x/89-654-x2013002-eng.pdf.

Statistics Canada. (2013e). *Generation status: Canadian-born children of immigrants.* Retrieved from https://www12.statcan.gc.ca/nhs-enm/2011/as-sa/99-010-x/99-010-x2011003_2-eng.cfm.

Statistics Canada. (2013f). *Immigration and ethnocultural diversity in Canada: National Household Survey, 2011.* Ottawa, ON: Minister of Industry. Retrieved from http://www12.statcan.gc.ca/nhs-enm/2011/as-sa/99-010-x/99-010-x2011001-eng.pdf.

Statistics Canada. (2014). Canada's population estimates: Age and sex, 2014. Retrieved from http://www.statcan.gc.ca/daily-quotidien/140926/dq140926b-eng.htm.

Statistics Canada. (2015a). *Disability in Canada: Initial findings from the Canadian Survey on Disability.* Retrieved from https://www150.statcan.gc.ca/n1/pub/89-654-x/89-654-x2013002-eng.htm.

Statistics Canada. (2015b). *Police-reported hate crime in Canada, 2013.* Ottawa, ON: Minister of Industry. Retrieved from http://www.statcan.gc.ca/pub/85-002-x/2015001/article/14191-eng.pdf.

Statistics Canada. (2015c). *Population projections by Aboriginal identity in Canada, 2006 to 2031.* Retrieved from http://www.statcan.gc.ca/pub/91-552-x/2011001/hl-fs-eng.htm.

Statistics Canada. (2015d). *Visible minority of person.* Retrieved from https://www23.statcan.gc.ca/imdb/p3Var.pl?Function=DEC&Id=45152.

Statistics Canada. (2017). *Immigration and ethnocultural diversity: Key results from the 2016 Census.* Retrieved from https://www150.statcan.gc.ca/n1/daily-quotidien/171025/dq171025b-eng.htm?indid=14428-1&indgeo=0.

Statistics Canada. (2018). *Population projections for Canada (2018 to 2068), provinces and territories (2018 to 2043).* Retrieved from https://www150.statcan.gc.ca/n1/pub/91-520-201x/2019001/sect02-eng.htm.

Sue, D. W. (2010). *Microaggressions in everyday life: Race, gender, and sexual orientation.* Hoboken, NJ: Wiley.

Tervalon, M., & Murray-Garcia, J. (1998). Cultural humility versus cultural competence: A critical distinction in defining physician training outcomes in multicultural education. *Journal of Health Care for the Poor and Underserved*, *9*(2), 117–125. https://doi.org/10.1353/hpu.2010.0233.

Truth and Reconciliation Commission of Canada. (2015). *Honouring the truth, reconciling for the future: Summary of the final report of the Truth and Reconciliation Commission of Canada.* Retrieved from http://www.trc.ca/websites/trcinstitution/index.php?p=890.

Tuck, E. M., & Yang, K. W. (2012). Decolonization is not a metaphor. *Decolonization: Indigeneity, Education, and Society*, *1*(1), 1–40. Retrieved from https://jps.library.utoronto.ca/index.php/des/article/view/18630.

Turner, D. (2006). *This is not a peace pipe: Towards a critical Indigenous philosophy.* Toronto, ON: University of Toronto Press.

Van Herk, K., Smith, D., & Andrew, C. (2011). Examining our privileges and oppressions: incorporating an intersectionality paradigm into nursing. *Nursing Inquiry*, *18*(1), 29–39. https://doi.org/10.1111/j.1440-1800.2011.00539.x.

Varcoe, C., Browne, A. J., Wong, S., et al. (2009). Harms and benefits: Collecting ethnicity data in a clinical context. *Social Science & Medicine*, *68*, 1659–1666. https://doi.org/10.1016/j.socscimed.2009.02.034.

Villarruel, A., Bigelow, A., & Alvarez, C. (2014). Integrating the 3Ds: A nursing perspective. *Public Health Reports*, *129* (1 Suppl. 2), 37–44. https://doi.org/10.1177/00333549141291S208.

Wesp, M., Scheer, M., Ruiz, M., et al. (2018). An emancipatory approach to cultural competency: The application of critical race, postcolonial, and intersectionality theories. *Advances in Nursing Science*, *41*(4), 316–326. https://doi.org/10.1097/ANS.0000000000000230.

Wilson, A. (1996). How we find ourselves: Identity development and two-spirit people. *Harvard Educational Review*, *66*, 303–317. https://doi.org/10.17763/haer.66.2.n551658577h927h4.

Wood, L., Kamper, D., & Swanson, K. (2018). Spaces of hope? Youth perspectives on health and wellness in indigenous communities. *Health and Place*, *50*, 137–145. https://doi.org/10.1016/j.healthplace.2018.01.010.

World Health Organization. (n.d.). *Social determinants of health.* Retrieved from http://www.who.int/social_determinants/sdh_definition/en/.

World Health Organization. (2008). *Closing the gap in a generation: Health equity through action on the social determinants of health.* Geneva, Switzerland: Author. Retrieved from http://apps.who.int/iris/bitstream/10665/43943/1/9789241563703_eng.pdf.

World Health Organization. (2015). *Disability and health: Fact Sheet No. 352.* Retrieved from http://www.who.int/mediacentre/factsheets/fs352/en/.

World Health Organization. (2020). Noncommunicable Diseases. Retrieved from https://www.who.int/health-topics/noncommunicable-diseases#tab=tab_1.

Yeung, S. (2016). Conceptualizing Cultural Safety: Definitions and Applications of Safety in Health Care for Indigenous Mothers in Canada. *Journal for Social Thought*, *1*(1), pp. 1–13. Retrieved from https://ir.lib.uwo.ca/jst/vol1/iss1/3/.

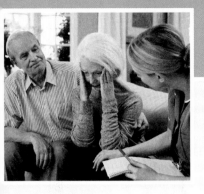

Ethical Issues and Dilemmas in Nursing Practice

Joyce K. Engel

(e) http://evolve.elsevier.com/Canada/Ross-Kerr/nursing

LEARNING OBJECTIVES

After reading this chapter, you will be able to:

- Explain the concept of everyday ethics in nursing.
- Discuss foundational concepts associated with the field of ethics.
- Explain traditional and contemporary ethical frameworks, concepts, and principles.
- Critique issues associated with the principles of autonomy, beneficence, and justice.
- Discuss everyday and broader ethical issues that impact nursing practice and patient care.
- Describe the importance of codes of ethics in professional practice.
- Describe strategies for ethical practice.

OUTLINE

KEY TERMS

active euthanasia
applied ethics
autonomy
beliefs
beneficence
consequentialism
deontology
dignity
doctrine of double effect
embodiment
engagement

euthanasia
everyday ethics
ethical awareness
ethical dilemma
ethics
fidelity
fiduciary relationship
justice
moral distress
morality
mutuality

noncoercion
nonmaleficence
normative ethics
paternalism
passive euthanasia
palliative sedation
social justice
therapeutic lying
values
virtue ethics
veracity

PERSONAL PERSPECTIVES

In the initial seminar in nursing ethics, the leader asks whether students have encountered ethical situations in their clinical rotations. Raja considers this question and concludes that he has yet to encounter anything that was unethical or that posed an ethical concern. Two weeks later, Raja is working with a patient in the surgical clinical setting who is very confused, and although confined to a chair, the patient frequently tries to get up and asks repeatedly as to when her husband and daughter are coming. From the chart, Raja learns that the patient's husband died a few months ago and that the daughter lives hundreds of miles away. Raja initially tries to distract the patient, but the patient returns again and again to attempts to get out of the chair and to pleas to see her husband. Raja observes that other staff tell the patient that her husband is coming in a few minutes. With this reassurance, the patient briefly settles, and so the staff encourage Raja to do the same thing. Raja is uncomfortable about lying to the patient because, like Kant, whose ideas were presented in ethics class, Raja believes that it is important to do what is right. Raja thinks "doing right" involves telling the patient some portion of the truth, especially because it has been stressed since year one of his nursing program that honesty is important. However, Raja wonders whether utilitarian ethics might suggest that lying will serve the greatest good if the patient settles and thus is less likely to get out of the chair and fall. Raja recognizes that he is liable to face similar patient situations in the future, and the idea of everyday ethics finally fits for him.

INTRODUCTION

Closely related to the issues pertaining to legal aspects of nursing practice are issues concerning nursing **ethics**. Nurses encounter ethical questions daily in practice in a health care environment that is becoming increasingly complex. Factors that contribute to this complexity are knowledge about health and illness, new technologies, finite and insufficient resources to meet all needs, and workload and stress among nurses. Societal values have increased the recognition of individual rights, freedoms, and responsibility for protecting those rights, including control over dying and concern for cultural competency and safety. Information on the Internet and social media is freely available, which means that the public asks more questions and expects more involvement in decisions about their health. Eradication and control of many diseases and technological advances mean that people are living longer, sometimes with diminished quality of life or great suffering. A longer lifespan has led to options in dying, such as medical assistance in dying (MAID). Because of these interacting factors, nurses face many ethical questions on a frequent basis. Who decides what is right for the person or family involved? Is there always a right answer? While legal aspects lay out social expectations and the consequences of actions and what one must do, ethics is about what one ought to do (Elster & Elliott, 2018) and involves choosing and justifying from among possible actions (Carper, 1978) that involve patients, colleagues, and the system.

FOUNDATIONAL CONCEPTS IN ETHICS

The field of ethics is a branch of philosophy that consists of several schools of thought, the purpose of which is to bring about good in society. Ethics include several divisions such as descriptive ethics (describes how persons behave), metaethics (explores why persons hold and interpret ideas of right and wrong), and **normative ethics** (provides principles and rules). **Applied ethics** (also termed practical ethics) involves the consideration of applying ethics to specific situations such as those in medicine or nursing (Oberle & Raffin Bouchal, 2009).

Some authors differentiate between ethics and **morality,** whereas others use the terms interchangeably. Ethics has been differentiated from morality in that ethics is sometimes considered to be the formal study of right and wrong and what ought to be, whereas morality is considered to be how individual persons decide and act on what they think is right or wrong, in accordance with their **beliefs** and **values.** Beliefs are what we believe to be true. Values are ideals or core beliefs of significance or importance and can be held by individual persons, groups, and societies. For example, the Canadian Nurses Association (CNA, 2017a) has outlined seven key values in its code of ethics that indicate what Canadian nurses believe to be especially important. Nurses need to be aware of their own personal values and beliefs and how these influence decisions in practice or conflict with the values and beliefs of other team members. This awareness is helpful in working through ethical concerns and issues.

Many studies are emerging in nursing that involve conflicts between (1) the beliefs acquired through early learning and through formal education; (2) the values or core beliefs held by nurses; and (3) the issues, expectations, and care situations in the workplace. For example, Ford and Austin (2018), in a study of the experiences of nurses in neonatal intensive care units, suggested that being required to carry out interventions for profoundly ill and suffering neonates sets up a conflict of conscience for some nurses, leading to guilt and burnout. The distress that is felt when nurses are unable to do what they think is right is termed **moral distress,** which can lead to low job satisfaction (McAndrew, Leske, & Schroeder, 2018).

Although the term **ethical dilemma** is frequently used to describe conflicts between right and wrong in nursing practice and in the literature, Jameton (1984) points out that dilemmas—which involve the need to make decisions where there are mutually exclusive choices of actions or choices and conflicts in principles—are rare in nursing practice. Nurses, for example, are not required to make decisions as to whether to withdraw treatment from profoundly ill neonates; these are the decisions of physicians. However, in everyday practice, nurses encounter, for example, the need to decide whether to use deception to elicit cooperation from a confused patient to take antipsychotic medications intended to control aggressive behaviours. These actions, which involve choices of right or wrong, often go unrecognized by nurses as ethical decisions because they are so ordinary. The notion of **everyday ethics** emerged as a predominant field of ethical inquiry in nursing and is foundational to the CNA *Code of Ethics for Registered Nurses* (CNA, 2017a). Everyday ethics refers to the day-to-day ethical choices made by nurses in relationship with patients, families, colleagues, communities, and the environment at large (Engel & Prentice, 2013; Wright & Brajtman, 2011).

As suggested in the definition, relationships are the foundation of everyday ethics, especially those that nurses have with patients, which are different from the relationships between nurses and physicians. Everyday ethics also involves **ethical awareness,** the recognition that every nursing action has the potential to impact the patient. Nurses often lack awareness that routine actions such as administering medications or taking vital signs can involve ethical decisions and implications (Milliken, 2018). This highlights the need for nurses to be aware of why and how they make choices in practice. These perspectives have challenged the popularity of bioethics, a discipline that arose in response to the dilemmas presented by advances in biology and medicine and was popular in nursing ethics in the 1980s and 1990s (Oberle & Raffin Bouchal, 2009).

There is considerable discussion in the nursing literature as to whether nursing ethics is a separate discipline or a subset of another, such as bioethics. There is also discussion as to whether health disciplines such as medicine and nursing should hold distinct perspectives on ethics or whether, in the context of collaborative person-centred care, there needs to be an overarching interprofessional ethics (Engel & Prentice, 2013). As nursing ethics broadens in its inquiry, nurses are exploring various ethical theories and concepts, including bioethics, to understand how these can guide nurses to understand how nurses make decisions and how to make ethical decisions relevant to their practice. Regardless of the theories or concepts chosen, it is clear that the issues dealt with by nurses are unique to nursing and cannot be subsumed under another discipline (Engel & Prentice, 2013; Wright & Brajtman, 2011). Additionally, it is clear that moral action in nursing begins with mindfulness of the potential impact that nursing activities can have on patients and the need for ethical awareness.

ETHICAL THEORIES AND FRAMEWORKS

Knowledge of several types of ethical theory is helpful to understand how individual and societal ethical decisions are made. These theories provide different lenses through which nurses can examine ethical issues and situations and assist in helping to clarify the values and beliefs that they and others bring to practice and the health care setting.

Normative Ethics

Normative ethics is concerned with providing a moral framework of values, principles, virtues, and ideals that can be used to work out what kinds of action are good and bad, right and wrong, and what persons ought to do. There are three main traditions in normative ethics: **virtue ethics, deontology,** and **consequentialism.**

Virtue Ethics

Virtue ethics stems from the work of Aristotle and focuses on the character of the person who is taking the action rather than the action itself. Virtues are character traits that are easily identified with and by nurses as consistent with nursing practice. Compassion, trustworthiness, integrity, wisdom, and conscientiousness (Beauchamp & Childress, 2013) make one a good person who will take good actions. Virtue ethics fell out of favour because of the emphasis on evidence and rationality, as well as concerns as to whether good character, even if it was required for moral action, could be taught. After many years of being ignored, virtue ethics is making a comeback in recent years, and character traits such as honesty and trustworthiness are reflected in the 2017 CNA *Code of Ethics* (CNA, 2017a). For example, the *Code of Ethics* contains statements such as "[n]urses are honest . . ." (p. 8) and statements about trustworthiness and having integrity. Virtue ethics has some advantages over the rule-based theories of ethics that have been more prominent. The main strengths of virtue theory are that it gives a central role to character rather than action or obligation and acknowledges emotion and intention in moral judgement.

Other ethical theories neglect these aspects of morality. Kantian ethics, for example, holds that it is important to act out of duty rather than inclination, which is decided through objective thought and rationality. Whether or not you want to do the right thing is irrelevant; all that matters is whether or not you do it. Could a nurse be ethical and do what is right if the nurse was not a good person? (See Applying Content Knowledge.) It could be argued that nurses could be of poor character and yet maintain excellent technical and organizational competence, know ethical rules and principles, and make decisions that were fully competent, safe, and ethical in accordance with good practice. Virtue ethics, however, maintains that it is not sufficient for persons to be technically competent and to know rules and principles of moral behaviour; the motivation to carry out those rules and principles comes from being of good character.

🔍 APPLYING CONTENT KNOWLEDGE

Your classmate is one of the top academic students in your class and excels at technical skills in clinical practice, although patients sometimes complain about your classmate's lack of interpersonal skills. In your nursing ethics course, this classmate wrote an outstanding paper on the need for ethics in nursing practice. Recently, however, you discovered that your classmate has frequently cheated on examinations and papers, including the one in the nursing ethics course. According to Aristotle, could this colleague, while unethical in academic matters, still be an ethical nurse?

Deontology

The second tradition of normative ethics is deontology, which holds the belief that certain acts are intrinsically right or wrong and are the product of reason. When we know this, we can set forth consistent rules to follow to ensure ethical actions. Immanuel Kant is the foremost deontology theorist. He stressed that persons have intrinsic worth and that they must never be treated as a means to an end, which is a basis for respect of others. Furthermore, Kant believed that persons are capable of reason and thus of freedom to make choices and autonomous decisions, providing that reason is used to make decisions and the choices do not interfere with the freedom of others (Yeo & Moorhouse, 2003). This thinking is reflected in later theories and in health care practices such as informed consent. Kant also stressed the importance of obligation, which means acting according to one's duty without emotion or concern for consequences. An action that is performed with goodwill or with the intent to do one's duty is considered right. If the act and intention are right, then the act is considered good in and of itself. Consider a situation in which a student or a graduate nurse is attentive to performing procedures correctly and safely for patients to avoid negative evaluation or a reprimand from an instructor or manager. Is that person acting morally? Although doing the right thing, which in this instance is fulfilling the duty to provide safe care, Kantian ethics would only consider doing the right thing worthy of praise if it was done out of good intention and not self-interest, such as fear. Kantian ethics places emphasis on doing what is right, rather than on consideration of context-laden consequences (Beauchamp & Childress, 2013; Oberle & Raffin Bouchal, 2009).

The idea of duty is reflected in professional standards, guidelines, and literature, where the duty of nurses is seen as that of putting patients first and ahead of the needs or desires of the nurses themselves (Jensen & Lidell, 2009), especially when the safety or well-being of patients is jeopardized (College of Nurses of Ontario, 2018).

According to Kant, duty arises out of maxims or logical principles that are derived from reason. These principles have an abstract foundation that is independent of current circumstances, intuition, or usefulness. Kant's categorical imperative, a rule that has no exceptions, maintains that if an act is morally right, then it must be right in all circumstances. An advantage of deontology and Kantian thought is that it promotes the ideas of impartiality and consistency, as well as the use of reason to determine what is right, which fits with objectivity of empiricism. The assumptions in deontology would disallow treating certain patients or populations differently than others, an attitude that could facilitate perceptions of fairness and consistency. However, a criticism of Kant's ideas is that they were inflexible and disallowed the capacity to act out of kindness in response to the unique needs of the person. A further criticism is that the theory does not provide guidance as to the right act when two duties are in conflict. For example, what duty would be followed if a woman is protected from the severe abuse of a partner, and so is prevented from harm, and the partner shows up, demanding to know the whereabouts of the woman? Both duties are relevant; the duty to be truthful and the duty to provide protection. According to Kant, both duties must be performed, which offers little assistance to resolve this dilemma (Beauchamp & Childress, 2013; Keatings & Adams, 2020).

Consequentialism

Consequentialism is the theory that the moral status of an act is determined by its consequences or the end result and thus is future oriented. No action is of itself either right or wrong. In order to achieve moral right, it is necessary to project the various consequences of actions and select the action that will maximize good. The moral imperative in consequentialism is that of maximizing good consequences and minimizing the bad (Burkhardt, Nathaniel, & Walton, 2018; Yeo & Moorhouse, 2003). Consequentialism thus rejects both the virtue ethicist's view that the moral status of an act is determined by the moral character of the agent performing it and the deontologist's view that the moral status of an act is determined by the type of act that it is. According to consequentialism, each of these factors is morally irrelevant.

The most well-known of consequentialist theories is utilitarianism. John Stuart Mill, who proposed utilitarianism, maintained that good is determined by the usefulness or utility of an action. According to Mill, utility, and thus moral action, requires doing the greatest good for the greatest number, although he also cautioned that this could not be at the expense of violating the rights of a few (Burkhardt, Nathaniel, & Walton, 2018). The highest good, according to Mill's principle of utility, is that of happiness, and thus utilitarianism is grounded in the pursuit of the greatest happiness for the greatest number of people and the avoidance of pain. Importantly, the happiness in question is not that of the agent or person performing the action, but that of all concerned. According to Mill, an action is moral when the utility or value of an act is higher than any other action that a person could have taken.

The distribution of health care frequently uses this type of reasoning to determine who will most benefit from health care resources. Utilitarianism is also evident in daily care when nurses are required to determine priorities among sometimes competing patient needs, and to distribute time and care to patients whose needs are greatest or most urgent; therefore, nurses are responsible for determining which patients will benefit the most. In this case, the happiness of the nurse is not what matters but that of the patients through the relief of their pain or discomfort.

Critics of utilitarianism point out several difficulties with utilitarianism. For example, how do we measure happiness? Who should decide what happiness means? Who makes decisions as to what options to pursue? One danger of utilitarian thinking is that the majority could decide on a definition of happiness and enact this for many, with limited or no concern for other definitions of happiness or the concerns of the minority. A further difficulty is that of accurately predicting consequences, particularly in complex and dynamic situations, where several factors may impact on outcomes.

There are several historical and recent examples of the limits to decisions that reflect utilitarian ethics as their basis. For example, in the early and mid twentieth century, the provinces of British Columbia and Alberta enacted legislation that enabled forced sterilization—without consent—of women who were deemed mentally incompetent to prevent the possibility of their giving birth to similarly affected children. Recent concerns have been raised about Indigenous women who were sterilized through this legislation, presumably to reduce the size of the Indigenous population, but also in response to reports that Indigenous women have experienced coerced sterilization in Saskatchewan, Alberta, Manitoba, and Ontario (Collier, 2017). The impacts of these decisions, made in the interests of benefitting society or of generating the greatest good, illustrate the difficulties in projecting morally defensible ends and in protecting the interests and rights of those who are in the minority, vulnerable, or without a voice.

Bioethics

Medical ethics emerged in the 1970s, specifically from a need to provide medicine with practical guidance in moral questions (Oberle & Raffin Bouchal, 2009). This discipline gave rise to bioethics, or principled reasoning, which is widely used within medicine, nursing, health care, and other disciplines. The most famous bioethical theory, developed by Thomas Beauchamp and James Childress, reflects ideas from deontology and utilitarianism. For example, this theory stresses duty to the patient and the importance of obtaining the best outcome for the patient. Additionally, bioethics assumes that ethical action can be determined through use of reason and application of generalist principles to clinical situations. The four principles included in bioethics include **autonomy, beneficence, nonmaleficence,** and **justice.** These principles were not initially developed by Beauchamp and Childress, but were first included in the *Belmont Report* to address issues in research (Oberle & Raffin Bouchal, 2009) and have been very influential in health care as a result of inclusion in bioethics. Two other principles, **veracity** and **fidelity,** were later added to bioethics by Michael Yeo and Anne Moorhouse (Oberle & Raffin Bouchal, 2009).

Autonomy

The principle of autonomy assumes that a capable and competent person has the right to self-determination or to act in accordance with their own wishes and goals if the exercise of these choices does not interfere with the rights and freedoms of others. This principle is heavily influenced by Kantian ethics and assumes that persons have worth and that they are capable of reason, which is the basis of informed consent—a principle that would have been violated in the coerced sterilization of Indigenous women. Respect for autonomy also grants patients the right to expect that information shared for the purposes of competent and compassionate care will remain confidential and will only be shared within the parameters included in the consent to care (Keatings & Adams, 2020). This right can become blurred when technology and social connections overlap; for instance, posting photos, videos, and other information on social media sites, even without identifying information, does not protect the confidentiality of patients (British Columbia College of Nursing Professionals, 2019).

Critics of the principle of autonomy suggest that it reflects the dominance of Western individualistic thinking, in which the person is considered self-determining, and therefore this principle is not applicable to all cultures or settings. For example, self-determination or individual autonomy is a contrary concept to that in Asian and African cultures, where community interests and rights come ahead of those of the individual and autonomy is interdependent rather than independent. In Ubuntu, or the African worldview, any decision that does not consider the community would be unethical. Procreation is considered crucial for the good of the community, and community members must each take their places in the chain of procreation or else be considered rebellious and a curse (Ekmekci & Arda, 2017); communal precedence overrides autonomy, even in the personal act of deciding to bear a child. Under Ubuntu philosophy, informing a patient as to the seriousness of a medical diagnosis without informing the family would be considered offensive, a perspective that is also shared in Japanese culture (Ekmekci & Arda, 2017). In another context, such as in Iran, the male head of household is expected to make decisions related to health care, which can cause concern for care providers who are accustomed to the rights of individual women or others to make decisions for themselves.

Beneficence

Beneficence is the obligation to act in the best interests of the patient and to do good. Prior to the development of bioethics and the preeminence of autonomy, beneficence was considered the primary goal of health care. Beneficence is arguably the basis of nursing practice because of close links with the concept of caring and is the foundation for the high level of trust that is placed in nurses. As a duty or obligation of nurses, it is included in practice standards and guidelines of regulatory bodies that direct nurses to put the interests of the patient first. For example, "Nurses, as self-regulated professionals, implicitly promise to provide safe, effective, and ethical care. Because of their commitment to clients, nurses try to act in the best interests of the client…" (College of Nurses of Ontario, 2018, p. 10).

Determination of what is good or what is in the best interests of the patient can potentially set up moral conflicts for the nurse. Who determines *the good*? What happens when the patient wants something different than what the nurse or other care providers think would be of benefit? (See Case Study.) In the case study, the beliefs of the family and of the patient as to what is best, as well as those of the nurse, are different from those of the physician and, perhaps, of other nurses.

Nonmaleficence

The principle of nonmaleficence refers to avoiding harm or doing no harm. 'The concept of doing no harm'? is included in various professional codes of ethics. Its inclusion in the Hippocratic oath and in the history and culture of medicine has presented ethical dilemmas for some physicians who would see the deliberate termination of death as contrary to the tenets of medicine. This conflict highlights the difficulty in defining harm or even good and also raises the question as to who should define what is good or harmful.

Nursing codes of ethics and practice standards and guidelines obligate nurses to practice in a manner that is safe, competent, and therefore avoids harm to patients. Nonetheless, some procedures, such as wound debridement or insertion of an intravenous line, can cause temporary harm. In such situations, the benefits of promoting healing outweigh the risks of infection and pain, and the harm is temporary. In other situations, the balance between benefit and harms may be less clear or even contentious, such as the harms or benefits of therapeutic abortions. Keeping persons on prolonged life support produces suffering and thus moral conflict for nurses. To alleviate this suffering, communication with families and patients about complex life decisions is important. Nurses can facilitate decision making by using neutral language such as "appropriateness of treatment" rather than "futility of treatment" and

CASE STUDY

John, an 88-year-old man, is admitted to hospital in end-stage renal failure. On admission, he is lethargic, his urine output is limited, and the skin on his legs is shiny and tight. Fluid seeps from where the skin on his legs has begun to crack. The physician has met with John and his family, and they are all aware that the prognosis for John is poor and that death is likely within a few days. Nonetheless, the physician orders fluid and sodium restrictions with the reasoning that this will reduce the load on the renal system and some of the build-up in edema. The family visit often, and because they are deeply concerned about John, they comply with the fluid and sodium restrictions, offering him ice chips to alleviate his thirst. On the third day in hospital, John begs his family for soup from the downstairs kiosk. The family checks with the nurses and are told that John can only have ice chips because he has reached his fluid allotment for that time in the day. John continues to ask for the soup. After weighing his need for comfort from food that he enjoys and the possibility that not having this minimal relief will cause more discomfort than the distressing symptoms from his renal failure, the family finally gives in and gets the soup for him. The next day, a sign is placed on the door of the room advising that visitors must check with staff before providing any food or fluids to John. The family is upset and speak to the nurse who is on duty. The nurse says she agrees that John's wishes are important, especially given his prognosis, but the physician has decided that fluid restrictions will be in John's best interest and that she must support the physician's orders at present by not allowing John to have additional fluids. However, she states that she will speak with the physician about more flexible fluid options when the physician makes his rounds.

by encouraging persons at the end of life to be clear about their wishes. Nurses must not only facilitate decisions about personal or advance directives, but also ensure that open discussion and sensitive listening occur (Storch, 2015) and that patient wishes and goals are documented and communicated to the rest of the team.

Justice

The principle of justice is concerned with fairness. It focuses on how individuals and groups within society are treated, and how benefits (such as health care) and burdens are distributed. The distribution of benefits and burdens at a societal level are culturally and socially determined and may be enshrined in laws and policies. Justice raises two particularly relevant questions: What criteria should be used to decide on fair outcomes for distribution of benefits and burdens and by what process should these decisions be made (Yeo & Moorhouse, 1996)? These questions remain especially challenging in the Canadian health care system, where many see public access to health care for all as a difficult aspiration (see Chapter 1). In everyday practice, nurses are frequently confronted with decisions about where and how to allocate their time and expertise when caring for groups of patients. Thus, nurses need to be conscious of biases and preferences for certain types of patients that can affect the distribution of their care and attention.

Justice can also refer to retribution or punishment for wrongdoing. Consider the issue of nurses whose substance abuse problems have affected their practice. This situation provokes debate about whether regulatory bodies and employers ought to punish nurses through disciplinary action, which can interfere with their seeking help, or instead require rehabilitative measures (Kunyk, 2015).

Veracity

Veracity refers to the value of truth-telling and is linked to respect for autonomy and the **dignity** of others. Truth-telling is also linked to trust, open communication, and shared responsibility and is promoted in codes of ethics and practice standards. Lying implies making decisions for another as to what that person should or should not know and communicates a difference in power between the person who tells the lie and the person who receives the lie. Furthermore, lies and deception can prevent patients from fully sharing in decisions related to their own care. Veracity refers to an approach to practice in which nurses continually strive to provide accurate, truthful, and objective information in communications between patients and other care providers (Burkhardt, Nathaniel, & Walton, 2018).

Fidelity

Fidelity refers to keeping promises and is foundational to creating and maintaining trust in nurse–patient relationships. In everyday practice, it can mean returning with pain medication when it is promised and maintaining the confidentiality of information that is shared in the nurse–patient relationship. This commitment, however, can create conflicts for nurses when patients ask to share information with a nurse that could be harmful to the patient or others. For example, if a patient shares their suicidal intent and asks the nurse to keep this a "secret," the nurse may worry that the patient will lose trust in the nurse if this information is subsequently shared. Similarly, an elderly person may share information with a nurse that indicates elder abuse is occurring and ask for confidentiality. While there are no consistent and specific laws regarding reporting of elder abuse in Canada, there is nonetheless an ethical argument to be made for breaking the promise of confidentiality (Burkhardt, Nathaniel, & Walton, 2018). When persons ask that "secrecy" be maintained, nurses should identify whether reporting is necessary if they suspect that the information to be shared could hurt the person in care or others.

Feminist Ethics

Feminist ethics grew out of a concern that traditional theories supported a male perspective in ethics, as these theories were concerned primarily with objectivity, reason, and virtues such as courage, traits that are commonly associated with men (Oberle & Raffin Bouchal, 2009). Feminist theorists believed that virtues frequently associated with women, such as nurturing and caring, tended to be ignored, as were issues of concern to women such as social context or questions about power and power differentials, gender bias, oppression, and **social justice** (Oberle & Raffin Bouchal, 2009). Further, feminist approaches suggest that ethical deliberations involve a collaborative approach in which persons work together to find shared understanding and meaning. Ethical decisions arise out of the context of relationships, rather than adhering to an objective, rational view or a concern with the greater good. Feminist approaches have given rise to care theories, in which moral weight is given to caring (Oberle & Raffin Bouchal, 2009), a trait that is considered feminine, as opposed to *being cared for*, which is considered masculine (Osuji, 2018). Care is considered a response to a need and is an act that builds relationships. As such, care theories are necessarily relational in which the particularity of the relationship, rather than rules or principles, is the dominant concern. For care theorists such as Joan Tronto, care and caring need to be considered within a web of bodies, ourselves, and the environment (Osuji, 2018), an influence that is reflected in relational ethics. Care theories stress the importance of the voice of the patient, the impact of power in relationships, and context, which is inescapable. According to care theories, ethical deliberations emphasize process rather than compliance with universal laws, principles, or overriding concern with outcomes. Rather than informed consent, agreement to procedures and care might better be conceptualized as shared decision making, wherein meanings are negotiated rather than assumed or universally determined and the inclusion of others, such as family, is emphasized.

Relational Ethics

Relational ethics builds on the assumptions inherent in feminist and care ethics, such as the importance of a negotiated understanding and the meaning of illness and health. Moral actions arise out of and within the context of the patient and care provider relationship and also within the context of institutional structures (Oberle & Raffin Bouchal, 2009). Within the framework of relational knowing, autonomy, which has often been considered the most important principle in health care, is reframed as involving interdependent rather than independent choices and decision making. In relational ethics, consent to a "do not resuscitate" (DNR) order, for example, goes beyond the question of whether DNR should be performed or not, based on the procedure, risks, and benefits for the patient. It also means engaging in detailed conversations with patients and families about their true intent in consenting or not consenting to DNR, seeing the patient as a unique person, imagining other morally acceptable options, and understanding the implications of elements such as deteriorating health and futility (Bjorklund & Lund, 2019). Bergum and Dossetor (2005), through extensive research on ethics in health care, have suggested that relational ethics involves **embodiment, mutuality, engagement, noncoercion,** freedom, and choice. Embodiment is the recognition that mind and body are one; pain, for example, is known not only through objective observation and science but also through the intimacy of the nurse–patient relationship and understanding how it is experienced and known by the patient. Mutuality refers to a reciprocal relationship of trust, in which neither patient nor caregiver is harmed. Engagement refers to the capacity to connect with others openly, respectfully, and away from "I respect your wishes" to "I respect you." Engagement means finding a way to look at things together, acknowledging the experiences and knowledge of each. Noncoercion means not forcing choice, but instead creating environments in which persons are free to make choices. The emergence of relational ethics in contemporary nursing as a significant approach to moral activity is congruent with the concept, within nursing, that relationship is the core of practice.

Understanding and Choosing Ethical Actions

Working through ethical questions and conflicts is part of everyday nursing practice. It is not always possible to find a single solution for an ethical problem, and nurses may experience ethical uncertainty when they are confronted with situations in which they are unsure of their values or where the moral problem resides. Furthermore, there may be system or team constraints that make it difficult to do what is right. What assists ethical practice is identifying

TABLE 15.1 Summary of Ethical Theories and Frameworks

Theory or Framework	Selected Proponents	Main Assumptions	Focus
Deontology	• Kant	• Persons have worth • Reason gives freedom to choose • Duty determined by logical principles derived from universal imperatives	• Right actions
Consequentialism	• Mill	• Greatest good for the greatest number • Maximization of happiness	• Outcomes or consequences
Virtue ethics	• Aristotle	• Persons of good character make moral choices • Golden mean (avoid excesses)	• Character
Bioethics	• Beauchamp • Childress • Yeo • Moorhouse	• Moral decisions guided by principles (autonomy, beneficence, nonmaleficence, justice, veracity, fidelity)	• Principles
Feminist/care ethics	• Noddings • Gilligan • Tronto	• Need to include context • Values include social justice, community, uniqueness of persons • Power differentials, collaboration important • Caring has moral worth	• Context • Caring
Relational ethics	• Bergum • Dossetor	• Moral decisions occur within relational spaces • Ethical relationships involve embodiment, engagement, mutuality, choice, freedom, noncoercion	• Relationships

ethical situations or ethical awareness; showing curiosity and commitment; and developing a moral community where open discussion and mentorship can occur in perplexing ethical situations. Additionally, knowledge of ethical frameworks and concepts (Table 15.1) supports nurses to gain additional perspectives and approaches to ethical concerns.

ETHICAL PRINCIPLES AND ISSUES IN CARE

Although ethical theory does not provide a formula for deciding whether certain behaviours are morally acceptable, the tradition of deontology provides principles that can help nurses take consistent positions on certain issues. Three of these principles—autonomy, beneficence, and justice—are particularly useful in nursing ethics.

Respect for Autonomy

Being autonomous implies the freedom to decide and act and is the key principle involved in informed consent. In bioethics, many issues stem from failure to respect autonomy or failure to recognize a person's rights to hold their own views on issues and to make decisions voluntarily based on their own perspectives. Issues of autonomy can range from whether a person has the right to refuse treatment to whether a person can decide to end their life. Many elements of health care erode a person's autonomy and serve to disregard their personal preferences or self-care knowledge. This issue is of especial concern in long-term care settings, where older adults may be given little or no control over their bathing or choices in food and may be given medications that they might otherwise refuse (Engel, Salfi, Micsinszki, & Bodnar, 2017). Codes of ethics for physicians and nurses all specifically address the principle of respect for autonomy. Problems arise when we try to interpret this principle when it conflicts with other principles, such as justice, which involves respecting the rights of others, and beneficence, which refers to acting in the best interests of the patient (Oberle & Raffin Bouchal, 2009). When can the principle of autonomy be overridden? An example may be when a person with serious mental health issues threatens serious harm to others or self and is admitted to hospital despite their refusal (see Applying Content Knowledge).

APPLYING CONTENT KNOWLEDGE

Consider a situation in which a person who has been threatening to harm others and kill themselves is admitted to hospital involuntarily. During admission, the patient's partner discloses to the nurses that the patient has a history of anger and violence. The patient is highly agitated and angry upon admission and refuses all medication. Shortly after admission, the patient attacks another patient verbally and pushes them into the wall. The newly admitted patient is restrained and given medication. Identify the ethical principles that apply in this situation. What ethical principles might be in conflict?

Autonomy in health care means that the patient has the right to accept or refuse treatment, except in situations where harm is imminent or there are legal restraints on autonomy. However, when the consequence of respecting this right is the death of the patient, other values come into play for health care providers, such as respect for life itself. It is relatively easy for nurses to respect patients' decisions about treatment when these decisions agree with what the nurse believes to be the right decision.

In Canada, the case of Nancy B. brought the issue of self-determination into prominent view (*Nancy B. v. Hôtel-Dieu de Québec* [1992]). Nancy B. was a young woman with Guillain-Barré syndrome who was paralyzed and living on a respirator. She requested to be disconnected from the respirator. Her request created a moral dilemma for most of the nurses and physicians involved in her care. This case became a legal battle between lawyers for Nancy B. and the Hôtel-Dieu hospital in Québec. The major issue was whether this was a question of Nancy B.'s right to refuse treatment or a question of assisted suicide or homicide, both of which are illegal (the MAID law came into effect in 2016). The Superior Court of Quebec determined the issue to be an ethical one of the right to refuse treatment. This case clarified the right of Canadians to refuse treatment, even when that treatment is sustaining life.

Self-determination is not limited to life and death matters—it also involves making decisions about lifestyle. For example, individuals make decisions to continue with lifestyles and behaviour patterns that are known to be detrimental to their health and well-being, such as smoking, overeating, excessive drinking, driving while high, and engaging in unprotected sexual activity. Efforts to educate the public about the hazards of such habits have met with some success, although many people continue to choose actions that are harmful to their health.

Informed Consent

Because health care providers possess significant knowledge about health and disease, the functioning of the human body, and various treatments for illnesses—knowledge that is not possessed by most members of the public—some difficult ethical issues are bound to arise. Lack of knowledge affects the ability of patients to make good decisions or choices regarding their treatment and to exercise their autonomy. Yet, complete knowledge of all the issues may be impossible for the average patient to achieve, no matter how much information the nurse or physician imparts. What are the ethics governing this imbalance of knowledge?

In the past, health care providers were mainly concerned with doing good for the benefit of the patient, a situation fraught with beneficence and **paternalism**, or deciding what is best for the patient, without necessarily gaining informed consent. Truth-telling did not play a large role in professional practice. Professionals were likely to decide that the truth would be harmful to the patient, and thus they would conceal facts that they believed were likely to cause distress. This attitude has changed, however, and in the present day, it is believed that patients have a right to know the truth, which includes giving patients appropriate information so that they can exercise their autonomy. Even though there may be a large knowledge gap between patients and health care providers, the truth can be told in a way that is helpful to the patient. That means a communication in which the patient will understand what the health care provider knows and believes to be true about the situation.

The right to be informed has increased the need for obtaining informed consent before medical interventions are implemented and before patients are asked to participate in research. Until the 1970s, there was no expectation or requirement for obtaining informed consent for participation in research, and people were sometimes exploited. There are many historical examples in the literature of unethical research practices. For example, in an experiment at the Allen Memorial Institute in Montreal in the late 1940s, patients were given mind-altering drugs, such as lysergic acid diethylamide (LSD), which had far-reaching effects on their mental health.

Beneficence

Beneficence refers to the obligation to take positive action to effect good for the patient and to protect patients from harm. Acts of beneficence are required by the **fiduciary relationship** between nurse and patient. Nurses know that the risks of harm must be weighed against the possible benefits to patients and that as nurses they have a duty to benefit others. Failure to do so can result in sanctions of nurses by provincial and territorial regulatory bodies or criminal charges through the criminal justice system. The recent case of Elizabeth Wettlaufer, an Ontario nurse who was convicted of causing the deaths of eight people in her care, highlights the responsibility of both individual nurses and regulatory bodies to ensure that nurses are acting in the best interests of patients and avoiding harm to them.

Justice

Justice implies treatment that is fair, due, or owed. The principle of justice is based on the idea that everyone has certain rights. When these rights are met, justice has been served. The term "distributed justice" refers to fair, equitable, and appropriate distribution of justice in society as determined by norms of distribution. Usually, distributive justice applies to such matters as political rights and economic goods, but it can also apply to health care services. The *Canada Health Act* requires equal access to health care for all Canadians, which means that unequal access is an injustice. Beauchamp and Childress (2013) identified guiding principles for distribution of resources, including distribution according to equal share, individual need, effort, contribution, merit, and free market exchange.

Deciding Among Conflicting Principles

Most societies use more than one of these principles of justice, with the acknowledgement that different situations require different approaches (Beauchamp & Walters, 2003). When conflicts arise among ethical principles, theorists have attempted to devise ways of determining which principle should prevail. Much of the discussion centres on the emergence of the idea that there are certain universal human rights. These are both moral and legal, but moral rights are the subject of ethics, whereas legal rights belong to the judiciary. The freedom of persons to choose or to exercise autonomy is frequently considered the most important of the ethical principles, but it is recognized that liberty has limits that commonly involve restrictions on the right to choose to harm oneself or others.

The question of justice presents ethical issues that are frequently described in the literature today. These issues concern inadequate staffing due to shortages in the nursing workforce, which causes nurses to make difficult decisions about apportioning care when all needs cannot be met, as well nurses' moral distress. The complexity of intensive care environments and their contribution to the moral distress of nurses were highlighted in a recent study conducted in Alberta. Opgenorth, Stelfox, Gilfoyle et al. (2018) identified that inappropriate utilization of beds, physician-related factors, patient and family factors (e.g., lack of advance planning), and provider factors contributed to this distress. Significantly, the primary provider factor was nursing

workforce related and included high attrition of nurses and high nurse-to-patient ratios. While this study considered only the complexities of critical care settings, nurses practising in all types of health care settings need a knowledge base in ethical concepts, theories, and principles. Nurses also need support and expert resources to assist them in ensuring that ethical issues are recognized and addressed, such as threats to patient safety related to staffing issues.

ETHICAL ISSUES IN NURSING AND HEALTH CARE

Choosing Options for Death

Medical aid or assistance in dying (MAID) presents various legal and ethical issues not only for health care systems but also for nurses, physicians, and other health care providers who might be called upon to assist with the act of dying. The decision to enact legislation and regulations that enable those who live with serious conditions to choose MAID also introduced emotional, moral, and professional complexities that are further complicated by various terminologies and conditions of participation in the process of dying (Government of Canada, 2020).

On June 17, 2016, the Canadian federal government enacted Bill C-14, a statute that enables those who are 18 years of age or older and who experience a "grievous and irremediable condition" (Government of Canada, 2020) to voluntarily request and agree to medical assistance in dying. This statute was a response to the earlier decisions (*Carter v. Canada, 2015; Rodriguez v. British Columbia, 1993*) of the Supreme Court of Canada. The Supreme Court held that laws preventing physician assistance with dying interfered with the rights of persons under the *Canadian Charter of Rights and Freedoms*, because not having the liberty to freely make decisions as personal as whether or not to end intolerable suffering threatened a person's security (*Carter v. Canada, 2015*). Furthermore, the justices of the court held that traditional means of suicide were more threatening to the security of person than enabling self-determined death under medical supervision or euthanasia (Attaran, 2015).

The word "euthanasia" is derived from Greek and means good or pleasant death. Is death ever preferable to life? That question is difficult to answer because there is always a context to be considered. **Euthanasia** is the putting to death, by painless method, of a terminally ill or severely debilitated person through omission (intentionally withholding a lifesaving medical procedure, or **passive euthanasia**, such as the withholding of intravenous or tube feedings) or through commission of an act (**active euthanasia**), such as intentional administration of an excessive dose of barbiturates (Attaran, 2015). Medically assisted dying in Canada, which permits a person to self-administer medication to cause their own death as well as administration of medication by a physician or nurse practitioner to a person to cause death, is a form of active euthanasia.

Some experts suggest that **palliative sedation,** or the practice of lowering consciousness in those near death to relieve refractory symptoms, such as pain and dyspnea, is a form of active euthanasia. Others argue that intention separates palliative sedation from active euthanasia, because the aim of palliative sedation is relief and not death. Palliative sedation is therefore ethically justifiable because it achieves good while doing no harm (Menezes & de Assis Figueiredo, 2019). The **doctrine of double effect**, a moral principle taken from the teachings of Saint Thomas Aquinas, is sometimes evoked to further distinguish between active euthanasia and palliative sedation. This doctrine asserts that some actions have both good and bad effects and relies on four conditions:

- The action itself is good or at least indifferent;
- A good, and not evil, effect is intended;
- The good effect cannot be produced by the evil effect; and
- There must be sufficiently grave reasons to permit the evil effect.

In the case of palliative sedation, it can be argued that the action of administering sedation to relieve pain is itself good, that the intent is to relieve refractory symptoms, refractory symptoms are relieved (good effect) without shortening life (evil effect), and that relief of pain (good effect) outweighs the possibility of ending life (evil effect). Some experts argue that euthanasia, however, would not satisfy the doctrine of double effect because the action of intentionally causing death is evil, and relief of symptoms (the good) occurred because of the evil effect (death) (Wholihan & Olson, 2017).

In Canada, unlike in some jurisdictions such as the United States, MAID is inclusive of health care providers (physicians and nurse practitioners) supplying medications for self-administration by persons who desire to die or of health care providers directly administering medications to persons with the intent of terminating life. This has been made possible by exemptions from the offence of culpable homicide in relevant sections of Canada's *Criminal Code, 1985* for medical and nurse practitioners so that persons can receive MAID (Government of Canada, 2019a). Under the provisions of Bill C-14, physicians and nurse practitioners (in provinces where allowed) can provide MAID, and pharmacists, other health care providers, and family members can help provide MAID. To be eligible for assistance in dying (Government of Canada, 2020), a person must

- Be eligible for either federal or provincial health services;
- Be at least 18 years old and capable of competent decision making immediately prior to the provision of medical assistance in dying;
- Have a grievous and irremediable medical condition;
- Make a request for medical assistance voluntarily; and
- Provide informed consent. ("Eligibility criteria," section 2)

A grievous and irremediable medical condition is considered one in which decline cannot be reversed, there is unbearable physical or mental suffering, and natural death is reasonably foreseeable (Government of Canada, 2020). A written request for MAID must be signed by two witnesses who will not benefit from the death and who are not involved in the person's care. Once this request is submitted, a physician or nurse practitioner confirms that the person meets all criteria, and a second physician or nurse practitioner, independent of the first, also confirms that eligibility for MAID has been met. A person must wait 10 days between submission of the written request and the service to allow time to consider the request, unless there is rapid deterioration in health status or in capacity to provide informed consent. Consent to MAID may be withdrawn up to and including immediately prior to the service (Government of Canada, 2020). Reporting of medically assisted deaths, as required by Bill C-14, indicates that 6,749 Canadians have received this service up to October 31, 2018, and that most deaths were administered by the clinician rather than the individual seeking MAID (Government of Canada, 2019b).

In 2016, an expert panel of 43 experts was asked to consider evidence and submissions related to MAID for mature minors, advance requests, and requests where mental illness was the sole underlying condition. The report, which was tabled in 2018, suggests that there is need for additional safeguards in these situations. With regards to mature minors, the report concluded that while they may have the necessary cognitive ability, requests from mature minors must take into account, case by case, the relational context of their decision making and the influences and impacts of MAID on the minor, family, and health care providers. The primary concern with advance requests was the uncertainty for health care providers in gauging when the suffering had become sufficiently intolerable that the person, who no longer had capacity, would have desired death. The issue of providing MAID to those for whom mental illness was the sole underlying condition was seen as particularly complex and contentious because of the implications of stigmatization, particular vulnerabilities, and the capacity of persons with profound illness to make rational decisions related to dying; as a result, no clear conclusions were reached by the panel (Council of Canadian Academies, 2018).

Nurses are the health professionals who are the most constant providers of care in various settings. With the uptake of MAID in Canada, it is likely that nurses in everyday practice may be asked about options to end suffering or to participate in MAID. This raises potential moral issues for nurses. Can a nurse agree with the principle of autonomy and yet be morally uncomfortable with intentionally ending a person's life? The CNA *Code of Ethics for Registered Nurses* suggests that dignity is preserved by encouraging those at the end of life to express their wishes and goals (CNA, 2017a) and advocates for capable persons to be able to make informed decisions about end of life options, including MAID. When nurses have a conscientious objection to MAID, they can consult their provincial and territorial nursing regulatory bodies for guidance (see Research Focus box). In general, nurses are directed to notify their employers as soon as possible of their conscientious objection and to ensure that the care of clients is not compromised, which may mean transferring care in a "respectful way" to an alternative provider (CNA, 2017b). Despite the implication that conscientious objection is allowed, nurses may still experience difficulty in expressing their objections to participating in MAID and other morally distressing situations (see Research Focus box).

RESEARCH FOCUS

Lamb and colleagues conducted this interpretive phenomenological study to explore the meaning of conscience for nurses in the context of conscientious objection in clinical practice. Through iterative analysis of in-depth interviews with eight nurses in Ontario, key themes were identified that suggested that conscientious objection is consistent with voicing one's beliefs about what is right or wrong. Despite the complexity of health care, the experience of the nurses who made conscientious objections suggested a lack of concrete support and a need for public and professional awareness of nurses' moral autonomy to decide, for example, whether or not to participate in assisted dying. The study recommended inclusion of conscience protection clauses in professional and organizational contexts.

Source: Lamb, C., Evans, M., Babenko-Mould, Y., et al. (2019). Nurses' use of conscientious objections and the implications for conscience. *Journal of Advanced Nursing, 75,* 594–602. http://doi.org/10.1111/jan.13869.

Choosing Quality End-of-Life Care

The emergence of interventions that prolong life (and potentially a patient's suffering) has raised a number of issues related to quality of end-of-life care, including the possibility of options other than MAID. Advocating for excellence in end-of-life care is identified in the CNA *Code of Ethics* as an important ethical endeavour and includes consideration of these options. Advocacy also requires that nurses engage in conversations in which the wishes and goals of the patient are respected, as well as assist families to understand patient decisions related to end-of-life care that may be in conflict with the family's own (CNA, 2017b). The creation of a personal directive (also termed advance directive or living will) enables a person, in advance of incapacity or serious illness or injury, to name a personal agent who will enforce the person's health care preferences and to outline values and beliefs that affect treatment and care. Additionally, a personal directive, which is a legal document, enables a person to outline preferences for life support, tube feeding, cardiopulmonary resuscitation, specific treatments, management of pain, organ donation, and living arrangements (Government of Alberta, 2019). Forms and information are available on provincial and territorial websites to guide the development of a personal directive (Dalhousie University, n.d.). A personal directive or living will, which can be updated to reflect current patient wishes, guides families, nurses, and physicians in providing care that is consistent with what the person would want if capacity was present.

As trusted care providers, nurses may be involved in conversations with persons who are contemplating a personal directive. Through dialogue and listening, nurses can help patients clarify their goals and wishes and refer patients to others in their relational network, such as physicians and families, who can assist in this process. Furthermore, nurses should advise patients to make family, friends, and care providers aware that a personal directive exists in the event that they are unable to speak for themselves. This enables nurses and other care providers to ensure that the wishes of the person are respected.

Hebert and Selby (2014) emphasize the importance of including discussion and consideration of DNR orders when developing an end-of-life treatment plan, especially in situations where death would not be a surprise. They suggest that while the use of DNR orders is increasingly widespread, broad or narrow interpretation of DNR orders can result in the application of basic or advanced life support in ways that may be inconsistent with patient and family wishes and their expectations about the value and importance of DNR. Additionally, Bjorklund and Lund (2019) suggest that dialogue is important to understand the context and relationships of the person when decisions are made regarding DNR and that this is an important area of advocacy for nurses.

Despite personal directives and clear DNR orders, nurses can find themselves sometimes caught between patient goals, family wishes, physician directives, best practices, and their own moral values and beliefs. In a study of experiences with next of kin, Ramvi and Ueland (2018) suggested that the vulnerabilities of the patient, family, and nurse intersect in end-of-life decisions and can result in decreased trust in one another. This can lead to conflict over whose wishes to follow (the patient's or the family's), with increased moral distress experienced when nurses feel compelled to act in ways that are consistent with family wishes and not necessarily in the best interests of the patient. The study also highlighted that nurses themselves experience fear of death and need confidence and competence in psychological and spiritual care, which they sometimes lack. This contributes to the vulnerability of nurses in relationships with family, who are sometimes engaged in a tension between their hope and the patient's wish for peaceful death. In such situations, it may be important for nurses to view next of kin separately from the patient and to engage in ethical reflection to understand how the responses of kin, such as anger or control of treatment decisions, threaten moral identity.

Dementia and Autonomy

Despite the use of personal directives and awareness of the need to consult, inform, and collaborate with patients and families, there is growing recognition that persons with dementia may have limited or no involvement in decisions affecting their health, daily care needs, or end-of-life care (Miller, Whitlach, & Lyons, 2016). This lack of involvement involves significant life changes such as relocation to residential care or refusal of hydration and food at the end of life. It also involves everyday decisions such as what to eat, what to wear, whether to accept medications, and how to respond emotionally to the failure of friends or partners to visit. Lack of meaningful engagement with persons with dementia has been a longstanding issue. It comes out of nurses' experiences and beliefs related to the decision-making capacity of persons with dementia, as well as care practice issues, including lack of time to consider preferences or opinions or accommodate slowed mobility, cognitive deficits, or difficulties in hearing and seeing. This can result in what Branelly (2011) has termed social death, as the person with dementia is avoided or experiences the deception or lying of care providers, and subsequently, diminished worth.

Dignity captures the idea that every person has unique value and worth and is therefore deserving of respect (Oberle & Raffin Bouchal, 2009). Dignity has been a matter of theoretical, religious, and philosophical discussion for centuries but again assumed prominence following the atrocities of the Second World War. Gastmans (2013) suggested that dignity is the ethical essence of nursing because

of the recognition that those in care are worthy but vulnerable and thus are deserving of our respect and protection. This extends to persons for dementia and their families and the need to respect their right to make decisions about care. It means establishing environments in which choices are encouraged and welcomed and that acknowledge cultural backgrounds, cognitive abilities, patient and family values, and how or when patients and families wish to be engaged in decision making. Miller, Whitlach, & Lyons (2016) have pointed out that shared decision making about everyday care, medical interventions, and placement between family carers and patients with dementia is important in validating the personhood of persons with dementia, regardless of outcomes.

Supporting shared decision making may mean questioning the practice of whether or not **therapeutic lying,** or the "practice of deliberately deceiving patients for reasons considered to be in their best interests" (Sperber, 2015, p. 43), protects the patient or others from harm or creates harm and therefore erodes dignity. Should, for example, medication be hidden in food to control behaviour in a person with dementia who strikes out at staff and other patients? Is manipulating cooperation morally justified if it achieves a greater good in reducing agitation or the likelihood that this person might harm staff and other patients? Should we protect the person with impaired cognitive capacity from the distress of knowing that a partner is deceased when the person asks whether the partner is coming to visit? Such decisions are morally complex and need to be made within the context of perspectives that consider family carer, patient, care provider expertise, and evidence. Sperber (2015) has suggested, for example, that the assumption that those with dementia will not be aware of deception is a mistaken one, and thus lying may affect the trust relationship between the patient and care provider. Instead, techniques such as validation of feelings can enable the person with dementia to share their underlying feelings and avoid mistrust. Erosion of dignity and social death (Branelly, 2011) are less likely to occur when persons with impaired cognitive capacity can feel that their preferences matter—even if they choose not to or are unable to make final decisions (Miller, Whitlach, & Lyons 2016)—and if we ensure that assumptions about a person's capacity to make decisions do not bleed over into each and every choice that they may be called upon to make.

Mental Illness

Many complex ethical questions derive from the care of persons with mental illness, largely because mental health nursing involves an intersection of legal, ethical, social, professional, and personal influences. Those who live with mental illness experience many challenges that arise from the illnesses themselves, including higher suicide rates and higher rates of certain physical illnesses. They also encounter social biases that result in marginalization and stigmatization, which affects where and how they are able to work, housing, relationships, and economic security, as well as access to health care (Pachkowski, 2018). Court-ordered treatments and legally mandated admissions for assessment can place nurses in a conflict between respect for the right of persons to make their own decisions and understanding that restrictions may benefit those with severe illnesses. Nurses can be placed in advocacy roles when the proposal of harm reduction programs (e.g., safe needle exchange or injection sites) face resistance from communities and assist others to understand the benefits versus the risks of such programs.

Mental health is also an issue for individual nurses and regulatory bodies. Fitness to practice means that nurses must have qualities and capabilities that enable them to practice safely and competently. This includes the requirement to be free from cognitive, physical (including fatigue), psychological, and emotional conditions that would place patients, colleagues, or themselves at risk in practice settings. If unable to satisfy this requirement, then nurses need to withdraw from practice until they are able to provide care that is safe and competent (College and Association of Registered Nurses of Alberta, 2019; Nurses Association of New Brunswick, 2013). A study by Kunyk (2015) has suggested that 3.8% of the nurses responding to a survey abused alcohol, a rate that is higher than the general population, and 1.0% of nurses abused drugs, a rate that is higher than for the general population of women. Professional associations and regulatory bodies direct peers to speak with colleagues who they suspect may be abusing drugs or alcohol, and if this does not result in resolution, then they should follow up with other appropriate persons. The study by Kunyk (2015) suggested that many colleagues may be unaware of the abuse, and that when abuse is active and hidden, it significantly threatens the safety of patients. Early detection and encouragement of self-identification are important measures in addressing this problem. Regulatory bodies and individual nurses need to advocate for approaches that avoid stigmatization of nurses with substance abuse and other mental disorders. Substance abuse disorders among nurses benefit positively from monitoring and treatment (Kunyk, 2015), and this approach is likely to have better outcomes than those resulting from punitive justice.

Ethical Concerns Related to Reproduction

Technological advancements have introduced options for reproduction such as cloning and the use of hybrids. These issues have been the focus of both research and much debate about ethics, legal issues, and funding. These are not necessarily nursing issues per se, because the technology involves medical procedures, but nurses are often in relational spaces with women and their partners where they address questions about options, clarify terms, and support women and their partners who are deciding the right course of action or choice. Nurses also provide technical support during procedures and genetic counselling and other care that places them in a position of trust or potential advocacy when it is clear that further information or referral may be necessary to make deeply personal, but sometimes financially burdensome decisions, related to reproduction and pregnancy. The issue of reproduction involves professional but also personal sensibilities, and it is important that nurses reflect on their own values and beliefs in the care of these women and their partners to identify potential biases that may unduly influence decisions that women or couples need to make.

Assisted reproductive technology (ART) is is the use of medical and laboratory procedures and treatments to establish pregnancy and also refers to a range of services related to medical assistance with pregnancy (National Cancer Institute, n.d.; College of Physicians and Surgeons of Saskatchewan, 2012). ART includes human and therapeutic cloning, use of hybrids or transplantation of nonhuman reproductive material into a human being, in vitro fertilization, and surrogacy. Many of these activities remain federally unregulated, such as restrictions on the number of embryos transferred into an in vitro fertilization (IVF) cycle, number of offspring from the same sperm donor, and genetic testing and screening; others are prohibited under federal law (or in the case of Quebec, provincial law), such as sex selection (except for prevention of sex-linked disorders), payment for surrogacy, creation of an embryo for purposes other than to create a human, and cloning (Davis, 2018).

While some activities associated with ART are regulated under provincial legislation, and thus may resolve legal concerns, the existence of options through ART nonetheless presents various ethical questions. For example, should women of advanced childbearing age have access to ART in order to bear children, given evidence that pregnancy beyond 35 or 36 years of age suggests increased risks to the fetus and to women themselves? Provincial governments have considered banning IVF in women who are too old to bear a child (De Simone, 2019). How old is too old? How many public resources should be directed toward ART and how much of the burden should women and partners bear? Should unrestricted funding be offered to curtail the transfer of multiple embryos and reduce fetal and maternal risks, which can impose further burdens on families and result in additional costs for the health care system? Current funding practices in Canada attempt to balance the greater or public good with that of individual families, with provinces such as Ontario providing funding for one cycle of IVF and unlimited rounds of intrauterine insemination to women under 43 years of age. Others such as Manitoba, New Brunswick, and Quebec offer tax credits for infertility treatments. The fully funded IVF program in Quebec was eliminated in 2015, despite its success in reducing multiple pregnancy rates from 30% to 5%, and replaced with a sliding scale of tax credits (Snow, 2018).

The right to reproduce and have a family is considered a basic human right, and this right applies to infertile couples or couples who have experienced miscarriage as well as those who are able to reproduce. Although the basic right to reproduce is widely recognized, does this imply unlimited access to available technology for women who wish to have a child? Some say yes, because they believe that the right to form a family is a concept woven into the fabric of society. However, the issue remains regarding who should be able to access such technology and whether it should be publicly funded.

Allocation of Health Care Resources

Ethical issues pertaining to the allocation of health care resources can be encountered at several levels. Policies that influence the use of health care resources are established at governmental, system, institutional, and unit levels. At the government level, public policies are established that determine what type of health care can be provided. Nurses and other health care providers have a responsibility to communicate with legislators to influence these policies, such as balancing the priorities of care and financial burdens in ART or the safe composition of the nursing workforce. As the largest sector of the health workforce, nurses have considerable potential to be influential voices as demonstrated through past initiatives such as the *Canada Health Act*, where the participation of nurses was instrumental in setting out the current framework for health care in Canada.

Despite their potential influence, nurses too often have little influence on health policies. Consequently, nurses need to take action to influence decision making and priority setting that impact the care and safety of patients and their own work lives. For example, decisions about staffing and staffing mixes can affect nurses' ability to respond to the demands placed on them and result in unsafe environments that make safe patient care difficult and lead to moral distress for nurses. Fortunately, nurses have become more vocal in expressing their concerns and in providing facts that can influence decision making, rather than merely responding to the decisions made by physicians and hospital administrators.

In addition to fair distribution of resources to ensure safe health care at system and unit levels, consideration of resource allocation includes access to care. The Canadian health care system is based on accessibility, or reasonable access to care, but how much access is available for those who live in poverty or in rural and remote areas of Canada? How much effort and funding ought to be expended to ensure that underserved areas in our population have the same benefits and health care as the rest of Canada? What is reasonable?

Cohen, Schultz, McGibbon et al. (2013) suggest that the distribution of health care resources is necessarily unequal and thus health equity rather than equality is a relevant consideration. Justice within the framework of bioethics is primarily concerned with the fair division of scarce resources or equal shares; social justice and equity take into consideration whether there are structural and systemic issues that affect the distribution of resources and the cases for unequal shares of resources. For example, how have government policies contributed to the poor housing conditions and lack of clean water supply for Indigenous peoples living on reserve? Do those in long-term care settings receive less than adequate care because of attitudes towards elders? Although social justice and equity are foundations of public health in Canada

GENDER CONSIDERATIONS

In June 2019, the House of Commons Standing Committee on Health presented its report on LGBTQ2 health in Canada (House of Commons, 2019). This report, while acknowledging that each LGBTQ2 community experiences health inequities differently, stated that LGBTQ2 persons experience poorer physical and mental health than heterosexual Canadians. These health issues are compounded by determinants of health and identity issues, as well as by stigmatization and discrimination, including that by health care providers. Fowler (2017) has pointed out that from its very beginnings, modern nursing has engaged in social change and policy as an essential component of its broad orientation toward ethics. As such, nursing continues to have a mandate to effect changes where health and human dignity are harmed and to address structures that promote disparities and prejudice for those in LGBTQ2 communities, such as those found by the Standing Committee.

Sources: Fowler, M. (2017). "Unladylike commotion': Early feminism and nursing's role in gender/trans dialogue. *Nursing Inquiry, 24*(1), 1–6. https://doi.org/10.1111/nin.12179; House of Commons. (2019). *Committee report No. 28-HESA (42-1).* Retrieved from https://www.ourcommons.ca/Committees/en/HESA.

(Cohen, Schultz, McGibbon et al., 2013), experts such as Elizabeth McGibbon suggest that health outcomes are worsening for several vulnerable and historically disadvantaged groups, such as LGBTQ2 people (see Gender Considerations box), Indigenous peoples, women, persons with disabilities, and African Canadians (St. Francis Xavier University, 2017).

The findings and recommendations of the Truth and Reconciliation Commission of Canada have highlighted the historical disparities in income, education, and health between Indigenous peoples and the non-Indigenous population in Canada (Truth and Reconciliation Commission of Canada, 2015). These disparities have their roots in colonization, residential schools, and systemic racism in which the difficulties of Indigenous peoples were treated as a social and economic problem and blamed for poverty and high rates of suicide and addiction in their communities. The Truth and Reconciliation Commission's recommendations call for medical and nursing students to be educated about the impact of residential schools and government policies on the health and well-being of Indigenous peoples. By becoming aware of the harmful legacy of these systems, health care providers can work respectfully with Indigenous peoples to correct historical and existing disparities. The commission's recommendations for health care providers include identifying the distinct health needs of Indigenous peoples and using culturally appropriate interventions; using traditional healing practices (see Cultural Considerations box); advocating for funding for Indigenous health centres; and increasing the number of Indigenous health care providers (Truth and Reconciliation Commission of Canada, 2015). Nurses have important roles to play, collectively and individually, in ensuring that health care and health promotion for Indigenous peoples follow these recommendations and that resources respect the priorities of Indigenous peoples.

🌐 CULTURAL CONSIDERATIONS

In her article about cultural safety and the appropriateness of relational ethics in practice with Indigenous persons, Monique Bearskin (2011) recounted the story of a young Indigenous woman named Nicole. Nicole was seriously injured in a motor vehicle accident and transferred from her community to a tertiary care facility. Nicole's biological family, the family who raised her, and a community Elder soon arrived in the ICU, where Nicole was being treated. The Elder requested permission for a smudging ceremony and the use of traditional medicines, but the requests were denied because of staff concerns about safety. The distressed family, recognizing the seriousness of Nicole's health status, continued to try to incorporate their traditions into Nicole's care. They pinned a medicine pouch under her gown and next to Nicole's heart to protect her as she transcended into the spirit world. They returned on various occasions to find the pouch removed and pinned to the wall or tied to other areas of the body. Tensions between the family and staff increased to the point where an interdisciplinary meeting was held, during which the attending physician informed the family that Nicole would be transferred home upon her recovery. With this assurance, the family returned home. Nicole died the next day.

Monique Bearskin shared this narrative to illustrate how the nurses and other health care providers, by deferring to Western ethical principles (i.e., beneficence and nonmaleficence), failed to recognize the ethical perspectives of Nicole's family background, and in doing so, humiliated and distressed the family. The use of a relational ethics framework may have enabled nurses and other staff to connect with the family in such a way that they could have understood the importance of relation, respect, holism, and the interconnectedness of persons with each other and with their environment, including the spiritual world, for Nicole and her family as Cree. Facilitation of the smudging ceremony would have created a moral intersection between the beliefs of the family and nursing care. For the family, there would have been the means to honour Nicole's spirit and to connect her living spirit with the spirit world as death approached; for the nurses, it would have been an opportunity to bring comfort and dignity to Nicole and her family. Failure to engage in relationships without acknowledging the unique culture, history, and the structural, economic, and political dimensions that influence access to health care serves to increase the burden of health disparities experienced by Indigenous peoples. In Nicole's case, this failure prevented the family from participating in Nicole's health care decisions and process of dying and kept them from accessing the support that they may have required.

Source: Bearskin, M. (2011). A critical lens on culture in nursing practice. *Nursing Ethics, 18,* 548–559. https://doi.org/10.1177/0969733011408048.

CODES OF ETHICS

Chan (2006) has offered principles of just health care allocation. It is understood that health care rationing or limiting the availability of potentially beneficial treatments is a necessity that is both practical and moral. These principles can be useful to policymakers who are responsible for the allocation of resources and who are subject to significant pressure from special-interest groups.

The first principle of resource allocation is that a basic level of health care must be provided to everyone. This requirement does not mean that everyone must have access to all potentially beneficial treatments or all the treatments that individuals request. Rather, it means that if safe, ethical, and effective treatments are available, a caring society should provide them through the health care system.

The second principle is that if treatment is expected to be futile, it should not be provided. This principle ensures that limited resources are not wasted on nonbeneficial treatments. Therefore, if the effectiveness of a particular treatment cannot be proven, then an individual cannot claim it as a right.

The third and final principle of just allocation is that allocation criteria for potentially beneficial treatments should be established in a public and democratic process. In this category, society must make decisions about what should be available to whom. This process may result in a priority listing for costly procedures when there are limited resources available (see Applying Content Knowledge). In this case, treatments that provide significant benefits take priority over treatments that provide only marginal benefit; treatments that can benefit many take priority over treatments than can benefit only a few; and treatments that are less expensive take priority over treatments that are more expensive.

👤 APPLYING CONTENT KNOWLEDGE

A person who is dying of liver disease and who has continued to engage in heavy consumption of alcohol is refused a life-saving liver transplant. Agency policies related to organ donation generally require that a person with liver damage caused by alcohol consumption must remain dry for at least 6 months prior to receiving an organ transplant. The family of the patient challenge this policy, arguing that the policy is discriminatory and violates constitutional rights to equality and life. What is fair in this situation? What principles of just allocation might be relevant?

Although some nurses have taken the Florence Nightingale pledge (which did not originate with Florence Nightingale but with Harper Hospital School of Nursing in Detroit), this pledge does not provide ethical direction for the

issues and dilemmas encountered in practice. In 1954, the CNA adopted the code of ethics, developed in 1953 by the International Council of Nurses (ICN), as its first code of ethics and replaced it in 1973 with the *ICN Code for Nurses—Ethical Concepts Applied to Nursing*. At its 1978 annual meeting, the CNA made the development of a new national code a priority, and in 1980, the CNA approved its own code of ethics, although revisions were deemed necessary. An ad hoc committee was established and sought input from nurses across Canada. After lengthy deliberations, the *Code of Ethics for Nursing* was published in 1985 (CNA, 1985). Since that time, the code has been reviewed on an ongoing basis, with revisions published in 1991, 1997, 2002, 2008, and 2017. The latest version reflects emerging professional and social contexts such as MAID, inequity, safe staffing, bullying, and environmental stewardship (CNA, 2017a). The code is available on the CNA website along with teaching learning modules that are helpful in becoming familiar with values and responsibilities in nursing practice and their application to practice. The latest version of the code (CNA, 2017a) has the following preamble:

> The Canadian Nurses Association (CNA) Code of Ethics for Registered Nurses (herein called the Code) is a statement of the ethical values of nurses and of nurses' commitments to persons with health-care needs and persons receiving care.
>
> The Code is both aspirational and regulatory. It is an aspirational document designed to inform everyone about the ethical values and subsequent responsibilities and endeavours of nurses. It is also a regulatory tool. Nursing in Canada is a self-regulating profession; thus, nurses are bound to a code of ethics as part of a regulatory process that serves and protects the public . . .
>
> The Code provides guidance for ethical relationships, behaviours and decision-making and is used in conjunction with professional standards, best practice, research, laws and regulations that guide practice . . .
>
> The Code is intended for nurses in all contexts and domains of nursing practice (clinical practice, education, administration, research and policy (CNA, 2015a) and at all levels of decision-making. It is not based on a particular philosophy or ethical theory but arises from different schools of thought, including relational ethics, an ethic of care, principle-based ethics, feminist ethics, virtue ethics and values. The Code is developed by nurses for nurses, and it has a practical orientation supported by theoretical diversity. It is a means for self- evaluation, feedback and peer review and is a basis for advocacy. (p. 2)

The *Code of Ethics* sets out the specific values and ethical behaviour expected of registered nurses, including those

---

BOX 15.1 Actions to Address Unethical or Incompetent Practice

- Address problem as directly as possible
- Maintain confidentiality
- Review all relevant information
- Separate personal and professional issues
- Seek information directly from the colleague whose actions have raised concerns, if feasible
- Consider risks of action or inaction and impact on others

---

in extended roles, in Canada. It educates not only nurses about their ethical responsibilities, but also informs other health care providers and members of the public about the moral commitments expected of nurses. Codes of ethics also provide guidelines for health care institutions to assess policy for its appropriateness to professional nursing practice. In addition, professional organizations and regulatory bodies use the *Code of Ethics* extensively when reviewing cases in which nurses have been charged with malpractice.

The *Code of Ethics* is organized into two parts. The first part describes the core responsibilities central to ethical nursing practice. It is organized around seven values or broad ideals. Each value is accompanied by responsibility statements that are intended to clarify its application in practice. These values are as follows:

- Providing safe, compassionate, competent, and ethical care;
- Promoting health and well-being;
- Promoting and respecting informed decision making;
- Preserving dignity;
- Maintaining privacy and confidentiality;
- Promoting justice; and
- Being accountable.

The values that make up the Canadian *Code of Ethics* stem from the heart of the professional nurse–patient relationship. The values illustrate what nurses believe to be important in that relationship and are one of the reasons why the Canadian *Code of Ethics* is considered by many to be the gold standard for nursing worldwide.

The second part of the code describes applications of the code in situations such as job action, disasters, and communicable disease outbreaks. A specific section under applications of the code provides guidance about actions that can be taken to address unethical or competent practice or practices that compromise the capacity to provide safe, compassionate, competent, and ethical care (Box 15.1). These actions reflect values expressed in the code, such as confidentiality and preservation of dignity for affected colleagues and others who are impacted by the situations and potential outcomes, as well as providing a solution-based focus.

The applications section of the second part of the code includes a section devoted to conscientious objection, an issue generating considerable interest in nursing research and practice. The passage of legislation to allow MAID and uses of advanced biotechnology to prolong life as well as personally and professionally sensitive practice situations such as abortion can lead to intense conflict between what nurses believe to be right and what they may be compelled to do (see Research Focus box). The conflict between duty, which the code directs nurses to observe in the best interests of the patient, and conscience can produce feelings of powerlessness, sadness, and loss of respect for self, especially if nurses experience a lack of organizational support or ambiguous guidance regarding options for ethical action.

RESEARCH FOCUS

Ford and Austin (2018) conducted this interpretative descriptive study to explore individual conflicts of conscience among neonatal nurses in Alberta. Five nurses with at least 1 year of experience in a neonatal intensive care unit were interviewed by telephone for the study. Interviews were guided by a semi-structured interview format and were recorded and transcribed. Three themes were identified in the findings: unforgettable conflict with pain and suffering; finding the nurse's voice; and the proximity of the nurse. These results have suggested that experienced nurses found more ways to deal with situations in which they experienced a conflict between their convictions and what was being asked of them, which included requesting reassignment. Conflict of conscience often involved feelings of powerlessness and failure to stop the pain and suffering of neonates under care, as well as a sense that refusal to provide care was not an option. The implications are that the moral residue from situations involving a conflict of conscience is long lasting, supports are needed at the unit level and from codes of ethics, and further research is required to understand the sources of these conflicts and barriers to declaring a conflict of conscience.

Source: Ford, N., & Austin, W. (2018). Conflicts of conscience in the neonatal intensive care unit: Perspectives of Alberta nurses. *Nursing Ethics, 25*, 992–1003. https://doi.org/10.1177/0969733016684547.

Nursing is not the only health profession to have a code of ethics. Medicine also has codes of ethics. For many years, physicians, upon graduation, have taken the Hippocratic Oath, which was derived from the time of Hippocrates. Although the oath provides some ethical guidance, it commits physicians to saving lives at all costs, which can be problematic in decisions to prolong lives when there is no hope. The orientation toward cure also differentiates physician and nursing practice and has led to differences of opinion regarding the prolongation of life and about whose decision, the physician's or the patient's, should lead care at end of life. Nonetheless, codes of ethics and ethical values in health professions are often very similar and reflect a concern with the need for honesty, trustworthiness, and respect. It is the interpretation of these statements into practice that differentiates one set of ethical values from another (Wright & Brajtman, 2011).

Codes of ethics are necessary and valuable both in terms of how they guide public perceptions and promote trust and in how they guide ethical decision making for nurses. Earlier codes of ethics were prescriptive in nature and essentially consisted of rules to govern the personal and professional conduct of members of a profession; recent codes are more similar to guidelines for practice that provide a framework for nurses to make ethical decisions and fulfill their responsibilities to the public and the profession. Although codes of ethics may or may not be part of statutory regulations, in most provinces there is a statutory requirement within the Act governing the nursing profession that mandates that nurses uphold ethical standards as defined by the nursing profession. This means that not only are individual nurses expected to uphold the precepts contained in codes of ethics, but they are also obliged to hold colleagues accountable for adhering to them. However, codes of ethics do have limitations. One criticism is that they offer broad normative statements that may not offer sufficient guidance in specific context-laden situations (Oberle & Raffin Bouchal, 2009). Codes must be considered in conjunction with relevant laws, legislation, provincial and territorial practice guidelines and standards, institutional policies, and nursing evidence, along with the values, wishes, and goals of persons and their families.

STRATEGIES FOR ADDRESSING ETHICAL DILEMMAS IN PRACTICE

Ethical concerns arise in everyday nursing practice, and the ensuing moral distress can lead to burnout, decreased communication, poor-quality patient care, and the failure of nursing and health care colleagues to work together in the interests of patients. Particularly troublesome is that nurses may be unaware of the ethical concerns that arise in everyday practice or how to deal with moral distress when it arises. Despite advances in many other areas of nursing practice and health care, the phenomena identified by Woods (2005) persist and have been affirmed in recent studies (Engel, Salfi, Micsinszki, & Bodnar, 2017):

- Nurses feel concerned about ethical issues that they face in the practice setting, but take no action, are uncertain about what to do, or feel unable to overcome barriers to action;
- Nurses who take ethical action, or advocate on behalf of their patients, find themselves ostracized by other personnel and then seek covert or subversive ways to promote their own moral survival;
- Newly graduated nurses do not assert themselves when faced with moral distress, opting instead to find other ways to cope with their distress, sometimes at the expense of compromising what they have learned is the right thing to do. (Woods, 2005, p. 7)

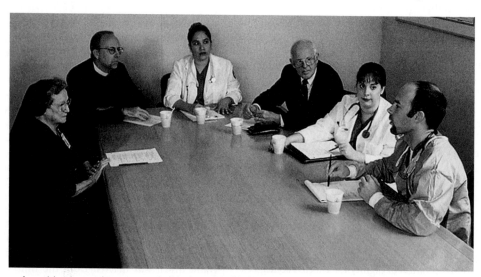

An ethics committee at work. (Harkreader, H., Hogan, M. A., & Thobaben, M. (2007). *Fundamentals of nursing: Caring and clinical judgment* (3rd ed.). St. Louis, MO: Saunders.)

Health care agencies attempt to address ethical questions and dilemmas through ethics committees, and in large teaching hospitals, an ethicist may be employed to provide expert assistance and guidance. Most hospitals now have institutional ethics committees that provide assistance to professional staff and set institutional guidelines for ethical practice.

Proactive strategies to avert moral distress and promote moral well-being among nurses have included teaching ethics as an official part of nursing curricula in undergraduate and graduate education rather than leaving ethics to chance. This approach acknowledges evidence suggesting that nurses and physicians who are formally taught ethics may be better prepared to address and cope with ethical issues and dilemmas in practice (Pachkowski, 2018). Thompson and Thompson (1989), who were early advocates of ethics education in basic and graduate nursing education, identified the goals of teaching ethics to students and health care providers as stimulation of the "moral imagination," recognition of "ethical issues," elicitation of "a sense of moral obligation," development of "analytical skills," and tolerance and reduction in "disagreements and ambiguity" (p. 86). These learning experiences can be facilitated through the formal presentation of ethical frameworks and concepts and their application to real-life case studies and scenarios involving everyday issues in nursing and broader issues in health care, as well as the exploration of personal and professional values and beliefs. Debates assist nursing students with honing skills of analysis and encourage involvement in ethical dialogue about issues and questions of interest to nurses and to health care, in general. These strategies require expert guidance to avoid the tendency of application and analysis to evolve into discussions that are more technical than ethical in nature and to facilitate differentiation between legal and ethical aspects of issues. The development of moral awareness and reasoning is appropriately continued in nonpunitive and open clinical learning environments for students, where observations about care and potential compromises in ethical care can be contextualized and vigorously analyzed, providing that instructional leaders themselves have the necessary background to guide discussions of an ethical nature.

Importantly, students need to explore strategies and tools to either address troubling situations or ameliorate moral distress. Without this guidance, students, as graduate nurses, may be left with the ability to identify morally troubling situations or with moral awareness, but without a means to process and deal with the situations. A potential consequence of the lack of strategies and application to the everyday realities of nursing practice is that students, either in their program or as graduates, may experience greater moral distress than those without exposure to ethics in their education (Pachkowski, 2018). In addition, ethical awareness without integration of ethical knowledge and tools can lead to strategies to resolve the discomfort of this dissonance, such as rationalization of bad care. Rationalization can become so habitual that when nurses encounter inadequate care or organizational failures to establish structures that support compassionate and ethical care, these situations are rationalized to resolve the discomfort of negative feelings (Engel, Salfi, Micsinszki, & Bodnar, 2017).

For Woods (2005), the use of appropriate role models in clinical settings is essential. The most effective approach is to use morally competent preceptors who are prepared to carry out vigorous ethical discussions with students in the clinical setting. The subsequent valuing of knowledge from the classroom combined with student values has the potential to create a whole new experience in which students "discover what they intuitively know alongside other nurses" (Woods, 2005, p. 13). This type of educational strategy endeavours to give ethical idealism a sense of realism and thus bridges the gap between the classroom and clinical setting.

The role of faculty, clinical instructors, and clinical staff in the development of ethical awareness, reasoning, and action is critical in the development of ethically prepared graduates. Paley (2013) has pointed to the importance of the nonaction of participants, which could include faculty or staff, in ethical or distressing circumstances as critical factors in the promotion of nonaction by others, which can include students. The hesitancy of students to report abuse, either of patients or themselves, and inappropriate or unethical care is related to a lack of knowledge of reporting structures, but also to perceptions that no action would be taken. Furthermore, students can fear reprisal if they bring forward concerns about issues with care that they have witnessed, either from clinical staff or their faculty, which is intensified if students have a poor relationship with their faculty or clinical supervisor (Graj, Sheen, Dudley, & Sutherland-Smith, 2019). The World Health Organization (2016) has identified the knowledge of legal and ethical principles as a key competence of nursing educators and highlighted the importance of role modelling in ethical actions and thinking by clinical instructors, faculty, and preceptors and ethically knowledgeable and supportive relationships between these persons and students.

For practising nurses who face ethical questions each day, the discussion of ethics should be included in workplace training and continuing education. The development of moral communities is important. Nurses need the opportunity to openly debrief morally difficult situations with mentors and colleagues and to reflect on values and beliefs that underscored decisions or activities. Ethics rounds, which are organized to address issues encountered in the care of specific patients, offer opportunities for nurses to openly discuss and consider ethical issues from the perspectives of various professionals, another strategy that can increase ethical knowledge and reasoning. This approach to teaching ethics was developed by the John Dossetor Centre for Health Care Ethics at the University of Alberta (Bergum & Dossetor, 2005). The project was originally the result of a collaborative effort to address ethical dilemmas and had equal representation from medicine, nursing, and philosophy through directors who planned and conducted bioethics rounds and were responsible for joint teaching in ethics for nursing and medical students. Such a collaborative approach facilitates addressing issues involving both professions, and decisions are reached that are in the best interests of the patients and the health care providers. This approach is based on the belief that collaboration in the delivery of health care is required to address complex ethical dilemmas; there are no right or wrong answers, but decisions must be made that will meet the needs of the consumers of health care.

CONCLUSION

This chapter has highlighted a few important ethical issues and dilemmas; many more are addressed in books and journals for nurses and other health care providers. Although there are no easy answers to ethical questions, ethical dialogues, moral communities, and ethical frameworks and concepts are valuable resources in dealing with ethical issues in everyday care and more complex issues.

SUMMARY OF LEARNING OBJECTIVES

- Nurses encounter issues daily in their nursing practice that have ethical implications, which has led to the emergence of the importance of everyday ethics in nursing practice.
- Everyday nursing practice is impacted by workload, technology, decisions by others, the knowledge and experiences of patients, and the beliefs and values of nurses themselves. Nurses are required to negotiate these factors in and through relationships with patients, families, communities, and the health system and come to decisions that lead to safe, compassionate, and ethical care, which is the aim of everyday ethics.
- The emergence of everyday ethics in nursing practices offers a lens through which to consider issues in practice that are of interest to nurses.
- Nursing ethics belongs to the field of applied ethics.
- Traditional ethical theories, such as deontology, consequentialism, virtue ethics, and bioethics, have made important contributions to nursing ethics and have been highly influential in areas of practice such as duty, freedom of choice and autonomy for patients, character and the importance of honesty and trustworthiness, the obligation to do what is right by the patient, and justice, such as the fair distribution of resources, including health care resources.
- Principles of bioethics have been hugely influential in areas such as informed consent and the fair distribution of resources, and nurses can encounter conflicts between principles such as autonomy and beneficence, which can lead to moral distress.
- Contemporary ethical theories such as feminist, care, and relational ethics acknowledge the importance of relationship, the uniqueness of persons, and power differentials.
- Knowledge of various ethical theories and frameworks provide different perspectives through which to view situations and to inform decisions.

- Specific issues that can involve nurses in everyday practice include decisions that persons make about dying or end of life (which have been captured in legislative changes) or in the right of persons to make their wishes known through personal directives.
- An emerging issue in ethical decision making is how those with dementia are involved in their own care and life decisions.
- Persons with mental health issues present multiple ethical issues in care because of the overlap of legal, social, and ethical issues and debates about how this care can best be provided.
- Mental health affects nurses personally and professionally. The appropriate approach for nurses affected by addiction has challenged regulatory bodies as well as colleagues and systems.
- Reproductive technology offers many options for those who have been unable to conceive or to bear an infant to viability, but also engenders many ethical, financial, and social debates.
- Funding and socially constructed decisions affect the distribution of health care resources and can contribute to the vulnerability and health disparities among LGBTQ2 persons and Indigenous peoples.
- Codes of ethics are common to professions and provide normative guidance in ethical decision making. The 2017 *Canadian Code of Ethics for Registered Nurses* reflects contemporary ethical concerns such as MAID, equity, and workplace bullying and offers guidance in conscientious objection for registered nurses who are faced with difficult matters of conscience when confronting complex issues.
- Strategies to address ethical issues include education about ethical frameworks and concepts, strong mentorship, ethical dialogue, rounds, and continuing education for practising nurses.

CRITICAL THINKING QUESTIONS

1. What factors would you take into consideration when deciding whether or not to deceive a confused patient about taking a medication to decrease agitation and potential aggression?
2. How can the CNA's *Code of Ethics* be of help to a nurse practising in a rural hospital who finds that staffing levels in her agency are at unsafe levels?

3. If reproduction is considered a basic human right, how would you advocate for a recommendation to make unlimited public funding for in vitro fertilization available to infertile couples over the age of 40?

REFERENCES

Attaran, A. (2015). Unanimity on death with dignity—Legalizing physician-assisted dying in Canada. *New England Journal of Medicine, 372*, 2080–2082. https://doi.org/10.1056/NEJMp1502442.

Beauchamp, T., & Childress, J. (2013). *Principles of biomedical ethics.* Belmont, CA: Wadsworth.

Beauchamp, T. L., & Walters, L. (2003). *Contemporary issues in bioethics* (6th ed.). Belmont, CA: Thompson/Wadsworth.

Bergum, V., & Dossetor, J. (2005). *Relational ethics: The full meaning of respect.* Hagerstown, MD: University Publishing Group.

Bjorklund, P., & Lund, D. (2019). Informed consent and the aftermath of cardiopulmonary resuscitation: Ethical considerations. *Nursing Ethics, 26*, 84–96. https://doi.org/10.1177/0969733017700234.

Branelly, T. (2011). Sustaining citizenship: People with dementia and the phenomenon of social death. *Nursing Ethics, 18*, 662–671. https://doi.org/10.1177/0969733011408049.

British Columbia College of Nursing Professionals. (2019). *Using social media responsibly.* Retrieved from https://www.bccnp.ca.

Burkhardt, M., Nathaniel, A., & Walton, N. (2018). *Ethics and issues in contemporary nursing.* Toronto, ON: Nelson.

Canadian Nurses Association. (1985). *Code of ethics for nursing.* Ottawa, ON: Author.

Canadian Nurses Association. (2017a). *Code of ethics for registered nurses.* Retrieved from https://www.cna-aiic.ca/~/media/cna/page-content/pdf-en/code-of-ethics-2017-edition-secure-interactive.

Canadian Nurses Association. (2017b). *National nursing framework on medical assistance in dying.* Retrieved from https://www.cna-aiic.ca/~/media/cna/page-content/pdf-en/cna-national-nursing-framework-on-maid.pdf.

Carper, B. (1978). Fundamental patterns of knowing in nursing. *Advances in Nursing Science, 1*(1), 13–23. https://doi.org/10.1097/00012272-197810000-00004.

Carter v. Canada (Attorney General), [2015] S.C.C.5 (CAN).

Chan, C. (2006). Infertility, assisted reproduction and rights. *Best Practice and Research Clinical Obstetrics and Gynaecology, 20*, 369–380. https://doi.org/10.1016/j.bpobgyn.2006.01.001.

Cohen, B., Schultz, A., McGibbon, E., et al. (2013). A conceptual framework of organizational capacity for public health equity action (OC-PHEA). *Canadian Public Health Association, 104*(2), 262–266. https://doi.org/10.17269/cjph.104.3735.

College and Association of Registered Nurses of Alberta. (2019). *Fitness to practice.* Retrieved from https://www.nurses.ab.ca.

College of Nurses of Ontario. (2018). *Practice standard: Ethics.* Retrieved from http://www.cno.org/globalassets/docs/prac/41034_ethics.pdf.

College of Physicians and Surgeons of Saskatchewan. (2012). *Standard: Assisted Reproductive Technology.* Retrieved from https://www.cps.sk.ca/imis/CPSS/Legislation__ByLaws__Policies_and_Guidelines/Legislation_Content/Policies_and_Guidelines_Content/Assisted_Reproductive_Technology.aspx.

Collier, R. (2017). Reports of coerced sterilization of Indigenous women in Canada mirrors shameful past. *Canadian Medical Association Journal, 189*(33), E1080–E1081. https://doi.org/10.1503/cmaj.1095471.

Council of Canadian Academies. (2018). *State of knowledge on medical assistance in dying for mature minors, advance requests, and where a mental disorder is the sole underlying medical condition: Summary of reports.* Retrieved from https://scienceadvice.ca/wp-content/uploads/2018/12/MAID-Summary-of-Reports.pdf.

Dalhousie University. (n.d.). *End-of-life law and policy in Canada: Health Law Institute.* Retrieved from http://eol.law.dal.ca/?page_id=231.

De Simone, A. (2019). *Delisting full coverage for in vitro fertilization in Quebec.* Retrieved from https://mjmmed.com/article?articleID=57.

Ekmekci, P., & Arda, B. (2017). Interculturalism and informed consent: Respecting cultural differences without breaching human rights. *Cultura (Iasi), 14*(2), 159–172. https://doi.org/10.3726/CUL.2017.02.09.

Elster, N., & Elliott, T. (2018). Distinguishing between law and ethics. *Journal of the American Dental Association, 149*(12), 1005–1006. https://doi.org/10.1016/j.adaj.2018.08.018.

Engel, J., & Prentice, D. (2013). The ethics of interprofessional collaboration. *Nursing Ethics, 20*, 426–435. https://doi.org/10.1177/0969733012468466.

Engel, J., Salfi, J., Micsinszki, S., & Bodnar, A. (2017). Informed strangers: Witnessing and responding to unethical care as student nurses. *Global Qualitative Nursing Research, 4*. https://doi.org/10.1177/2333393617730208.

Gastmans, C. (2013). Dignity-enhancing nursing care: A foundational ethical framework. *Nursing Ethics, 20*, 142–149. https://doi.org/10.1177/0969733012473772.

Graj, E., Sheen, J., Dudley, A., & Sutherland-Smith, W. (2019). Adverse health events associated with clinical placement: A systematic review. *Nurse Education Today, 76*, 178–190. https://doi.org/10.1016/j.nedt.2019.01.024.

Ford, N., & Austin, W. (2018). Conflicts of conscience in the neonatal intensive unit: Perspectives of Alberta. *Nursing Ethics, 25*, 992–1003. https://doi.org/10.1177/0969733016684547.

Government of Alberta. (2019). *Personal directives: Choosing now for the future.* Retrieved from https://open.alberta.ca/dataset/122d8cc6-d3a8-42d2-90f9-1e3c7979814d/resource/c13fdedb-c840-4033-9b39-37d801f68048/download/opg-personal-directives-publication-opg1645.pdf.

Government of Canada. (2019a). *An Act to amend the Criminal Code and to make related amendments to other Acts (medical assistance in dying).* Retrieved from https://laws-lois.justice.gc.ca/PDF/2016_3.pdf.

Government of Canada. (2019b). *Fourth interim report on medical assistance in dying in Canada.* Retrieved from https://www.canada.ca/en/health-canada/services/publications/health-system-services/medical-assistance-dying-interim-report-april-2019.html.

Government of Canada. (2020). *Medical assistance in dying.* Retrieved from https://www.canada.ca/en/health-canada/services/medical-assistance-dying.html.

Hebert, P., & Selby, D. (2014). Should a reversible, but lethal incident, not be treated when a patient has a do-not-resuscitate order? *Canadian Medical Association Journal, 186*, 528–530. https://doi.org/10.1503/cmaj.111772.

Jameton, A. (1984). *Nursing practice: The ethical issues.* Englewood Cliffs, NJ: Prentice Hall.

Jensen, A., & Lidell, E. (2009). The influence of conscience in nursing. *Nursing Ethics, 16*, 31–42. https://doi.org/10.1177/0969733008097988.

Keatings, M., & Adams, P. (2020). *Ethical and legal issues in Canadian nursing* (4th ed.). Toronto, ON: Elsevier.

Kunyk, D. (2015). Substance use disorders among nurses: Prevalence, risks, and perceptions in disciplinary jurisdictions. *Journal of Nursing Management, 23*, 54–64. https://doi.org/10.1111/jonm.12081.

McAndrew, N., Leske, J., & Schroeder, K. (2018). Moral distress in critical care nursing: The state of the science. *Nursing Ethics, 25*, 552–570. https://doi.org/10.1177/0967333016664975.

Menezes, M., & de Assis, Figueiredo (2019). The role of end-of-life palliative sedation: Medical and ethical aspects—Review. *Revista Brasileira de Anestesiologia, 69*(1), 72–77. https://doi.org/10.1016/j.bjane.2018.03.002.

Miller, L., Whitlach, J., & Lyons, S. (2016). Shared decision-making in dementia: A review of patient and family carer involvement. *Dementia, 15*, 1141–1157. https://doi.org/10.1177/1471301214555542.

Milliken, A. (2018). Ethical awareness: What it is and why it matters. *Online Journal of Issues in Nursing, 23*(1), 2. https://doi.org/10.3912/OJINVOL23No01Man01.

Nancy B. v. Hôtel-Dieu de Québec, [1992], 86 D.L.R. (4th) 385 (Quebec Superior Court).

National Cancer Institute. (n.d.). *Assistive reproduction technologies.* Retrieved from https://www.cancer.gov/publications/dictionaries/genetics-dictionary/def/assisted-reproductive-technology.

Nurses Association of New Brunswick. (2013). *Ask a practice consultant.* Retrieved from www.nanb.nb.ca/media/resource/APA-Vol44-No1-E.pdf.

Oberle, K., & Raffin Bouchal, S. (2009). *Ethics in Canadian nursing practice: Navigating the journey.* Toronto, ON: Pearson.

Opgenorth, D., Stelfox, H., Gilfoyle, E., et al. (2018). Perspectives on strained intensive care unit capacity: A survey of critical care professionals. *PLOS ONE, 13*(8), e0201524. https://doi.org/10.1371/journal.pone.0201524.

Osuji, P. (2018). Relational autonomy in informed consent (RAIC) as an ethics of care approach to the concept of informed consent. *Medicine, Health Care, and Philosophy, 21*(1), 101–111. https://doi.org/10.1007/s11019-017-9789-7.

Pachkowski, K. (2018). Ethical competence and psychiatric and mental health nursing education. Why? What? How? *Psychiatric and Mental Health Nursing, 25*, 60–66.

Paley, J. (2013). Social psychology and the compassion deficit. *Nurse Education Today, 33*, 1451–1452. https://doi.org/10.1016/j.nedt.2013.05.011.

Ramvi, E., & Ueland, V. (2018). Between the patient and the next of kin in end-of-life care: A critical study based on feminist theory. *Nursing Ethics, 26*, 201–211. https://doi.org/10.1177/09697016688939.

Rodriguez v. *British Columbia (Attorney General),* [1993] 3 SCR 519.

Snow, D. (2018). *Assisted reproduction policy in Canada: Framing, federalism, and failure.* Toronto, ON: University of Toronto Press.

St. Francis Xavier University. (2017). *Nursing professor awarded national grant to study health equity in Canadian public policy.* Retrieved from https://www.stfx.ca.

Sperber, M. (2015). Therapeutic lying: A contradiction in terms. *Psychiatric Times, 32*(4), 43–47.

Storch, J. (2015). Ethics in practice: At end of life—Part 2. *Canadian Nurse, 111*(7), 20–22.

Thompson, J. E., & Thompson, H. O. (1989). Teaching ethics to nursing students. *Nursing Outlook, 37*(2), 84–88.

Truth and Reconciliation Commission of Canada. (2015). *Honouring the truth, reconciling for the future: Summary of the final report of the Truth and Reconciliation Commission of Canada.* Winnipeg, MB: Author. Retrieved from http://nctr.ca/assets/reports/Final%20Reports/Executive_Summary_English_Web.pdf.

Wholihan, D., & Olson, E. (2017). The doctrine of double effect: A review for the bedside nurse providing end-of-life care. *Journal of Hospice and Palliative Nursing, 19*(3), 205–211. https://doi.org/10.1097/NJH.0000000000000348.

World Health Organization. (2016). *Nurse educator competencies.* Geneva, Switzerland: Author.

Woods, M. (2005). Nursing ethics education: Are we really delivering the good(s)? *Nursing Ethics, 12*(1), 1–18. https://doi.org/10.1191/0969733005ne754oa.

Wright, D., & Brajtman, S. (2011). Relational and embodied knowing; nursing ethics within the interprofessional team. *Nursing Ethics, 18*, 20–30. https://doi.org/10.1177/0969733010386165.

Yeo, M., & Moorhouse, A. (2003). *Concepts and cases in nursing ethics.* Peterborough, ON: Broadview Press.

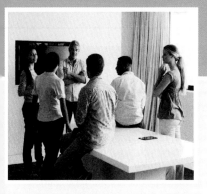

Collaboration in Nursing Practice

Dr. Kelly A. Lackie and Dr. John H.V. Gilbert

ⓔ http://evolve.elsevier.com/Canada/Ross-Kerr/nursing

LEARNING OUTCOMES

After reading this chapter, you will be able to:
- Understand the language of collaboration to inform the practice of teamwork.
- Examine the concept of collaboration in nursing practice.
- Understand the history of interprofessional education in Canada.
- Distinguish the macro, meso, and micro levels of interprofessional education, interprofessional collaborative practice, and interprofessional care.
- Understand the components of the Canadian Interprofessional Competency Framework.
- Compare patient, provider, and system outcomes related to interprofessional collaborative practice.

OUTLINE

KEY TERMS

interprofessional collaboration
interdisciplinary collaboration
interprofessional education
interprofessional learning

intraprofessional collaboration
micro-level factors
meso-level factors
macro-level factors

PERSONAL PERSPECTIVES

Imagine that you are a newly registered family practice nurse beginning your shift in a primary health care clinic. The first patient that you are about to see today is a 60-year-old man, newly diagnosed with type 1 diabetes. He is accompanied by his partner of 35 years. How will you proceed with initiating the appointment? Will you ask his partner to wait in the waiting room? Is there any reason why the partner should be in the examination room with the patient? You decide to ask the partner to accompany the patient. What kind of information do you want from the patient? Will you ask the partner any questions? Should they be included in the conversation?

During your initial assessment, you learn that the patient had a myocardial infarction 5 years ago, which has prevented him from working since then. He is on medical disability pension and his partner does not work. The patient lives a relatively sedentary lifestyle, occasionally taking walks around the block with his partner. His partner shares that they are trying to make new and interesting meals but that the patient is just not interested; he wants the food that he has been used to eating for most of their married life.

The patient has brought his latest blood work and medications to the appointment. When asked whether he has also brought his glucose monitoring results, he appears sheepish and his partner shares that he doesn't check his glucose every day. What do you do with this information? What other information do you want to obtain? Who should you approach to get the information you require?

You proceed to develop a care plan for this patient, discuss it with the patient and his partner, and end the appointment. Later in the day, you are approached by the diabetes educator, who is quite upset that you did not include them in the development of the care plan. You explain that you developed the patient care plan from a nursing perspective. You have not met everyone who works in the clinic and as a result you did not consider who else might need to be involved. The diabetes educator tells you that not only are they upset but the other members of your clinic team (dietician, family physician, nurse practitioner, pharmacist, and a social worker) may also be concerned that they were not included. How will you address this potential conflict? How do you get to know the various roles and responsibilities of each member of your team? How do you access the other members of the team? How will you communicate with everyone on the team? What types of information do you share? What type of information do you want from the other team members? How can the team support this patient's self-management? As you read through the following chapter, consider the questions posed above.

INTRODUCTION

The World Health Organization (World Health Organization [WHO], 2016) has highlighted a health workforce crisis with disastrous implications for the health and well-being of millions of people. It might be surmised that the crisis is due to a shortage of health care providers, which is true in part. However, the shortage is more far-reaching, since it encompasses all health and social care providers—those whose primary focus is to improve the health and well-being of others, including those who promote and preserve health, diagnose and treat diseases, manage and support workers—as well as regulated and nonregulated providers roles and conventional and complementary care providers (WHO, 2010).

While not enough health and social care providers are being educated to close this shortfall, there is also a growing mismatch between health workforce requirements, the supply of health and social care providers, and the health needs of the population. At a time when the world is facing a measurable shortage of health and social care providers, policymakers are looking for innovative strategies that can help to develop programs that optimize the various knowledge and skills of the global health and social care workforce. It has become clear that such strategies must be firmly based in **interprofessional education** (IPE) for collaborative patient/client/family- and community-centered practice.

The Royal Commission on the Future of Health Care in Canada advocated for changes in education to support health care providers to practice collaboratively (Romanow, 2002). Since the publication of that report, reforms in health system design and delivery have been articulated in a range of national reports (Canadian Nurses Association [CNA], 2011, 2012; Conference Board of Canada, 2012; Dinh & Bounajm, 2013; Dinh, Stonebridge, & Thériault, 2014; Donato, 2015; Suter, Deutschlander, Mickelson et al., 2012). New models of care built on the principles and competencies of interprofessional collaboration (IPC) are beginning to be developed globally. Many of these new models propose unique mixes of health and social care providers to meet the needs of the population and address health care disparities while focusing on value and sustainability (Elliot Rose & Lackie, 2014; Lackie, 2016).

This chapter introduces the language of collaboration to better understand collaborative interprofessional practice (IPP) and interprofessional care. The concept of collaboration both within nursing (intraprofessional) and between other professions (interprofessional) will be explored. Understanding the history of IPE and its link in the continuum of IPP and IPC will emerge, as will insight into the micro-, meso-, and macro-level factors associated with both. Examples of the interprofessional competencies that underpin IPP and IPC will be discussed. Finally, this chapter will address patient, provider, and system outcomes related to IPP and IPC.

THE LANGUAGE OF COLLABORATION

It is important to understand the language used in any occupation or profession. Without a common language, miscommunication and misunderstanding may arise. The terms used in a profession must be defined and understand in order to conduct sound research, advance theory, and strengthen and reinforce evidence-informed IPP and IPC.

Intraprofessional Collaboration

Intraprofessional collaboration refers to collaboration between two or more disciplines of the same profession (Bainbridge & Nasmith, 2011). For example, in the nursing profession, intraprofessional collaboration may occur among the various disciplines of nursing professionals—registered nurse, licensed or registered practical nurse, registered psychiatric nurse, and nurse practitioner—and the strategies that foster healthy work environments while maintaining the awareness that collaboration must align with the needs of the patient or client (Registered Nurses' Association of Ontario [RNAO], 2016). Similarly, intraprofessional collaboration in the medical profession can relate to the interactions between generalist medical practitioners and specialists (Meijer, de Groot, Blaauw-Westerlaken, & Damoiseaux, 2016).

Interprofessional Collaboration

Interprofessional collaboration (IPC) is often used synonymously with the term IPP. It is described as occurring ". . . when practitioners from two or more professions work together with a common purpose, commitment and mutual respect" (Center for the Advancement of Interprofessional Education [CAIPE], 2017, p. 30) to provide health and social care services. In IPC, there is shared accountability, interdependence, role clarity, mutual goal setting, and knowledge and skills that are translated into competencies for IPP (Khalili, Thistlethwaite, El-Awaisi et al., 2019). When learners/practitioners, patients/clients/families, and communities develop and maintain interprofessional working relationships that enable optimal health

outcomes, they experience IPC. IPC is meant to simplify access to other health care providers, enhance communication, promote **interprofessional learning** (IPL) and evidence-informed practice, and support health care providers to work to their full scope of practice (Gilbert, 2014). The term interprofessional pertains to the relationship that forms when two or more professional disciplines interact and collaborate to achieve some desired outcome; for example, when medicine and nursing collaborate on surgical procedures. By contrast, intraprofessional refers to a collaboration between subspecialties within a profession; for example, when pathology and dermatology in medicine collaborate to arrive at a diagnosis of cancer.

Interdisciplinary Collaboration

The word "interdisciplinary" is often mistakenly used as a synonym for "interprofessional." To clarify, a discipline is a field of study (e.g., sociology, anthropology, psychology, computer sciences, etc.) (Cambridge Dictionary, 2019; Gilbert, 2014), whereas a profession is any type of work requiring specialized knowledge and skills that are often gained through long and intensive higher-level academic preparation (Cambridge Dictionary, 2019). **Interdisciplinary collaboration** refers to different disciplines working together on the same project, requiring them to analyze, blend, and complement their distinctive attributes, thereby reaching a coherent and coordinated whole (Khalili, Thistlethwaite, El-Awaisi et al., 2019).

Multidisciplinary and Multiprofessional Collaboration

The Centre for the Advancement of Interprofessional Education (CAIPE) (CAIPE, 2017) defines the term multidisciplinary as ". . . individuals from two or more disciplines working in parallel, coming together only for specific issues and problems" (p. 30). When working in a multidisciplinary team, health care providers are working independently (i.e., in parallel with each other) rather than interdependently, as in IPP and IPC. Most health services have been provided in this way based on the siloed academic structures in which health care providers are traditionally taught and practice environments that are similarly siloed.

Interprofessional Education

Interprofessional education (IPE) is defined as ". . . occasions when members or students of two or more professions learn with, from, and about each other, to improve collaboration, and the quality of care and services" (CAIPE, 2016, p. 1). IPE is the beginning of a continuum of collaboration that spans **interprofessional learning** (IPL) and is continuously interwoven into IPP and IPC. Preferably, the continuum of IPE begins in prelicensure health and social care education and moves forward, in the postlicensure years, through the various mechanism of continuing professional development and lifelong learning (Khalili, Thistlethwaite, El-Awaisi et al., 2019).

THE CONCEPT OF COLLABORATION IN NURSING PRACTICE

Now that the language of interprofessional collaboration is clearer, we can turn to the concept of collaboration in nursing practice. Collaboration has two basic but contrasting definitions. The first is favourable and refers to people working together to achieve an outcome. The second has a negative connotation, such as when people work with an enemy who has taken control of their country (Cambridge Dictionary, 2019). It is interesting that a word used so freely in health care can have such different meanings. When the definition is deconstructed, it does not delineate who is working with whom nor for what purpose they are working. For this reason, the concepts of *intra*professional collaboration and *inter*professional collaboration should be explored.

Collaboration Within Nursing

Health care is delivered in teams and rarely by one person, even though only one person may attend to a patient or client at any given time. Nurses, being the largest provider group of health care services, typically are involved as team members. However, as in interprofessional collaboration, intraprofessional collaboration is crucial to safe, efficient, and effective care of the public.

As noted earlier, intraprofessional collaboration occurs when two or more professions of the same discipline collaborate in the pursuit of quality person-centered care. The Registered Nurses' Association of Ontario (RNAO, 2016) identifies intraprofessional collaboration as occurring between registered nurses, registered practical nurses (or licensed practical nurses), registered psychiatric nurses, and nurse practitioners. Each type of nurse has specific knowledge and skills that circumscribe their roles and responsibilities and inform their scope of practice. Intraprofessional collaboration is not unique to nursing, as medicine consists of different categories of professionals who also need to collaborate.

Much like interprofessional collaboration, intraprofessional collaboration should be a systemic and organizational imperative. When a lack of understanding of another team member's role and/or scope of practice exists, it is difficult to understand how to work collaboratively. Furthermore, a lack of understanding may lead to conflict and result in horizontal or lateral violence. Understanding what intraprofessional collaboration is provides progress toward safe and effective patient care.

For example, the guiding principles for intraprofessional collaboration within nursing include:
- All categories of nurses work together in a holistic model to facilitate continuity of care;
- The College of Nurses of Ontario outlines the competencies for each category of nurse;
- The respective environment is a factor that must be considered when guiding nursing assignments;
- Respecting and understanding the roles of each nursing category facilitates effective intraprofessional collaborative practice among nurses;
- Nursing assignments are guided by the acuity (stability, predictability, risk of negative outcome, and complexity) of the patient's or client's condition;
- Nursing is based on the relationship with patients or clients and team members; and
- Effective teams produce better outcomes for patients or clients and team members. (RNAO, 2016, p. 7)

The remainder of this chapter focuses on interprofessional collaboration within the health care team.

Collaboration Between Nursing and Health/Social Care Providers

Members of the public, particularly the patients that nurses serve every day, have clearly articulated their expectations for a seamless health care experience. They want health and social care providers to work together more effectively and efficiently, with clear communication pathways enabling integration of safe care across health and social care sectors (Elliot Rose & Lackie, 2014). Understanding that no single health or social care provider can, or will, meet all the complex needs of any individual is the first step to ensuring that those expectations are met.

Many health and social care providers, including nurses, claim that they work in teams, and they more than likely they do. However, working alongside other health and social care providers does not necessarily mean working collaboratively—in most instances, such work is multidisciplinary (i.e., parallel working). In multidisciplinary teams, there are distinct professional roles, designated leadership that does not change, independent practice and decision making, and little emphasis on group processes (Banfield & Lackie, 2009). Their functioning is very different from that of interprofessional collaborative teams, where individuals integrate their efforts, competence, and skills to work toward a common goal (Elliot Rose & Lackie, 2014; Lackie, 2016). In an interprofessional collaborative team, leadership is shared and flexible based on complementary knowledge, expertise, and skill, and team members strive to improve team functioning while engaging patients and families as team members (Bridges, Davidson, Odegard et al., 2011; Canadian Interprofessional Health Collaborative

[CIHC], 2010; Ellerby, Lockwood, Palin et al., 2010; Elliot Rose & Lackie, 2014; Banfield & Lackie, 2009; Oandasan & Reeves, 2005a). In IPC, "it is no longer about what *I* perceive to be patient-centered care; it is now about how *we* define and enact patient-centered care" (Lackie, 2016). As the popular business saying goes, there is no *I* in the word *team*.

Among the numerous descriptions of IPC, the most appropriate might be the one developed by Way, Jones, and Busing (2000), who state that IPC is an "inter-professional process for communication and decision making that enables the separate and shared knowledge and skills of care providers to synergistically influence the client/patient care provided" (p. 3). In 2003, Health Canada (Oandasan, D'Amour, Zwarenstein et al., 2004) used the language of "collaborative patient-centered practice" to describe IPC, focusing on the active contributions of each health worker while considering patient-centered goals and values. In both descriptions, robust communication and clinical decision making is envisioned among and between professions.

The WHO (2010) definition of IPC includes health care providers from different backgrounds who may or may not be regulated and who may not even come into direct contact with patients or families, but are still considered to be an integral part of any health care team. From this perspective, health care providers use their different yet complementary knowledge and skills to create shared understanding that could not have been realized were they working in isolation (WHO, 2010). The WHO (2010) has emphasized that while coordination and cooperation are important for team functioning, by themselves they are not enough to ensure or even sustain IPC. However, when combined with mutual respect, trust, autonomy, responsibility, communication, and assertiveness, IPC is possible (Lackie, 2016). In a collaborative team, there is shared leadership and *inter*dependence between members, and all members take responsibility to improve team performance (Lackie, 2016; Oandasan & Reeves, 2005a).

InterprofessionalResearch.Global, a worldwide network for IPE and collaborative practice research, describes IPC as an interprofessional work environment in which health or social care professions regularly team up to provide collaborative services, where IPC is distinguished by clear goals and roles, shared accountability, and interdependence (Khalili, Thistlethwaite, El-Awaisi et al., 2019).

Interprofessional communication is believed to be the cornerstone of IPC, yet research has shown that

GENDER CONSIDERATIONS

The way in which health care providers understand and use the word "interprofessional" and behave in interprofessional settings is compounded by gender and its influences on language. Gender differences in speaking, which we learn in childhood, can contribute to misunderstanding and a resulting lack of coherent approaches to learning. In turn, these differences affect IPE, which is the foundation of IPC.

Men's and women's communication styles can be differentiated by language and interactional factors like pronunciation, choice of words and grammatical constructions, and voice quality and smiling. Gender-related speaking patterns create and maintain asymmetries in interactions, with men's style associated with power and status and women's style associated with social connectedness (Tannen, 1990). The effect of such asymmetries on interprofessional interactions and education can be exacerbated when particular health professions are dominated by men or women.

Systematic gender-related patterns of speaking interact with what is called institutional dialogue, patterns of speaking related to individuals' orientations to their professional roles and identities and management of institutionally relevant activities (Drew & Sorjonen, 2001). As with gender-related

language use, lexical and grammatical choices, along with pragmatic factors such as turn-taking behaviours, construct individuals' identities in interactions as certain kinds of health care providers and frame how they fulfil their professional roles and tasks (Drew & Sorjonen, 2001). Students begin to learn these language patterns in school.

Institutional dialogue, which often overrides gender differences, can set up differential power and status relations in interactions involving a variety of health care providers. One asymmetry perpetuated by language use is the way we frequently refer to health professions when we speak of medicine, nursing, and allied health professions. Combining all other health professions other than physicians and nurses under a single umbrella term diminishes the status and autonomy of the professions lumped together as "allied health." Such asymmetries create barriers that must be overcome in a well-functioning interprofessional care-providing or learning environment. As protocols for IPE are developed, these differences in language use and understanding present numerous barriers that are frequently externalized through stereotypes. The language of stereotypes then perpetuates power differentials, which can in turn lead to noncoherent teaching approaches.

Sources: Drew, P., & Sorjonen, M. L. (1997). Institutional dialogue. In T. A. Van Dijk (Ed.), *Discourse as social interaction, Vol. 2* (pp. 92–118). London, UK: SAGE Publications; Tannen, D. (1990). *You just don't understand: Women and men in conversation.* New York, NY: Ballantine Books.

communication within teams is strained owing to power differentials and inefficient organizational communication structures (Gotlib Conn, Lingard, Reeves et al., 2009). A lack of good interprofessional communication hampers shared decision making, respect, and valuing the contributions of others in providing safe quality care (Lackie, 2016; Power, 2019). Studies have established that the inability of workers to talk with each other in a common language negatively impacts team performance, resulting in frequent adverse events (Gilbert, 2014). If this is the case, then there is a compelling reason to explore how profession-specific communication is navigated, which styles are valued by each profession, and which strategies are most useful within the team (Gotlib Conn, Lingard, Reeves et al., 2009; Lackie, 2016).

Essential elements of IPC include the ability to be both a team leader and a team player while also understanding one's role and being able to articulate it, possessing conflict resolution skills, having confidence in oneself and others, demonstrating mutual respect, and sharing responsibility for team outcomes regardless of whether or not they are positive (Lackie, 2016; WHO, 2010). Also critical to effective IPC is the establishment of strong interpersonal relationships that frequently emerge only when health care providers have had the opportunity to build these relationships outside of professional clinical practice, where they can get to know one another on a personal level (Culver Clark & Greenawald, 2014).

IPC strategies are needed that reflect local contexts and conditions. IPC may be set in motion by patient safety issues, limited health resources, a shift of focus from acute to primary care, job dissatisfaction, or the need for greater role clarity among health care providers. Irrespective of the reason, IPC has been shown to capitalize on the knowledge and skills of each health care provider, which improves work culture and thus job satisfaction, continuity of care, and collaborative decision making while decreasing duplication of services, inappropriate referrals, and, quite possibly, health worker migration (WHO, 2010).

APPLYING CONTENT KNOWLEDGE

1. What types of collaboration are you most familiar with?
2. What factors would you use to facilitate collaboration within and between nursing and other health/social care providers at your institution?

INTERPROFESSIONAL EDUCATION AS THE FOUNDATION

IPE has been promoted as one of the most effective ways to advance IPC, as it ensures that health care providers gain the knowledge, training, and tools necessary to promote the active participation of each care provider in patient care (Accreditation of Interprofessional Health Education, 2009, 2011; Lackie, 2016; WHO, 2010). Figure 16.1 depicts the interplay between education and health systems to effect health outcomes (WHO, 2010).

There are many ethical reasons for moving toward IPE for collaborative person-centred practice and care. The need for IPE has been occasioned by changes taking place in the ways that health and social care services are delivered based on findings from research on the social determinants of health, population health and safety, and quality of health care systems. The ability to collaborate requires a fundamental shift in how health care providers are educated and how care is organized and delivered so that the focus shifts from being provider to person centric (Elliot Rose & Lackie, 2014). During IPE's development over the past 30 years, it has addressed key issues identified by the WHO for transforming education for health care providers, recognizing that the patient or client is not only the focus of interprofessional attention but also a member of the collaborative care team (WHO, 2013).

Health care providers' attitudes and behaviours change when they have opportunities to learn about, from, and with one another through IPE (Lackie, 2016). IPE is viewed as foundational for collaborative practice–ready health and social care providers, preparing them to deliver comprehensive services in a wide variety of practice settings (WHO, 2010). Yet, despite general consensus about the utility of IPE, the debate continues as to when to bring students together to experience IPE. Should it be early on in their education or much later, after students have achieved firm footing in their own profession? Should it happen in prelicensure or postlicensure education? The research related to these questions is varied and somewhat confusing. Some would recommend bringing students together later in their programs so as not to confuse specific roles, while others endorse introducing IPE early to decrease negative stereotypes of other professions (Barksdale, Christy, & Kobal, 2019). Despite these debates, it is agreed that IPE should focus on helping students understand each other's knowledge, skills, abilities, and roles before graduation, as it is significantly easier to train *for* IPC before entering practice than it is to change *to* IPC when in practice (Blue, Mitcham, Smith et al., 2010; Gilbert, 2014).

The multivariate complexity of transforming health provider education through the continuum of IPE is obvious from its definition. There has been continuous and continuing work to ensure that the three parts of the IPE definition—*with, from,* and *about*—are well understood and agreed on and that teaching, learning, research, and evaluation recognize the need to show how the parts are interwoven. Attempts to understand the relationships

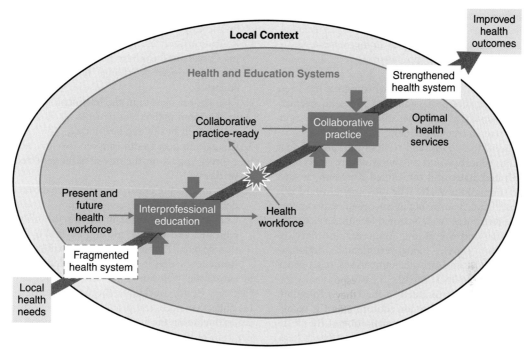

Fig. 16.1 The interplay between education and health systems. (**Source:** World Health Organization. (2010). *Framework for action on interprofessional education & collaborative practice.* Geneva, Switzerland: Author.)

among and between the various parts of the definition continue in research and evaluation programs that have roots in academic disciplines such as anthropology, sociology, and linguistics and are based on an understanding of the social determinants of health and population health. Case-, simulation-, and experiential-based learning have been found to support the effectiveness of IPE, and combining these methods could result in improved student competence (Riskiyana, Claramita, & Rahayu, 2018).

IPE initiatives have been successful to date because champions have recognized the following nine principles (Gilbert, 2010):

- One size does not fit all;
- Resources are required, both from a top-down approach as well as operationally;
- Curricula changes are essential;
- IPE must be introduced at the right time;
- Collaborative learning environments must be created;
- Structures must be modified to support collaboration;
- IPE should be embedded in the system;
- Evidence makes the best case for IPE; and
- Interprofessional players must engage the community.

These principles are not all inclusive, as those in the field can no doubt identify others that are required to support IPE. Nevertheless, to address these nine principles successfully, each requires a leadership style that is open, inclusive, and comprehensive; recognizes the complexity of each principle; and applies unique strategies in addressing them (Gilbert, in press).

The History of Interprofessional Education

IPE has had a long history in Canada, beginning with the revolutionary vision of Dr. John F. McCreary, Dean of Medicine at The University of British Columbia (UBC). In 1964, McCreary published an article in the *Canadian Medical Association Journal*, stating that, "All of these diverse members of the health team should be brought together during their undergraduate years, taught by the same teachers, in the same classrooms and on the same patients" (McCreary, 1964, p. 1220). Three years later, under the direction of Dr. George Szasz, the Division of Interprofessional Education at UBC was established. Szasz (1969) remarked,

> It appears that, among other problems, the health professionals employ their talents inappropriately, and, as a consequence, scarce human resources are wasted. Evidence also indicates fragmentation and

compartmentalization, both of scientific investigation and the approach to human problems, and of poor communication between those who provide different components of the health services. (pp. 449–450)

In the ensuing 40-plus years, much progress has been made in realizing interprofessionalism in health sciences education; yet many of the issues discussed by Szasz four decades ago remain true to this day.

Throughout the 1970s and 1980s, interprofessional approaches to education and collaborative care emerged in both the United States and the United Kingdom, as well as globally, through the WHO. The movement toward IPE for IPC has included some highly successful experiments funded by government (e.g., National Health Service, UK; Health Canada; and the Health Resources and Services Administration, USA); nongovernmental organizations (e.g., WHO); and private foundations (e.g., Macy Foundation, USA) (Gilbert, 2014).

In 1987, CAIPE was founded in the United Kingdom to provide a central resource for educators and is recognized with developing the accepted definition of IPE. With an international membership of educators and researchers, CAIPE remains active and relevant in the advancement of IPE to this day. During the same time period, the WHO (1988) advocated for shared learning to complement profession-specific programs and recommended that students should learn together during certain periods of their education to acquire the skills necessary for solving the priority problems of individuals and communities. In 1992, one of the first IPE courses in Canada was offered by the University of Alberta. Shortly thereafter, and well into the 2000s, offices of IPE began to turn up at many universities. The Centre for Collaborative Health Professional Education was established at Memorial University of Newfoundland in 1999; in 2001, UBC established the College of Health Disciplines; and, in 2006, the Office of Interprofessional Education was founded at the University of Toronto (Banfield & Lackie, 2009). Since then, other IPE offices have emerged in universities across Canada.

In the early 2000s, IPE began to take more of a foothold on the national stage in Canada. In 2001, the federal government established the commission to review Medicare, Canada's universally accessible, publicly funded health care system. The commission's mandate was to recommend policies and measures to improve the health care system and its long-term sustainability. The report made various observations and recommendations supporting the need for a coordinated approach to health human resources planning, noting that:

1. Initiatives in primary health care highlight the need for providers to work together in integrated teams, and across institutional provider networks, that are focused on meeting patients' needs;
2. Education and training of providers falls short of meeting Canadians' health care needs;
3. There is a need to change how health workers are educated;
4. Changes are needed in the relationship between health workers and patients, as patients take a more proactive role in their health and health care;
5. Changes in how health care services are delivered have a direct impact on the mix of skills expected of health workers;
6. New models are needed to reflect the different ways of delivering health care services; and
7. Changes must be made in the way health workers are educated and trained, moving beyond a siloed education system. (Romanow, 2002, pp. xxiii–xxxiv)

Romanow's report (2002) also pointed out the need to substantially improve the base of information about Canada's health workforce through concerted efforts to (1) collect, analyze, and provide regular reports on critical issues, including the recruitment, distribution, and remuneration of health workers; and (2) establish strategies for addressing the supply, distribution, education, training, and changing skills and patterns of practice for Canada's health workforce. Commissioner Romanow further stressed the importance of IPE for patient-centered care, advocating for new approaches to education and training as well as how health care providers' roles and responsibilities change when patterns of care change. He noted the need to develop new models of care to reflect different ways of delivering health services, stating ". . . corresponding changes must be made in the way health care providers are educated and trained . . . If health care providers are expected to work together and share expertise in a team environment, it makes sense that their education and training should prepare them for this type of working arrangement" (Romanow, 2002, p. 109).

Following the release of the Romanow commission's report, a meeting of Canada's First Ministers in 2003 identified the need to change the way health care providers were educated in Canada, leading to a budgetary commitment to health human resource planning, recruitment and retention, and IPE. This led to the announcement of two major Health Canada initiatives that would invest approximately $60 million over the subsequent 5-year period (2003–2008): the first initiative would examine and recommend ways to establish coherent policies with respect to health human resources planning; the second initiative would examine new ways to conduct IPE and its correlate, patient-centered collaborative care. This initiative led to the establishment of the Pan-Canadian Health Human Resources Strategy, which was intended (among other goals) to facilitate and support the implementation of a strategy for Interprofessional Education for Collaborative Patient-Centered Practice (IECPCP) across all health care sectors. The National Expert Committee (NEC) on IECPCP, established under that strategy, was designed to be a forum for innovative forward-thinking and broad strategic advice to Health Canada. During the same time period, the Canadian Interprofessional Health Collaborative (CIHC) was established and funded by Health Canada for a 5-year term (2003–2008) through a contribution agreement with UBC. In 2008, CIHC became a nongovernmental organization and remains the national voice for IPE and IPC in Canada.

The IECPCP initiative had a clear set of objectives that served as its guide across the life of its funded projects (Health Council of Canada, 2005):

- Promote and demonstrate the benefits of IECPCP;
- Increase the number of educators prepared to teach from an IECPCP perspective;
- Increase the number of health professionals trained for collaborative patient-centered practice before, and after, entry-to-practice;
- Stimulate networking and sharing of best educational approaches for collaborative patient-centered practice; and
- Facilitate interprofessional collaborative care in both education and practice settings. (pp. 40–41; 91–93)

In 2004, further work emerged in support of the IPE movement in Canada. A model that delineated the macro-, meso-, and micro-level factors associated with IPE and IPC was developed by D'Amour and Oandasan (2005). Moreover, the first (and at the time, only) national interprofessional student association in the world—National Health Sciences Students' Association—was incorporated as a society.

The IECPCP initiatives that have developed across Canada, which have been largely funded by Health Canada, have shown that IECPCP should be a coherent and integrated component of prelicensure education that centres the patient. It should provide opportunities for students from at least three different health and human service educational programs to work collaboratively in teams on matters of mutual clinical concern. At base, IECPCP is largely about curricular change in the widest possible domain and, like all curricular change, is both painful and slow to bring about. As we tackle the immensely complex task of entrenching IPE as the norm rather than the exception, it is worth bearing in mind the words variously ascribed to Calvin Coolidge and Woodrow Wilson: "Changing a college curriculum is like moving a graveyard—you never know how many friends the dead have until you try to move them."

The benefits to IPE for IPC are numerous. Health care providers are said to experience enhanced personal and professional confidence, increased reflective practice, increased respect for other professions, awareness of ways to support each other, and appreciation of the pressures experienced by other professions. IPE promotes mutual understanding between health and social care providers and better intraprofessional and interprofessional communication, fostering a greater understanding of other health providers' roles. From a patient/family perspective, there are reports of improved patient care, patient satisfaction, safety, and access to health care. Improved recruitment and retention of health care providers, more effective employment of health human resources, and improved population health are important system outcomes (Banfield & Lackie, 2009).

FACTORS THAT IMPACT INTERPROFESSIONAL EDUCATION AND INTERPROFESSIONAL COLLABORATION

IPE for IPC should consider the various influences that impact both the education system (academia) and the professional system (health care sector) and which ultimately affect learner and patient outcomes, respectively. Figure 16.2 illustrates these interconnected influences, or factors, that have been situated in the micro, meso, and macro levels and will be discussed later. But first, we must examine what lies at the heart of each system—what is their main focus?

Learner-centredness characterizes the IPE system based on constructivist and democratic principles that require collaborative approaches to learning (Serin, 2018). In a learner-centred environment, students develop personal responsibility for learning by playing an active role. In doing so, they relate what they are learning to their prior knowledge and make meaning through discussion with students from other health education programs. The educator acts as a facilitator to student learning; the interface between the two is critical to the success of IPE. It is within this interface that the values and beliefs of one's profession emerge; without reflecting upon, examining, and challenging these profession-specific socialized beliefs, the development of interprofessional relationships may be blocked (Stanley, Dixon, Warner, & Stanley, 2016). In the health system, professional cultures differ owing to generations of social positioning, class, power, and gender disparities (Price, Doucet, & McGillis Hall, 2014). In fact, students entering health professional programs do so often favouring one profession over another, further

Interprofessional Education for Collaborative Patient-centered Practice: A Model

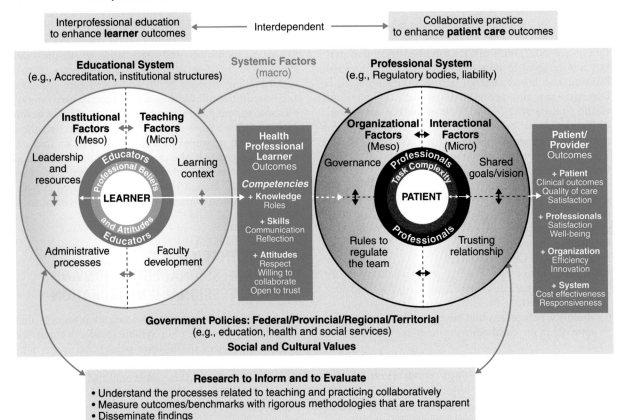

Fig. 16.2 Interprofessional education for collaborative patient-centred practice: An evolving framework. (**Source:** D'Amour, D., & Oandasan, I. (2005). Interprofessionality as the field of interprofessional practice and interprofessional education: an emerging concept. *Journal of Interprofessional Care, 19*(Suppl. 1), 8–20.)

entrenching hierarchies that have been in place for ages (Price, Doucet, & McGillis Hall, 2014). Students and practitioners must be socialized not only within their own profession but between professions so that a dual professional–interprofessional identity can be cultivated to foster IPC (King, Orchard, Khalili, & Avery, 2016). Educators, as role models, shape learner thinking about the "other," acting as either a barrier or an enabler to IPL and IPC (D'Amour & Oandasan, 2005).

Likewise, in the health care system, patient-centredness is the focus of attention, where emphasis is on caring for patients and families in ways that are meaningful to them. To do so, health care providers must incorporate patients' preferences, needs, and values to guide mutual clinical decision making. In IPC, patients are listened to, informed, and involved in their own care (Institute of

Medicine, 2001) and are central to the collaborative process. Patients must be active members of their team, and their needs determine the interactions between health/social care providers, where the composition of each team is dependent on the needs of patients (D'Amour & Oandasan, 2005). The Patient Voices Network (BC Patient Safety and Quality Council, n.d.) is one example of ongoing efforts to engage patients, families, and caregivers so that their perspectives about how to improve the quality of care are heard. The Strategy for Patient-Oriented Research strives to engage patients, families, and caregivers in the research process by changing their roles from passive receptors to proactive partners. Both initiatives help to shape health care services.

There are micro-, meso-, and macro-level factors that impact both the academic and health care systems.

Foundational work by D'Amour and Oandasan (2005) and Oandasan and Reeves (2005a, 2005b) has informed the following discussion because these works clearly delineate key considerations of IPE and IPC, noting that there is interdependency between the two. Without this interdependency, implementation and sustainability are threatened. Since the work of D'Amour and Oandasan (2005), the field has moved to develop an interprofessional competency framework (CIHC, 2010; Interprofessional Education Collaborative [IPEC] Expert Panel, 2011), in which the various factors outlined by D'Amour and Oandasan (2005) are encapsulated as principles on which to develop interprofessional curricula.

Micro-Level Factors

Micro-level factors refer to connections between students, educators, and health care providers that influence IPE and IPC. Micro-level factors in education relate to teaching, whereas micro-level factors in the practice setting refer to interactions.

Interprofessional Education: Teaching Factors

Interprofessional education and learning (IPE/IPL) are the mechanisms used to establish IPP and IPC as the foundations for change in the systems of health and social care. The IPE/IPL curriculum is designed and developed to establish IPP and IPC as significant influences on learners' attitudes, knowledge, skills, and behaviours as they move to being true interprofessional collaborators. At the micro level, there are two major considerations: faculty development and learning context.

IPE/IPL must be thoughtfully and repeatedly facilitated by educators who have the requisite knowledge and skills to guide students through the "about, from, and with" of IPE (Hall & Zierler, 2015). Lack of interprofessional facilitator development can lead to learner dissatisfaction and undermine future collaborative working relationships (Banfield & Lackie, 2009). Educators at all levels of instruction are urged to gain the competencies required to develop, facilitate, and evaluate IPE along with evaluating the learning outcomes associated with interprofessional groups of learners (Lackie, 2016; WHO, 2010). Interprofessional facilitators must understand the elements of group dynamics—forming, storming, norming, performing, and adjourning (Tuckman & Jensen, 1977)—and be confident in managing interprofessional teams of students as they move through each component. Facilitators must be role models for interprofessional communication, reflection, and shared leadership, using a variety of educational principles and interactive methods to lead the group processes

required for successful IPE/IPL (Davis, Clevenger, Posnock et al., 2015).

Unfortunately, studies have highlighted several problems related to the preparation of educators to teach interprofessionally, such as uncertainty about how best to prepare IPE facilitators for their new role (Egan-Lee, Baker, Tobin et al., 2011); identification of challenges in teaching in an IPE environment (Buring, Bhushan, Brazeau et al., 2009); proposals for innovative approaches to meet IPE program goals (Abu-Rish Blakeney, Pfeifle, Jones et al., 2016); and lack of practice guidelines for faculty development to effectively facilitate IPE (Hall & Zierler, 2015). Other faculty-related barriers to effective IPE include negative attitudes and lack of perceived value, lack of rewards, turf wars between professions, and bias toward own profession (Lawlis, Anson, & Greenfield, 2014).

The learning context—who, what, how, when, and where—of IPE is equally important to its success. Significant barriers to successful IPE include pedagogical barriers; logistical challenges; allocation (and lack of) resources; deep-rooted hierarchical philosophies and culture; and resistance to change (Gilbert, 2005; De Los Santos, Degnon McFarlin, & Martin, 2014). Also important are consideration of the theories that inform IPE, teaching and learning strategies, settings in which IPL will take place, competencies, and timing. Curricular change is essential and needs to be built and supported across all postsecondary institutions and health and human service programs. Maintaining a psychologically safe environment, where learners feel safe openly expressing ideas and opinions and are willing to engage in interpersonal risk taking in the workplace (Newman, Donohue, & Eva, 2017; Edmondson & Lei, 2014), can result in improved attitudes of students who learn interprofessionally (Oandasan & Reeves, 2005a). A psychologically safe environment is characterized by colleagues

> who will not reject others for being themselves or saying what they think; respect each other's competence; are interested in each other as people; have positive intentions to one another; engage in constructive conflict or confrontation; and feel that it is safe to experiment and take risks. (Newman, Donohue, & Eva, 2017, p. 522)

The benefits of a psychologically safe environment cannot be understated, for when it is in place, there is enhanced individual and team learning; improved performance; increased creativity and innovation; use of learning activities to implement new practices; increased knowledge exchange; and increased engagement and commitment (Newman, Donohue, & Eva, 2017; Edmondson & Lei, 2014).

CASE STUDY

Recall the personal perspective at the beginning of this chapter. You were caring for a 60-year-old man who had been newly diagnosed with type 1 diabetes. That encounter did not go particularly well—the other members of the health care team felt left out because they were not included in the development of the patient's plan of care.

Since your first week in this clinic, you have made it a priority to get to know the other members of your team and understand how their knowledge and skills complement yours. You have participated in interprofessional education sessions held in the clinic, where you have learned about the roles and responsibilities of all the different members of the team; discussed diabetes care from their perspectives—what their main priorities are and the skills they have that are different, and the same, as yours; and learned about novel diabetes practices together, where active learning has taken place with your colleagues. You have learned that there are competencies that overlap between professions but also that there are distinct differences in your scopes of practice. Your team comes together daily to discuss patients and families under their care and the services they need. From there, each member of the team shares what they can offer to address patient/family needs, and robust plans of care emerge. Leadership is shared in your team, and decisions are made interprofessionally based on patient/family needs.

It has now been many weeks since you began working in the diabetes clinic. Today, you are meeting with another patient newly diagnosed with type I diabetes. During the interview, they disclose that they are not doing well financially and struggle with buying the proper food and supplies needed to manage their diabetes. Thinking about the members of your team, you offer to arrange a meeting with the social worker and dietician, as you know that they have knowledge and skills that you do not and which would benefit this patient's plan of care.

Interprofessional Collaboration: Interactional Factors

IPC is accomplished through interactions—those between patients/families and health care providers, those between health care providers of various backgrounds, and those with the organization in which all health care providers reside. These interactional micro-level factors in the professional (health care) system fall within two categories: shared goals and vision and a sense of belonging.

Without either, collaboration is not possible (D'Amour & Oandasan, 2005).

Having a shared vision and goals is of paramount importance to IPC. It is imperative to identify a professionally diverse base of champions within practice—even just a few at first—who have a clear interest in IPE and IPC and who have access to all levels of senior administration within the practice setting. The connection to senior administration is important, as it is through this conduit that IPE is best promoted and endorsed. Patients, who can be engaged as teachers and who understand the importance of team-based care, should be integral members of the champion team. From the outset, students must also be part of the planning, for in countries where IPE is flourishing, it has done so because students have conveyed its importance to their professional development (Gilbert, 2014).

To build trusting relationships, health care providers must know each other personally and professionally to become familiar with each other's conceptual models, roles, and responsibilities (D'Amour & Oandasan, 2005). Working within collaborative teams is proposed to enhance people's belongingness. Belongingness, a sense of who you are and your social worth, is considered one of the most basic human needs for psychological well-being (Cockshaw, Shochet, & Obst, 2014; Colyer, 2008; Mohamed, Newton, & McKenna, 2014). When a person believes that they are valued, needed, and accepted and that their unique qualities blend with the system or environment they are in, they feel that they belong and hence become engaged in the success of the team (Lackie, 2016; Mohamed, Newton, & McKenna, 2014).

A willingness to collaborate and the existence of mutual trust, respect, and communication are also important interactional factors that facilitate IPC. Willingness to collaborate depends on one's professional education, previous experience working collaboratively, personal maturity, and common objectives. Trust in oneself develops when health care providers are confident in their own abilities; they also need to trust others by allowing for time, effort, and patience to build these relationships. Sharing knowledge, communicating, and negotiating openly and actively leads to a collective understanding about how everyone's work contributes to positive outcomes and to team objectives, ultimately supporting IPC (San Martin-Rodriguez, Beaulieu, D'Amour, & Ferrada-Videla, 2005). IPC is successful when team members can effectively communicate so that individual and team goals are balanced, communal resources are negotiated, and decision-making is shared (WHO, 2010). Strategies, such as communication protocols, must be put in place that enhance communication processes among health care providers to support collaborative practice.

A major challenge confronting any leader of IPE is to understand and assess the multiplicity of identities and cultures (Harper & Leicht, 2006) that are interwoven in the workforce of postsecondary education and health and social care. Culture encompasses shared ways of being, living, and thinking. Culture consists of symbols, languages, knowledge, values, norms, and techniques. Each person in the workforce comes from a culture that defines their individual identity. Each comes gendered. Each comes as part of a community that is unrelated to their work site or professions/occupation. Currently, many health care providers identify as members of a siloed profession, but also carry an identity as a member of a siloed professional community. Each comes with an identity as a care provider (in the sense of providing a professional service). Each carries an identity as a sometime(s) patient/client/customer/service user. Every day, the interplay of these various identities contributes to the larger complex culture of their workplace which is, itself, most frequently siloed and deeply rooted in personal values. These challenges must be addressed every day by leaders who are developing interprofessional collaborative practice.

Source: Harper, C. L., & Leicht, K. T. (2006). *Exploring social change: America and the World* (5th ed.). New York, NY: Pearson.

Meso-Level Factors

Meso-level factors refer to connections at the organizational level that influence interprofessional education and collaborative practice, such as connections between teaching and health organizations.

Interprofessional Education: Institutional Factors

Over the course of many years, barriers to effective IPE programs have been identified. These barriers include variable geographical locations; inadequate and unsustainable funding; scheduling challenges; rigid and/or condensed curriculums; differing degree timetables; concerns that IPE will not meet professional requirements; lack of recognition of IPE workload for tenure and promotion; and varying knowledge bases of the educators and students involved (Barksdale, Christy, & Kobal et al., 2019; Gilbert, 2014; Lawlis, Anson, & Greenfield, 2014). IPE initiatives are usually undertaken on top of a normal workload by a committed few and can inhibit the development and sustainability of IPE (D'Amour & Oandasan, 2005; Oandasan & Reeves, 2005b). The persistence of these barriers is having a significant negative impact on the advancement of interprofessionalism in academia and practice.

IPE requires an organizational structure and strong leadership committed to ensuring that reasonable human and nonhuman resources are in place and that there are strategic directions and infrastructure that advise on logistical decisions, dedicated administrative assistance, and operating funds (D'Amour & Oandasan, 2005; Grymonpre, Ateah, Dean et al., 2016; Oandasan & Reeves, 2005b). Success will depend on getting commitment from both institutional and political leadership. It is essential that senior administrators are in place with the power to move the IPE agenda forward so that champion faculty can carry the IPE vision forward (D'Amour & Oandasan, 2005; Oandasan & Reeves, 2005b). A strategic plan, IPE policy, adequate distribution of resources, curricular mapping and modification, support for faculty champions, and recognition of IPE for tenure and promotion are critical enablers of IPE that rely on strong leadership (D'Amour & Oandasan, 2005; Grymonpre, Ateah, Dean et al., 2016).

Interprofessional Collaboration: Organizational Factors

Leadership plays as important a role in the health care sector as it does in postsecondary education. An organizational philosophy that understands that collaboration exists not only within teams but also within the organization as a whole will unequivocally support IPC, inspire health care providers to think about ways of working together that are innovative, encourage the development of common goals, and rise above resistance (Oandasan, Ross Baker, Barker et al., 2006). How an organization is governed reflects the efforts used to shift away from a medical model to one of collaboration among all health care providers. This shift will then be reflected in how clinical care is structured.

The dominance of the medical model of health and the resultant territoriality, power struggles, and hierarchy is a significant barrier to teamwork (Bihari Axelsson & Axelsson, 2008; Chong, Aslani, & Chen, 2013; Clements, Dault, & Priest, 2007; Dinh, Stonebridge, & Thériault et al., 2014; Orchard, King, Khalili, & Bezzina, 2012; McNeil, Mitchell, & Parker, 2015). Leaders that support IPC must steer the development of team processes, set clear goals, establish the right mix of health care providers to meet patient needs, and create conditions for team success (Goldman Meuser, Rogers et al., 2010; Oandasan, Ross Baker, Barker et al., 2006).

An organizational culture (i.e., assumptions, values, norms, and customs) that endorses IPC is crucial, as innovative models of care can thrive and staff are encouraged to work together in new ways (Dinh, Stonebridge, & Thériault et al., 2014; Lackie, 2016; Suter et al., 2007; Tataw, 2012). There is an imperative to create formal structures for IPC that demonstrate openness for change and support shared learning. To create organizations in which IPC is the model for patient-centred practice, all workers need to have a clear sense of the institution's shared values, goals, and objectives, and these must be reinforced by clearly defined tasks, procedures, and protocols (Gilbert, 2014). Sustaining these facilitators requires regular appraisal and reflection on progress and informed feedback on performance (Gilbert, 2014).

Organizations must consider the context in which health care providers practise, the capacity of leaders to make IPC possible, as well as the availability of resources to support collaboration (Lackie, 2016). Each health care setting is unique, and therefore strategies used to establish IPC must consider where teams are situated (i.e., in community, rehabilitation, or tertiary care settings) and local requirements and challenges (WHO, 2010). Clinical care should be structured so as to establish and maintain IPC. Time and space-sharing opportunities must be provided for health care providers on the same team to facilitate information sharing, develop interpersonal relationships, and reduce professional territoriality (San Martin-Rodriguez, Beaulieu, D'Amour, & Ferrada-Videla, 2005).

Organizations also need to consider how traditional siloed learning impacts health services delivery. With duplication in learning comes duplication in practice. When health care providers repeat, for strictly professional reasons, the same skills, interventions, or processes as their colleagues, valuable time, effort, and energy are lost (Gilbert, 2014). IPE has a significant role in developing senior and mid-level management as well as health care providers to work collaboratively (Lackie, 2016; Morano & Damiani, 2018).

Macro-Level Factors

Macro-level factors refer to system-level connections that influence IPE and collaborative practice, such as politics, socioeconomics, and culture. With the ongoing development of accreditation guidelines and interprofessional competencies, it is apposite to briefly review the macro lessons that have been learned through the Health Canada IECPCP initiative. There is a pronounced disconnect between policies developed separately, and frequently without consultation, across ministries of health and postsecondary education. This lack of policy coherence (and congruence) seriously impacts attempts to build joint health human resource strategies that encompass the ideals of IECPCP. It also prevents a good idea from becoming one that is widely recognized, accepted, and implemented in all policy decisions. If it were possible to improve policy coherence and congruence between ministries of health and advanced education across Canada, then perhaps it might afford IECPCP the permanent status in the health and educational system that it deserves.

Interprofessional Education: Systemic Factors

The health education system is on its way to helping students understand the expertise, responsibilities, competencies, values, and differing philosophical perspectives of others, but more work is required at a system level to sustain this momentum. Structural and financial segregation of postsecondary health and social care provider programs must be alleviated, as this divide can be an insurmountable barrier to IPE. Unless there is funding allocated to faculties, human resources, and the built environment, the necessary infrastructure will be nonexistent, and any IPE initiative will ultimately fail. It is necessary to fund and formally recognize practice-based research and evaluation strategies that build evidence that IPE improves outcomes (Ho, Jarvis-Selinger, Borduas et al., 2008).

Some universities have made IPE mandatory, while others have established courses with an elective status. This optional choice in and of itself does not authenticate the importance of IPE for IPC. This is the stage where accreditation and accreditors can influence decisions about how to embed IPE in curricula. Accreditation of health professional education can act as a strong lever for advancing IPE if the accrediting agency chooses to monitor for collaborative practice and structured IPE activities (Accreditation of Interprofessional Health Education, 2009). Mandated and accredited IPE for all health care providers (both those in training and those in practice) is required to support the attainment and mastery of IPC competencies. Policy must support such transition to address individual, practice, and system-level barriers (Dinh, Stonebridge, & Thériault et al., 2014).

Strategies are needed to help health policymakers around the world to implement the continuum of IPE that will be most beneficial in their own jurisdictions and within their local contexts. Building on what is readily and currently available as well as developing, maintaining, and nurturing strong partnerships within the community will provide a sound platform for strategies to contextualize IPE. These strategies include:

- Agreeing on why interprofessional education and collaborative practice can benefit the local community and how key stakeholders in local regional facilities and organizations can work together to achieve this aim;
- Considering how to structure processes in a way that promotes shared decision making, regular communication, and community involvement; and

- Introducing integrated workforce capacity and capability planning across the health and education systems at regional, national, and local levels. (WHO, 2010, p. 38)

Interprofessional Collaboration: Systemic Factors

The systemic factors related to IPC in practice settings are multifaceted. Partnerships must be established between the health sector and academia; not only would such a reciprocal relationship grow, but it would also increase capacity for IPE and IPC in both settings, thereby advancing collaborative learning environments for staff and students and helping to institute different models of care (CNA, 2012; MacMillan, 2013).

There is an urgent need to modify institutional and management structures and policies to support IPC. One of the most difficult tasks for advancing IPC is building models of collaboration. Middle managers require support from senior leadership to facilitate innovation among their staff and encourage experimentation with new interprofessional models of care. IPE for managers is crucial if they are to act as role models and facilitate IPC (Begun, White, & Mosser, 2011). Health care providers must also participate in IPE within the practice setting and be introduced to the competencies that are required to work collaboratively; without it, IPC will not become a reality. There is also an urgent need to recognize and promote the role of all agencies—from acute to community care—as equal partners. In Ontario, the RNAO has created best practice guidelines to address both interprofessional (RNAO, 2013) and intraprofessional (RNAO, 2016) collaboration.

Health care providers also have a role in effecting change through regulatory bodies, which are responsible for defining scopes of practice and dealing with issues of liability (D'Amour & Oandasan, 2005; Oandasan & Reeves, 2005b; Lahey, Hutt, Hopkins, & Hobson, 2009). Laws establish the standards and scopes of practice for regulated health care providers and thus can support or inhibit interprofessional practice; the perceptions and attitudes of health care providers toward these laws can determine the success or failure of IPC (Ries, 2017). As each province/territory is responsible for regulating its health care providers, provinces/territories are also integral to changing outdated restrictions and moving professions away from siloed care practices (Ries, 2017).

With the advent of new roles and new ways of working comes fear and uncertainty of legal liability among regulated health care providers. Who is responsible for patient care and outcomes in collaborative teams? Certainly, there has been the belief that physicians bear the legal brunt for the actions of all other professions. But is this fear grounded in truth? According to Ries (2017), "Canadian courts do not adopt a traditional view of a healthcare hierarchy where legal liability automatically flows up to a doctor at the top of a pyramid" (p. 418). Each regulated health worker is responsible to practice in a manner that meets a reasonable standard of competence within their profession. There is an expectation that health care providers communicate with one another regarding their roles, responsibilities, scopes of practice, and areas of expertise. It is also the organization's responsibility to ensure that there are polices and procedures reflective of IPC. If they do not, they also may be legally culpable (Ries, 2017).

In select Canadian provinces, some regulatory agencies have statutory duties to implement IPE and IPC, and they are working together to develop joint standards and guidelines. For example, in 2007, regulated health professions in Nova Scotia agreed to an informal yet structured forum whereby they could share information and best practices on regulation. Such an entity is unique in that it is a single point of contact for numerous regulators for discussion and consultation of health professional regulation. One of their main foci, in the public's best interest, is to advance IPC teams by exploring collaborative regulatory processes. In doing so, they have implemented policies for collaborative investigations, registration appeals, and decision-making frameworks (Nova Scotia Regulated Health Professions Network, 2018, 2019). In 2013, Nova Scotia enacted the *Regulated Health Professions Network Act* and concomitant bylaws were approved by council in 2018.

INTERPROFESSIONAL COLLABORATIVE COMPETENCIES

Many functions in health care are guided by a core set of knowledge, skills, attitudes, and behaviours (i.e., competencies). IPC is no different. These distinct competencies are required and must be shared with all learners and health care providers if a new model of working together is to be realized. In fact, at a time of heightened risk management, increased attention from consumers about their rights, and needs-based health human resources planning, there are many professions, regulatory bodies, and health care and government organizations advocating for the use of competencies because they provide performance predictors and delineate standards of practice (Reeves, Fox, & Hodges, 2009).

Competencies, and their associated descriptors and performance criteria, identify broad performance requirements that workers use to complete a required work task or function (Lackie, 2016; Wood, Flavell, Vanstolk et al., 2009). Competencies also inform lifelong learning, accreditation standards, scopes of practice, and curricular development (CIHC, 2010; IPEC Expert Panel, 2011). For this reason, a clear understanding of the characteristics of the

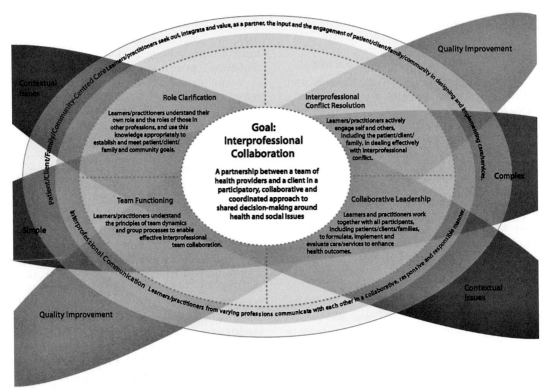

Fig. 16.3 CIHC national interprofessional competency framework. (**Source:** Canadian Interprofessional Health Collaborative. (2010). *A national interprofessional competency framework*. Vancouver, BC: Author.)

ideal collaborative practitioner, as described by competencies, was required to inform curriculum and professional development IPE, thereby advancing professional practice for IPC. These IPC competencies form the basis of collaboration and facilitate understanding of what is essential to actualize team-based care (Reeves, 2012; Thistlethwaite, Forman, Matthews et al., 2014). Three frameworks of IPC competencies in three different jurisdictions will be highlighted next.

Canada

The National Interprofessional Competency Framework, developed by the CIHC (CIHC, 2010), is supported by many underlying assumptions, including:

- Robust, comprehensive competency statements stand the tests of time;
- Competency descriptors delineate the knowledge, skills, attitudes, values, and judgments that are "dynamic, developmental, and evolutionary" (CIHC, 2010, p. 9);
- IPL is cumulative, along a continuum;
- IPC is vital for improved health outcomes;

- The degree of collaborative practice competence is contingent on the breadth of, and opportunities for, IPE and IPC practice;
- The adoption of IPC competencies depends on the level of the learner and the complexity of learning;
- Execution of IPC competencies necessitates a change in how learners, health care providers, educators, and practice environments conceptualize IPC; and
- For IPC to thrive, the learning and practice cultures must support IPC competencies. (CIHC, 2010, pp. 8–9)

The six CIHC (2010) IPC competency domains are patient/client/family/community-centred care; IP communication; role clarification; team functioning; collaborative leadership; and IP conflict resolution. Figure 16.3 shows a schematic representation of the CIHC interprofessional collaborative competencies.

The first two competency domains, patient/client/family/community-centred care and IP communication, influence and support the remaining four competency domains (Bainbridge, Nasmith, Orchard, & Wood, 2010). Complexity, contextual issues, and quality improvement influence how the framework is applied. The skill level required to perform the competencies is contingent upon the complexity of the situation and therefore the complexity of the collaborative process. Fairly simple patient cases may only require collaboration between two health care providers, whereas more complex situations will require more health care providers and thus more intricate collaboration. The health care setting and the comfort and skill sets of health care providers (i.e., contextual considerations) will also impact integration of the IPC competencies. Differences will be observed between comprehensive and consistent teams (i.e., in long-term care, pediatrics), teams and/or patients that only come together for short periods of time (i.e., emergency or high-turnover areas), and community settings where nontraditional workers merge with the team (i.e., community health and school health). Quality improvement underpins each competency and impacts the approach to collaboration (Bainbridge, Nasmith, Orchard, & Wood, 2010; CIHC, 2010; Lackie, 2016).

USA

In a similar body of work, the IPEC Expert Panel (2011) identified four core competency domains and associated behavioural learning outcomes for IPC practice. Figure 16.4 shows the schematic representation of IPEC's interprofessional collaboration competency domain. The IPEC Expert Panel— represented by dentistry, medicine, nursing, osteopathic medicine, pharmacy, and public health—envisioned IPC as the means to achieving safe, accessible, quality patient-centered care. The IPEC IPC competencies were based on the following principles:
- Patient/family-centered care;
- Community/population and relationship focused;
- Process oriented;
- Associated with developmentally suitable learning educational strategies and behavioural assessments;
- Ability to be incorporated across the learning continuum;
- Sensitive to various contexts and professions;
- Written in common and meaningful language; and
- Outcome driven. (IPEC Expert Panel, 2011, p. 2)

Building on general professional competencies, the IPEC Expert Panel (2011) identified the four core IPC competencies as values/ethics for interprofessional practice; roles and responsibilities for collaborative practice; interprofessional communication practices; and interprofessional teamwork and team-based practice. In the performance of the competencies, health care providers must be reflective, flexible, and adaptive to variable care contexts and goals (Association of American Medical Colleges, 2011). The competency statements "reflect the endpoint of initial health professional education (pre-licensure or pre-credentialling)" (IPEC Expert Panel, 2011, p. 30); however,

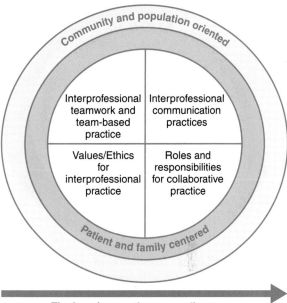

Interprofessional Collaboration Competency Domain

Community and population oriented

| Interprofessional teamwork and team-based practice | Interprofessional communication practices |
| Values/Ethics for interprofessional practice | Roles and responsibilities for collaborative practice |

Patient and family centered

The learning continuum pre-licensure through practice trajectory

Fig. 16.4 Core competencies for interprofessional collaborative practice. (**Source:** Interprofessional Education Collaborative. (2016). Core competencies for interprofessional collaborative practice: 2016 update. Washington, D.C.: Author.)

the competencies were constructed to facilitate the uptake of IPL beyond the prelicensure level. The IPEC core competency framework was updated in 2016 to reaffirm its value, organize the competencies under the domain of collaborative practice, and broaden the competencies to encompass the Triple Aim (i.e., improved patient care experiences, improved population health, and reduced per capita health care costs) (Interprofessional Education Collaborative, 2016).

Thailand

The IPE Guideline represents the first step in Thailand's medical and health science IPE vision. It recognizes that there will be future opportunities to further develop subject matter and methods that are suited to Thailand's geographic, cultural, and social contexts (Chuenkongkaew, 2018). It is intended that the guideline can be applied in both prelicensure and postlicensure settings so that health care providers can acquire the knowledge and skills necessary for IPC. The guideline identifies five competency domains: ethics and shared values; roles and responsibilities; teamwork and leadership; learning and reflection; and

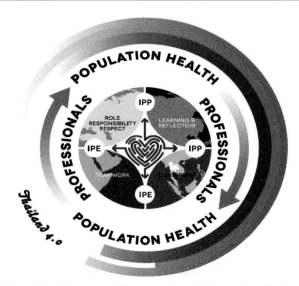

Fig. 16.5 Conceptual framework of interprofessional education. (**Source:** Chuenkongkaew, W. (Ed.). (2018). *Interprofessional education guideline.* Nonthaburi, Thailand: The National Health Professional Education Foundation. Retrieved from http://www.healthprofessionals21thailand.org.)

interprofessional communication. Figure 16.5 shows the schematic representation of Thailand's IPE/IPC competency domains.

Each of the domains consists of a general competency statement, subcompetencies, teaching and learning methodologies, and assessment strategies. The Interprofessional Collaborator Assessment Rubric (Curran, Casimiro, Banfield et al., 2011), developed in part as a response to increasing calls for a competency-based approach to IPE (Lackie, 2016), is also offered as a means to assess IPC performance. The bilingual (English and French) competency-based assessment rubric consists of six competency categories with descriptors, competency statements, and associated behavioural indicators. The competency categories are as follows:

- Communication;
- Collaboration;
- Roles and responsibilities;
- Collaborative patient/client/family-centred approach;
- Team functioning; and
- Conflict management/resolution. (Curran, Casimiro, Banfield et al., 2011, p. 342)

As can be seen in the highlighted frameworks, in Figures 16.3, 16.4, and 16.5, there is general consensus as to the knowledge, skills, behaviours, and attitudes that health care providers require to be collaborative practice–ready.

OUTCOMES OF INTERPROFESSIONAL EDUCATION AND INTERPROFESSIONAL COLLABORATIVE PRACTICE

When implementing a "new way" to educate health care providers and transform practice in the health care system, the impact of said changes should be examined. Stakeholders, including faculty and educators, academic and health system leaders, funders, and policymakers need to know how IPE and IPC impact patient, health care provider/worker, and system outcomes in order to make informed decisions. Strong evidence supports the notion that IPE has improved health worker knowledge, skill, and insight in IPC practice; however, it is far more challenging to ascertain whether there is an empirical relationship between IPE and patient, population, and health system outcomes (Cox, Cuff, Brandt et al., 2016). Underpinning the difficulties associated with generating evidence related to the relationship between IPE and outcomes are lack of a commonly agreed upon taxonomy and conceptual models that guide education. Despite, or maybe because of, these difficulties, it is imperative that research produces generalizable and transferrable findings through rigorous qualitative, quantitative, and mixed-methodological research that focuses on outcomes at all levels.

Patient Outcomes

At the heart of IPE and IPC is the patient. As such, there must be repeated and constant focus on the patient/family by both health care providers and educators (Gilbert, 2014). When interprofessional teams care for patients as though they were at the centre of care and full team members, patient outcomes are improved. Improved clinical outcomes have been reported in the literature in relation to access to care, patient safety, and satisfaction, but there is more work to do. There is an imminent need to establish a clear link between IPE and patient and population outcomes; to do so requires different methodological approaches and the inclusion of service users (patient, family, and community) as research team members.

Provider Outcomes

Positive outcomes associated with IPE have been established, including better attitudes about others, enhanced role understanding, improved communication, optimized clinical decision making, establishment of mutual respect, increased job satisfaction, improved retention rates and productivity, and improved team functioning (Baker, Egan-Lee, Martimianakis, & Reeves, 2011; Chong, Aslani, & Chen, 2013; Evans, Henderson, & Johnson, 2012; Gausvik, Lautar, Miller et al., 2015; McNeil, Mitchell, & Parker, 2015; Nayeri, Negarandeh, Vaismoradi et al., 2009; Reeves, Fletcher, Barr et al., 2016; Tataw, 2012). Although IPE has been shown to improve the adoption of IPC competencies by health care providers, more objective measures to evaluate IPE are needed to provide reliable conclusions about program success (Riskiyana, Claramita, & Rahayu et al., 2018).

System Outcomes

From a systems standpoint, governments want health care services to be timely, appropriate, and financially judicious. It is proposed that when IPC is put into full effect, timely access to care, reduced duplication of services, more effective and efficient use of health human resources, and increased integration of care can be achieved (Lackie, 2016). John Gilbert (personal communication, 2019) made the following observations about the complexities associated with the learning identified in the first part of the CAIPE definition of IPE, that is, the "learning with, from, and about".

ⓘ APPLYING CONTENT KNOWLEDGE

1. What is the continuum of IPE?
2. How are the parts of the continuum interrelated, and why is the interrelationship important to understanding interprofessional collaborative practice and care?
3. What factors would you use to facilitate a curriculum that addresses the continuum of IPE/IPL/IPP/IPC at your institution?

Examining the concepts of collaboration in nursing practice and the competencies necessary for collaboration provides firm footing for you to begin to practice in a team-based model of care. Understanding the history of IPE elucidates the long journey that has been taken to improve collaborative practice so that patient, provider, and system outcomes are of better quality. The micro/meso/macro-level factors of both IPE and IPC explain the many elements necessary to change how we learn and how we practice, always with the understanding that the student and patient must be at the centre of each. Although much has been learned from the research undertaken thus far, much more research is required to advance the practice of both IPE and IPC.

⚑ RESEARCH FOCUS

There is a need for more scientific evidence that IPE and IPC lead to meaningful outcomes for patients, providers, populations, and systems. Improvements are needed in the evaluation of IECPCP, including the types of questions asked, theoretical perspectives, methodologies and research designs, resources, and dissemination of evaluation results (Reeves, Boet, Zierler, & Kitto, 2015).

InterprofessionalResearch.Global (IPR.Global) is a newly formed research collaborative designed to advance the science of IECPCP. Composed of distinguished and emerging scholars, leaders, service providers, decision makers, administrators, service users, and health and social care students, the intent of this research collaborative is to advance and facilitate theory-driven, methodologically rigorous IPECP research through promotion and advocacy of evidence-informed policies and practices. In order to answer the questions that need to be answered regarding the efficacy of IPE and IPC, research teams must be diverse (i.e., health, medical, social, education, business, economic, and other related fields) and include patients while employing a range of research methodologies (i.e., quantitative, qualitative, and/or mixed methods) (Khalili, Thistlethwaite, El-Awaisi et al., 2019).

Sources: Reeves, S., Boet, S., Zierler, B., & Kitto, S. (2015). Interprofessional education and practice guide No. 3: Evaluating interprofessional education. *Journal of Interprofessional Care, 29* (4), 305–312. https://doi.org/10.3109/13561820.2014.1003637; Khalili, H., Thistlethwaite, J., El-Awaisi, A., et al. (2019). *Guidance on global interprofessional education and collaborative practice research: Discussion paper.* A joint publication by InterprofessionalResearch.Global & Interprofessional.Global. Retrieved from https://research.interprofessional.global/.

SUMMARY OF LEARNING OBJECTIVES

- The practice of health care collaboration has its own language and key concepts. A common language decreases miscommunication and confusion. At times, the words interprofessional, interdisciplinary, and multidisciplinary have been used interchangeably, adding to the confusion around the practice of collaboration. Key terms in the common language of collaboration in health care are intraprofessional collaboration, interprofessional collaboration (IPC), interprofessional care, interprofessional education (IPE), interdisciplinary collaboration, and multidisciplinary collaboration.

- The concept of collaboration within nursing practice relates to intraprofessional collaboration—collaboration between different types of the *same* profession, such as between registered nurses, registered practical nurses (or licensed practical nurses), registered psychiatric nurses, and nurse practitioners. Each type of nurse has specific knowledge and skills that circumscribe their roles and responsibilities and inform their scope of practice; however, they are all within the profession of nursing.

- The concept of IPC relates to collaboration between *different* professions, such as when nurses collaborate with physiotherapists, occupational therapists, or social workers.

- The history of IPE in Canada began in 1964, at The University of British Columbia. Dr. John F. McCreary, Dean of Medicine, published an article that called for members of different health care professions to be taught together in their undergraduate education. In subsequent years, there has been much growth internationally and nationally in IPE, with the first IPE program established in Alberta in 1992.

- There are micro, meso, and macro factors associated with IPE and IPC. System-level factors (macro), such as politics, accreditation, regulation, socioeconomics, and culture, influence IPE and IPC. Meso-level impacts occur at the level that directly influences IPC and IPC, such as the academic organizational level (e.g., teaching) and health care organizations. Micro-level influences occur between students, educators, and health care providers; in education, micro-level factors relate to teaching, whereas in the practice setting, micro-level factors refer to interactions between patients, families, and health care providers.

- The interprofessional collaboration competencies identified by the Canadian Interprofessional Competency Framework are patient/client/family/community-centred care; IP communication; role clarification; team functioning; collaborative leadership; and IP conflict resolution.

- Patient outcomes related to IPC include improved access to care, patient safety, and satisfaction. Provider outcomes include better attitudes about others, enhanced role understanding, improved communication, optimized clinical decision making, establishment of mutual respect, increased job satisfaction, improved retention rates and productivity, and improved team functioning. System outcomes have been less visible but should relate to timely access to care, reduced duplication of services, more effective and efficient use of health human resources, and increased integration of care. This would require better integration of IPE system wide.

CRITICAL THINKING QUESTIONS

1. What is the relationship between the continuum of IPE, patient safety, and quality of care?

2. What kind of research methodology is needed to demonstrate improved clinical practice and outcomes along the continuum of IPE?

REFERENCES

Abu-Rish Blakeney, E., Pfeifle, A., Jones, M., et al. (2016). Findings from a mixed-methods study of an interprofessional faculty development program. *Journal of Interprofessional Care, 30*(1), 83–89. https://doi.org/10.3109/13561820.2015.1051615.

Accreditation of Interprofessional Health Education. (2009). *Principles and practices for integrating interprofessional education into the accreditation standards for six health professions in Canada.* Ottawa, ON: Health Canada. Retrieved from https://casn.ca/wp-content/uploads/2014/12/AIPHEPrinciplesandPracticesGuidev2EN.pdf.

Accreditation of Interprofessional Health Education. (2011). *AIPHE interprofessional health education accreditation standards guide. Phase 2.* Ottawa, ON: Health Canada. Retrieved from https://www.peac-aepc.ca/pdfs/Resources/Competency%20Profiles/AIPHE%20Interprofessional%20Health%20Education%20Accreditation%20Standards%20Guide_EN.pdf.

Association of American Medical Colleges. (2011). *Core competencies for interprofessional collaborative practice. Pre-publication recommendations from the IPEC Expert Panel.* Washington, D.C.: Author. Retrieved from https://www.umassmed.edu/globalassets/office-of-educational-affairs/ipeg/collaborativepractice.pdf.pdf.

Baker, L., Egan-Lee, E., Martimianakis, M. A., & Reeves, S. (2011). Relationships of power: Implications for interprofessional education. *Journal of Interprofessional Care, 25*(2), 98–104. https://doi.org/10.3109/13561820.2010.505350.

Bainbridge, L., & Nasmith, L. (2011). *Inter- and intra-professional collaborative patient-centred care in postgraduate medical education*. Vancouver, BC: Members of the Future of Medical Education in Canada Postgraduate Consortium. Retrieved from https://icre2011.files.wordpress.com/2011/11/inter-and-intraprofessional-education-in-postgraduate-medical-education.pdf.

Bainbridge, L., Nasmith, L., Orchard, C., & Wood, V. (2010). Competencies for interprofessional collaboration. *Journal of Physical Therapy Education, 24*(1), 6–11. https://doi.org/10.1097/00001416-201010000-00003.

Banfield, V., & Lackie, K. (2009). *ICE C². Interprofessional and contributor education for collaborative care*. Halifax, NS: Registered Nurses Professional Development Centre & Nova Scotia Department of Health.

Barksdale, E. M., Christy, K., & Kobal, N. (2019). Evolution and current practice of interprofessional education (IPE): A review. *Current Surgery Reports, 7*(3), https://doi.org/10.1007/s40137-019-0222-4.

BC Patient Safety and Quality Council. (n.d.). *Patient Voices Network*. Retrieved from https://patientvoicesbc.ca/.

Begun, J. W., White, K. R., & Mosser, G. (2011). Interprofessional care teams: The role of the healthcare administrator. *Journal of Interprofessional Care, 25*, 119–123. https://doi.org/10.3109/13561820.2010.504135.

Bihari Axelsson, S., & Axelsson, R. (2008). From territoriality to altruism in interprofessional collaboration and leadership. *Journal of Interprofessional Care, 23*(4), 320–330. https://doi.org/10.1080/13561820902921811.

Blue, A. V., Mitcham, M., Smith, T., et al. (2010). Changing the future of health professions: Embedding interprofessional education within an academic health center. *Academic Medicine, 85*, 1290–1295. https://doi.org/10.1097/ACM.0b013e3181e53e07.

Bridges, D. R., Davidson, R., Odegard, P., et al. (2011). Interprofessional collaboration: Three best practice models of interprofessional education. *Medical Education Online, 16*, 1–10. https://doi.org/10.3402/meo.v16i0.6035.

Buring, S., Bhushan, A., Brazeau, G., et al. (2009). Keys to successful implementation of interprofessional education: Learning location, faculty development, and curricular themes. *American Journal of Pharmaceutical Education, 73*(4), 60.

Cambridge Dictionary. (2019). *Collaboration*. Retrieved from https://dictionary.cambridge.org/dictionary/english/collaboration.

Cambridge Dictionary. (2019). *Discipline*. Retrieved from https://dictionary.cambridge.org/dictionary/english/discipline.

Canadian Interprofessional Health Collaborative. (2010). *A national interprofessional competency framework*. Vancouver, BC: Author. Retrieved from http://ipcontherun.ca/wp-content/uploads/2014/06/National-Framework.pdf.

Canadian Nurses Association. (2011). *Position statement: Interprofessional collaboration*. Ottawa, ON: Author.

Canadian Nurses Association. (2012). *A nursing call to action: The health of our nation, the future of our health system*. Retrieved from http://www.cna-aiic.ca/~/media/cna/files/en/nec_report_e.pdf.

Centre for the Advancement of Interprofessional Education. (2016). *Statement of purpose*. Retrieved from https://www.caipe.org/resource/CAIPE-Statement-of-Purpose-2016.pdf.

Centre for the Advancement of Interprofessional Education. (2017). *Interprofessional education guidelines 2017*. Retrieved from https://www.caipe.org/download/caipe-2017-interprofessional-education-guidelines-2/.

Chuenkongkaew, W. (Ed.). (2018). *Interprofessional education guideline*. Nonthaburi, Thailand: The National Health Professional Education Foundation. Retrieved from http://www.healthprofessionals21thailand.org.

Chong, W. W., Aslani, P., & Chen, T. F. (2013). Shared decision-making and interprofessional collaboration mental healthcare: A qualitative study exploring perceptions of barriers and facilitators. *Journal of Interprofessional Care, 27*(5), 373–379. https://doi.org/10.3109/13561820.2013.785503.

Clements, D., Dault, M., & Priest, A. (2007). Effective teamwork in healthcare: Research and reality. *Healthcare Papers, 7*(Spec. No.), 26–34. https://doi.org/10.12927/hcpap.2013.18669.

Cockshaw, W. D., Shochet, I. M, & Obst, P. L. (2014). Depression and belongingness in general and workplace contexts: A cross-lagged longitudinal investigation. *Journal of Social and Clinical Psychology, 33*(5), 448–462. https://doi.org/10.1521/jscp.2014.33.5.448.

Colyer, H. M. (2008). Embedding interprofessional learning in pre-registration education in health and social care: Evidence of cultural lag. *Learning in Health and Social Care, 7*(3), 126–133. https://doi.org/10.1111/j.1473-6861.2008.00185.x.

Conference Board of Canada. (2012). *Improving primary health care through collaboration. Briefing 1—Current knowledge about interprofessional teams in Canada*. Ottawa, ON: Author. Retrieved from http://www.integrationresources.ca/wordpress/wp-content/uploads/2013/09/D36_PrimaryHealthCare-Briefing1.pdf.

Cox, M., Cuff, P., Brandt, B., et al. (2016). Measuring the impact of interprofessional education on collaborative practice and patient outcomes. *Journal of Interprofessional Care, 30*(1), 1–3. https://doi.org/10.3109/13561820.2015.1111052.

Culver Clark, R., & Greenawald, M. (2014). Nurse–physician leadership: Insights into interprofessional collaboration. *The Journal of Nursing Administration, 43*(12), 653–659. https://doi.org/10.1097/NNA.0000000000000007.

Curran, V. R., Casimiro, L., Banfield, V., et al. (2011). Development and validation of the Interprofessional Collaborator Assessment Rubric (ICAR). *Journal of Interprofessional Care, 25*(5), 339–344. https://doi.org/10.3109/13561820.2011.589542.

D'Amour, D., & Oandasan, I. (2005). Interprofessionality as the field of interprofessional practice and interprofessional education: An emerging concept. *Journal of Interprofessional Care, 19*(Suppl. 1), 8–20. https://doi.org/10.1080/13561820500081604.

Davis, B. P., Clevenger, C. K., Posnock, S., et al. (2015). Teaching the teachers: Faculty development in inter-professional education. *Applied Nursing Research, 28,* 31–35. https://doi.org/10.1016/j.apnr.2014.03.003.

De Los Santos, M., Degnon McFarlin, C., & Martin, L. (2014). Interprofessional education and service learning: A model for the future of health professions education. *Journal of Interprofessional Care, 28*(4), 374–375. https://doi.org/10.3109/13561820.2014.889102.

Dinh, T., & Bounajm, F. (2013). *Improving primary health care through collaboration: Briefing 3—Measuring the missed opportunity.* Ottawa, ON: Conference Board of Canada.

Dinh, T., Stonebridge, C., & Thériault, L. (2014). *Getting the most out of health care teams: Recommendations for action.* Ottawa, ON: Conference Board of Canada.

Donato, E. (2015). *The importance of interprofessional collaboration in health care in rural and northern settings.* Thunder Bay, ON: Northern Policy Institute. Retrieved from https://www.northernpolicy.ca/upload/documents/publications/briefing-notes/briefing-note-interprofessional-care-in-.pdf.

Edmondson, A., & Lei, Z. (2014). Psychological safety: The history, renaissance, and future of an interpersonal construct. *Annual Review of Organizational Psychology and Organizational Behavior, 1,* 23–43. https://doi.org/10.1146/annurev-orgpsych-031413-091305.

Egan-Lee, E., Baker, L., Tobin, S., et al. (2011). Neophyte facilitator experiences of interprofessional education: Implications for faculty development. *Journal of Interprofessional Care, 25*(5), 333–338.

Ellerby, N., Lockwood, A., Palin, G., et al. (2010). *Working relationships for the 21st century: A guide for authentic collaboration.* Retrieved from http://www.oasishumanrelations.org.uk/resources/books/a-guide-to-authentic-collaboration.

Elliot Rose, A., & Lackie, K. (2014). From me to we and back again: Creating health system transformation through authentic collaboration within and beyond nursing. *Nursing Leadership, 27*(1), 21–25. https://doi.org/10.12927/cjnl.2014.23762.

Evans, J. L., Henderson, A., & Johnson, N. W. (2012). Interprofessional learning enhances knowledge of roles but is less able to shift attitudes: A case study from dental education. *European Journal of Dental Education, 16*(4), 239–245. https://doi.org/10.1111/j.1600-0579.2012.00749.x.

Gausvik, C., Lautar, A., Miller, L., et al. (2015). Structured nursing communication on interdisciplinary acute care teams improves perceptions of safety, efficiency, understanding of care plan and teamwork as well as job satisfaction. *Journal of Multidisciplinary Healthcare, 8,* 33–37. https://doi.org/10.2147/JMDH.S72623.

Gilbert, J. H. V. (2005). Interprofessional learning and higher education structural barriers. *Journal of Interprofessional Care, 19*(Suppl. 1), 87–106. https://doi.org/10.1080/13561820500067132.

Gilbert, J. H. V. (2010). The status of interprofessional education in Canada. *Journal of Allied Health Supplement, 39*(Suppl. 1), 216–223.

Gilbert, J. H. V. (2014). Interprofessional education (IPE): Learning together to practice collaboratively. In J. Daly, S. Speedy, & D. Jackson (Eds.), *Leadership and nursing: Contemporary perspectives* (2nd ed., pp. 213–229). Chatswood, NSW: Elsevier Australia.

Gilbert, J.H. V. (in press). Leadership challenges when creating and sustaining cultural change for interprofessional collaboration. In D. Forman, M. Jones, & J. Thistlethwaite (Eds.,) *Leadership, resilience and sustainability in interprofessional collaboration.* New York, NY: Palgrave Macmillan.

Goldman, J., Meuser, J., Rogers, J., et al. (2010). Interprofessional collaboration in family health teams. An Ontario-based study. *Canadian Family Medicine, 56,* e368–e374. Retrieved from https://www.cfp.ca/content/56/10/e368.long.

Gotlib Conn, L. G., Lingard, L., Reeves, S., et al. (2009). Communication channels in general internal medicine: A description of baseline patterns for improved interprofessional collaboration. *Qualitative Health Research, 19*(7), 943–953. https://doi.org/10.1177%2F1049732309338282.

Grymonpre, R. E., Ateah, C. A., Dean, H. J., et al. (2016). Sustainable implementation of interprofessional education using an adoption model framework. *Canadian Journal of Higher Education, 46*(4), 76–93. Retrieved from https://journals.sfu.ca/cjhe/index.php/cjhe/article/view/186571/pdf.

Hall, L., & Zierler, B. (2015). Interprofessional education and practice guide No. 1: Developing faculty to effectively facilitate interprofessional education. *Journal of Interprofessional Care, 29*(1), 3–7. https://doi.org/10.3109/13561820.2014.937483.

Health Council of Canada. (2005). *Health care renewal in Canada: Accelerating change.* Ottawa, ON: Author. Retrieved from https://healthcouncilcanada.ca/files/2.48-Accelerating_Change_HCC_2005.pdf.

Ho, K., Jarvis-Selinger, S., Borduas, F., et al. (2008). Making interprofessional education work: The strategic roles of the Academy. *Academic Medicine, 83*(10), 934–940. https://doi.org/10.1097/ACM.0b013e3181850a75.

Institute of Medicine. (2001). *Crossing the quality chasm: A new health system for the 21st century.* Washington, D.C.: National Academy Press.

Interprofessional Education Collaborative Expert Panel. (2011). *Core competencies for interprofessional collaborative practice: Report of an expert panel.* Washington, D.C.: Author.

Interprofessional Education Collaborative. (2016). *Core competencies for interprofessional collaborative practice: 2016 update.* Washington, D.C.: Author.

Khalili, H., Thistlethwaite, J., El-Awaisi, A., et al. (2019). *Guidance on global interprofessional education and collaborative practice research: Discussion paper.* A joint publication by Interprofessional Research.Global & Interprofessional.Global. Retrieved from https://research.interprofessional.global/.

Khalili, H., Gilbert, J., Lising, D., et al. (2019). *Proposed lexicon for the interprofessional field.* A joint publication by InterprofessionalResearch.Global, & Interprofessional.Global. Retrieved from https://research.interprofessional.global/.

King, G., Orchard, C., Khalili, H., & Avery, L. (2016). Refinement of the Interprofessional Socialization and Valuing Scale (ISVS-21) and development of 9-item equivalent versions. *Journal of Continuing Education in the Health Professions, 36*(3), 171–177. https://doi.org/10.1097/CEH.0000000000000082.

Lackie, K. (2016). *Examination of the effects of interprofessional collaboration on health care provider and team productivity in primary health care: An important consideration in health human resources planning* [Doctoral dissertation, Dalhousie University]. OCLC Accession No. 1033180335. Retrieved from https://www.bac-lac.gc.ca.

Lahey, W., Hutt, L., Hopkins, A., & Hobson, T. (2009). *Collaborative self-regulation and professional accountability in Nova Scotia's health care system. A report from the Working Group on Collaborative Regulation of the Nova Scotia Health Professions Regulatory Network to the Nova Scotia Health Professions Regulatory Network.* Halifax, NS: Nova Scotia Health Professions Regulatory Network. Retrieved from https://cdn.dal.ca/content/dam/dalhousie/pdf/law/HLI/HLI_WG_Document_Nov2009.pdf.

Lawlis, T. R., Anson, J., & Greenfield, D. (2014). Barriers and enablers that influence sustainable interprofessional education: A literature review. *Journal of Interprofessional Care, 28*(4), 305–310. https://doi.org/10.3109/13561820.2014.895977.

MacMillan, K. (Ed.). (2013). *Proceedings of a think tank on the future of undergraduate nursing education in Canada.* Halifax, NS: Dalhousie University School of Nursing.

McCreary, J. F. (1964). The education of physicians in Canada. *Canadian Medical Association Journal, 90*(21), 1215–1221.

McNeil, K., Mitchell, R., & Parker, V. (2015). The paradoxical effects of workforce shortages on rural interprofessional practice. *Scandinavian Journal of Caring Sciences, 29*(1), 73–82. https://doi.org/10.1111/scs.12129.

Meijer, L., de Groot, E., Blaauw-Westerlaken, M., & Damoiseaux, R. (2016). Intraprofessional collaboration and learning between specialists and general practitioners during postgraduate training: a qualitative study. *BMC Health Services Research, 16*(1), 1–8. https://doi.org/10.1186/s12913-016-1619-8.

Mohamed, Z., Newton, J. M., & McKenna, L. (2014). Belongingness in the workplace: A study of Malaysian nurses' experience. *International Nursing Review, 61*, 124–130. https://doi.org/10.1111/inr.12078.

Morano, C., & Damiani, G. (2018). Interprofessional education at the meso level: Taking the next step in IPE. *Gerontology & Geriatrics Education, 40*(1), 43–54. https://doi.org/10.1080/02701960.2018.1515739.

Nayeri, N. D., Negarandeh, R., Vaismoradi, M., et al. (2009). Burnout and productivity among Iranian nurses. *Nursing and Health Sciences, 11*(3), 263–270. https://doi.org/10.1111/j.1442-2018.2009.00449.x.

Newman, A., Donohue, R., & Eva, N. (2017). Psychological safety: A systematic review of the literature. *Human Resource Management Review, 27*, 521–535. https://doi.org/10.1016/j.hrmr.2017.01.001.

Nova Scotia Regulated Health Professions Network. (2018). *By-laws relating to the activities and operations of the Nova Scotia Regulated Health Professions Network.* Halifax, NS: Author. Retrieved from https://www.nsrhpn.ca/wp-content/uploads/2014/08/238664183-NSRHPN-By-Laws.pdf.

Nova Scotia Regulated Health Professions Network. (2019). *FAQs.* Halifax, NS: Author. Retrieved from https://www.nsrhpn.ca/faqs/.

Oandasan, I., D'Amour, D., Zwarenstein, M., et al. (2004). *Interdisciplinary education for collaborative, patient-centred practice. Research and findings report.* Ottawa, ON: Health Canada.

Oandasan, I., & Reeves, S. (2005a). Key elements for interprofessional education. Part 1: The learner, the educator and the learning context. *Journal of Interprofessional Care, 19*(Suppl. 1), 21–38. https://doi.org/10.1080/13561820500083550.

Oandasan, I., & Reeves, S. (2005b). Key elements of interprofessional education. Part 2: Factors, processes, and outcomes. *Journal of Interprofessional Care, 19*(Suppl. 1), 39–48. https://doi.org/10.1080/13561820500081703.

Oandasan, I., Ross Baker, G., Barker, K., et al. (2006). *Teamwork in healthcare: Promoting effective teamwork in healthcare in Canada. Policy synthesis and recommendations.* Ottawa, ON: Canadian Health Services Research Foundation.

Orchard, C. A., King, G. A., Khalili, H., & Bezzina, M. B. (2012). Assessment of Interprofessional Team Collaboration Scale (AITCS): Development and testing of the instrument. *Journal of Continuing Education in the Health Professions, 32*(1), 58–67. https://doi.org/10.1002/chp.21123.

Power, A. (2019). Interprofessional education: Shared learning for collaborative, high-quality care. *British Journal of Midwifery, 27*(2), 1280129. https://doi.org/10.12968/bjom.2019.27.2.128.

Price, S., Doucet, S., & McGillis Hall, L. (2014). The historical social positioning of nursing and medicine: Implications for career choice, early socialization and interprofessional collaboration. *Journal of Interprofessional Care, 28*(2), 103–109. https://doi.org/10.3109/13561820.2013.867839.

Reeves, S. (2012). The rise and rise of interprofessional competence. *Journal of Interprofessional Care, 26*, 253–255. https://doi.org/10.3109/13561820.2012.695542.

Reeves, S., Fox, A., & Hodges, B. (2009). The competency movement in the health professions: Ensuring consistent standards or reproducing conventional domains of practice. *Advances in Health Sciences Education, 14*, 451–453. https://doi.org/10.1007/s10459-009-9166-2.

Reeves, S., Fletcher, S., Barr, H., et al. (2016). A BEME systematic review of the effects of interprofessional education. BEME Guide No. 39. *Medical Teacher, 38*(7), 656–668. https://doi.org/10.3109/0142159X.2016.1173663.

Registered Nurses' Association of Ontario. (2013). *Developing and sustaining interprofessional health care: Optimizing patients/clients, organizational, and system outcomes.* Retrieved from https://rnao.ca/bpg/guidelines/interprofessional-team-work-healthcare.

Registered Nurses' Association of Ontario. (2016). *Intra-professional collaborative practice among nurses.* Retrieved from https://rnao.ca/bpg/guidelines/intra-professional-collaborative-practice-among-nurses.

Ries, N. M. (2017). Law matters: How the legal context in Canada influences interprofessional collaboration. *Journal of Interprofessional Care, 31*(4), 417–419. https://doi.org/10.1080/13561820.2017.1310495.

Riskiyana, R., Claramita, M., & Rahayu, G. R. (2018). Objectively measured interprofessional education outcome and factors that enhance program effectiveness: A systematic review. *Nurse Education Today, 66*, 73–78. https://doi.org/10.1016/j.nedt.2018.04.014.

Romanow, R. (2002). *Commission on the future of health care in Canada. Building on values. The future of health care in Canada. Final report.* Retrieved from http://publications.gc.ca/collections/Collection/CP32-85-2002E.pdf.

San Martin-Rodriguez, L., Beaulieu, M., D'Amour, D., & Ferrada-Videla, M. (2005). The determinants of successful collaboration: A review of theoretical and empirical studies. *Journal of Interprofessional Care, 19*(Suppl. 1), 132–147. https://doi.org/10.1080/13561820500082677.

Serin, H. (2018). A comparison of teacher-centered and student centered approaches in educational settings. *International Journal of Social Sciences & Educational Studies, 5*(1), 164–167. https://doi.org/10.23918/ijsses.v5i1p164.

Stanley, K., Dixon, K., Warner, P., & Stanley, D. (2016). Twelve possible strategies for enhancing interprofessional socialisation in higher education: Findings from an interpretive phenomenological study. *Journal of Interprofessional Care, 30*(4), 475–482. https://doi.org/10.3109/13561820.2016.1159186.

Suter, E., Arndt, J., Lait, J., Jackson, K., Kipp, J., Taylor. E., & Arthur, N. (2007). How can frontline managers demonstrate leadership in enabling interprofessional practice? *Healthcare Management Forum, 20*(4), 38–43. https://doi.org/10.1016/S0840-4704(10)60090-7.

Suter, E., Deutschlander, S., Mickelson, G., et al. (2012). Can interprofessional collaboration provide health human resources solutions? A knowledge synthesis. *Journal of Interprofessional Care, 26*(4), 261–268. https://doi.org/10.3109/13561820.2012.663014.

Szasz, G. (1969). Interprofessional education in the health sciences: A project conducted at the University of British Columbia. *Milbank Quarterly, 67*, 449–475.

Tataw, D. (2012). Toward human resource management in interprofessional health practice: Linking organizational culture, group identity and individual autonomy. *International Journal of Health Planning and Management, 27*(2), 130–149. https://doi.org/10.1002/hpm.2098.

Thistlethwaite, J. E., Forman, D., Matthews, L. R., et al. (2014). Competencies and frameworks in interprofessional education: A comparative analysis. *Academic Medicine, 89*(6), 1–7. https://doi.org/10.1097/ACM.0000000000000249.

Tuckman, B. W., & Jensen, M. A. C. (1977). Stages of small group development revisited. *Group and Organization Studies, 2*(4), 419–427.

Way, D., Jones, L., & Busing, N. (2000). *Implementation strategies: Collaboration in primary care—Family doctors and nurse practitioners delivering shared care.* Ottawa, ON: Ontario College of Family Physicians.

Wood, V., Flavell, A., Vanstolk, D., et al. (2009). The road to collaboration: Developing an interprofessional competency framework. *Journal of Interprofessional Care, 23*(6), 621–629.

World Health Organization. (1988). *Learning together to work together for health. Report of a WHO Study Group on Multiprofessional Education for Health Personnel: The Team Approach.* Technical Report Series 769: 1-72. Geneva, Switzerland: Author.

World Health Organization. (2010). *Framework for action on interprofessional education & collaborative practice.* Geneva, Switzerland: Author.

World Health Organization. (2013). *Transforming and scaling up health professionals' education and training. World Health Organization Guidelines 2013.* Geneva, Switzerland: Author.

World Health Organization. (2016). *Global strategy on human resources for health: Workforce 2030.* Geneva, Switzerland: Author.

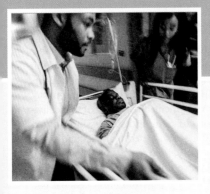

Shortage or Oversupply?
The Registered Nursing
Workforce Pendulum

Tammie R. McParland

http://evolve.elsevier.com/Canada/Ross-Kerr/nursing

LEARNING OBJECTIVES

At the end of this chapter, you will be able to:
- Examine trends in the employment of registered nurses and nurse practitioners in Canada.
- Compare registered nurses with other regulated nurses in Canada such as licensed practical nurses and registered psychiatric nurses.
- Discuss the trends in supply and demand for registered nurses.

- Examine the imbalances between the supply of and demand for registered nurses.
- Articulate the challenges facing the nursing profession in the context of health human resources.
- Discuss the implications of the shortage of registered nurses for the health care of the future.
- Identify recommendations to address questions about health human resources.

OUTLINE

KEY TERMS

inflow
Organisation for Economic Co-operation and
    Development
outflow

regulated nurses
skill mix
vacancy rates

PERSONAL PERSPECTIVES

Alyssa lives in a small city in northern Manitoba (population 50,000). The hospital there has a small maternity ward and a neonatal intensive care unit (NICU) that can admit babies who are born at 32 weeks gestation or older. Alyssa is 32.5 weeks pregnant with twins when she starts to experience premature labour and a suspected premature rupture of membranes. Upon being admitted to the labour and delivery triage unit, Alyssa is informed that even though there are beds available in the NICU, she will be flown to another hospital in the province that has both specialized nurses and space for her twins, since her local NICU has no specialized nurses to care for her babies. After the medical team spends several hours trying to slow down Alyssa's contractions and find a place to send her, she is finally transferred to a large tertiary hospital in Winnipeg, a 4.5-hour drive from her home. Alyssa remains there until her twins are born 1 week later, and the twins stay in Winnipeg for 2 more weeks after their birth. In telling her story, Alyssa often mentions her concern for her babies' return to her community, especially in the event that they develop complications as premature infants.

INTRODUCTION

The beginning of the twenty-first century has seen health care systems worldwide change and evolve under continuing cost-containment pressures, new technologies, and shifting health care demands. The situation in Canada is no different. Despite these changes, nurses continue to play a major role in delivering health services and are recognized as invaluable to the health of individuals in Canada and globally (World Health Organization [WHO] & International Council of Nurses [ICN], 2018). Studies have documented trends in registered nurse (RN) shortages (McGillis Hall, MacDonald-Rencz, Peterson et al., 2013; Registered Nurses' Association of Ontario [RNAO], 2016). Professional nursing associations and others have studied the importance of recruiting and retaining nurses and made recommendations to mitigate the nursing shortage (Canadian Nurses Association [CNA], 2019a; George, 2015; RNAO, 2016). Governments recognize that nursing workforce shortages have serious, negative repercussions on the availability of, access to, and scope of health services—precisely those attributes of the Canadian health system on which we pride ourselves. One of the most challenging tasks for nursing, hospital administrators, governments, and society is to ensure that enough nurses are available to provide care now and in the future.

Many studies in Canada and internationally (Littlejohn, Campbell, & Collins-McNeil, 2012; CNA, 2019; McGillis Hall, MacDonald-Rencz, Peterson et al., 2013; RNAO, 2016; Rondeau & Wagar, 2016) have indicated that autonomy, authority, workplace environment, and quality of work environment, including access to continuing professional development, need to be addressed in order to attract and retain nurses. In Canada, as of 2019, there were 439,975 **regulated nurses,** of which 303,146 were RNs (including 5,697 nurse practitioners), 122,600 licensed practical nurses (called registered practical nurses in Ontario), and 6,023 registered psychiatric nurses (Canadian Institute for Health Information [CIHI], 2020). While the number may seem to be large, and the nursing workforce has increased in tandem with the annual population growth rate of 1.2% (CIHI, 2020), it is not easy to determine whether or not there are enough nurses to care for the population of Canada. Global workforce research indicates that there have never been as many doctors and nurses as there appear to be now, with 3.6 million doctors and 10.8 million nurses employed in **Organisation for Economic Co-operation and Development** (OECD) countries (Organisation for Economic Co-operation and Development [OECD], 2016). However, current statistics show that Canada, like other countries, is facing a shortage of health professional resources, with 50% of the shortfall in health care workers belonging to the nursing and midwifery professions. This trend of a shortage in health care workers (including nurses) is expected to increase in African and Middle Eastern countries by 2030 (WHO, 2016). Clearly, health human resources are an important strategic mandate of the nursing profession as well as of governments globally. Human health resources planning for health care must be considered in the context of the historical development of the nursing profession.

Nursing shortages have been a historical reality since the profession gained legitimacy in the earlier part of the twentieth century. After the First World War, many nurses found work in hospitals and rehabilitation centres caring for the wounded until the Great Depression ended discretionary cash and there were massive job losses, including those for nurses and other health care providers. In Canada in particular, the funding of community public health nurses provided some employment, but not enough to meet the demand for work. The Second World War, however, again saw an exponential increase in the need for health human resources, so much so that training for nurses became shorter and classifications of nurses were created to meet the burgeoning demand from the war (Toman, 2005). The war effort also sent women into nontraditional roles on assembly lines and in office environments—traditionally male-dominated areas—further decreasing the availability of women who might have wanted to pursue nursing and contributing to a postwar nursing shortage.

TABLE 17.1   Nurses and Other Selected Health Care Occupations in the Canadian Labour Force

	2009	2018
Registered nurses	282,642	297,449
Nurse practitioners	2,048	5,697
Licensed practical nurses	85,277	122,600
Registered psychiatric nurses*	5,321	6,023
Total nurses	**375,288**	**431,769**
Pharmacists	23,082	42,844
Physiotherapists	16,847	22,391(2016[†])
Occupational therapists	9,141	17,034(2016[†])

*Registered psychiatric nurses are in the four Western provinces only.
[†]Latest data for these professionals from CIHI.
Sources: Canadian Institute for Health Information. (2018). *Nursing in Canada, 2018: A lens on supply and workforce.* Ottawa, ON: Author. Retrieved from https://secure.cihi.ca/free_products/regulated-nurses-2018-report-en-web.pdf; Canadian Institute for Health Information. (2019). *Health workforce: Pharmacists 2018.* Retrieved from https://www.cihi.ca/en/pharmacists; Canadian Institute for Health Information. (2017). *Health workforce: Physiotherapists 2016* [Data tables]. Retrieved from https://www.cihi.ca/en/physiotherapists; Canadian Institute for Health Information. (2017). *Health workforce: Occupational therapists, 2016* [Data tables].

TRENDS IN EMPLOYMENT OF NURSES

As of 2018, regulated nurses remain the largest occupational group in Canada. There had been a steady increase in the nursing workforce in Canada from the 1960s until 2014, when a downward trend began (CIHI, 2020). In the 1960s, there was a 33% increase in the number of RNs. In the 1970s, the rate of growth in the RN workforce doubled to 68%, returning to about 3.3% per year between 1981 and 1993, before a period of limited growth began in the 1990s, reflecting a period of fiscal restraint (Ross, 2003). In the 2010s, the number of RNs, licensed practical nurses (LPNs), registered psychiatric nurses (RPNs), and nurse practitioners (NPs) increased. Table 17.1 shows human resources data for 2009 and 2018 for selected health occupations.

In addition, human resources in other allied health occupations have increased. The world population more than doubled between 1960 and 2018, from 3 billion to over 7 billion people. Projections for population growth indicate that the world's population will increase to 10 billion in 2083 (Rosenberg, 2019). Clearly, a bigger population will necessitate an increased number of health care providers, including RNs, to address people's health care needs.

PLACES WHERE NURSES WORK

Hospitals

Most regulated nurses still work in a hospital setting. In 2018, 63.6% of RNs and 45% of LPNs worked in hospitals (Table 17.2). In 2009, 62.7% of RNs who were employed and 42.5% of LPNs who were employed worked in a hospital. There has been a small increase in RNs who work in a hospital, and a larger percentage increase in the proportion of LPNs who do, which is illustrated by the percent growth—LPNs have increased overall by 3.1% since 2014, while RNs have increased by 1.5% (Figure 17.1). As a percentage of health care employees in hospitals, there has been a decline in the percentage of RNs from 83.3% in 2005 to 78.7% in 2014.

Community Health Agencies

Community agencies include community health agencies, public health, home care, and nursing stations. The proportion of RNs working in the community has remained virtually unchanged—15.6% in 2018 versus 15.7% in 2009—while the proportion of LPNs working in the community has increased from 9.8% to 14.3%. For example, RNs in Ontario have declined to 70.2% of those working in health care, compared with 82% in 2014 (Grinspun, Harripal-Yup, Jarvi, & Lenartowych, 2016). The bigger concern is the decline of both RNs and LPNs in rural and remote areas (CIHI, 2020).

Nursing Homes and Long-Term Care

The majority of regulated nurses who work in long-term care (LTC) facilities are from the LPN category of nurses, representing 58% of nurses working in LTC in 2018 (CIHI, 2020). This represents 31.7% of the LPN population, whereas the population of LPNs working in 2009

TABLE 17.2   Where Regulated Nurses* Work in Canada, 2009 and 2018

	2009	% of Type of Nurse	2018	% of Type of Nurse
Hospitals				
RNs and NPs	161,096	60.4%	183,107	63.6%
LPNs	32,707	42.5%	49,388	45.1%
RPNs	2,275	43.6%	2,516	43.7%
Community Health				
RNs and NPs	42,031	15.7%	45,161	15.6%
LPNs	7,599	9.8%	15,729	14.3%
RPNs	1,258	24.1%	1,792	31%
Nursing Home or Long-Term Care Facility				
RNs and NPs	25,432	9.9%	25,869	8.9%
LPNs	28,055	36.4%	34,767	31.7%
RPNs	971	18.6%	601	10%
Other (Not Identified/Not Stated)				
RNs and NPs	37,782	13.2%	37,599	9.2%
LPNs	8,588	2.4%	9,550	2.3%
RPNs	469	8.1%	410	7.1%
Total	**348,263**		**406,487**	
	(375,288 reported)		**(431,769 reported)**	

*Regulated nurses included registered nurses (RNs), nurse practitioners (NPs), licensed practical nurses (LPNs) (which are called registered practical nurses [RPNs] in Ontario), and registered psychiatric nurses (RPNs). Registered practical nurses are members of the LPN category, while registered psychiatric nurses are members of the RN category.
Source: Adapted from Canadian Institute for Health Information. (2018). *Healthcare providers employed in direct care by place of work and type of provider, selected provinces and territories 2009–2018* [Data tables]. Ottawa, ON: Author. Retrieved from https://www.cihi.ca/en/nursing-in-canada-2018.

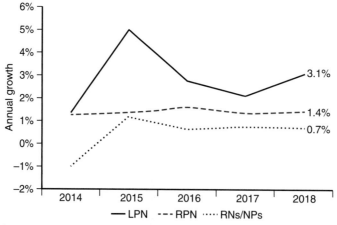

Fig. 17.1 Annual growth rate of regulated nurses by year, 2014–2018. (**Source:** Canadian Institute for Health Information. 2019. *Nursing in Canada, 2018: A lens on supply and workforce.* Ottawa, ON: Author. Retrieved from https://secure.cihi.ca/free_products/regulated-nurses-2018-report-en-web.pdf.)

in LTC was 36.4% (CIHI, 2020). The percentage of RNs working in LTC was 42% in 2018, with most in administrative roles having minimal patient contact. The percentage of RNs who worked in LTC was 9.9% of the RN workforce in 2009 and has since declined to 8.9% in 2018 (CIHI, 2020). As an example, in Ontario, RNs who work in LTC have declined from 49.4% to 37% of those employed in health care in LTC (Grinspun, Harripal-Yup, Jarvi, & Lenartowych, 2016). Given that the Canadian population is steadily aging, increasing the population aged 65 and

over, this decline in regulated nurses is concerning. LPN and RN numbers have both declined, with some of their duties taken on by nonregulated health care providers like personal support workers.

AREAS OF RESPONSIBILITY

Nurses have several areas of responsibility in their day-to-day work. Table 17.2 identifies where nurses were working (hospital, community, and LTC) in Canada in 2009 and

---

RESEARCH FOCUS

Letting Go: How Newly Graduated Registered Nurses in Western Canada Decide to Exit the Nursing Profession

Despite an increasing number of students choosing nursing education since 2007, the Canadian Nurses Association forecasts a shortage of RNs by 2022 (Canadian Nurses Association, 2014). One of the trends that impacts the availability of nurses is the exit of nurses from the profession. Chachula, Myrick, and Yonge (2015) conducted a qualitative grounded theory study that examined what factors influenced newly graduated nurses (5 years or less after graduation) to leave the profession, and the psychosocial processes involved. Benner's novice to expert theory postulates that nurses do not become proficient until they have spent 3 to 5 years in the profession (Benner, 1984), and this formed the theoretical framework of the study. Nurses who met the inclusion criteria (a sample size of 8) were recruited from the three Western provinces in Canada.

The psychosocial process involved in the participants' decision to leave nursing was identified as "letting go" and was acknowledged to be a difficult journey. Four integrated activities contributed to the process:

1. Navigating constraints of the health care system and workplace;
2. Negotiating social relationships, hierarchies, and troublesome behaviours;
3. Facing fears, traumas, and challenges; and
4. Weighing competing rewards and tension. (Chachula, Myrick, & Yonge, 2015, p. 914)

Contributing factors that determined whether the nurse was going to "let go" were coined as those that "dampened the spirit" or "fanned the flame" (Chachula, Myrick, & Yonge, 2015, p. 915). Behaviours that dampened the

spirit included workload and shift work; feeling unwelcomed; lateral and/or horizontal violence; paternalism; lack of support; own feelings of inadequacy or fear of not knowing enough; disconnect between education and reality; and not feeling prepared for patient acuity and/or patient workload. Factors that fanned the flame included reasonable workloads; support from management to mitigate fatigue; opportunities for life-long learning; meaningful orientations; ability to work as part of a team in interprofessional activities; feeling informed; feeling valued, respected, and accepted; existence of emotional support and time to debrief experiences; caring and friendly atmosphere; and constructive feedback. The presence of transformational and authentic leadership was also highlighted.

The findings of this research will inform education, policy development, and workplace settings and reinforce previous research on the need for and recognition of the value of healthy workplace environments. The authors also recommended quality orientation, mentorship programs while the new hire is a novice, and preceptorship during the transition from student to new grad. The use of transformative leadership practices, role modeling, supportive communication, and emancipatory education practice can help reinforce socialization to the profession and help the novice nurse develop confidence, proficiency, and competency. Finally, the increasing acuity of patients should indicate the use of an appropriate skill mix and nurse-to-patient ratio to permit new nurses to have a safe workload when they are starting out, with senior staff available to provide support.

Sources: Benner, P. (1984). *From novice to expert: Excellence and power in clinical nursing practice.* Menlo Park, CA: Addison-Wesley; Chachula, K. M., Myrick, F., & Yonge, O. (2015). Letting go: How newly graduated registered nurses in Western Canada decide to exit the nursing profession. *Nurse Education Today, 35*(7), 912–918. https://doi.org/10.1016/j.nedt.2015.02.024; Canadian Nurses Association. (2014). *Tested solutions for eliminating Canada's RN shortage.* Retrieved from https://www.cna-aiic.ca/-/media/cna/page-content/pdf-en/rn_highlights_e.pdf.

CULTURAL CONSIDERATIONS

Working in Rural and Remote Indigenous Communities: The Role of Nurses and Health Care Providers

The nurse in a remote Indigenous community is often the only primary health care provider. Rahaman and colleagues conducted a qualitative critical discourse analysis with 25 health care workers, including nurses, who worked in remote Northern Saskatchewan (Rahaman, Holmes, & Chartrand, 2017). The themes identified in the study were structural health care systems, public portrayal of "Native" peoples, public portrayal of "Native" communities, and colonizing nursing practice.

The work done by nurses in rural and remote areas in Canada is hampered by limited and possibly restricted resources. Nursing practice in remote areas is diverse, shaped by "land and climate, isolation, community needs, available resources, degree of vulnerability, and nurses' professional integrity" (Rahaman, 2017, p. 188). The lack of organizational structure (policies, etc.) also caused challenges, but more support from the organization resulted in fewer feelings of isolation and being "stuck." As well, colonialization of the Indigenous patient had continued to occur, as nurses may see patients as "Native," a label that is then used as a lens to care for the population; for example, nurses may label patients as an "ill Native" rather than a First Nations person who is ill. Culture became the favoured explanation for etiology or for more severe conditions, such as substance abuse, mental health issues, and chronic conditions, among Indigenous populations compared with non-Indigenous populations. Overall, nurses were aware of the challenges being experienced by the population but were unsure about what to do to address it. The authors suggested that it is important for nurses to reflect on their role in the continued colonialization of the Indigenous population as well as identification of the supports that would assist in their work.

Source: Rahaman, Z., Holmes, D., & Chartrand, L. (2017). An opportunity for healing and holistic care: Exploring the roles of health care providers working within Northern Canadian Aboriginal communities. *Journal of Holistic Nursing, 35*(2), 185–197. https://doi.org/10.1177/0898010116650773.

2018. Nurses have increased their employment in all sectors as a result of the overall growth of the profession, but the gain is modest in some areas. RNs continue to have more workers in hospital and community settings, but the majority of regulated nurses in LTC are LPNs.

Inflow and **outflow** of nurses describe the number of regulated nurses who enter and leave the profession. In 2018, there was a 7.4% net inflow of regulated nurses nationally. The only provinces/territories that did not have a positive inflow of regulated nurses were Newfoundland and Labrador, Northwest Territories, and Nunavut (CIHI, 2020). After the 2017 registration year, 26,020 regulated nurses did not renew their registration in the same province or territory. This represents an outflow of 6.1%. Of the positive inflow, LPNs represented 61.8% of the net gain of 5,817 nurses, and RNs represented 36.7% of the net gain (CIHI, 2020). With respect to the outflow, the proportion of outflow of regulated nurses was higher in rural and remote areas (7.4%) than in urban areas (5.9%), with Newfoundland and Labrador, Northwest Territories, and Nunavut experiencing the outflow loss (CIHI, 2020). The increased outflow of regulated nurses from rural and remote areas should be a cause for concern for nurse leaders, given that there is already a shortage of nurses in these regions.

The urban–rural distribution of the workforce is a major challenge for the health care sector in each province and territory. In 2018, 87.8% of the RN workforce worked in urban areas in Canada, ranging from highs of 98.4% in the Yukon and 93.9% in Ontario to lows of 57.1% in the Northwest Territories and Nunavut and 67.9% in Newfoundland and Labrador (CIHI, 2020). Since many of these nurses are in the 50 and over age group, there is concern as to how health care will be provided in the rural and remote areas of Canada in the future.

Of the RNs employed in Canada who reported their location of graduation in 2018, 93% graduated from a nursing program in Canada and 8.5% (20,319) graduated from an international nursing program. In 2018, the number of internationally educated nurses (IENs) in the Canadian RN workforce was 36,189, or 8.5%, an increase from 7.8% in the 5 years since 2013 (CIHI, 2020). International nurses make a significant contribution to our supply of nursing graduates.

TRENDS IN DEMAND

The review of where nurses work and the number of RNs employed illustrates the increasing demand for nursing knowledge and skills. The national and international trends

BOX 17.1 Factors Driving the Demand for Nursing Knowledge

- Increasing specialization
- Reduction in bed-to-nurse ratio
- Technological advances in health care
- Fluctuation in part-time employment
- New and evolving roles for nurses

in health care are shorter hospital stays; more complex diseases, resulting in increased acuity of care; a shift from hospital to ambulatory, home, and community care; new infectious and reemerging diseases; an aging population; globalization; increased acts of terrorism; a growing private sector; and technology. In general, all the specialized roles of nurses in hospitals have increased, although the number of RNs employed to teach employees and patients has declined.

The factors driving the increasing need for RN knowledge and skills (Box 17.1) include (1) the increase in the specialization of nurse employment in hospitals and the community; (2) the reduction in the bed-to-RN ratio because of the increasing acuity and complexity of patients; (3) the continuing number of nurses working part-time; and (4) the new and emerging RN roles, such as NP, telehealth, and self-employment.

Increasing Specialization

Although the number of RNs in 2019 compared with 2018 increased only slightly (1.1%), the percentage of RNs in the hospital setting did not proportionally increase, with only a 0.3% growth rate recorded for these dates (CIHI, 2020). The number of RNs in the hospital setting increased by only 1.1%, despite the overall increase in the RN population of 8.8% (from 210,666 in 2010 to 229,503 in 2018) (CIHI, 2020). Hospital beds have been reduced, and many patients have a shorter stay. The use of new technologies allows for procedures and major surgeries to be done on an outpatient basis and for care to be delivered in the community. The proportion of Canadians over age 65 is increasing, and the resultant comorbidities indicate that in coming years patients will be sicker and thus require more complex care. Part of the strategy employed by both nurses and health care agencies to respond to these changing demographics has been increasing the specialization of nurses in the hospital setting. Chapter 22 identifies where specialization in nursing has occurred in the past two decades.

Statistics indicate that LPN numbers increased between 2009 and 2018. The LPN workforce grew by 3.1% from 2014 to 2018, in contrast to a 1.4% increase for RNs and less than 1% for RPNs. In the 1980s, the increasing use of

RNs instead of LPNs was explained by the fact that hospitalized patients were sicker and required more care than in years past; in reality, RNs were paid a relatively low wage and were highly adaptable. RNs could perform a wide variety of other roles, including clerical positions and therapists; substitute for physicians under some circumstances; and assume hospital management roles after regular work hours. Nurses required little supervision and took responsibility for a myriad of duties. By 1993, however, nurses'

CASE STUDY

Nursing Positions Eliminated in Alberta in 2020

In 2019, the Government of Alberta announced its plan to eliminate 300 FTE (full-time equivalent) RN and RPN positions. The job elimination started with the removal of currently unfilled positions and continued with the removal of any positions not filled by April 1, 2020. In May 2020, layoffs of bedside nursing positions were expected to take effect. Alberta Health Services sent a letter to the United Nurses of Alberta outlining several steps the government believed would "address savings and efficiencies in the healthcare system, and/or changes in services to better serve patients and families." The proposed strategies included eliminating 500 FTE positions over 3 years, starting in April 2020, with potential contracting out of homecare services, nursing, and pediatric and palliative care; closing of acute care beds as chronic care beds become available; and reducing hospital clinic visits to nonhospital areas in the community such as outreach clinics, and so on.

The nurses' union indicated that they believed health care services in Alberta were undergoing privatization. They also expressed concern about the impact of the lost positions on the care of the population, especially since there has been an increase in both patient age and acuity. There have been several public outcries about the impact of these cuts on the health care of Albertans should the government proceed. The United Nurses of Alberta began contract talks with the government in 2020, but the COVID-19 pandemic has halted bargaining and job cuts for the time being (Dryden, 2020).

Sources: Mertz, E. (2019, November 29). *Alberta Health Services cutting hundreds of nursing positions: UNA and NDP*. Global News. Retrieved from https://globalnews.ca/news/6234684/alberta-health-services-cuts-ndp-nurses/; Dryden, J. (2020, March 18). *Cuts to Alberta nurses, public-sector jobs paused amidst COVID-19 outbreak*. CBC News. Retrieved from https://www.cbc.ca/news/canada/calgary/covid-19-coronavirus-alberta-public-sector-nurses-union-1.5502084.

salaries in Canada had increased because of pay equity legislation and negotiated salary increases. Now nurse salaries across Canada are comparable to those of other well-paying jobs (Canadian Federation of Nurses Unions [CFNU], 2018). During the 1990s, hospitals began downsizing, and major layoffs occurred following decentralization, regionalization, and strategic alliances. Layoffs involved middle management and frontline nurses. The cost of the significant amount of overtime and absenteeism that occurred among nurses was due, in part, to the conditions resulting from the layoffs and cost-containment measures (Burke, Ng, & Wolpin, 2016; Jacobson Consulting, 2017). Nursing layoffs continue in this decade, with media reports of wards being closed due to a lack of staff, or staff layoffs being implemented as a cost-containment measure. Now, the biggest increase in hiring among nurses seems to be among LPNs, a group that has witnessed a four-fold growth over RNs within the 1-year timeframe of 2017–2018 (CIHI, 2020).

Reduction in Bed-to-Nurse Ratio

The second factor that has led to an increased number of employed RNs is the reduction in the bed-to-RN ratio, meaning the number of RNs employed on a unit per number of beds available. Historically, the number of RNs per bed had increased over time (Meltz & Marzetti, 1988). However, between 1999 and 2018, hospital beds have declined from 3.92 beds per 1000 people to 2.55 beds per 1000 people (Elflein, 2020). This reduction was due in part to a shift from acute care to community care along with cost-cutting measures imposed by health care institutions, resulting in fewer hospital beds being available. A strategy espoused by the RNAO and other nursing associations in Canada for quality patient care is the use of an adequate **skill mix** and the appropriate caregiver (RNAO, 2016), meaning the use of the best health care provider for the task at hand. Currently, nurses spend nearly 36% of their jobs in hospitals on non-nursing tasks, such as assisting with the activities of daily living and making lab, linen supply, and pharmacy trips (Berlin, English, Higgins, & Lapointe, 2014). The decline in the bed-to-RN ratio through the replacement of RNs with less costly nursing personnel has added to the complexity of the situation (RNAO, 2017).

The research evidence supports the importance of sufficient, well-qualified RNs in relation to patient outcomes and cost effectiveness (Aiken, Clarke, Sloane, et al., 2009; Hugonnet, Chevrolet, & Pittet, 2007; Kieft, de Brouwer, Francke, & Delnoij, 2014; Armstrong, Laschinger, & Wong, 2009). The use of the most appropriate level of skill for a given area of work was a cornerstone of the 2016 RNAO publication *Mind the Safety Gap in Health System Transformation* (RNAO, 2016). This report indicated that

effectively matching health human resources to the needs of patients should be the driver of what level of provider is used.

Although much discussion has ensued about new models of care, such as total patient care and patient-focused care, it is difficult to find evidence of much change in where and how services are delivered. Data about the health care aide or personal service worker are not captured in available reports. Only the regulated professions are tracked and documented. It is uncertain how much the system and hospitals have changed in delivering care in hospitals vis-à-vis the use of nonregulated help such as personal support workers. The growth of LPNs has been outpacing the growth of RNs in 2017 to 2018 (CIHI, 2020). Replacement of the RN at the bedside by the LPN has been identified as an issue by RN leadership (RNAO, 2016). Appropriate skill mix is a nursing resource issue that can enhance job satisfaction and increase patient outcomes (Driscoll, Grant, Carroll et al., 2017; Duffield, Diers, O'Brien-Pallas et al., 2011). In addition, generic or personal support workers have become a staple in the care of individuals in LTC facilities (Saari, Patterson, Killackey et al., 2017).

Fluctuation in Part-Time Employment

The third factor leading to an increase in the number of employed RNs is the increase in the proportion of nurses working part-time. Almost half of the RNs in Canada were working part-time by 1985 (Meltz & Marzetti, 1988), an increase from 27% of RNs working part-time in 1971. This trend then reversed, with 36.7% of RNs working part-time (see Table 17.3). In 2009, 58.7% of RNs were working full time; in 2018, that percentage was 56.7% (CIHI, 2020). Nursing associations and governments in Canada have focused on increasing the number of full-time positions in the last 5 to 10 years; there is a dearth of research to confirm whether this has indeed happened. However, few studies clarify whether the majority of RNs continue to work part-time and casually by choice because of workplace issues and/or work–life balance.

New and Evolving Roles for Registered Nurses

The fourth factor that has increased RN employment is new and expanding roles for RNs in the health care system. There are currently two advanced practice roles for nurses in Canada: the NP and the clinical nurse specialist. Clinical nurse specialists, an idea that arose in the 1940s after World War Two and came into being in the 1960s, was created to "provide clinical consultation, guidance and leadership to nursing staff managing complex and specialized client care to improve the quality of care and to promote evidence-informed practice" (CNA, 2019, p. 7). The NP, like the clinical nurse specialist, is not a new role for nurses but is

TABLE 17.3   Demographics of Part-Time and Full-Time Regulated Nurses in Canada, 2009 and 2018

	2009	2018
No. of Nurses Across Canada		
RNs and NPs	284,690	303,146
Regulated nurses	348,499	431,769
No. of Nurses Per 100,000 People		
RNs	787	707
Regulated nurses	696	825
Average Age (Years)		
RNs and NPs	45.2	44.6
LPNs	43.4	41.1
RPNs	47.6	44.6
No. of Full-Time Nurses		
(% of Regulated Nurses*)		
RNs and NPs	156,178 (44.8%)	171,084 (39.6%)
LPNs	38,623 (11%)	54,386 (12.5%)
RPNs	3,479 (0.9%)	2,887 (0.6%)
No. of Part-Time Nurses (incl. Casual)		
(% of Regulated Nurses*)		
RNs and NPs	109,975 (31.5%)	116,498 (26.9%)
LPNs	38,308 (10.9%)	54,984 (12.7%)
RPNs	1,707 (0.04%)	1,889 (0.04%)

*Regulated nurses included registered nurses (RNs), nurse practitioners (NPs), licensed practical nurses (LPNs) (which are called registered practical nurses [RPNs] in Ontario), and registered psychiatric nurses (RPNs). Registered practical nurses are members of the LPN category, while registered psychiatric nurses are members of the RN category.
Sources: Canadian Nurses Association. (2011, May). *2009 Workforce profile of registered nurses in Canada.* Retrieved from https://www.cna-aiic.ca/-/media/cna/page-content/pdf-en/2009_rn_snapshot_e.pdf; Canadian Institute for Health Information. (2018). *Nursing in Canada, 2018: A lens on supply and workforce* [Data tables]. Retrieved from https://www.cihi.ca/sites/default/files/document/regulated-nurses-2018-report-en-web.pdf; Canadian Institute for Health Information. (2010, December). *Regulated nurses: Canadian trends, 2005 to 2009.* Retrieved from https://secure.cihi.ca/free_products/nursing_report_2005-2009_en.pdf.

an example of an evolving role for RNs. NPs are employed in a variety of positions in hospitals and the community in primary, secondary, and tertiary settings. NPs have existed in Canada since the 1960s to service rural and remote locations (CNA, 2019). NPs can now lead clinics in an interprofessional model of primary care. Also, new telehealth networks and telephone advice and information centres (Goodwin, 2007) require the knowledge and skills of RNs. These have expanded as technology has improved to include items such as chatlines and online counseling sessions for people who cannot access these services where they live. Nurses are not linked to a specific setting, such as a hospital, but to a community or population (Robert Wood Johnson Foundation, 2015).

In Canada, RN prescribing is also being explored and has received government support. Currently, only NPs can order tests for the purpose of diagnosing a condition to prescribe medication. In Ontario, along with changes to the *Nursing Act* in 2018 that allowed NPs to prescribe narcotics, RNs in the general class in Ontario will be allowed

to prescribe certain medications and communicate a diagnosis for the purpose of prescribing (College of Nurses of Ontario [CNO], 2019a). The scope of medications that RNs will be allowed to prescribe is outlined in Table 17.4.

In 2019, the Government of Ontario announced that it had instructed the province's regulatory college, the College of Nurses of Ontario, to explore legislative changes that would allow RN prescribing following completion of a postgraduate certificate. This change will introduce RN prescribing for those RNs who are not extended-class NPs and introduces a new role for RNs on the front line in certain areas. At the same time, the scope of practice of registered practical nurses (RPNs) was also opened to allow the RPN to practise the same types of skills as the RN (CNO, 2019b), thus allowing new roles to evolve for these nurses as well. The requisite skills and abilities that will need to be taught and the length of time that RPNs will spend in their undergraduate training may change. This change to the scope of practice of the RPN (in Ontario only) is in the exploratory phase, and the impact remains to be seen.

TABLE 17.4	Proposed Medications for Registered Nurse Prescribing in Ontario
Immunization	• Vaccines for prevention of bacterial and viral disease
Contraception	• Hormonal contraceptives for systemic use
	• Intravaginal contraceptives
	Excludes intra-uterine contraceptive
Travel Health	• Aminoquinolines for malaria prevention
	• Biguanides for malaria prevention
	• Methanolquinolines for malaria prevention
	• Anti-bacterials for systemic use for malaria prevention
	• Anti-bacterials for systemic use for traveller's diarrhea
Topical Wound Care	• Corticosteroids, plain for topical use
	• Antibiotics for topical use
	• Metronidazole for topical use
	• Anesthetics for topical use
	• Medicated dressings
Smoking Cessation	• Bupropion for smoking cessation
	• Varenicline
Over-the-Counter Medication	• Any drug or substance that may lawfully be purchased or acquired without a prescription and is available for self-selection in a pharmacy or retail outlet.
	• Although these medications do not legally require a prescription, some patients can only access them if they are prescribed by an authorized prescriber. For example, a patient who receives Ontario Drug Benefits.
	• This excludes any medication available "behind" the pharmacy counter (i.e., where consultation with a pharmacist is necessary to obtain the medication).
Miscellaneous	• Epinephrine for anaphylaxis

(© 2020 College of Nurses of Ontario. Reproduced with permission of the College of Nurses of Ontario (CNO). At the time permission was granted to reproduce this content, the proposed medications had not been approved by government and are subject to change. If approved, the information and location on the CNO website may change over time. For current information on RN prescribing in Ontario, readers are advised to visit cno.org.)

TRENDS IN SUPPLY

The supply of nurses in Canada comes from recent graduates of baccalaureate programs; immigrants from other countries who have received nursing education and meet the required competencies to work in Canada; and former nurses returning to the workforce. In 2018, 14,354 regulated nurses who were not employed in the profession sought a job as a nurse, which represents an increase over the past 5 years (CIHI, 2020). Of the regulated nurses seeking to reenter the workforce, more were LPNs (5,908) than RNs (4,967).

In educating new nurses for the future, the current educational model for RNs includes collaborative models with community colleges that allow graduates to achieve a baccalaureate in nursing. Several colleges deliver the RN curriculum as outlined by the degree-granting university. At this time, colleges do not have authority to grant baccalaureate degrees in nursing, but they can grant applied and honours degrees in other professions such as accounting, information technology, behavioural

sciences, and technology. Colleges also educate LPNs and RPNs (practical nurses) as well as other allied health care providers, such as respiratory therapists, physiotherapy assistants, dental hygienists, and occupational therapy assistants. Universities deliver postbaccalaureate education such as master's and doctoral degrees in nursing and other disciplines.

Since 2003, the percentage of nurses educated internationally has varied from 7% to 8% and currently sits at 8.5% (CIHI, 2020). Support for IENs to bridge their education to Canadian standards is seen as a major strategy to increase the retention of this group (Covell, Primeau, & Kirkpatrick, 2017). Enrollment in nursing programs in Canada and the United States fluctuated in the 1980s and 1990s (Aiken & Mullinix, 1987). Interest in nursing as a career declined for many reasons, including increased career opportunities for women; rigid and capped salary structures for staff nurses; layoffs during the 1990s; and lack of economic return for degrees in nursing at the time. The decrease in the number of students enrolling was also due to changes in RN education in Canada and a declining number of 18-year-olds and fewer young adults entering the workforce. In Canada, in response to the resultant shortage that began in the 1990s, nursing schools increased their enrollment. The number of graduates from entry-to-practice baccalaureate programs crested at 9,000 in 2007 and has been above 10,000 since 2010 (CIHI, 2020). The number of nursing graduates continued to rise. There were 12,283 graduates in 2018, a decline from 2017 and 2016. In 2018, there were 9,527 candidates who wrote the NCLEX-RN; 89% were educated in Canada and 10.7% were educated internationally (Canadian Council of Registered Nurse Regulators, 2019). It should be noted there is a discrepancy in writers to graduates in 2018 (12,283). The reason may be that several students did not write the NCLEX-RN and that Quebec nurses do not write the NCLEX-RN. However, in 2018, the year for which the latest data are available on the ratio of RNs to population, the average ratio was 831 RNs per 100,000 people in Canada (Ontario Nurses' Association, 2019); in 2019, this number decreases to 812 when the ratio of RNs in Canada is calculated as directed by the CIHI (2019).

Historically, as the shortages became more pronounced, some hospitals focused on recruiting unemployed nurses or nurses who had left the profession. However, a review of unemployment and employment data does not support these nurses as a major source of RNs. Over 93% of actively registered RNs were working in 2006 (CNA & Canadian Association of Schools of Nursing [CASN], 2008), similar to the 94% employed in 2018 (CNA, 2019).

SUPPLY–DEMAND IMBALANCES

The actual imbalance between supply and demand is complex. From the 1970s until today, the supply of RNs has varied according to the number of graduates. Meanwhile, the demands have continued to expand and increase over this same period. Imbalances in a labour market can occur through unfilled vacancies or unemployment and underemployment (Meltz & Marzetti, 1988). Vacancies indicate an inability to recruit people or to retain them for a particular position. Although job **vacancy rates** had been reported in some areas across Canada in the 1980s, the rates varied tremendously. Meltz and Marzetti (1988) found that critical care and LTC positions consistently had high vacancy rates, and vacancy rates for chronic care, psychiatric care, and active teaching hospitals were also well above the provincial average. By 1993, the vacancy rate was virtually zero because of funding cutbacks and downsizing in the 1990s. Recent data do not reveal vacancy rates. Individual workplaces may have such data, but no central registry could be found. Nurse researchers looked at vacancy rates in the early part of this new century and recommended a standard methodology that would better quantify vacancy rates and provide a more accurate assessment of nurse utilization and shortage (Fisher, Baumann, & Blythe, 2007). It is uncertain at this time whether this recommendation has been implemented.

Unemployment

A low unemployment rate can indicate a shortage, while a high rate can indicate a potential supply source of RNs. The Statistics Canada Labour Force Survey in 2017 (Martel, 2019) indicated that the unemployment rate for health occupations was 6.1% and unemployed-to-job-vacancy ratio in health care and social assistance was 0.9. This number meant that there were more job vacancies than unemployed persons in that sector, which could point to a shortage of skilled personnel. This pertains to all health care professions.

Canada has had consistently low rates of unemployment for nurses; these rates are 50% or less of the general labour force unemployment rates. In 2019, the proportion of RNs who were employed in nursing remained the same (94%) as that in 2007 (CIHI, 2019). Across Canada, of RNs employed per 100,000 people, 707 were in direct care, 77 were in jobs other than direct care, and 16 were unemployed (CIHI, 2020).

Overtime and Absenteeism

Despite the low unemployment rate among nurses, there are four areas of growing concern in the profession: the amount of overtime worked by nurses, nursing absenteeism, nursing turnover, and the aging nursing population (Jacobson Consulting, 2017). Canadian nurses have the highest rates of overtime and absenteeism (9%) among public-sector workers (an overall average of 5.7%) (Jacobson Consulting, 2017). The rate of overtime worked by nurses equaled 10,000 FTEs in 2005, and in 2017, overtime reached 15,900 FTEs. In Canada, researchers are examining what factors contribute to healthy workplaces (Enns, Currie, & Wang, 2015; Magnavita & Garbarino, 2017; Rondeau & Wagar, 2016; Steege & Rainbow, 2017; Stone & Gershon, 2006; Stone, Mooney-Kane, Larson et al., 2007; Hall, Doran, & Pink, 2008). Sufficient staffing ratios of RNs, LPNs, and NPs with the appropriate skill mix can reduce the workload and stress on RNs and would also improve patient care outcomes and the efficiency and cost effectiveness of the health system (Aiken, Clarke, & Sloane, 2002; Aiken, Clarke, Sloane et al., 2002; Aiken, Clarke, Sloane et al., 2009; Armstrong, Laschinger, & Wong, 2009; Griffith, Ball, Drennan et al., 2016; RNAO, 2016; Nelson, Hearld, & Wein, 2018; Tourangeau, Doran, McGillis Hall et al., 2007).

Turnover

Turnover is a major challenge for health human resources planning in nursing, as high turnover has been considered an indicator of nurse dissatisfaction. Factors that have been identified as contributing to turnover are heavy workload, work stress, schedules, and staff burnout (Labrague, McEntroe-Petitte, Gloe et al., 2016; Steege & Rainbow, 2017). Retention has been an area of study and recommendations over the past 20 years (Chang, Chu, Liao et al., 2018; Laschinger, Wong, & Greco, 2006; Leners, Wilson, Connor et al., 2006; Pendry, 2007; Twigg & McCullough, 2014; Zeytinoglu, Denton, Davies et al., 2006). Modifying the work environment by implementing participative management, career development, and continuing education opportunities has been recommended (O'Brien-Pallas, Duffield, & Hayes, 2006; Wilson, 2005). Research is still required to evaluate the impact of these strategies. Some units in some institutions may have successfully implemented strategies to attract and retain nurses, but these efforts are not well documented. An accreditation program introduced by Accreditation Canada (2019), Qmentum Workforce, includes worklife as one of the six required organizational practices in patient safety.

Aging and Retirement of Nursing Faculty

The RNs educating the next generation of nurses are the oldest group of nurses, with 41% of nurses over 55 years of age (CASN, 2018). They represent a large group of nurse educators will be retiring over the next 10 years. Despite an increasing in the number of postgraduate students who will finish either a master's or doctoral degree in the next few years, the numbers will still be inadequate to completely replace upcoming nursing faculty retirements, if the postgraduate enrollment numbers do not change (CASN, 2018). Please see Chapters 9 and 22 for a more in-depth discussion about postgraduate education.

In summary, the supply–demand imbalance is complex. These data emphasize the need to view supply as being more than just a function of the number of new graduates. The retention of RNs, the quality of the workplace environment, and the number of full-time positions are all important factors that must be considered in addressing the supply–demand imbalance.

> ### APPLYING CONTENT KNOWLEDGE
>
> With all the published research related to workplace environment, why has so little change taken place in acute care facilities, where the majority of RNs still work?

 CULTURAL CONSIDERATIONS

Challenges Faced by Internationally Educated Nurses Migrating to Other Countries

As a strategy to address the nursing shortage, nurses who have been educated in one country are allowed to migrate to a host country. IENs make up around 8.5% of the Canadian nursing workforce (CIHI, 2019). Pung and Goh (2017) conducted an integrative literature review to identify the challenges faced by IENs who went to work in another country. Twenty-four articles from 2005 to 2015 were reviewed using Cooper's five-stage integrative process and the Joanna Briggs Institute appraisal checklists for interpretive and critical research and descriptive/case series (Cooper, 1989; Joanna Briggs Institute, 2013). Challenges identified related to the following issues: (1) communication barriers; (2) difficulty orienting; (3) longing for what is missing; (4) professional development and devaluing; (5) discrimination and marginalization;

(6) personal and professional differences; and (7) a meaningful support system.

Interventions that could address these challenges were identified, including cultural workshops, sharing sessions among international nurses, orientation programmes that involve procedures and protocols, and language lessons that could be implemented to assist international nurses with adapting to their new host countries. A "buddy program" whereby local nurses were paired with the IEN to mentor them could also be introduced to reduce discrimination and assist with their adaptation to the new country. The authors also emphasized the importance of involving both IENs and nurses from the host country in developing and implementing new strategies.

Sources: Canadian Institute for Health Information. (2019). *Nursing in Canada, 2018: A lens on supply and workforce.* Retrieved from https://www.cihi.ca/sites/default/files/document/regulated-nurses-2018-report-en-web.pdf; Cooper, H. (1989). *Integrating research: A guide for literature review.* Newbury Park, CA: Sage Publications; Joanna Briggs Institute. (2013). *Evidence-based practice resources and publications.* Retrieved from https://joannabriggs.org/ebp#tools; Pung, L. X., & Goh, Y. S. (2017). Challenges faced by international nurses when migrating: An integrative literature review. *International Nursing Review, 64,* 146–165. https://doi.org/10.1111/inr.12306.

CHALLENGES FACING THE PROFESSION

Major challenges continue to face the nursing profession (see Box 17.2). Canada's health care system depends overwhelmingly on the work of women, as the majority of nurses are women. Ryten (1988) identified that 4 of 5 workers in health-related occupations are women, and 4 of 10 workers overall are women. The gender balance among health workers has not changed despite the increase in the number of male nurses by 17% since 2014 (CIHI, 2020). During the past 40 years, women have entered traditionally male occupations, such as medicine, veterinary medicine, and engineering; however, men have not entered traditionally female occupations, such as nursing, at the same rate. This phenomenon is explored in depth in Chapter 6.

In the United States, since 2014, more women than men have graduated from university (Duffin, 2019). Women have also made great strides in pursuing higher education, but their participation has benefited fields of study that are not predominantly female (Ryten, 1988).

A key Canadian labour market trend that began in the 1980s and 1990s and continues to this day is the continually increasing demand for well-educated and skilled workers. This trend reflects changes both in the occupational "mix" of employment toward business services in areas of professional, scientific, and technical service industries and in the administrative and support, waste management, and remediation service industries. The computer and telecommunications sector, which has grown very fast in the late twentieth century, continues to evolve. This sector is changing the work of RNs worldwide. This trend in the general labour market is also evident in the health care industry, in hospitals, and in the nursing profession. Nurses are being taught in increasingly technological contexts; for example, the use of simulation in nursing education is a well-established learning strategy involving technology; most documentation is done electronically in developed countries; and machines now do the work of nurses that was manual as little as 10 years ago (e.g., IV therapy delivery, such as mixing medications in IV bags; insulin mixing and delivery; phlebotomy; and moving and lifting patients). The use of informatics and artificial intelligence in health care delivery has been increasing, and there is much debate about its pros and cons (Susskind & Susskind, 2018). Core entry-to-practice competencies, including those for informatics, have also been developed for nurses by the Canadian Association of Schools of Nursing and Canada Health Infoway (CASN, 2012).

The mid-1990s witnessed a more turbulent, chaotic, and challenging economic and health care environment, and after a relatively quiet period in the first decade of this century, the economic and health care landscape is turbulent once again. Reorganization and decentralization were key principles of the many institutional changes back then and are again being used. Program management, case management, and patient focus remain the values driving health care decisions. Although many studies have highlighted that nursing issues are related to lack of recognition, lack of professionalism, and lack of authority or responsibility, these management structures have not necessarily addressed the empowerment of nurses or the need for the nurse to be a professional knowledge worker. Organizational and technological support for their work, however, remains as low as it has been in past decades (Bower & McCullough, 2004). Susskind and Susskind (2015) identified the use of technology as fundamental to the future work of the professions.

Nurses continue to face several challenges in the new millennium. First, the continued need to restructure the Canadian health care systems—to enhance nurses' value, knowledge, and roles—should be considered. Nurse prescribing and enhancing the role of NPs are two initiatives currently being implemented in Ontario. NP-led clinics are also addressing the need for accessibility while using the skill set of the NP in more appropriate ways (CNA, 2019; Government of Ontario, 2015). These new ways of delivering care should enhance nurses' work–life balance and create more efficient work patterns. Second, there needs to be a continued focus on implementing recommendations for recruitment and retention that will deal with the aging nursing population as well as the younger generations (Kwok, Bates, & Ng, 2016; Widger, Pye, Cranley et al., 2007). Higher efficiency and productivity are required as we move toward an era of reduced birthrates, resulting in a smaller, aging population (Statistics Canada, 2018).

BOX 17.2 Challenges Facing the Nursing Profession

- Continued casualization of the workforce
- Aging workforce and decline in experienced nurses
- Reorganized health care systems that are slow to recognize and support nurses' need for additional knowledge and skills
- Continued reorganization of health care systems to provide cost-efficient care
- Continued lack of coordinated recruitment and retention strategies
- Continued lack of structural changes to address working conditions and quality of work–life balance in nursing

RESEARCH FOCUS

Intent to Stay in Rural and Remote Nursing Positions

In 2015, nurses who worked in a rural or northern area made up 11.8% of the population of all nurses in Canada and cared for 17.4% of the Canadian population (MacLeod, Stewart, Kulig et al., 2017). The challenge of recruiting nurses to work, and stay, in rural and remote communities contributes to health care inequities for patients (Nowrouzi, Rukholm, Larivière et al., 2016). Researchers conducted a cross-sectional survey of nurses employed in direct and indirect care in rural and remote communities in Northern Ontario, Canada, to assess nurses' intent to stay in their nursing positions and to identify any factors that contributed to their intent to leave their positions. Using logistic regression analysis, the researchers considered two factors: (1) demographics and (2) occupation and career satisfaction.

There were 459 respondents (28% response rate), with a mean age of 48 years. The findings indicated that respondents aged 46 to 56 years had the most statistically significant finding for intent to stay. Factors that contributed to intent to stay include available staff development from the employer, greater career and educational advancement opportunities, quality of lifestyle, and work–life balance (as evidenced by less than 1 hour of overtime per week).

As part of future work, the researchers suggested examining how nurses' quality of work and retention of nurses are influenced by factors such as organizational size, size and location of the community, continuing education opportunities, and organizational structure and leadership (Nowrouzi, Rukholm, Larivière et al., 2016, p. 56).

Sources: Nowrouzia, B., Rukholm, E., Larivière, M., et al. (2016). An examination of retention factors among registered nurses in Northeastern Ontario, Canada: Nurses' intent to stay in their current position. *Work, 54*, 51–58. https://doi.org/10.3233/WOR-162267; MacLeod, M. L. P., Stewart, N. J., Kulig, J. C., et al. (2017). Nurses who work in rural and remote communities in Canada: A national survey. *Human Resources for Health, 15*(34), 1–11. https://doi.org/10.1186/s12960-017-0209-0.

RESEARCH FOCUS

A National Survey of Nurses in Rural and Remote Communities in Canada

The nursing workforce in rural and remote parts of Canada is already smaller than that in urban settings. To help identify trends and issues in rural workforce planning, MacLeod and colleagues (2017) undertook a national study—the Nursing Practice in Rural and Remote Canada II—to better understand the regulated nursing workforce (registered nurses, RNs; nurse practitioners, NPs; licensed or registered practical nurses, LPNs; and registered psychiatric nurses, RPNs) working in rural and remote communities in Canada. They posed two research questions: What is the nature of nursing practice in rural and remote Canada? How can the capacity of nursing services and access to nursing care in rural and remote Canada be enhanced?

A questionnaire was sent to nurses who worked in an area identified as a "rural or small town-Canada" location (as defined by Statistics Canada). Sampling was achieved by sending the survey to nursing associations to forward to their member nurses, using postal code stratification, and identifying those geographic locations that were rural or remote. The initial target sample was 10,072 nurses, of which 9,622 nurses were deemed eligible after an initial mailout. From this group, the return sample was 3,822, or a 40% response rate.

The authors found that the average age of nurses working in rural or remote locations is 55, well above the national average of 44. Casualization of the workforce continues to be a concern, with 52% working in full-time positions, mostly as NPs. Research on why physicians move to small locales has discovered a link between where one grew up and where one practices, in that physicians are more likely to work in places that are of a similar size to where they spent their formative years. This trend was also confirmed for nurses in this study; working in a remote or rural location correlated to growing up in a similar-sized community. Reasons to stay in a remote location were identified as location, practice setting, and income. RNs and NPs were more likely to be satisfied with work–life balance and opportunities for career advancement, whereas LPNs and RPNs reported that income was more important to them.

Indications for future research were suggested, including more discourse with each group to identify factors that support them in their practice and further examination of recruitment and retention predictors of RNs' intent to stay or go.

Source: MacLeod, M. L. P., Stewart, N. J., Kulig, J. C., et al. (2017). Nurses who work in rural and remote communities in Canada: A national survey. *Human Resources for Health, 15*(34), 1–11. https://doi.org/10.1186/s12960-017-0209-0.

Partly in response to these challenges, the nursing profession has become more vocal in its advocacy efforts, with strong support from unions (see Chapters 18 and 19). Nurses first participated in illegal strikes in the 1980s and 1990s. Although there was much anger and unrest among nurses at the time, leading to better salaries, systemic changes did not come to pass. Today, nurses continue to fight for systemic change, voicing their collective opinions on the profession, health care, and health policy, and engaging in political activism. For instance, for several years now, provincial/territorial and national nursing associations have identified key priorities in upcoming elections.

The aging of RNs also remains a major concern. Although the average age of nurses has declined somewhat over the past 5 years, it remains in the 40s. The youngest group of nurses continues to be the LPN group, while the oldest continues to be nursing faculty. However, despite nearing retirement age, some RNs, like the general population, might choose to continue working. Strategies to assist and encourage nurses to continue working need to be considered (Kwok, Bates, & Ng, 2016). Studies in Canada and globally since the 1980s have recommended structural changes that would address unsatisfactory working conditions and quality of worklife in nursing. However, these recommended changes have yet to be fully adopted by the health care system.

RECOMMENDATIONS FOR CHANGE

A review of trends in nursing employment, supply and demand, and supply imbalances indicates that Canada has not seen a real "shortage" of RNs when only the numbers are considered. However, with the number of part-time and casual RNs remaining, over 40% of the total RNs working, and the high rate of absenteeism, there is indeed a shortage. The increasing number of aging nurses is a concern. Despite the seemingly large number of students who graduated from entry-to-practice programs in 2016 (12,484) and the continuous increases in nursing graduates since 2009, there was a decline of 1.6% in the number of graduates in 2017 (12,282) (CIHI, 2020). In fact, 2016 also witnessed a decline in the number nursing graduates (0.8%) from 2015 numbers. Two consecutive years of decline in RN nursing graduates should be a concerning trend to the nursing profession and those in administration and policy.

Back in 1989, some specialties, hospitals, and other nursing areas in Canada had large RN position vacancy rates, which had a negative impact on patient care. Then, during the early 1990s, there was greater employment for nurses, although this was negatively impacted following health care restructuring and layoffs, leading to a decline in nursing education seats (Kephart, Maaten, O'Brien-Pallas et al., 2004). In 2016, wait times and access to specialized care again became a concern (Barua & Ren, 2016). In 2019, the increase in hallway medicine and the number of RN vacancies is a growing concern (Devlin, 2019).

According to the Canadian Nurses Association, Canada could be facing a shortage of 60,000 nurses by 2022 (CNA, 2014). In order to address the continued challenge of recruiting RNs to maintain an adequate workforce that can meet the needs of the population, several strategies have been recommended: providing career opportunities and advancement and mentorship opportunities; maintaining the workforce of those employees who are eligible for retirement in the future to assist with knowledge transfer to the new generation of nurses; recruiting and supporting IENs; employing appropriate and efficient technology and automation; creating flexible work schedules; and supporting educational and professional development (Kwok, Bates, & Ng, 2016).

Because health care in Canada is a provincial/territorial matter, in planning for health care, the provincial/territorial governments need a coordinated health human resources strategy to address the imbalances in supply and demand for RNs. Many organizations and published reports have highlighted the human resources issues in health care and provided guidelines for human resources planning. In October 2000, Canada and the provincial/territorial governments developed a plan that addresses human resources planning in nursing over the long term (Government of Canada, 2011, p. 16). The need for an ongoing coordinated human resources plan for health care based on the health needs of Canadians cannot be overemphasized. To this end, the federal government created the Health Human Resources Strategy (Government of Canada, 2011) with the following four key strategic directions:

1. Supply of health providers—To increase the number of qualified providers entering the health workforce;
2. More effective use of skills—To increase the productivity of health care providers by making full use of their skills; and to improve access to health care services for all Canadians, particularly in underserved areas, by addressing the maldistribution of health human resources;
3. Creating healthy, supportive, learning workplaces—To enhance working and learning conditions to maintain an experienced, dedicated workforce with the skills to provide high-quality, safe, timely care; and
4. More effective planning and forecasting—To develop the capacity for more effective health human resources

planning and forecasting to support an affordable, sustainable health care system.

The last annual report about the Health Human Resources Strategy (2010–2011) outlined several initiatives that Health Canada had initiated and funded to develop, implement, and disseminate knowledge, best practices, and strategies for innovative health care delivery. However, the lack of an update since 2011 makes it difficult to assess progress.

Governments have a responsibility to review and update legislation that will enact structural changes to give nurses the authority to participate in decision making. This legislation is needed to ensure that nurses' participation in decision making occurs not simply by virtue of invitation, as it is at present in most provinces. Administrators of health care delivery organizations need to retain the nurses they have and preserve RNs' time for direct care of patients and families. Staffing ratios have been identified in the United States and the United Kingdom as being key to positive patient outcomes and RN work satisfaction (Griffith, Ball, Drennan et al., 2016; He, Staggs, Bergquist-Beringer, & Dunton, 2016; Shin, Park, & Bae, 2017).

Staffing affects quality and cost of patient care (Kieft, de Brouwer, Franke, & Delnoij, 2014). Organizations should design and implement innovative, cost-effective staffing methods that include job restructuring, use of support personnel, flexible scheduling plans, and labour-saving technology (Susskind & Susskind, 2015). Management must continue to introduce incentives to encourage experienced nurses to remain in clinical care. Wage structures and benefit packages that recognize experience and advanced education are needed. Artificial intelligence and other advanced technology such as robots, as noted previously, continue to replace the heavy work of nurses—these changes are happening around the world. Robots can be programmed to deliver medications to patients with the push of a button. Phlebotomy can now be done by machine to ensure the correct position. Even delicate surgeries such as neurosurgery or microsurgery are performed by robots.

Although many new management models emerged in the 1990s, the health care system continues to be a hierarchical and bureaucratically managed system. In response to rapid changes brought on by government cost-cutting initiatives, many agencies have downsized by reducing not only the number of beds but also the number of nurses. The balancing of government budgets through the elimination of health care positions, and especially RNs—who often make up the largest workforce in a health care institution—is a common strategy used from the last century to this one.

The need for innovation, creativity, and entrepreneurial acts has never been greater. The need to maximize every nurse's skill and knowledge is paramount. Technology and delivery models must be designed to best use nurses' knowledge (Archibald & Barnard, 2017; Bower & McCullough, 2004; Twigg & McCullough, 2014). Every unit or agency likely requires a different system of delivering care based on the needs of a specific population of patients.

Nurses also bear the responsibility for addressing some of these issues. Each nurse must value and recognize the importance of nursing care and be able to articulate that value. Nurses should realize the strength of nursing, as it includes many different groups, organizations, and specialties. External groups have suggested that a major problem in nursing is the lack of unity or a unified voice. However, this may be a "blame the victim" phenomenon, like those seen in commentary on other women's issues. Such comments by government and administrators maintain the status quo; they need not do anything about the nursing problems, since they are "nursing's problems." Therefore, systemic and legislative changes that would deal with quality of worklife and workplace issues are avoided. Nurses should take pride in their differences and recognize that some among their number perceive the "shortage" issue to be the result of work–life balance and workplace problems common to nurses everywhere. Nurses have become more politically aware and should be advocating for legislation and policies developed by nurses that direct how decisions are made and who makes them.

CONCLUSION

The retention and recruitment of nurses is critical to addressing the ongoing nursing workforce pendulum. According to the OECD, Canada does have enough nurses (OECD, 2016). But numbers alone do not indicate whether a problem exists in health human resources planning for nursing. The problems are non-numerical and persistent, including lack of respect; limited autonomy and authority in clinical situations; lack of technological and management support; lack of educational opportunities; and an inability to participate in management decisions about resource allocation (which affects support services and staffing). The demand for nursing skills and knowledge continues, and new and expanded roles for nurses are being implemented. Collaboration among government, administrators, and nurses must continue to be a priority to deal adequately and comprehensively with the various quality of worklife issues facing nurses in Canada today.

SUMMARY OF LEARNING OBJECTIVES

- While the number of RNs has increased in the past 5 years, there has been a decrease in the rate of growth. It has gone from a 2.2% increase in 2014 to 1% annually between 2017 and 2018. It matches the population growth of 1.2% from 2017 to 2018.
- The average age of regulated nurses has declined from 45.2 to 43.8 years. In 2018, the average age of RNs was 44.6 years, the average of LPNs was 41.1 years, and the average age of RPNs was 44.6 years. Nurse educators are the group with the highest average age—58% are over age 50, while 34.1% of the RN workforce is over age 50.
- Regulated nurses continue to be the biggest health care workforce, with RNs still the largest subgroup. However, the trend shows that the growth of LPNs is outpacing that of RNs and NPs. LPNs are being used to replace RNs in certain settings, such as LTC and community care.
- According to a numerical-only approach, the supply of RNs may be seen to be enough to meet demand. The reasons for imbalances in the supply of and demand for RNs include lack of respect; limited autonomy and authority in clinical situations; lack of technological and management support;

lack of educational opportunities; continued casualization through increasing part-time and casual positions, causing increased absenteeism and turnover; and an inability to participate in management decisions about resource allocation (which affects support services and staffing).
- Challenges facing the nursing profession due to shortages include burnout, younger RNs leaving the profession due to a lack of work–life balance, increased turnover costs, implications for patient safety, and declining enrollment due to a lack of nursing faculty.
- According to the Canadian Nurses Association, Canada could be facing a shortage of 60,000 nurses by 2022. Strategies to address such a shortage include providing career opportunities and advancement and mentorship opportunities; maintaining the workforce of those employees who are eligible for retirement in the future to assist with knowledge transfer to the new generation of nurses; recruiting and supporting IENs; employing appropriate and efficient technology and automation; creating flexible work schedules; and supporting educational and professional development.

CRITICAL THINKING QUESTIONS

1. Is the shortage of RNs caused by demand or supply factors?
2. Is there a "real" shortage of RNs?
3. What do you see as the most pressing issue in health human resources for governments, nursing associations, administrators, and nurses to address?
4. What might your role be as a member of the profession in helping to address the imbalance and challenges facing nursing resources, now and in the future?

REFERENCES

Accreditation Canada. (2019). *Qmentum.* Retrieved from https://accreditation.ca/accreditation/qmentum/.

Aiken, L., & Mullinix, C. (1987). Special report: The nurse shortage—myth or reality? *New England Journal of Medicine, 317*(10), 641–646. https://doi.org/10.1056/NEJM198709033171030.

Aiken, L. H., Clarke, S. P., Sloane, D. M., et al. (2002). Hospital staffing, organization, and quality of care: Cross-national findings. *International Journal for Quality in Health Care, 14*(1), 5–14. https://doi.org/10.1093/intqhc/14.1.5.

Aiken, L. H., Clarke, S. P., Sloane, D. M., et al. (2009). Effects of hospital care on patient mortality and outcomes. *Journal of Nursing Administration, 38*(5), 223–229. https://doi.org/10.1097/NNA.0b013e3181aeb4cf.

Archibald, M. M., & Barnard, A. (2017). Futurism in nursing: Technology, robotics and the fundamentals of care. *Journal of Clinical Nursing, 27*(11–12), 2473–2480. https://doi.org/10.1111/jocn.14081.

Armstrong, K., Laschinger, H., & Wong, C. (2009). Workplace empowerment and magnet hospital characteristics as predictors of patient safety climate. *Journal of Nursing Care Quality, 24*(1), 55–62.

Barua, B., & Ren, F. (2016). *Waiting your turn: Wait times for healthcare in Canada.* Fraser Institute. Retrieved from https://www.fraserinstitute.org/sites/default/files/waiting-your-turn-wait-times-for-health-care-in-canada-2016-execsum.pdf.

Berlin, G., English, C.R., Higgins, H., & Lapointe, M. (2014, May 1). *Optimizing the nursing skill mix: A win for nurses, patients, and hospitals.* Retrieved from https://healthcare.mckinsey.com/optimizing-nursing-skill-mix-win-nurses-patients-and-hospitals.

Bower, F. L., & McCullough, C. (2004). Nurse shortage or nursing shortage: Have we missed the real problem? *Nurse Economics, 22*(4), 200–203.

Burke, R. S., Ng, E. S., & Wolpin, J. (2016). Effects of hospital restructuring and downsizing on nursing staff: The role of union support. *Journal of Health Management, 18*(3), 473–488. https://doi.org/10.1177/0972063416651598.

Canadian Association of Schools of Nursing. (2012). *Nursing informatics entry-to-practice competencies for registered nurses.* Canadian Association of Schools of Nursing & Canada Heath Infoway. Retrieved from https://www.casn.ca/wp-content/uploads/2014/12/Infoway-ETP-comp-FINAL-APPROVED-fixed-SB-copyright-year-added.pdf.

Canadian Association of Schools of Nursing. (2018). *Registered nurses education in Canada statistics: 2016–2017.* Retrieved from https://www.casn.ca/wp-content/uploads/2018/12/2016-2017-EN-SFS-FINAL-REPORT-supressed-for-circulation-r.pdf.

Canadian Council of Registered Nurse Regulators. (2019). *NCLEX-RN 2018: Canadian and international results.* Retrieved from http://www.ccrnr.ca/nclex---data.html.

Canadian Federation of Nurses Union. (2018). *Overview of key nursing contract provisions.* Retrieved from https://nursesunions.ca/contract-comparison/.

Canadian Institute for Health Information. (2006). *Health personnel trends in Canada, 1995 to 2004.* Retrieved from https://secure.cihi.ca/free_products/Health_Personnel_Trend_1995-2004_e.pdf.

Canadian Institute for Health Information. (2019). *Nursing in Canada, 2018: A lens on supply and workforce.* Retrieved from https://www.cihi.ca/sites/default/files/document/regulated-nurses-2018-report-en-web.pdf.

Canadian Institute for Health Information. (2020). *Nursing in Canada, 2019.* Retrieved from https://www.cihi.ca/en/nursing-in-canada-2019.

Canadian Nurses Association. (2014). *Tested solutions for eliminating Canada's registered nurse shortage.* Retrieved from https://cna-aiic.ca/-/media/cna/page-content/pdf-en/rn_highlights_e.pdf.

Canadian Nurses Association. (2018, March 21). *CNA network advisory committee's definition of specialty nursing practice.* Retrieved from https://www.cna-aiic.ca/-/media/cna/page-content/pdf-en/specialty-nursing-practice-definition-2018_e.pdf.

Canadian Nurses Association. (2019). *Advanced practice nursing: A Pan-Canadian framework.* Ottawa, ON: Author. Retrieved from https://www.cna-aiic.ca/-/media/cna/page-content/pdf-en/advanced-practice-nursing-framework-en.pdf.

Canadian Nurses Association & Canadian Association of Schools of Nursing. (2008). *Nurse education in Canada statistics, 2006–2007.* Ottawa, ON: Author. Retrieved from https://www.cna-aiic.ca/-/media/cna/page-content/pdf-en/education_statistics_report_2006_2007_e.pdf.

Chang, H., Chu, T., Liao, Y., et al. (2018). How do career barriers and supports impact nurse professional commitment and professional turnover intention? *Journal of Nursing Management, 27*(2), 347–356. https://doi.org/10.1111/jonm.12674.

College of Nurses of Ontario. (2019a). *FAQ: RN prescribing.* Retrieved from https://www.cno.org/en/trending-topics/journey-to-rn-prescribing/qas-rn-prescribing/.

College of Nurses of Ontario. (2019b). Scope of practice for NPs and RPNs to expand. *The Standard.* Retrieved from http://www.cno.org/en/learn-about-standards-guidelines/magazines-newsletters/the-standard/july-2019/Scope-of-practice-NPs-and-RPNs-expand/.

Devlin, R. (2019). *Premier's Council on improving healthcare and ending hallway medicine: Interim report.* Retrieved from http://www.health.gov.on.ca/en/public/publications/premiers_council/docs/premiers_council_report.pdf.

Driscoll, A., Grant, M. J., Carroll, D., et al. (2017). The effect of nurse-to-patient ratios on nurse-sensitive patient outcomes in acute specialist units: A systematic review and meta-analysis. *European Journal of Cardiovascular Nursing, 17*(1), 6–22. https://doi.org/10.1177/1474515117721561.

Duffield, C., Diers, D., O'Brien-Pallas, L., et al. (2011). Nursing staffing, nursing workload, the work environment and patient outcomes. *Applied Nursing Research, 24*(4), 244–255. https://doi.org/10.1016/j.apnr.2009.12.004.

Duffin, E. (2019, August). *Percentage of the U.S. population with a college degree, 1940–2018, by gender.* Retrieved from https://www.statista.com/statistics/184272/educational-attainment-of-college-diploma-or-higher-by-gender/.

Elflein, J. (2020, July 24). *Density of hospital beds in Canada from 1976 to 2019.* Retrieved from https://www.statista.com/statistics/831668/density-of-hospital-beds-canada/.

Enns, V., Currie, S., & Wang, J. L. (2015). Professional autonomy and work setting as contributing factors to depression and absenteeism in Canadian nurses. *Nursing Outlook, 63*(3), 269–277. https://doi.org/10.1016/j.outlook.2014.12.014.

Fisher, A., Baumann, A., & Blythe, J. (2007). The effects of organizational flexibility on nurse utilization and vacancy statistics in Ontario hospitals. *Canadian Journal of Nursing Leadership, 20*(4), 48–64. https://doi.org/10.12927/cjnl.2007.19471.

George, C. (2015). Retaining professional workers: What makes them stay? *Employee Relations, 37*(1), 102–121. https://doi.org/10.1108/ER-10-2013-0151.

Government of Canada. (2011). *Health human resource strategy.* Retrieved from https://www.canada.ca/en/health-canada/services/health-care-system/health-human-resources/strategy.html.

Government of Ontario. (2015). *Nurse practitioner led clinics.* Ministry of Health and Long-Term Care. Retrieved from http://health.gov.on.ca/en/common/system/services/npc/.

Goodwin, S. (2007). Telephone nursing: An emerging practice area. *Canadian Journal of Nursing Leadership, 20*(4), 38–46.

Griffith, P., Ball, J., Drennan, J., et al. (2016). Nurse staffing and patient outcomes: Strengths and limitations of the evidence to inform policy and practice. A review and discussion paper based on evidence reviewed for the National Institute for Health and Care Excellence Safe Staffing guideline development. *International Journal of Nursing Studies, 63,* 213–225. https://doi.org/10.1016/j.ijnurstu.2016.03.012.

Grinspun, D., Harripal-Yup, A., Jarvi, K., & Lenartowych, T. (2016). *Mind the safety gap in health system transformation: Reclaiming the role of the RN.* Retrieved from https://rnao.ca/sites/rnao-ca/files/HR_REPORT_May11.pdf.

Hall, L. M., Doran, D., & Pink, L. (2008). Outcomes of interventions to improve hospital nursing work environments. *Journal of Nursing Administration, 38*(1), 40–46. https://doi.org/10.1097/01.nna.0000295631.72721.17.

He, J., Staggs, V. S., Bergquist-Beringer, S., & Dunton, N. (2016). Nurse staffing and patient outcomes: A longitudinal study on trend and seasonality. *BMC Nursing, 15,* 60. https://doi.org/10.1186/s12912-016-0181-3.

Hugonnet, S., Chevrolet, J. C., & Pittet, D. (2007). The effect of workload on infection risk in critically ill patients. *Critical Care Medicine, 35*(1), 296–298. https://doi.org/10.1097/01.ccm.0000251125.08629.3f.

Jacobson Consulting. (2017). *Trends in own illness- or disability-related absenteeism and overtime among publicly employed registered nurses.* Ottawa, ON: Canadian Federation of Nurses Unions. Retrieved from https://nursesunions.ca/wp-content/uploads/2017/05/Quick_Facts_Absenteeism-and-Overtime-2017-Final.pdf.

Kephart, G., Maaten, S., O'Brien-Pallas, L., et al. (2004). *Building the future: An integrated strategy for nursing human resources in Canada.* Simulation analysis report. Retrieved from https://www.cna-aiic.ca/~/media/cna/page-content/pdf-fr/simulation_analysis_report_e.pdf.

Kieft, R. A. M. M., de Brouwer, B. B. J. M., Franke, A. J., et al. (2014). How nurses and their work environment affect patient experiences of the quality of care: A qualitative study. *BMC Health Services Research, 49*(249), 1–10. https://doi.org/10.1186/1472-6963-14-249.

Kwok, C., Bates, K. A., & Ng, E. S. (2016). Managing and sustaining an ageing nursing workforce: Identifying opportunities and best practices within collective agreements in Canada. *Journal of Nursing Management, 24*(4), 500–511.

Labrague, L. J., McEnroe-Petitte, D. M., Gloe, D., et al. (2016). Organizational politics, nurses' stress, burnout levels, turnover intention and job satisfaction. *International Nursing Review, 64*(1), 109–116. https://doi.org/10.1111/inr.12347.

Laschinger, H. K. S., Wong, C. A., & Greco, P. (2006). The impact of staff nurse empowerment on person–job fit and work engagement/burnout. *Nursing Administration Quarterly, 30*(4), 358–367. https://doi.org/10.1097/00006216-200610000-00008.

Leners, D. W., Wilson, V. W., Connor, P., & Fenton, J. (2006). Mentorship: Increasing retention probabilities. *Journal of Nursing Management, 14,* 652–654. https://doi.org/10.1111/j.1365-2934.2006.00641.x.

Littlejohn, L., Campbell, J., & Collins-McNeil, J. (2012). Comparative analysis of nursing shortage. *International Journal of Nursing, 1*(1), 21–26. Retrieved from https://www.ijnonline.com/index.php/ijn/article/view/21.

Martel, L. (2019, March). *The labour force in Canada and its regions: Projections to 2036.* Catalogue No. 75-006-X. Ottawa, ON: Statistics Canada. Retrieved from https://www150.statcan.gc.ca/n1/pub/75-006-x/2019001/article/00004-eng.htm.

Magnavita, N., & Garbarino, S. (2017). Sleep, health and wellness at work: A scoping review. *International Journal of Environmental Research and Public Health, 14*(11), 1347–1365. https://doi.org/10.3390/ijerph14111347.

McGillis Hall, L., MacDonald-Rencz, S., Peterson, J., et al. (2013). *Moving to action: Evidence-based retention and recruitment policy initiatives for nursing.* Ottawa, ON: Canadian Foundation for Healthcare Improvement.

Meltz, N., & Marzetti, J. (1988). *The shortage of registered nurses: An analysis in a labour market context.* Toronto, ON: Registered Nurses' Association of Ontario.

Nelson, D., Hearld, L., & Wein, D. (2018). The impact of emergency department RN staffing on ED patient experience. *Journal of Emergency Nursing, 44*(4), 394–401. https://doi.org/10.1016/j.jen.2018.01.001.

O'Brien-Pallas, L., Duffield, C., & Hayes, L. (2006). Do we really understand how to retain nurses? *Journal of Nursing Management, 14,* 262–270. https://doi.org/10.1111/j.1365-2934.2006.00611.x.

Organisation for Economic Co-operation Development. (2016). *Health workforce policies in OECD countries: Right jobs, right skills, right places.* OECD Health Policy Studies. Paris, France: OECD Publishing. http://dx.doi.org/10.1787/9789264239517-en.

Ontario Nurses' Association. (2019). *Last again—Ontario has the most dismal RN-to-population ratio in the country.* Retrieved from https://www.ona.org/news-posts/ontario-last-ratio-2019/.

Pendry, P. S. (2007). Moral distress: Recognizing it to retain nurses. *Nursing Economics, 25*(4), 217–221.

Registered Nurses' Association of Ontario. (2016). *Mind the safety gap in health system transformation: Reclaiming the role of the RN.* Retrieved from https://rnao.ca/mind-the-gap.

Registered Nurses' Association of Ontario. (2017). *70 years of RN effectiveness. Policy and political action report.* Retrieved from https://rnao.ca/policy/reports/70-years-rn-effectiveness.

Rondeau, K. V., & Wagar, T. (2016). Human resource management practices and nursing turnover. *Journal of Nursing Education and Practice, 6*(10), 101–109. https://doi.org/10.5430/jnep.v6n10p101.

Robert Wood Johnson Foundation. (2015). Patient-centered care. *Nurses take on new and expanded roles in health care.* Retrieved from https://www.rwjf.org/en/library/articles-and-news/2015/01/nurses-take-on-new-and-expanded-roles-in-health-care.html.

Rosenberg, M. (2019). Current world population and future projections. Retrieved from https://www.thoughtco.com/current-world-population-1435270.

Ross, E. (2003). From shortage to oversupply: The workforce pendulum. In J. C. Ross & M. J. Wood (Eds.), *Canadian nursing* (4th ed., pp. 229–243). Toronto, ON: Elsevier Science Canada.

Ryten, E. (1988, June). *Women as deliverers of healthcare.* Unpublished speech presented at the Canadian Association of Schools of Nursing Annual Conference. Windsor, ON: University of Windsor.

Saari, M., Patterson, E., Killackey, T., et al. (2017). Home-based care: Barriers and facilitators to expanded personal support worker roles in Ontario, Canada. *Home Health Care Services Quarterly, 36*(3–4), 127–144. https://doi.org/10.1080/01621424.2017.1393482.

Shin, S., Park, J.-W., & Bae, S. H. (2017). Nurse staffing and nurse outcomes: A systematic review and meta-analysis.

Nursing Outlook, 66(3), 273–282. https://doi.org/10.1016/j.outlook.2017.12.002.

Statistics Canada. (2018). *Fertility overview: 2012–2016.* Retrieved from https://www150.statcan.gc.ca/n1/pub/91-209-x/2018001/article/54956-eng.htm.

Steege, L. M., & Rainbow, J. G. (2017). Fatigue in hospital nurses—"Supernurse" culture is a barrier to addressing problems: A qualitative interview study. *International Journal of Nursing Studies, 67*, 20–28. https://doi.org/10.1016/j.ijnurstu.2016.11.014.

Stone, P. W., & Gershon, R. R. (2006). Nurse work environment and occupational safety in intensive care units. *Policy, Politics, & Nursing Practice, 7*(4), 240–247.

Stone, P. W., Mooney-Kane, C., Larson, E. L., et al. (2007). Nurse working conditions and patient safety outcomes. *Medical Care, 45*(6), 571–578. https://doi.org/10.1097/MLR.0b013e3180383667.

Susskind, R., & Susskind, D. (2018). *The future of the professions: How technology will transform the work of humans.* Oxford, UK: Oxford University Press.

Toman, C. (2005). Body work, medical technology, and hospital nursing practice. In C. Bates, D. Dodd, & N. Rousseau (Eds.), *On all frontiers: Four centuries of Canadian nursing* (pp. 89–106). Ottawa, ON: University of Ottawa Press.

Tourangeau, A. E., Doran, D. M., McGillis Hall, L., et al. (2007). Impact of hospital nursing care on 30-day mortality for acute medical patients. *Journal of Advanced Nursing, 57*(1), 32–44. https://doi.org/10.1097/mlr.0b013e3182763284.

Twigg, D., & McCullough, K. (2014). Nurse retention: A review of strategies to create and enhance positive practice environments in clinical settings. *International Journal of Nursing Studies, 51*, 85–92. https://doi.org/10.1016/ijnurstu.05.015.

Widger, K., Pye, C., Cranley, L., et al. (2007). Generational differences in acute care nurses. *Canadian Journal of Nursing Leadership, 20*(1), 49–61. https://doi.org/10.12927/cjnl.2007.18785.

Wilson, A. A. (2005). Impact of management development on nurse retention. *Nursing Administration Quarterly, 29*(2), 137–145.

World Health Organization. (2016). *Global strategy on human resources for health: Workforce 2030.* Geneva, Switzerland: Author. Retrieved from https://www.who.int/hrh/resources/global_strategy_workforce2030_14_print.pdf.

World Health Organization & International Council of Nursing. (2018, February 27). *Nursing Now campaign.* Retrieved from https://www.who.int/hrh/news/2018/NursingNow_launch_press_release.pdf.

Zeytinoglu, I. U., Denton, M., Davies, S., et al. (2006). Retaining nurses in their employing hospitals and in the profession: Effects of job preference, unpaid overtime, importance of earnings and stress. *Health Policy, 79*(1), 57–72. https://doi.org/10.1016/j.healthpol.2005.12.004.

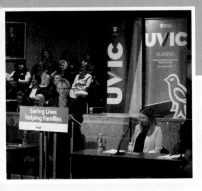

Political Influence in Nursing

Susan M. Duncan

(e) http://evolve.elsevier.com/Canada/Ross-Kerr/nursing

LEARNING OBJECTIVES

After reading this chapter, you will be able to:

- Recognize the significance of political influence in professional practice.
- Understand nursing's political imperative in the twenty-first century.
- Understand the relationship between the concepts of political influence, power, and policy.
- Identify the relationship between political influence and achieving goals in nursing, the health care system, and health and public policy.
- Understand the history of political action in nursing.
- Identify how nurses engage politically both as individuals and as members of collectives.
- Explain the importance of developing a base of support as a strategy for political influence.

OUTLINE

KEY TERMS

advocacy
critical perspective
feminist perspective
interprofessional collaboration

nursing organizations
policy influence
politics
power

PERSONAL PERSPECTIVES

Nurses can exert power and influence in political processes toward achieving health care goals. They do so both as individuals and as members of nursing organizations such as unions and professional associations. When nurses use a collective voice, they can effect change in health organizations in their local communities and globally. In order for nursing to have influence on health care policies, they must have a senior presence in government and health organizations that influence policy. Nurses in high-level government positions can bring about change by sharing their perspectives, informed by their knowledge and experience. The International Council of Nurses (ICN) had been concerned for many years that despite nurses' being the largest group of health professionals worldwide, they were not represented by a chief nursing officer at the World Health Organization (WHO). In 2017, the ICN publicly wrote to the three candidates for the position of Director General—a role held by a physician—to take a critical look at the issue and commit to appointing a chief nurse at the WHO. Following the appointment of Dr. Tedros Adhanom Ghebreyesus as Director General, the ICN met with him to advocate for nursing leadership. The ICN was successful in taking political action. In October 2017, Dr. Adhanom Ghebreyesus appointed Elizabeth Iro of the Cook Islands as Chief Nursing Officer at the WHO (International Council of Nurses [ICN], 2018a).

As of 2019, nurses in Canada remain concerned about the absence of a chief nursing officer. Through a growing advocacy initiative called Nursing Now Canada, launched in July 2019, Canadian nursing organizations are strategizing to urge the provincial/territorial governments and federal government to appoint chief nursing officers that would advise the ministries of health. The issues raised at the most recent ICN Congress in 2019 signal the importance of political action for Canadian nurses and nursing organizations (Duncan & Whyte, 2019).

INTRODUCTION

This chapter explores concepts of policy, **power,** and **politics** in relation to the current pressing issues in nursing and health. The core issue is determining how nurses can exert their influence to advance nursing care, health services, and the health of people on a broad and global scale. Nurses are being called to political action by organizations such as the WHO and the ICN as well as local and national governments; this level of influence is seen as a political imperative for nurses today. The rationale for harnessing nurses' collective power is that nurses accompany people at every stage of their journeys through life and therefore have firsthand knowledge of the human experience of care, health, and illness. Nursing students need to understand the dynamics of political influence—how to bring voice and influence policy directions for health while drawing on a nursing perspective. This chapter includes a discussion of perspectives, historical influences, and challenges and opportunities.

THE POLITICAL IMPERATIVE IN NURSING TODAY

The term **politics** has taken on many different meanings. For some, it might conjure up images of smoke-filled rooms, devious dealings, or power in the hands of a few. For others, it invokes images that are more generic. Among the earliest philosophers who attempted to understand the relationship between politics and people were Aristotle (384–322 BC) and Plato (428–348 BC). In his seminal work *The Republic*, Plato discussed the development of political leaders and the qualities of good leadership. For Aristotle, individuals were charged with the responsibility of supporting the common good through the domain of philosophy he called politics (Roberts, 2009). Politics can be viewed as the art of influencing others. In practical terms, political activity means influencing others for the purpose of allocating resources wisely.

One cannot engage in discussions about political influence without an understanding of its fundamental relationship to power. **Power** is the "ability to mobilize economic, social, or political forces to achieve a result" (Blackburn, 1994, p. 296). Some members or institutions in society are understood to have more power than others and therefore have more capacity to secure their own interests and goals. Understanding how power in society influences health care and health equity is fundamental to nurses' engagement with political processes in the twenty-first century. Nurses are encouraged to adopt **critical perspectives** and **feminist perspectives** on power to understand the dynamics of political influence on health (MacDonald & McIntyre, 2019; Peart & McKinnon, 2018). Critical and feminist perspectives assist nurses with understanding who has power over others and how nursing as a gendered profession can work to overcome hierarchical and patriarchal influences. These understandings are key to positioning the nursing profession for political influence.

A Historical Perspective

Historical is replete with stories of nurses who engaged in political action and did so successfully. In the early years

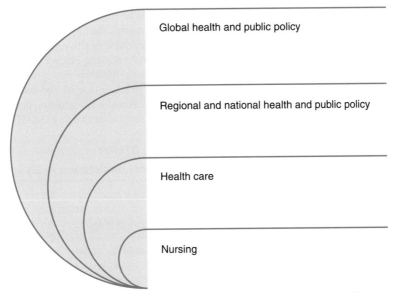

Global health and public policy

Regional and national health and public policy

Health care

Nursing

Fig. 18.1 "Bubble theory" and spheres of nursing influence—future goal. (**Source:** Shamian, J. (2014). Global perspectives on nursing and its contribution to healthcare and health policy: Thoughts on an emerging policy model. *Canadian Journal of Nursing Leadership, 27*(4), 44–50.)

of Canadian nursing, Jeanne Mance would have been considered a political activist par excellence, as she raised and sustained support for her hospital and for the colony in New France. Florence Nightingale's accomplishments are legendary, and the success of her nurses in ministering to sick and wounded soldiers in Crimea raised the potential contributions of well-prepared female nurses to the top of the public agenda (Dossey, 2010). Nightingale's skills as a researcher were impressive, and her interpretation of the statistics she collected led to important, lasting changes that positively impacted health and the organization of health services; her work continues to resonate with nurses taking on present-day nursing challenges to broadly influence health (Dossey, Rosa, & Beck, 2019). Nightingale demonstrated the positive effect of sanitation and nutrition on the health of soldiers; her principles now apply to health care in the general population. Her work had important offshoots for the British—and indeed for people in other nations—as the principles that Nightingale championed were carried far afield. For a more in-depth examination of the history of Florence Nightingale and her influence on nursing, please see Chapter 2.

Nurses in Canada argued strongly between 1900 and 1922 for the enactment of legislation that would govern the registration of nurses. The provincial campaigns were successful—every province had such legislation by 1922, when Ontario passed its first regulatory act for the nursing profession. More recent political activity by nurses has also

been successful. **Advocacy** by the Canadian Nurses Association (CNA) for the *Canada Health Act* of 1984 resulted in an amendment to the act, after it was tabled in Parliament, permitting federal funding for health practitioners. This legislation also made it possible for a provincial health plan to fund the services of nurses or other health care providers on a direct reimbursement basis, as the services of physicians and hospital dental surgeons had been financed since the passing of the *Medical Care Act* of 1968.

Power as Seen Through Critical and Feminist Perspectives and Their Impact on Nurses

Another term related to power and political influence is **policy**. In its broadest sense, public policy is "a course of action or inaction chosen by public authorities to address a given problem or set of interrelated problems" (Pal, 2006, p. 2). Nursing must use its political influence to target different levels of policy within nursing units, organizations, and governments while acting locally and globally. Figure 18.1 illustrates nursing's spheres of **policy influence** as envisioned by Dr. Judith Shamian, Canadian nurse leader and former president of the ICN (2013–2017). Dr. Shamian and others assert that nursing must extend political influence in and beyond the nursing sphere to the health care sphere, the regional and national health and public policy sphere, and the global health and public policy sphere (Cohen, Mason, Kovner et al., 1996; Shamian, 2014). Understanding the essential nature of nursing's contributions in each of the spheres constitutes the imperative for political influence.

Examples of political influence in the nursing sphere include the work of associations and unions to advocate for safe staffing and care delivery models and the advancement of nursing education and research. The health care sector has recognized for some time that the ability for the growth of care and treatment is limited. High-tech health care is expensive, and decisions will have to be made in some cases about health care priorities. Ensuring the most effective and efficient use of certain technologies increasingly means that not everyone can receive expensive care and treatment. Policymakers in organizations and governments are responsible for deciding how to allocate the available resources, while political leaders and health administrators must provide the rationale for allocating resources in one way or another. Nurses have a responsibility to evaluate the decisions that are made to allocate those resources and advocate for just decisions for the care of their patients, including the use of compelling evidence on safe nurse staffing models (International Council of Nurses [ICN], 2018b). Where nursing service is the primary activity, the politics of patient care may be less visible, but they are important and essential to good care. Nevertheless,

there can be no better reason for enhancing the political skills of nurses than to improve the care of patients wherever they receive health care (Box 18.1).

Recently, nursing extended its influence in the regional and national health policy sphere in the areas of harm reduction practices for opioid overdose prevention, access to health services for refugees, and the implementation of medical assistance in dying (MAID).

CASE STUDY
Medical Assistance in Dying

The CNA influenced the legislation that led to the legalization of medical assistance in dying (MAID). Prior to the passage of Bill C-14: An Act to Amend the *Criminal Code* and to Make Amendments to Other Acts (Medical Assistance in Dying), the CNA persuaded decision makers to change the name from "physician-assisted death" to the more inclusive "medical assistance in dying." This more inclusive title acknowledged the roles of nurse practitioners, registered nurses, and other health care providers in MAID.

The CNA used a variety of strategies to exert political influence, including distributing briefs to standing and special committees of government. A briefing note (Canadian Nurses Association, 2016) was developed to present a nursing perspective on ethics and human rights in end-of-life care and palliative care as options, with six priority requirements:
1. Safeguards to support individual decision making by patients;
2. Equitable and timely access to information about end-of-life options, including palliative care and physician-assisted death;
3. Support for patient choice through a person-centred approach;
4. Quality and safety mechanisms;
5. Equitable access to psychological support for health care providers; and
6. Protection of nurses and other health care providers under the *Criminal Code*. (p. 8–12)

Source: Canadian Nurses Association. (2016). *Physician-assisted dying: Brief for the Special Joint Committee on Physician-Assisted Dying (Based on CNA's Brief for the Government of Canada's External Panel on Options for a Legislative Response to Carter v. Canada).* Ottawa, ON: Author. Retrieved from https://www.cna-aiic.ca/-/media/cna/page-content/pdf-en/physician-assisted-dying-brief-for-the-special-joint-committee-on-physician-assisted-dying-january-2016.pdf.

For decades, nurses have exerted political influence for the delivery of primary care at a time when many

Canadians lack access to a primary care provider or team at the point of entry to a physician-dominated health system. Researchers have accumulated evidence demonstrating the effectiveness of services provided by nurses and the capacity for advancing their use (Aiken, Sloan, Bryneel et al., 2014; Chambers, Bruce-Lockhart, Black et al., 1977; Laurant, Reeves, Hermens et al., 2004; Hoey, McCallum, & LePage, 1982; Ramsay, McKenzie, & Fish, 1982). Despite barriers, nurse practitioners (NPs) and registered nurses (RNs) are now integrated at the point of entry within health systems across Canada. The CNA has worked with the Canadian Nurse Practitioner Association to remove barriers to NP practice and enable them to provide care in their full scope of practice (Canadian Nurses Association [CNA], 2016). Although physician numbers in Canada continue to rise at an ever-increasing rate, to the highest physician-to-population ratio in history, many Canadians lack access to a primary care provider. The increased use of NPs as an alternative to physicians is largely thanks to nursing's political influence with governments. It is critical that nurses embrace the fundamental tenets of team-based care, or **interprofessional collaboration**, consistent with nursing codes of ethics that place persons and communities as full partners in the design and delivery of nursing and health services (CNA, 2019). This collaboration extends to political action, with nurses collaborating with the public and other organizations to influence health and public policy (see Chapter 16).

The year 2020 marks the two-hundredth anniversary of Florence Nightingale's birth. In her honour, the WHO and the ICN have declared 2020 the Year of the Nurse and the Midwife, marking Nightingale's political influence and leadership in nursing and societal health. Both the WHO and ICN call for nurses to influence the directions of health care and health equity to meet the challenge of "health for all." As noted in the ICN Code of Ethics, "the need for nursing is universal," and nursing's political influence is key to ensuring that health for all is a human right (ICN, 2019). The Health for All framework depicts nursing's scope of influence, including nursing and health services, and the broad areas of public policy that determine health such as housing, income, and justice (ICN, 2019).

Nursing Now is a 3-year global campaign (2018–2020) jointly sponsored by the WHO, ICN, and Burdett Trust. Nursing Now aims to improve health globally by raising the profile and status of nursing worldwide—influencing policymakers and supporting nurses themselves to lead, learn, and build a social movement (Nursing Now, 2019). The premises underlying the campaign include the realization that nurses need more power to influence key decisions across the spectrum of nursing practice, health systems, and the broad public policy areas that determine health equity. This vision defines the most significant issues of the day and calls nurses to be politically engaged in transformational change for care delivery systems, universal health coverage, and human rights. The campaign is fundamentally about nurses bringing values-informed solutions to bear on the most pressing health and social issues of our time.

THE NURSING WORKFORCE AND HEALTH CARE SYSTEM CONTEXT IN CANADA

A significant component of any political strategy is to understand the broad context of trends in nursing and health workforce capacity as well as health system economics. In 2017, 48% of health care providers in Canada were regulated nurses (Canadian Institute for Health Information [CIHI], 2018). There is strength in numbers, and that is especially true where nursing is concerned: as the largest group of health care providers, nurses can maximize their power and influence by speaking and acting collectively.

Nurses have worked for over a century to advance their educational levels by obtaining baccalaureate, master's, and doctoral degrees. Nurses' educational attainment is rising relatively rapidly, with 52.3% of RNs in 2017 holding a baccalaureate degree (CNA, 2018). Nurses have also struggled against the gender stereotyping of their profession and the lack of value placed on care by a society that views it as women's work, with little to no recognition of its economic benefit nor of the emotional labour involved. Women made up 92% of the profession in 2017 and contributed 10.4% of the gross domestic product, or GDP (CIHI, 2018). In most medical schools, more than 50% of the students are women (CIHI, 2019). The gender stereotype in nursing remains firmly entrenched, with men not yet entering the nursing profession in rapidly increasing numbers—certainly not at the rate women are entering traditionally male-dominated professions. Nevertheless, changes are occurring because of the women's movement, increased recognition of human rights, and increased acknowledgement of nursing's valuable contribution to health and society. These factors bode well for nursing in the future, as arguments for restructuring and policy change in health and other areas of public policy are likely to engender considerable interest and support.

The Legislative and Economic Contexts of Health Care

Since the enactment of legislation establishing a national health insurance system for hospital and medical care, the philosophical basis of this system has been open to question. Historically, the proportion of private and public expenditures for health has remained relatively stable. Of health expenditures in 2019, 70.5% were funded from public sources, while 29.5% were privately funded (CIHI, 2019). Current categories of top health expenditures in Canada include hospitals (26%), prescribed drugs (13%), and physicians (15.1%) (CIHI, 2019). While overall spending on physicians and drugs continues to rise, public health spending remains low (5.4%) (CIHI, 2019). The public–private debate continues as more conservative elements of society argue for a system based entirely in the private sector, while those with socially democratic or liberal, equity-oriented views push for either maintaining the status quo or increasing the proportion of public-sector funding.

Since 10.7% of the GDP was attributed to health expenditures in Canada in 2018 (CIHI, 2019), any public-sector activity that involves a substantial expenditure of tax dollars provokes considerable debate and competition among providers of the service. This scenario is obvious in health care, where the various professions compete to increase their "share of the pie." Physicians have been extraordinarily successful in increasing income earned for services provided. Physicians' incomes have risen considerably over the past half century, attesting to the success they have had in the political arena. Nurses, through their unions and professional organizations, have demonstrated a growing ability to argue for proportionately greater compensation for their services. Significant gains have thus been made in past decades.

Although more men are joining the profession, nursing remains a gendered profession; gender plays a role in nursing's status, prestige, and ability to secure essential resources for the professional services provided. Members of the profession challenge the status quo assiduously and assertively, striving for higher salaries and better working conditions. Nurses have gained an understanding of the feminist processes involved in influencing others, becoming more powerful and exercising more control over the factors that influence their working lives through their unions and other organizations. Please refer to Chapter 5 for a more detailed discussion on gender in nursing.

As primarily public-sector employees, nurses find themselves within hierarchical and bureaucratized structures in health organizations. To achieve their goals, nurses must influence several levels within their organizations. Because health is a provincial responsibility at the level of the organized profession, nurses must approach provincial legislators with their ideas for change, as it is this level of government that is responsible for public health expenditures. At the national level, the professional association for nurses, the CNA, interacts with the federal government on national issues affecting health. Within each health agency, nurses must approach management with their ideas for systemic change. As most health agencies are unionized, the process for doing so at the agency level is usually clearly outlined.

 CULTURAL CONSIDERATIONS

Indigenous Nursing Leadership and Cultural Safety

Indigenous nurse leader Jean Goodwill led the development of the first national association for Indigenous nurses in 1975. The Aboriginal Nurses Association of Canada (ANAC) (now the Canadian Indigenous Nurses Association, or CINA) was a force in the development of nursing leadership and political action to promote health equity among Indigenous peoples. Goodwill's leadership style was one of serving as a leader and joining with other Indigenous and non-Indigenous organizations to promote health. She was recognized for her leadership with many awards and named an Officer of the Order of Canada in 1992 (Aboriginal Nurses Association of Canada, 2016).

It is important for all nurses to understand how Indigenous nurses—as both individuals and collectives—act politically to improve the **cultural safety** and **decolonization** of health care. With the recent history of residential schools and their legacy, it is critical that this decolonizing work continue and be supported by Canadian nursing as a whole. To this end, the CNA has identified an Indigenous pillar as one of the three pillars of the national Nursing Now campaign, with the goal of enabling culturally safe care by nurses and midwives. Specific strategies for action have yet to be identified. Culturally safe care will no doubt be one of the most important political advocacy issues of our time.

Source: Aboriginal Nurses Association of Canada/Canadian Indigenous Nurses Association. (2016). *Ninanâskomânânak Kâkînîkânohtêcik—We are grateful to the first leaders, 1975–2015*. Ottawa, ON: Author.

There are many other examples of nurses' political action for important public health measures. Nurses have campaigned to improve safety in the home, encourage governments to enact seat belt legislation, and promote the use of bicycle helmets. A review of websites of the various provincial and territorial nurses' associations gives an indication of the range of issues being addressed today by organized nursing in Canada.

Political Action by Nursing Students

Nursing students have also engaged in political activism to raise important issues. They have used a variety of strategies to champion their causes, including media advocacy, briefing notes and interviews, position statements, and letter writing. When the province-wide baccalaureate Nursing Education Program of Saskatchewan was developed in the 1990s (College of Nursing & University of Saskatchewan, 2009), the provincial government attempted to put a diploma exit in place. However, it was thwarted by nursing students, who protested at the legislature in Regina with suitcases in hand, threatening to leave the province if the proposal went ahead.

More recently, the Canadian Nursing Students' Association (CNSA) championed diversity and Indigenous health and cultural safety and sought to address critical issues in the NCLEX-RN exam (Canadian Nursing Students' Association, 2019). The CNSA promotes the development of political engagement skills among nursing students; the organization is a powerful vehicle for advancing the influence of the profession for years to come. In a letter to leaders of other **nursing organizations**, the students articulated their request for an open dialogue regarding their concerns about the exam; they noted that "the NCLEX-RN exam contains major omissions of Canadian nursing competencies including Indigenous health and cultural safety. . . [and its] power dimensions." Please refer to the CNSA website to review advocacy resources and events related to the NCLEX-RN exam.

> ### APPLYING CONTENT KNOWLEDGE
>
> 1. From your perspective, reflect on the argument that nursing makes a difference to health through political action. What is meant by a political imperative?
> 2. Discuss the role of power in nurses' and nursing's political action and strategy.
> 3. Identify issues of relevance to nursing in each of the four spheres of policy influence that you would anticipate in the coming decade.

CREATING POLITICAL AWARENESS

Understanding the Fundamentals of Political Action

Nurses can greatly enhance the achievement of their goals by learning how to work within the formal and informal systems in the workplace. Although understanding both is essential, comprehending the informal structures and processes of an organization is a more difficult and nebulous task than understanding formal ones. There is no substitute for understanding how an organization works or for thinking carefully about the nature and scope of problems and how they might be solved.

Although individual nurses may not see themselves as capable of taking political action to achieve a goal they have in mind, those who do venture forth are often amazed that elected officials are eager to hear what they have to say and show respect for their ideas. In fact, the informed nurse, whether a student or not, is capable of communicating ideas effectively and being a positive asset in a campaign to achieve health care goals. Nurses are among the most highly educated and trusted of professional and occupational groups and are skilled in working with people and the media, as well as expressing ideas. Thus, they tend to be highly effective communicators and command respect from others because of their knowledge and deep understanding of health needs.

Another way for individual nurses to become politically engaged is to understand the positions of political parties on health issues. Nurses might attend all-candidates' meetings during local, provincial, territorial, or national elections to bring voice to patient care and health care. In voicing their opinions and asking questions of political candidates, nurses can raise public awareness of issues and identify political agendas that might best lead to equity in access to essential health services and health public policy. For instance, in the 2016 and 2019 Canadian federal elections, the CNA identified the health agendas of all the political parties and raised awareness of the implications for nurses and the public (CNA, 2019; Whyte & Duncan, 2016).

Nursing organizations in Canada are currently undergoing significant transitions that alter their capacity for political and policy influence. Over the past decade, the political environment has led to the development of regulatory bodies or colleges in nursing, which in turn has affected how nursing associations can express collectivity and have influence in policy spheres. Nursing must ensure that it continues to develop its collective capacity to advocate for the most critical health issues of our time, especially because there is a growing critique that the former advocacy potential of nursing associations may be reduced in current contexts (Whyte & Duncan, 2016). It is time to examine how individual nursing students and nurses engage with and support their nursing organizations, as their participation is the foundation of the voice and influence of the profession.

Nurses also hold positions as governors of nursing and other organizations. As members of boards of directors, nurses have the power to set policy directions that determine resource allocation and the vision and contributions of organizations, including nursing associations. Developing the competencies to serve on boards of directors is deemed essential for nurses to be able to maximize their contributions to high-level policy directions. These competencies including an astute understanding of power relationships, emancipatory knowing, confidence in one's contribution, and ability to articulate values-informed policies; nurses are well positioned for these roles (Myrick & Pepin, 2019; Peart & McKinnon, 2018). Nurses are making concerted efforts to position themselves to play a role in organizational board governance, including at community agencies, financial institutions, school boards, and the array of organizations that influence individuals and communities (Benson & Harper, 2017). There is also growing awareness of the need for a feminist perspective on knowledge and power to fully enact nursing influence in board governance (Sundean & Polifroni, 2016).

A deep understanding of power in relationships is an essential pillar of political strategy. Those wielding substantial power within the organization should be identified as key individuals, and the development of working relationships with these people is essential. Informal groups and social contacts within the organization may also be important. And although they may be organized around activities unrelated to the organization, these networks may represent opportunities for exchange of information and political activity. It is essential that nurses hold positions in top administrative and governance roles in organizations, and it is critical that nurses in these leadership positions use their power to promote the nursing perspective—one that is inclusive of the values and knowledge needed for health—in policy and political processes.

Nurses must be risk takers. Timing is essential to achieving any goal. All sides of a policy problem, issue, or challenge must be understood in order to develop a more effective strategy; furthermore, negotiation and compromise may be required in determining solutions and directions. Consider the example provided by Linda Silas, President of the Canadian Federation of Nurses Unions. She has led a political initiative with nursing and other organizations calling for a national pharmacare strategy. The CFNU's advocacy for this national program has included political strategies such as developing an evidence-informed policy submission that contains clear recommendations for a pharmacare program, hosting consensus conferences with Canada's premiers, and joining a coalition of 75 national, provincial, and territorial organizations to sign onto a set of consensus principles that would form "the basis of a truly effective and equitable program" (Canadian Federation of Nurses Unions, 2019).

RESEARCH FOCUS

The origins of outreach nursing in Canada can be found in the work of Marguerite d'Youville, who founded the Grey Nuns in 1737. Other examples of social activism for health include Florence Nightingale in the United Kingdom in the nineteenth century; Lillian Wald in the United States in the twentieth century; and Lady Ishbel Aberdeen in Canada, who founded the Victorian Order of Nurses, also in the twentieth century. This unique work examines the origins of "street nursing" in Vancouver, Toronto, and Montreal and in doing so addresses a topic that has received little attention in the literature. Written by a nurse with a strong background in outreach nursing, this work underscores the need for political advocacy for vulnerable populations, in particular for those who are homeless and living in poverty. Indeed, a convincing case is made for political advocacy on behalf of the members of marginalized groups in Canadian society.

Source: Hardill, K. (2006). From the Grey Nuns to the streets: A critical history of outreach nursing in Canada. *Public Health Nursing, 24*(1), 91–97.

POLITICAL VOICE AND COMMUNICATION

Speaking with a persuasive and informed voice is key to successful advocacy in the political arena. Because politics involves influencing others, the ability to form effective relationships and engage in skilled communications is essential. It is impossible to influence others if interpersonal activity is not positive and dynamic. As discussed earlier in this chapter, communication is the fundamental skill in political action, as all other techniques build on it. By communicating effectively with others, goals can be enhanced and attained. Approaching others with respect and understanding increases the likelihood of effective political activity.

Cooperating with others in pursuit of collective goals is both an effective way to achieve those goals as well as an effective political strategy. Nursing has recently focused more attention on networking or joining together with others to achieve common goals. Networking is an important political strategy and can be personally rewarding. Students can develop these skills through informal means and through their nursing education. For instance, nursing curricula in baccalaureate and graduate programs contain courses designed to enhance persuasive communications, including teaching students how to write policy positions, briefs, and blog posts.

Because nurses are in close contact with their patients and other people virtually everywhere in the community, nurses are compelled to "paint a picture" of the ways that people experience health and illness and the contributions nursing makes to health care and health more broadly

(Buresh & Gordon, 2013). Narratives of nursing experiences from all walks of life and nursing are powerful influences in the development of political strategy.

The advent of social media as vehicles for communication in the twenty-first century is revolutionizing communication around the world. In the sphere of politics, legislators who ignore the power of digital media and technologies for communicating with their constituents do so at their peril. People are increasingly turning to web-based health resources and social media to help them understand their health issues. With a strong background in communication, nurses are well placed to assume prominent roles in developing and maintaining e-health and telehealth-based resources.

DEVELOPING A BASE OF SUPPORT

Consolidating and developing a base of support often takes considerable skill and time. Credibility must be established, and the desire to work in the best interests of the organization and its goals must be demonstrated. In professional associations, this means working with the public interest in mind. Nurses need to demonstrate that clear and careful thought preceded the development of a campaign for support on a particular issue, as it can be a powerful factor in convincing potential allies that the issue is worth supporting. As noted previously, there is power in numbers, and nursing has a great advantage in this respect. A political action initiative is more likely to be successful if many people are committed to working toward the goal. Although nurses have not always recognized the strength in their numbers, they have been successful in the past in mobilizing group support on crucial issues. Many nursing organizations now recognize this potent force and are using its power to their advantage, including working strategically with patients and communities to bring voice to health issues and solutions.

In a show of collective power, the CNA and CINA recently issued a joint statement of support for a motion introduced in the House of Commons in May 2019 for the creation of a national suicide prevention action plan. The nursing organizations' position recognizes how vital collaborative and community-informed processes are to addressing the incidence of suicide among young people in Indigenous communities. Joining their perspectives and strength in support of this motion undoubtedly contributed to the unanimous vote in favour of the action plan on May 9, 2019 (CNA & CINA, 2018). It is especially important for non-Indigenous nurses and Indigenous nurses and organizations to co-organize politically and advocate for the implementation of the Truth and Reconciliation Commission of Canada (2015) Calls to Action and for the United Nations Declaration on the Rights of Indigenous peoples (United Nations, 2007); advocating for Indigenous peoples is the most critical health equity movement of our time.

POLITICAL STRATEGY

Enacting an effective political strategy is a labor-intensive process that requires clear thinking and the ability to recognize factors, processes, and actors of importance. Identifying an issue or problem is crucial (Box 18.2), and its relative importance must be measured against that of other issues or problems that arise. Action cannot be taken in all matters, so it is wise to carefully choose one's priorities for policy agendas. Analysis is essential to determine whether pursuing the issue is reasonable. Once a decision has been made to pursue a particular goal, additional analysis determines what other resources might be helpful.

Because every issue is different, a plan of action should be outlined for the benefit of all those involved in a political campaign. The leaders of a campaign need to determine how the issue will be dealt with, both formally and informally. It is possible that many avenues will need to be taken to argue for or against the issue of concern. These need to be outlined at the outset and revised as necessary.

BOX 18.2   How Can Nursing Students and Registered Nurses Become Politically Involved?

- Join and maintain membership and engagement with professional and health associations
- Submit resolutions to professional organizations at annual meetings to take action on health issues
- Become informed and engage with the public in developing solutions and strategies for health advocacy
- Talk to your neighbours and co-workers about policy issues impacting health
- Speak out at organizational meetings or all-candidates' meetings during elections
- Never back down or apologize for bringing an informed nursing perspective to public policy
- Write to your federal or provincial representative about a health policy issue that is important to you
- Lend your expertise and voice as an RN, NP, or nursing student to a community issue
- Run for elected office
- Develop skills to serve as a board member of nursing and health organizations, bringing your voice and policy perspective on health.

Source: Adapted from Registered Nurses' Association of Ontario. (2015, April). *Taking action: A toolkit for becoming politically involved* (p. 8). Toronto, ON: Author. Retrieved from https://rnao.ca/sites/rnao-ca/files/Taking_Action_Political_Action_Toolkit_Final_0.pdf.

The Nursing Now campaign includes an advocacy tool-kit to assist nurses in developing political campaigns by following a five-step road map. The road map guides nurses in appropriately investing their time to define the policy problem, its root causes, and the desired outcome, as well conducting an analysis of power relationships for change. A strategic approach to political action and advocacy is essential to determining the success and failure of nursing initiatives on a global scale. Nursing Now also includes resources for social media campaigns and case studies illustrating how nurses are organizing politically for health around the world.

🔲 APPLYING CONTENT KNOWLEDGE

1. Visit the Nursing Now social media toolkit webpage. Consider how nursing students might launch a social media campaign on a global health issue to raise awareness among the public and politicians.
2. Visit the CNA and ICN websites to identify their policy advocacy and political action initiatives. Consider how these relate to your experiences as a nursing student in various practice settings. Consider the issues that you would like to see championed by nursing organizations and why.

NURSING'S POLITICAL IMPERATIVE AS ESSENTIAL TO HEALTH EQUITY IN THE TWENTY-FIRST CENTURY

In the current era of global health challenges, nurses around the world are called upon to ensure that health and access to universal health care is upheld as a basic human right. These global and public policy agendas require an intense commitment to a political strategy based on a nursing perspective. Political influence in nursing has never been more significant and never more challenging. Nurses must act politically as individuals and as members of collectives—through professional associations or unions, through governing boards of nursing and health care organizations—to effect changes within regional, national, and provincial/territorial health and global policy spheres.

Over the next decade until 2030, nurses and the organizations that represent them have a profound opportunity to contribute to the success of the United Nations Sustainable Development Goals for health equity. Expanded awareness, skilled communication, and joining with the public to influence policy and politics are essential elements of nursing practice. New models and theories of conceptualizing and enacting nursing's political imperative are needed to inform the call for action for global health and equity.

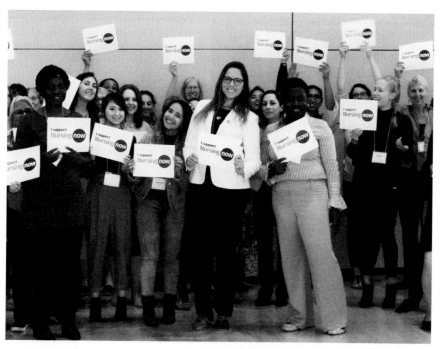

Nursing students launch a Nursing Now initiative at The University of British Columbia. (UBC Graduate Students in Nursing Association, © Gabriel Morosan)

SUMMARY OF LEARNING OBJECTIVES

- A political imperative constitutes a call to action for nurses and nursing to exert power and influence in the direction of health and health equity.
- A nursing perspective is an essential contribution to achieving each of the United Nations Sustainable Development Goals and in responding to the Truth and Reconciliation Commission of Canada's Calls to Action.
- Nurses must have a deep understanding of power and think critically about positions of influence in health policy.

- Nurses must understand the strategy of political action, including communications, social media, coalitions, and partnerships.
- Nurses must act politically with the support of others in community and organizations related to the health issue at hand.
- Nurses must influence political processes as individuals and as members of nursing and other organizations and collectives.

CRITICAL THINKING QUESTIONS

1. Discuss the role of professional associations and unions in political action.
2. What are some of the priority issues for national nursing associations to advocate on behalf of people in Canada and globally?
3. Identify ways that individual nurses can express themselves politically.

REFERENCES

Aiken, L., Sloane, D. M., Bryneel, L. M., et al. (2014). Nurse staffing and education and hospital mortality in nine European countries: A retrospective observational study. *Lancet, 383*(9931), 1824–1830. https://doi.org/10.1016/S0140-6736(13)62631-8.

Benson, L., & Harper, K. J. (2017). Why your nurses should serve on community health boards. *Boardroom Press, 28*(1). Retrieved from https://www.nursesonboardscoalition.org/resources/.

Blackburn, S. (1994). *Oxford dictionary of philosophy.* Oxford, UK: Oxford University Press.

Buresh, B., & Gordon, S. (2013). *From silence to voice—What nurses know and must communicate to the public* (2nd ed.). Ithaca, NY: ILR Press.

Canadian Federation of Nurses Unions. (2019). *CFNU's pharmacare recommendations.* Retrieved from https://nursesunions.ca/campaigns/pharmacare/.

Canadian Institute for Health Information. (2018). *Regulated Nurses, 2017.* Retrieved from https://www.cihi.ca/en/regulated-nurses-2017.

Canadian Institute for Health Information. (2019). *National health expenditure trends 1975 to 2019.* Retrieved from https://www.cihi.ca/sites/default/files/document/nhex-trends-narrative-report-2019-en-web.pdf.

Canadian Nurses Association. (2016, November). *Position statement: The nurse practitioner.* Ottawa, ON: Author. Retrieved from https://www.cna-aiic.ca/-/media/cna/page-content/pdf-en/the-nurse-practitioner-position-statement_2016.pdf.

Canadian Nurses Association. (2016, January). *Brief: Physician-Assisted Dying.* Ottawa, ON: Author. Retrieved from https://www.cna-aiic.ca/-/media/cna/page-content/pdf-en/physician-assisted-dying-brief-for-the-special-joint-committee-on-physician-assisted-dying-january-2016.pdf?la=en&hash=C1E135B9760551FCBACC78DB24EFCC0ED80AE0B8.

Canadian Nurses Association. (2018). *2005 workforce profile of registered nurses in Canada.* Ottawa, ON: CNA. Retrieved from https://www.cna-aiic.ca/en/nursing-practice/the-practice-of-nursing/health-human-resources/nursing-statistics/canada.

Canadian Nurses Association. (2019). *Position statement: Interprofessional collaboration.* Retrieved from https://www.cna-aiic.ca/-/media/cna/page-content/pdf-en/interprofessional-collaboration-ps-2019.pdf.

Canadian Nurses Association & Canadian Indigenous Nursing Association. (2018). *Joint statement of support for motion to create a national suicide prevention action plan.* Retrieved from https://www.cna-aiic.ca/en/news-room/news-releases/2018/joint-statement-of-support-from-cna-and-cina-for-motion-to-create-national-suicide-prevention-action-plan.

Canadian Nursing Students' Association. (2019). *About us.* Retrieved from http://cnsa.ca/about-us.

Chambers, L. W., Bruce-Lockhart, P., Black, D. P., et al. (1977). A controlled trial of the impact of the family practice nurse on volume, quality, and cost of rural health service. *Medical Care, 15*(12), 971–981.

Cohen, S. S., Mason, D. J., Kovner, C., et al. (1996). Stages of nursing's political development: Where we've been and where we ought to go. *Nursing Outlook, 44*(6), 259–266.

College of Nursing & University of Saskatchewan. (2009). *History of the College of Nursing*. Retrieved http://www.usask.ca/nursing/college/history.php.

Dossey, B. (2010). *Florence Nightingale: Mystic, visionary, healer.* Philadelphia, PA: FA Davis.

Dossey, B., Rosa, W. E., & Beck, D. (2019). Nursing and the sustainable development goals: from Nightingale to now. *American Journal of Nursing, 119*(5), 44–49.

Duncan, S., & Whyte, N. (2019, September 13). *Aligning our public policy influence with the international nursing community.* Retrieved from https://www.nnpbc.com/blog/aligning-our-public-policy-influence-with-the-international-nursing-community-by-susan-duncan-and-nora-whyte/.

Hoey, J. R., McCallum, H. P., & LePage, E. M. (1982). Expanding the nurse's role to improve preventive service in an outpatient clinic. *Canadian Medical Association Journal, 127*(1), 27–28.

International Council of Nurses. (2018a). *International Council of Nurses annual report 2016–2017.* Geneva, Switzerland: Author. Retrieved from https://www.icn.ch/who-we-are/icn-annual-reports.

International Council of Nurses. (2018b). *Position statement: Evidence-based safe nurse staffing.* Retrieved from https://www.icn.ch/sites/default/files/inline-files/ICN%20PS%20Evidence%20based%20safe%20nurse%20staffing.pdf.

International Council of Nurses. (2019). *Nurses—A voice to lead health for all.* Retrieved from https://2019.icnvoicetolead.com/wp-content/uploads/2017/04/ICN_Design_EN.pdf.

Laurant, M., Reeves, D., Hermens, R., et al. (2004). Substitution of doctors by nurses in primary care. *Cochrane Database of Systematic Reviews* (Issue 4). https://doi.org//10.1002/14651858.CD001271.pub2.

MacDonald, C., & McIntyre, M. (Eds.). (2019). *Realities of Canadian nursing—Professional, practice and power issues* (5th ed.). Philadelphia, PA: Wolters Kluwer.

Myrick, F., & Pepin, J. I. (2019). Governance education: Preparing nurses of influence in contemporary times. *Quality Advancement in Nursing Education, 5*(2), article 8.

Nursing Now. (2019). *Social media toolkit.* Retrieved from https://www.nursingnow.org/.

Pal, L. (2006). *Beyond policy analysis: public issues management in turbulent times.* Toronto, ON: Nelson.

Peart, J., & McKinnon, K. (2018). Cultivating praxis through Chinn and Kramer's emancipatory knowing. *Advances in Nursing Science, 41*(4), 351–358.

Ramsay, J. A., McKenzie, J. K., & Fish, D. G. (1982). Physicians and nurse practitioners: Do they provide equivalent health care? *American Journal of Public Health, 72*(1), 55–57.

Roberts, J. (2009). *Routledge philosophy guidebook to Aristotle and the politics.* New York, NY: Routledge.

Shamian, J. (2014). Global perspectives on nursing and its contribution to healthcare and health policy: Thoughts on an emerging policy model. *Nursing Leadership, 27*(4), 44–50. https://doi.org/10.12927/cjnl.2015.24140.

Sundean, L. J., & Polifroni, E. C. (2016). A feminist framework for nurses on boards. *Journal of Professional Nursing, 32*(6), 396–400.

Truth and Reconciliation Commission of Canada. (2015). *Honouring the truth, reconciling for the future: Summary of the final report of the Truth and Reconciliation Commission of Canada.* Retrieved from http://www.trc.ca/assets/pdf/Honouring_the_Truth_Reconciling_for_the_Future_July_23_2015.pdf.

United Nations (2007). *United Nations Declaration on the Rights of Indigenous Peoples.* Retrieved from https://www.un.org/development/desa/indigenouspeoples/wp-content/uploads/sites/19/2018/11/UNDRIP_E_web.pdf.

Whyte, N. B., & Duncan, S. (2016). Engaging nursing voice and presence during the federal election campaign 2015. *Nursing Leadership, 29*(4), 19–34. https://doi.org/10.12927/cjnl.2016.24986.

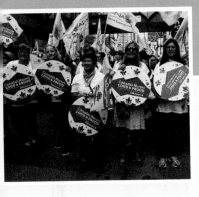

Nursing Unions as a Social Force in Canada: Advocating for Nurses, Patients, and Health Care

Linda Haslam-Stroud

LEARNING OBJECTIVES

After reading this chapter, you will be able to:

- Describe catalysts to the development of nursing unions in each jurisdiction in Canada.
- Describe the establishment, membership, and role of the Canadian Federation of Nurses Unions.
- Describe the gradual evolution of nursing unions in each province and territory in Canada and the impact of unions on the socioeconomic welfare and work life of nurses and health care quality.
- Describe the nature of professional responsibility clauses and their role in patient care advocacy.

- Discuss the impact of nursing unions on health and safety in the workplace.
- Explain the issue of the right to strike and its impact on nursing in certain provinces.
- Identify the juxtaposition of unions and professionalism and how they work together.
- Understand advocacy efforts of nurses' unions to preserve Medicare.

OUTLINE

KEY TERMS

bargaining agent
bargaining unit(s)
Canadian Federation of Nurses
    Unions

collective agreement
collective bargaining
duty of fair representation
labour relations legislation

neoliberalism
professional responsibility language
Rand formula

PERSONAL PERSPECTIVES

We as nurses have come a long way since the day I graduated from nursing at the age of 18. In 1977, we still wore nursing caps, and some nurses who had graduated before me still stood up when physicians entered the nursing station. I found it odd that we, as nurses, predominantly female, were not equal partners in the health care system. I knew we could be so much more by advocating for our patients and our profession. But at that point I wasn't sure how.

I didn't know what a union was when I graduated—until I needed one. The year before getting married, I requested to use a stat holiday so that I could take the day off for my wedding. I was denied that request because "stat holidays couldn't be taken on a weekend." The nurse beside me in the nursing station told me that the union could help me get my wedding day off—and they did!

The rest is history. I was invited to a bargaining unit meeting, agreed to take on a role on the union executive, and for the next 40 years was a union and health care leader. The union led me on a path to grow as a nursing leader, advocating for nurses, their professional practice, occupational health and safety, pay equity, reasonable workloads and schedules, vacation, education leaves, human rights and equity, including the rights of the LGBTQ2 community, persons with disabilities, Indigenous people, and racialized people. I was also proud to spearhead student–union liaisons and affiliate membership for nursing students in our union.

Who would have imagined that being denied my wedding day off would open the door to having the privilege of leading the Ontario Nurses' Association, the union representing over 65,000 registered nurses, nurse practitioners, registered practical nurses, and health professionals? It gave me the right to represent a group of respected nursing professionals who provide quality care, influence health policy, and serve as the foundation of health care in Canada.

INTRODUCTION

In the century following Florence Nightingale's championing of nursing as a legitimate and respectable profession for laywomen, it was never expected that nurses would engage in strike action. Indeed, it is unlikely that the rise of powerful and independent nursing unions could have been foreseen even at the midpoint of the twentieth century. Nurses were not looked upon as professional independent practitioners as they are today. There continues to be growing advocacy among nurses who believe that their skills and the essential nature of their contributions have been undervalued and overlooked. The new employment environment is characterized by a negotiation framework centered on skill-based remuneration (pay equity). The power of unions has been challenged by some provincial governments, and most unions have felt the impact of these threats to their hard-earned power base. However, the membership numbers of nursing unions have increased, unlike those of most other unions, and their relevance continues.

Although the majority of nurses are covered by union contracts, some groups of nurses are not represented by unions. Many nurse managers and nurses in private practice are not covered by union contracts. For nurses working in a unionized setting, under Canadian labour law, the **Rand formula** provides that any nurses covered under the union contract must pay dues. However, nurses' unions are not closed shops where nurses are required to belong to the union as a condition of employment. Accordingly, nurses can choose not to be union members. Even in those cases, nonmembers are covered by all the provisions of the **collective agreement** (including the right and obligation to pay union dues pursuant to the Rand formula). Nonmembers are also owed a **duty of fair representation** by the union in the event that their rights are violated. In addition, non-members may attend a ratification meeting to vote on a collective agreement.

Although provinces show considerable variation in the approach and achievements of unions, nursing unions have increasingly directed their energy to consolidating membership, withstanding threats to structural integrity, maintaining the right to negotiate collective agreements on behalf of members, and improving nurses' socioeconomic welfare. The impact of a worldwide climate of economic constraint and downsizing, both in the mid-1990s and again in the late 2000s, led to severe and almost overnight downsizing of the health care system. Widespread public-sector salary restraint in most provinces during each downturn has created an environment in which all unions struggle to preserve their mandates. These issues underscore the fact that economic conditions tend to be cyclical and exert a strong effect on nursing, health care, and the patients that nurses serve.

THE RISE OF NURSING UNIONS

The Catalyst for the Development of Nursing Unions in Canada

In Canada, as well as in other countries, professional nursing associations have played key roles in the development of nursing unions. However, everything changed in Canada in 1973 because of a Saskatchewan case that was appealed to the Supreme Court of Canada. At issue was a dispute between the Service Employees International Union and the Saskatchewan Registered Nurses' Association (SRNA) over the SRNA's application for certification as a **bargaining agent**. The union charged that the SRNA should not be permitted to act as a trade union because its board of directors included nursing managers. The Court ruled in favour of the union. This radically altered labour relations in nursing in Canada in little more than a decade. Because the rules governing the structure of the SRNA allowed for the election of nursing managers to its governing body, the association was presumed to have an inherent bias (or conflict of interest) that precluded participation in **collective bargaining**. Thus, the way was paved for establishing new organizations across the country to assume the collective bargaining function of the professional associations.

Stance of the Canadian Nurses Association

The Canadian Nurses Association (CNA) approved the principle of collective bargaining for nurses in the 1940s and affirmed that the bargaining agent at the provincial and territorial level should be the professional nursing association. The passage of the federal *Labour Relations Act* in 1944, which gave federal employees collective bargaining rights, was likely instrumental in the CNA's decision to support collective bargaining among its member associations. The CNA also supported a no-strike policy, a stand that became controversial two decades later and was subsequently repealed.

The First Bargaining Agent for Nurses in Canada

After the 1944 decision, nurses were concerned about possible management domination from the boards of directors of provincial associations (Rowsell, 1982). Because there was no formal collective bargaining at that time, the provincial associations struggled with the issues facing nurses in their work. Shortly after, member organizations informed the CNA that it was not legally possible for them to act as bargaining agents. The first breakthrough in provincial **labour relations legislation** appeared in 1946, when the Registered Nurses Association of British Columbia (RNABC) became the first provincial association to successfully apply for certification as a bargaining agent under the provincial labour relations act, beginning a movement that would eventually involve all provinces and territories.

The "Personnel Policies" Approach

Although they were not permitted to be formally involved in collective bargaining, the other nine provincial associations became engaged in promoting the social and economic welfare of their memberships in a less formal and proactive manner. It became customary in most provinces to publish annual personnel policies giving recommendations on salaries and working conditions. The associations then discussed the recommendations with employers or hospital associations. The personnel policies were not binding and often not implemented, leading to disillusionment with the process and its results. The failure to make progress using the personnel policy approach led to a search for a more effective way to influence salary and wage decisions.

Professional Associations Attempt to "Take Up the Torch"

During the expansionist decade of the 1960s, most of the provincial professional associations became more assertive in applying for the right to bargain collectively for the large groups of nurses employed by health care agencies. Several factors set the stage for this new phase of development in nursing organizations. The economy was finally booming after a slow recovery through the postwar period, and workers were making gains in financial status. The Royal Commission on the Status of Women in Canada (1967–1970) drew attention to the need for equal opportunity for women in society and for removing inequities in a system that inadequately remunerated women. Society's new optimism brought what had seemed impossible in the past into the realm of the possible.

Professional nursing associations in all provinces and territories except British Columbia could not be certified under provincial labour laws in the early 1960s. This restriction allowed professional associations within each province and territory to establish an important role for themselves: they began teaching staff nurses in hospitals and community health agencies about collective bargaining and helped them to organize staff nurses' associations. Except in PEI, these organizations became the **bargaining units** that were eventually certified under the various labour acts. By the time of the Supreme Court decision that led to the separation of professional associations and unions, nurses had gained some experience and expertise in collective bargaining. As of 1987, the process was complete, and the dual structure was then in place in all provinces and territories.

Changes in the Roles of Professional Associations Following Separation

Because professional nursing associations were no longer responsible for collective bargaining, their attention now centered more on health care policy. Instead, they focused on serving the public interest by improving standards of nursing education and practice, promoting nursing research, and, along with the unions, interacting with government and other health care professions.

In 1973, professional associations and regulatory bodies were still one entity in most provinces except Ontario (the organizations had separated in 1963). After 2010, the regulatory bodies in many other provinces and territories commenced a separation process from their nursing associations, thus creating three nursing bodies in each province: the union, the professional organization, and the provincial regulatory body. Provincial membership fees and dues in most provinces and territories were now paid to these three entities.

The provincial unions were founded between 1973 and 1987 (Silversides, 2019). The union dues voted on by the union members now supported the labour-intensive negotiations by unions—striving to achieve collective agreements that reflected the value and worth of nurses. As the unions evolved, they also became involved in government relations advocacy, professional issues, and public policy.

CANADIAN FEDERATION OF NURSES UNIONS

Parallel to the development of provincial nursing unions, there were those who directed their efforts at establishing a national voice for unionized nurses. The **Canadian Federation of Nurses Unions** (CFNU) is the national voice advocating for nurses and quality public health care. The CFNU has upheld its vision as a strong national voice for unionized nurses in Canada and is part of the world voice for unionized nurses. The CFNU acts as the collective voice

of Canada's frontline nurses, representing nurses to governments and the national media, in order to protect and improve the quality of health care for patients and to safeguard and enhance our public health care system.

With the implementation of wage and price controls by the federal government and the publication of a controversial professional code of ethics drafted by the CNA in the late 1970s—which implied nurses' strikes were unethical because they placed self-interest, high wages, and improved working conditions before the needs of patients—unionized nurses were increasingly convinced of the need for a more formal national structure to support their interests. In 1981, these discussions led to a founding convention in Winnipeg, and on May 1, 1981, International Workers' Day, the National Federation of Nurses Unions (NFNU) was established to represent unionized nurses across Canada. Founding member organizations were the New Brunswick Nurses Union, Newfoundland and Labrador Nurses' Union, Manitoba Organization of Nurses' Associations, Prince Edward Island Provincial Collective Bargaining Committee, and the Saskatchewan Union of Nurses. Some of the NFNU's first objectives included developing common bargaining goals, advocating for the standardization of working conditions for nurses across the country, and becoming a national voice to speak for nurses on major issues (Silversides, 2019; Canadian Federation of Nurses Unions [CFNU], 2019a).

Early on, the federation recognized that nurses were concerned about broader issues relating to the health care system and social justice. In 1982, the federation joined the Canadian Health Coalition. In 1987, the NFNU opened a national office in Ottawa with a full-time president. In 1998, it joined the Canadian Labour Congress. And in 1999, in recognition of its growing global outreach, the NFNU was formally renamed the CFNU. In 2007, the CFNU began representing nursing students through the Canadian Nursing Students' Association when it joined CFNU as an associate member. In 2013, the CFNU extended its international networks by helping to found Global Nurses United (GNU) along with the leaders of other major health care unions around the world. The GNU rapidly expanded to include representatives from 24 nations committed to the goal of safeguarding public health and quality patient care through safe staffing, in the face of global privatization efforts and climate change. The CFNU also promotes justice abroad via its International Solidarity Fund and, along with the CNA, is a member of the International Council of Nurses (ICN) International Workforce Forum, a federation of over 130 national nurses' associations representing more than 20 million nurses worldwide (Silversides, 2019; CFNU, 2019a).

As of 2019, CFNU member organizations include all provincial nurses' unions except those from Quebec and

British Columbia. The federation has close to 200,000 nurses and student nurse members from across Canada, including nurses working in hospitals, the community, home, industry, and long-term care. The foundation of CFNU's national advocacy campaigns is evidence-informed research presented in readily accessible materials to governments, decision makers, its membership, and the general public. CFNU's elected officials and National Executive Board members have met with premiers, federal cabinet ministers, and provincial health ministers and developed and released peer-reviewed research publications and position statements on a wide range of issues. These activities have helped the CFNU to advocate for shared health care approaches, such as safe staffing, occupational health and safety, universal pharmacare, and safe seniors care.

Advocacy Campaigns

Safe Staffing

A priority issue for the CFNU and its member affiliates is the issue of safe staffing. With many provinces experiencing nurse shortages, and some provinces reporting many vacant nursing positions, the CFNU's advocacy on this issue is becoming increasingly important. As Canada's population continues to age, an increasing number of people are living with long-term chronic diseases. Only the sickest patients are being admitted to hospitals—meaning higher patient acuity levels in acute care—but without an increase in staffing levels to meet the greater demand. High acuity levels can potentially contribute to an increased nursing workload, erosion of the quality of nurses' work environments, as well as diminished patient safety and public confidence in the health care system.

Research indicates that when hospitals have better nurse-to-patient ratios, meaning fewer patients per nurse or more direct nursing care hours per patient per day, there is a corresponding increase in patient satisfaction and a decrease in adverse outcomes (Berry & Curry, 2012; MacPhee, 2014; Canadian Nurses Association [CNA] & Canadian Federation of Nurses Unions [CFNU], 2015). Examples of adverse patient outcomes linked to inadequate staffing are higher mortality rates, death following preventable complications, postoperative and urinary infections, falls, and improper pain management (Aiken, Clarke, Sloane et al., 2002; Ball, Bruyneel, Aiken et al., 2017; Cimiotti, Aiken, Sloane, & Wu, 2012; Duffield, Diers, O'Brien-Pallas et al., 2011; Needleman, Buerhaus, Mattke et al., 2002; Needleman, Buerhaus, Pankratz et al., 2011; Rafferty, Clarke, Coles et al., 2007; Schubert, Clark, Aiken, & de Geest, 2012; Shindul-Rothschild, Flanagan, Stamp, & Read, 2017). The CFNU has produced several documents outlining how the cuts to nurse staffing affect patient care and

health outcomes, including *Nursing Workload and Patient Care* (Berry & Curry, 2012) and *Valuing Patient Safety: Responsible Workforce Design* (MacPhee, 2014). It also co-created, with the CNA, an online *Evidence-Based Safe Nurse Staffing Toolkit* (CNA & CFNU, 2015), an accessible resource meant to help frontline nurses and nurse managers make an effective case for safe staffing. The CFNU became involved with 12 interprofessional groups to develop strategies that would address the quality of work life of Canada's health care providers as a way to improve patient care and health system outcomes.

The CFNU has also explored health care innovations internationally to address nurse-to-patient ratios, nursing hours per patient day (NHPPD), and the Care Capacity Demand Management Programme (CCDM) of the New Zealand Nurses Organisation. The CFNU produced a series of information pamphlets, called *mythbusters*, to promote evidence-informed research around appropriate staffing mix and the resulting savings to the health care system. CFNU's work with international partners has identified the foundation of any safe staffing program: adequate base staffing that accounts for vacations and sick leave paired with accurate real-time data to identify the acuity level of patients (in all wards and all sectors) (MacPhee, 2014).

The CFNU has expressed concerns over the proportion of registered nurses within Canada. There has been a decline in the proportion of registered nurses relative to the number of regulated nurses in Canada. Chapter 17 further explores this issue in detail.

Another key workforce issue for the CFNU is the working conditions of nurses. The CFNU compared increases in overtime in 2016 versus 2014, estimating that public-sector health care nurses worked 20.1 million hours of both paid and unpaid overtime at a cost of $968 million in a single year (Jacobson Consulting Inc., 2017). This number is equivalent to 11,100 full-time positions, which may suggest that overtime is being used as a regular part of scheduling in health care facilities rather than filling vacancies or replacing staff when they are absent. Hours lost due to illness or disability in 2016 was equivalent to the annual workload of almost 15,900 nurses; looked at another way, replacement staff needed to be found to work 28.8 million hours for the absent staff (Jacobson Consulting Inc., 2017). This staff shortage continues to be a major issue in nursing in Canada.

Pharmacare

For more than two decades, the CFNU has advocated for a national pharmacare strategy that includes access to affordable prescription drugs. In 2014, the CFNU published groundbreaking research that calculated the potential savings of universal pharmacare to be an estimated $9 billion to $11 billion annually. These findings were presented to the provincial premiers at their annual summit in 2014, with the CFNU arguing for better access to affordable prescription drugs through a national pharmacare program (Gagnon, 2014).

In 2015 and 2016, when the national study on pharmacare had commenced at the federal level, the CFNU hosted breakfast discussions about pharmacare with parliamentarians. During the same period, the CFNU continued to provide evidence-informed outreach to the premiers at their summit, hosting national and international experts on the issue. Building on existing research, the CFNU published two resources that examined pharmacare (Mackenzie, 2016; Batt, 2019). In 2017, the Canadian Labour Congress joined the CFNU to bring more than 3 million members on board in support of a labour pharmacare campaign launched under the banner A Plan for Everyone (aplanforeveryone.ca) (Figure 19.1).

In 2018, the CFNU published *Body Count*, a report in which pharmacare researchers calculated the annual loss of life and premature decline resulting from patients' poor adherence to drug treatment regimens due to cost (Lopert, Docteur, & Morgan, 2018). That same year also saw two major national developments pharmacare: the Standing Committee on Health recommended universal single-payer pharmacare in Canada in its final report (House of Commons Standing Committee on Health, 2018), and the federal government launched the Advisory Council on the Implementation of National Pharmacare.

As the evidence for pharmacare has mounted, the public, the labour movement, and governments have lined up to support it. More than 80 organizations representing a diverse coalition of health care providers, nonprofit organizations, workers, seniors, patients, and academics came together to sign onto the five Pharmacare Consensus

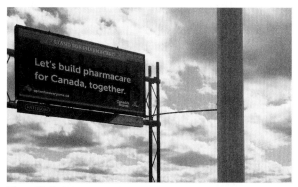
Fig. 19.1 Advocacy for universal pharmacare by the Canadian Federation of Nurses Unions. (© Canadian Federation of Nurses Unions)

Principles: universality; public, single-payer administration; accessibility; comprehensiveness; and portable coverage. The Advisory Council released their final report in June 2019, calling for a national, single-payer, public pharmacare program (Health Canada, 2019). The CFNU continues to work with its partners in nursing and other health care professions to bring universal pharmacare to Canadians.

 APPLYING CONTENT KNOWLEDGE

Reflect on the purpose of the CFNU and the relevance of its ongoing work to patients, the public, and nurses. Provide rationales for your thoughts and share with your peers either in discussion or a reflective writing assignment.

Occupational Health and Safety

The CFNU and its member nursing unions are committed to the occupational health and safety of nurses across Canada. They recognize that when a workplace is unsafe for nurses, it also poses risks for patient safety, leading to a decline in outcomes for both nurses and patients. Unsafe staffing and workload is associated with a number of negative outcomes for nurses, including burnout, dissatisfaction at work, musculoskeletal disorders, employment injuries, and aggression of residents toward staff (Aiken, Clarke, Sloane et al., 2002; Cohen, Village, Ostry et al., 2004; Robinson & Tappen, 2008; Sheward, Hunt, Hagen et al., 2005; Trinkoff, Johantgen, Muntaner, & Le, 2005).

Over the past 5 years, the CFNU has been a leader in addressing health and safety issues, especially workplace violence, which has become endemic in health care settings across the country. A recent survey found that over a 12-month period, 61% of nurses reported having a serious problem with workplace violence (Reichert, 2017). National data from the Workers' Compensation Board has indicated that the number of violence-related lost-time injuries for frontline health care workers increased by nearly 66% between 2006 and 2015, a rate three times that for police and correctional officers combined (Reichert, 2017).

The CFNU published their report on workplace violence, *Enough Is Enough* (Reichert, 2017), after which they brought together experts and stakeholders at a roundtable event in January 2018 to discuss the issue. In June 2018, the CFNU worked with Dr. Doug Eyolfson, Member of Parliament for Charleswood–St. James–Assiniboia–Headingley, to convince the Parliamentary Standing Committee on Health to study workplace violence in health care, a motion that was unanimously agreed to by the committee. A parliamentary petition (e-1902) subsequently launched by Dr. Eyolfson and the CFNU's president, calling for a national strategy to address workplace violence in health care, garnered 8,743 signatures. The petition was presented to Parliament shortly before the federal committee's study on workplace violence in health care commenced in 2019 (House of Commons, 2019). Linda Silas, president of the CFNU, presented to the committee on behalf of 200,000 nurses and nursing students. Silas proposed several strategies to deal with the issue of workplace violence:

- A comprehensive federal study into health human resources planning;
- Targeted federal funding to enhance protections for health care workers through violence-prevention infrastructure and programs, with community police included as an essential partner with Joint Health and Safety Committees;
- The application of best practices around violence prevention in federally regulated health care settings—to lead by example;
- The legislation of national minimum security training standards for health care environments;
- Support from this committee for Bill C-434, as well as promoting the use of the Westray bill among Crown prosecutors in cases involving health care workers; and
- Federal funding toward facility-level data collection and reporting on workplace violence-related data by the Canadian Institute for Health Information. (CFNU, 2019b, para. 7)

In addition, the CFNU created the *Workplace Violence Toolkit* (CFNU, 2019b), an online hub for members, the public, and the media that integrates both national and provincial resources, research, information, tools, and best practices related to violence in health care workplaces. Finally, in February 2019, in response to the lobbying efforts of the CFNU and other health care associations, Bill C-434 was introduced in Parliament. The bill amended the federal *Criminal Code* to require a court to consider the fact that the victim of an assault is a health care sector worker to be an aggravating circumstance for the purposes of sentencing; however, being a private member's bill, it received only first reading.

The CFNU has also raised the issue of occupational stress injuries, which are linked to high rates of workplace violence. One provincial union found that 25% of its members showed symptoms of post-traumatic stress disorder (PTSD) (Manitoba Nurses' Union [MNU], 2015). After 2 years of lobbying to include nurses in Bill C-211, an Act to establish a federal framework on PTSD, the Senate Committee on National Security issued a recommendation to the health minister in June 2018 to include nurses in the implementation of the legislation. Additional efforts by the CFNU related to workplace violence have included helping to plan a PTSD conference, held in spring 2019, and collaborating with the Public Health Agency of Canada.

UNIONS: HISTORY OF GROWTH AND IMPACT

The development of separate and unique provincial–territorial unions for collective bargaining occurred within a relatively short time after the Supreme Court's decision in 1973. Only 14 years elapsed between the inception of the first such organization, Ontario Nurses' Association (ONA), and the last, the PEI Nurses' Union, in 1987. The 1990s were characterized by cutbacks and health care restructuring, and nursing unions struggled to maintain what they had gained in the previous decade. It was a time of relative labour peace; rather than making big demands of employers, the unions strove to maintain staff positions. As the economic climate improved in the late 1990s, unions demanded higher wages, improved workloads, less overtime, and improved working environments (Archibald, 2004). Although the SARS crisis of 2003 impelled a period of consensus, labour strife was soon to follow a period of economic growth. Although union demands were loud and clear, governments were less than willing to grant concessions, fearing that the long-term costs would be too high (Archibald, 2004). With the sudden economic downturn in 2008, provinces began to slash their health care budgets in response to declining revenues, and unions had to do a quick turnaround to focus on nursing positions that were at risk.

Registered nurse (RN) unions, born out of the professional RN organizations, represent the bulk of RNs in Canada, including both registered nurses and nurse practitioners. Licensed practical nurses (LPNs), registered practical nurses (RPNs), and registered psychiatric nurses in some provinces are also represented by the same unions that represent registered nurses. Other unions also represent some RNs (and NPs), LPNs, and RPNs in various capacities, such as the Canadian Union of Pubic Employees (CUPE), Christian Labour Association of Canada (CLAC), United Steelworkers of America (USW), provincial public service unions, Service Employees International Union Healthcare, Unifor, Public Service Alliance of Canada, and The Professional Institute of the Public Service of Canada.

British Columbia

The RNABC was one of the first associations to be legally recognized as an official bargaining agent for nurses, and by 1956 it was the only organization negotiating for RNs in British Columbia. At first, the RNABC operated on the basis of annually approved personnel policies that were used to bargain with hospital boards. Although this process was also used in other provinces, the difference was the legal recognition of the RNABC as a bargaining agent.

Dissatisfaction arose with the personnel policies in all provinces. In 1959, many disputes went to conciliation, and strike votes were taken in several health care agencies, leading to the first province-wide collective bargaining for nurses in British Columbia. This approach was successful and was used until 1976, when the RNABC created a distinct and separate labour relations division to carry out collective bargaining.

After the Supreme Court's decision that the SRNA could not fairly represent point-of-care nurses on labour relations matters, momentum gathered to form a nurses' union in British Columbia. In 1980, the RNABC and its labour relations division formed a joint committee to study the issue and unanimously recommended that the two bodies separate completely. In February 1981, the labour relations division held a special founding convention where nurses voted unanimously to form the BCNU.

In 1973, the BC government introduced changes to the *Labour Relations Code*, which created the Labour Relations Board and gave police, firefighters, and hospital workers the right to strike with an option of binding arbitration. A decade later, new legislation revoked the right to strike for those deemed essential, including nurses. Hence, prior to any job action, the union and the employer would have to negotiate essential service levels to determine how many nurses were to remain at work in the event of a strike.

In 1989, bargaining began for a new contract to cover 17,500 hospital nurses. After years of government restraint, nurses were looking for compensation to counter what many saw as undervalued work. The union called for a 33% wage increase over 3 years, but the employers offered only 18% (Tatroff, 2006). Backed by a 94% strike vote, nurses walked off the job in all public hospitals in British Columbia (Tatroff, 2006). A 13-day strike resulted in an offer of a 29.5% increase in wages plus benefit improvements (Tatroff, 2006). This offer was rejected after two nurse leaders from Vancouver General Hospital, Debra MacPherson and Bernadette Stringer, travelled the province speaking to nurses about voting no. And vote no they did; 65% of nurses rejected the union's recommended settlement (Tatroff, 2006). The reasons were twofold. Nurses believed in equal pay for work of equal value and in being compensated as professionals. Of equal concern was the feeling that unelected union staff, who had led negotiations, were not communicating with members or adequately involving them in decisions or priority setting. At an impasse, the parties agreed to binding arbitration and a 2-year contract with a total wage increase of 20.9% awarded (Tatroff, 2006). While nurses were disappointed with this result, a sea change had occurred, and many innovations were subsequently implemented at the BCNU, making it a far more democratic, member-driven organization.

Several years later, the BCNU and other provincial unions representing health care workers negotiated a landmark employment security agreement. Across Canada, governments were downsizing hospitals, causing major job losses. When the BC government announced plans to close Vancouver's Shaughnessy Hospital, a campaign was mounted to prevent the closure. Nurses worked with a broad coalition to mobilize public support, but the campaign failed.

The BC government intended to proceed with hospital downsizing while minimizing loss of employment, so an agreement was negotiated between health care unions, health care employers, and the government. Under the Health Labour Accord, unions accepted the plan to eliminate 2,000 acute care beds in exchange for 3 years of job security while retraining a role in hospital decision making through the implementation of Labour Adjustment Committees and a reduction from 37.5 to 36 hours a week of work with no loss in pay. The Health Care Labour Adjustment Agency was formed to fund retraining programs, early retirement incentives, and job placement alternatives for laid-off employees. After March 31, 1996, unions, including the BCNU, negotiated the agreement provisions into their collective agreements. This unique arrangement remained in effect until a change in government in 2001.

In the aftermath of the health system restructuring that took place in the 1990s, BC nurses became disillusioned with their wages and benefits, which had not kept pace with those of nurses in other provinces. A bitter dispute between the BCNU and the Health Employers Association of British Columbia (HEABC) occurred in the spring and summer of 2001. The dispute took place in an unusual political context, as the government changed hands before final resolution. Shortly after the new government was elected, BC nurses voted to reject the deal. A cooling-off period was then imposed, which brought job action to an end. Subsequently, the last offer was imposed through legislation.

The following year, the government used Bill 29 to cancel existing health care union contracts, eliminating job security and union successorship rights, weakening bumping rights, and allowing for significant contracting out. The BCNU, along with the BC Government and Service Employees' Union and the Hospital Employees' Union, launched a lawsuit that claimed Bill 29 violated the *Canadian Charter of Rights and Freedoms* with respect to freedom of expression, freedom of association, and equality rights for women. In 2007, the Supreme Court of Canada sided with the unions, ruling that parts of Bill 29 were indeed unconstitutional.

From 2012 to 2014, the BCNU entered a time of significant growth. In 2012, more than 7,000 acute and long-term care LPNs voted to join. Later that year, 600 community

LPNs from various unions also transferred to the BCNU. And in 2014, more than 1,100 registered psychiatric nurses at the Union of Psychiatric Nurses voted to merge with the BCNU (MacDonald, 2014).

In 2012, the BCNU negotiated the first contract in Canada to give nurses a say in matching staff levels with patient care needs. Management resisted implementing that language, resulting in employers having to pay $10 million in damages to the union in 2015. The BCNU's safe staffing contract language was further strengthened in the 2019 contract.

Alberta

United Nurses Alberta (UNA) was established in 1977. Today, the union represents more than 30,000 RNs, registered psychiatric nurses, and allied health care workers throughout Alberta. UNA had its beginnings in a period of turmoil in labour relations and in the Alberta Association of Registered Nurses, which had acted both as a regulatory body and a bargaining agent for many Alberta nurses starting in 1965. By 1977, pressure was growing for the association to split into separate bargaining and regulatory organizations. On May 6, 1977, 1,300 nurses attended a contentious general meeting in Calgary; at the end of the meeting, the decision to form a new independent union was ratified.

Things soon began to change. By July that year, 2,500 UNA nurses went on strike at seven Alberta hospitals in Edmonton, Calgary, Lethbridge, and Grande Prairie for basic improvements in working conditions and pay. They were legislated back to work after 4 days, but the seeds of an effective and formidable nurses' union had been sown.

The new union's first annual general meeting was held in 1978, and soon after UNA negotiated a hospital collective agreement without having to resort to strike action. However, other strikes would follow. In 1980, 6,400 members at 79 hospitals defied a back-to-work order. And while they continued to walk picket lines, members negotiated a 39.8% wage increase over 2 years. That contract also included, for the first time, **professional responsibility language**, a key strategic goal of UNA then, and now.

A lockout and another strike followed in 1982. The next year, the Alberta government banned all strikes by hospital employees. But in 1988, 14,000 Alberta nurses illegally walked off the job at 98 hospitals, resulting in massive fines—but also solidarity and political sophistication among the membership and leaders of UNA.

Over the ensuing years, nurse members of UNA confronted decreased public funding for several provincial agencies and efforts to privatize public health care during the mid-1990s. When the provincial government decreased funding to public services across the board, instituted multiple reorganizations of the system, and attempted to introduce legislation that would open the door to increased health care privatization, nurses fought to protect their jobs, their patients, their profession, and, in coalition with other groups, publicly funded health care.

In 1997, the 2,400 members of the Staff Nurses' Associations of Alberta (a second nurses' union in Alberta) joined UNA, bringing the union's membership to 16,000. By the first years of the twenty-first century, growth in the provincial health care system and a provincial decision to consolidate public health care bargaining increased the size of UNA. With one voice, UNA was able to advocate more effectively for the concerns of its members about issues such as patient care, fair and just wages and working conditions, and a national pharmacare program.

Saskatchewan

Historically, Saskatchewan has seen a close relationship between the principle of collectivity and the provision of health care. In the same decade that the patients of the province benefitted from the *Saskatchewan Medical Care Insurance Act* of 1978 coming into existence, those professionally responsible for care faced increasingly challenging conditions in the practice environment. Workloads were high and workplaces were constrained by efforts to reduce costs in health care. The desire of a largely female-dominated occupation to have a voice for their own ability to provide care, and the need for some degree of wage parity across Saskatchewan's nursing workforce, led to the early stages of collective negotiations.

By the end of its first year, the Saskatchewan Union of Nurses (SUN) represented approximately 2,500 nurses. By the mid-1990s, this number had grown to 6,500. In 1998, SUN membership increased to 8,500 when the Dorsey Commission ruled that the union should represent all RNs, registered psychiatric nurses, and graduate nurses employed by health districts and their affiliates. SUN now represents over 10,000 members.

Defining moments in the organization's history came in 1988 and again in 1999, when nurses went on strike for their right to have traditional labour relations issues addressed through the collective agreement but also their right for their professional practice to be supported and upheld by their employers. These issues are further reflected in the role SUN has played as a member of both the Saskatchewan Federation of Labour and the CFNU.

Through tracking the evolution of SUN, what becomes apparent is the interconnectedness of workplace issues and nurses' ability to uphold their professional responsibilities. Ongoing issues that echo this tenet include the protection of Medicare, the implementation of pharmacare, advocacy for social determinants of health-based policies, and

BOX 19.1   A Public Relations Approach

SUN members are responsible for executing a holistic model of care across all areas of Saskatchewan's health system—emergency rooms and hospitals, rural facilities, long-term care and psychiatric facilities, schools, blood services, and community and primary health clinics. Given the depth of RNs' interactions with the physiological and psychological aspects of care for patients and families, they are uniquely positioned to understand the socioeconomic components that affect well-being and to contribute solutions for positive change.

Taking inspiration from members, who continuously rank safe patient care as their top priority, SUN's most recent public campaigns have centred on key issues that continue to challenge the province: access to care, HIV, addictions, and mental health. These issues cannot be meaningfully addressed without understanding the social determinants of health, nor can they be addressed in isolation.

To that end, SUN has made use of multifaceted communications and public relations tools in partnership with a wide variety of traditional and nontraditional stakeholders. These strategies have included creating documentary-style video content that highlights the work and experiences of patients, practitioners, and community partners; leveraging digital and social media; and engaging in events and face-to-face conversations with the goal of educating, raising awareness, reducing stigma, and improving health outcomes.

the formation of partnerships for sustainable solutions to community issues (see Box 19.1).

Manitoba

In the mid-twentieth century, faced with some of the lowest wages in Canada, long hours, and job insecurity, nurses in Manitoba began to call for better pay and working conditions. At the time, the Manitoba Association of Registered Nurses (MARN), the registering body for nurses in Manitoba, realized the need to address some of the challenges facing the profession in order to attract and retain nurses. In 1950, the MARN labour relations committee assembled and disseminated recommended hospital personnel policies. However, many hospitals did not adopt them, leading to growing dissatisfaction among nurses.

Some began to turn to collective action as a means of pressing their concerns, but it was not until 1953 that the first nurses in Manitoba became members of a union. At that time, nurses working for the City of Winnipeg realized, as a result of an automatic dues check-off, that they were

members of the Federation of Civic Employees. While these nurses had approached MARN to represent them as their bargaining agent, MARN's reluctance to support unionization inspired them to look for an alternative. As a result, the unionized City of Winnipeg nurses decided to start the first nurses-only union in Manitoba—the Winnipeg Civic Registered Nurses' Association. This effort was led by four nurses who were willing to mortgage their homes in order to cover the legal costs of establishing a nurses-only union. It was their courage that laid the groundwork for the wave of nurse unionization that followed. By the late 1960s, several nurses' unions had emerged in Manitoba. By 1974, the bylaws of the Provincial Staff Nurses' Council of MARN were amended to include LPNs in the nurse bargaining units that had emerged.

Then, in 1975, after successfully achieving significant wage increases for nurses through bargaining, the Provincial Staff Nurses' Council officially separated from MARN. The new organization, the Manitoba Organization of Nurses' Associations (MONA), quickly expanded and turned its attention to improving working conditions, protecting job security, and gaining better wages and benefits for Manitoba's nurses. Throughout the 1980s, MONA achieved several key improvements for its members, including better pay and extended health care, and expanded its influence to many more sites.

In 1990, MONA officially became the MNU. Concerned that Manitoba's nurses still significantly lagged behind many of their peers in other provinces, and determined to address these disparities, the MNU took a strong stance in negotiations in 1990. Unable to reach an agreement, nurses officially went on a month-long province-wide strike in January 1991. It was the longest and largest nurses' strike in Canadian history. This show of strength cemented the position of the MNU as the voice of Manitoba's nurses.

Manitoba's nurses faced many struggles in the 1990s under a government determined to make cuts and restructure the health care system. In 1995, the MNU launched a Yellow Ribbon campaign to try to keep emergency rooms open that were slated for closure by the government. They also launched the It's Raining campaign in 1999 to embarrass the government of the day for directing tax dollars into a pre-election fund instead of investing in health care. Nurses showed up in large numbers, with umbrellas in hand, at the provincial legislature on March 15, 1999, to make their point (MNU, 2010).

The election of a new government in 1999 did not diminish the MNU's efforts. Significant gains were made for Manitoba's nurses throughout the 2000s. In 2011, the MNU successfully convinced the government to include in its Workplace Safety and Health regulations a requirement for all health care facilities in the province to institute a

BOX 19.2 **Post-Traumatic Stress Disorder**
In 2014, amid a rising tide of awareness about PTSD in first responders, the MNU embarked on a research project to identify the prevalence of PTSD among nurses (MNU, 2015). The combined findings of a survey and focus groups demonstrated that PTSD and its symptoms were far more prevalent among nurses than many had expected (MNU, 2015). MNU released a report in 2015 outlining the findings of its research. The report provided the foundation for an MNU lobbying campaign advocating for nurses to be included in an amendment to workers' compensation legislation, which would allow for a presumption of PTSD under certain circumstances.
While the government had initially been considering an amendment to the legislation to include first responders under a PTSD presumption, the efforts of the MNU and other actors compelled the government to broaden its perspective. In June 2015, *The Workers Compensation Amendment Act* was passed by the Manitoba legislature. The act included language allowing for a PTSD presumption for all occupations, not just first responders. The law took effect January 1, 2016, representing a monumental step forward in the struggle to have psychological injuries among nurses recognized under the law. With the passage of this bill, Manitoba became the first province in Canada to include nurses under a PTSD presumption clause.

Source: Manitoba Nurses' Union. (2015). *Post-traumatic stress disorder (PTSD) in the nursing profession: Helping Manitoba's wounded healers.* Winnipeg, MB: Author.

violence prevention policy (MNU, 2019). Then, in 2015, the MNU released a groundbreaking report discussing the prevalence of PTSD among nurses (MNU, 2015). A lobbying campaign, geared toward persuading the government to cover nurses under presumptive PTSD legislation, followed the report's release. The campaign proved successful when Manitoba became the first province in Canada to include nurses in such legislation (MNU, 2019). See Box 19.2.

In 2018, the MNU released another report advocating for greater investment in long-term care in the province. The report highlighted the importance of increasing resident care hours as a means of providing better care (MNU, 2018).

Ontario

Events took a different course in Ontario. The regulatory function had been assumed by the Registered Nurses'

Association of Ontario (RNAO) until 1963, at which time the College of Nurses was formed and took over the regulatory role. As a result, the RNAO became a voluntary professional organization. Looking for new avenues to maintain and grow its membership base, the RNAO membership at the 1964 annual meeting passed a resolution to achieve collective bargaining for all nurses. Consequently, the Employment Relations Department (ERD) was established to focus on this mandate.

Collective bargaining rights were not, however, achieved easily in Ontario. The RNAO unsuccessfully lobbied for legislation to designate it as the bargaining agent for all registered nurses in Ontario. As a result, the RNAO had no other option but to seek unionization under the terms of the *Labour Relations Act*. With the assistance of the ERD, the RNAO organized nurses into independent trade unions called "nurses associations" on an agency-by-agency basis.

Many nurses were motivated to organize because of their substandard wages and benefits. Others were driven by the need to establish a grievance procedure to combat unfair discipline and discharge. Still others wanted a real say in the quality of care that they provided, to enhance job security, or to improve promotional opportunities— or a combination of any of these factors. Regardless of the motivation, it was important that a nurses' union be seen to be a professional union such as the ones that represented the teaching profession in Ontario.

Legislation passed in 1965 (the *Hospital Labour Disputes Arbitration Act*) prevented nurses in hospitals and long-term care homes from legally striking. The legislation did not, however, apply to community health nurses, certain retirement homes, or industry. As a result, public health nurses were the first to organize, followed by hospitals, schools of nursing, and an industrial unit at Chrysler Canada. By 1972, the ERD was servicing 78 nurses' associations—38 in hospitals, 33 in public health, 4 in schools of nursing, and the occupational health nurses at Chrysler Canada.

One example of the early hurdles faced by nurses in Ontario was the fact that section 89 of the *Labour Relations Act* allowed a municipality to exclude its employees from unionization by the passage of a bylaw invoking the section. As a result, several units in community health had to threaten to submit their resignations en masse in order to achieve collective agreements.

During the early 1970s, government and employer groups continued having ongoing discussions about province-wide collective bargaining. While there was widespread support for the concept, practical issues such as structure and representation needed to be addressed. ONA formed in 1973 with the expectation that a provincial union would help to achieve a province-wide collective agreement for all nurses. The existing 104 independent nurses' associations subsequently merged into the newly created ONA and became chartered locals of the union. Though achieving one collective agreement to cover all nurses in all sectors proved to be elusive, ONA ultimately negotiated separate sector agreements for all nurses.

The first form of central bargaining in the hospital sector occurred in 1974, when ONA called on all hospitals to meet to negotiate a collective agreement or face strike action that July. The employers came to the table. Although the bargaining initially resulted in an impasse, an interest arbitration award for nurses at the Ottawa Civic Hospital was released shortly after the impasse was announced and would ultimately form the basis of the first negotiated central agreement.

ONA reached a second central hospital agreement in 1975, but the central process was then abandoned by ONA until serious implementation issues could be addressed. As a result, the parties reverted to individual bargaining from 1976 to 1980—when the central process was completely revamped, remaining in place to this day. Figure 19.2 shows a visual representation of the hourly rates for staff RNs from 1973 to 2019.

While the government implemented the *Social Contract Act, 1993*, disallowing any compensation increases for a 3-year period, that same year ONA achieved pay equity settlements in many sectors, including hospitals. These settlements provided substantial wage increases but were not impacted by the social contract initiative of the government. Pay-equity work did not end with the initial settlement, and even today there is continued negotiation for achieving pay equity for members.

Most unionized nurses in Ontario do not have the right to strike, and there have been limited strikes among the sectors in Ontario where nurses can strike. The largest took place in 2015, when over 4,000 RNs and case managers in the Community Care Access Centres (CCAC) went on strike. During a very cold winter, RNs, nurse practitioners (NPs), RPNs, and health care providers walked the picket line for 6 weeks. The nurses had the public's support and were not willing to back down. Finally, the CCAC agreed to engage in "final offer selection arbitration," whereby the dispute would be mediated by an arbitrator whose decision would be final. The arbitrator awarded ONA all its positions.

Collective bargaining provided nurses with input into their wages and benefits. Doing the same for working conditions was a larger hurdle until 1989, when ONA helped to obtain an amendment to the *Public Hospital Act*. This amendment allowed an elected staff nurse to be included on the Hospital Fiscal Advisory Committee and the participation of staff nurses in decision making related to

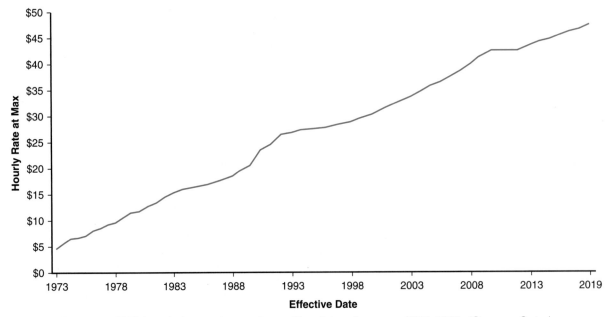

Fig. 19.2 ONA hospital central rates for staff registered nurses, 1973–2019. (**Source:** Ontario Nurses' Association)

administrative financial, operational, and planning matters in the hospital. This legislation contributed to changing the perception of nurses as autonomous professionals.

ONA now represents over 68,000 RNs, NPs, RPNs, and allied health professionals.

Collective Agreement Leading Provisions

In addition to the professional responsibility clause, ONA has negotiated other leading provisions to benefit its members, such as a wage grid, benefits, pensions, and job security for part-time nurses. In the early 1970s, for example, part-time nurses were without wage grids, any form of benefits, and had little to no job security. They were also ineligible to contribute to the employer's pension plan. Today, part-time compensation mirrors that of full-time positions with the same grids, percentage pay in lieu of benefits, pension eligibility, and job security. ONA has also negotiated the first weekend premiums, responsibly pay provisions, and student supervision and mentorship premiums for nurses in Canada. Health and safety provisions negotiated by ONA compare favourably to those of the Canadian health care sector.

Pensions

Prior to 1993, the Hospitals (now Healthcare) of Ontario Pension Plan (HOOPP) was governed solely by the Ontario Hospital Association (OHA). In 1989, the OHA granted hospitals a contribution holiday while requiring employees to maintain their contribution levels. The backlash from unions, including ONA, led to numerous appeals and lawsuits. While the contribution holiday stood, the protests ultimately led to joint union–employer governance of HOOPP and the inclusion of part-time employees in the plan. From that day forward, the newly appointed Board of Trustees for HOOPP has never wavered from its fiduciary duty to the plan members.

Government Relations

Politically, ONA, like other provincial nursing unions, provides input into provincial policy, appropriate health care funding, national issues such as pharmacare, and working conditions. The union encourages nurses to be vocal and politically active about their issues. They continuously run campaigns addressing employer funding, occupational health and safety, staffing, and the value of the RN role (Figure 19.3).

CASE STUDY

Keeping Nurses Safe: Occupational Health and Safety on the Front Line—The SARS and Ebola Epidemics

As part of their efforts to improve working conditions, nurses' unions advocate for occupational health and safety. In 2003, two ONA member nurses died after being exposed to severe acute respiratory syndrome (SARS) while caring for their patients. In September of that year, ONA made a submission to the Campbell Commission examining SARS. Their submission included emotional impact statements from ONA members, who detailed their experiences working in hospitals during the outbreak.

Justice Archie Campbell went on to make 83 sweeping recommendations in his final SARS Commission report. The central theme was the lack of health care sector knowledge of, and adherence to, occupational health and safety law and principles, and the need for public health and infection control to incorporate occupational health and safety in any response to outbreaks. Justice Campbell's (2006) main recommendation was that the precautionary principle, which states that action to reduce risk [like the use of a fitted N95 respirator] need not await scientific certainty, be expressly adopted as a guiding principle throughout Ontario's health, public health and worker safety systems. (p. 1158)

ONA has continued to advocate for occupational health and safety following Justice Campbell's advice to improve law, policy, funding, and system capacity to protect Ontario workers. Through their advocacy, the government and ONA now work together on infectious disease protocols, adapting them more recently with the threat of the Ebola virus. When Ebola was identified in 2015 as a severe infectious disease threat to the Western Hemisphere, ONA took the lead in the media and with policymakers to ensure that the experience of SARS was not repeated. To this end, and because of its experience and knowledge, ONA sat at the table with the ministries of Labour and Health to ensure that frontline health care providers were given the proper equipment and training needed to protect themselves should Ebola come to Ontario.

Source: Campbell, J. A. (2006). *The SARS Commission Executive Summary, Spring of Fear, Volume 1.* Toronto, ON: The SARS Commission. Retrieved from http://www.archives.gov.on.ca/en/e_records/sars/report/v1.html; Ontario Nurses' Association. (2015). ONA leading charge on Ebola preparedness. *Frontlines, 15*(1), 1, 3. Retrieved from https://www.ona.org/wp-content/uploads/ona_frontlines_201501.pdf.

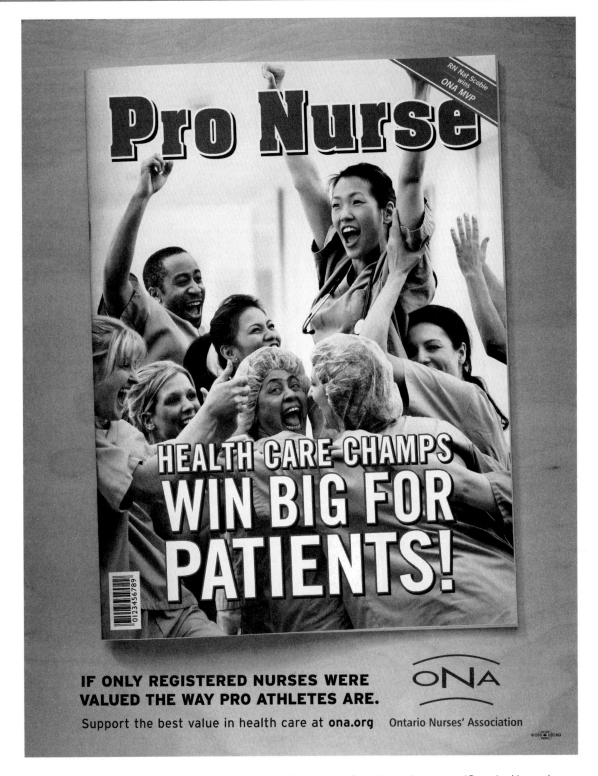

Fig. 19.3 Bus shelter campaign poster on the value of registered nurses. (Ontario Nurses' Association)

CASE STUDY

Workplace Violence: The Death of Lori Dupont, RN

Nursing unions have also led lobbying efforts to improve health and safety legislation by addressing the unsafe environments of their members. On November 12, 2005, Lori Dupont, an ONA member, was murdered by a physician while working in the recovery room of the Hôtel-Dieu Grace Hospital in Windsor. The physician subsequently took his own life. ONA pursued accountability from the employer and subsequently was a leading voice in the coroner's jury inquest.

ONA was one of the parties granted standing at the inquest. The 10-week inquest included testimony from Dupont's co-workers, who identified the assailant's past aggressive behaviour and resulting complaints. In 2007, the jury made 26 recommendations aimed at preventing similar incidents and supported the union's recommendation that there be a review of the *Occupational Health and Safety Act* to consider including emotional or psychological harm as a workplace safety issue.

ONA also filed a grievance that the hospital had failed to take the necessary steps to maintain a safe workplace free of violence, harassment, and discrimination. After a lengthy mediation between the two parties, the grievance was resolved in the summer of 2008. Both reaffirmed their mutual commitment to maintain a workplace free of violence and to support the hospital's new Workplace

Violence Prevention Program; both parties also agreed to recognize a broad definition of violence covering both physical and verbal conduct of an abusive nature. As part of the settlement, the hospital reaffirmed its commitment to implementing the recommendations of the coroner's inquest and to training and educating staff and physicians on preventing workplace violence.

After the release of the inquest report, ONA worked with other unions and, together with women's groups, the Dupont family, and other parties, convinced the government to add provisions to the *Occupational Health and Safety Act* in 2010 to prevent and respond to violence in the workplace, including domestic violence spillover from home to work. The amendments to the Act also extended the reach of law with respect to harassment at work (Government of Canada, 2009).

Other amendments to the legislation included the responsibilities of employers to assess risk when a person with a history of violent behaviour is in the workplace, to alert workers, to alert the Joint Health and Safety Committee (as required) when there is an injury from such a person, and to clarify that violence and threats are health and safety issues and should be covered by an employer's Occupational Health and Safety Committee.

Source: *Occupational Health and Safety Act*, RSO 1990, c. O.1, as amended by An Act to amend the *Occupational Health and Safety Act* with respect to violence and harassment in the workplace and other matters, SO 2009, c. 23. Retrieved from https://www.ola.org/en/legislative-business/bills/parliament-39/session-1/bill-168.

The Work of ONA

ONA continues to organize nurses and allied health professionals who are not members of a union. They negotiate and service collective agreements, represent members at grievances, arbitrations, regulatory body procedures and hearings, and Workplace Safety Insurance Board cases and appeals. It also addresses professional and workload issues, provides secondary malpractice coverage, and runs a Legal Expense Assistance Program for members who require representation at regulatory body and privacy hearings. ONA also develops commercials, print and electronic advertising, and branding strategies to ensure that the union addresses its members' issues and communication between members and the union remains relevant.

Quebec

Nurses' associations have been present in Quebec since the 1940s. They represented nurses at every hospital in

Quebec at a time when health institutions were controlled by religious communities. However, nurses did not truly gain the right to collective representation and bargaining until the early 1960s with the adoption of the *Labour Code, 1964*, which allowed public-sector employees to unionize. During that same period, the Quebec government took over the management and delivery of health care, which led to the public health and social services network. Nurses were thus represented by three labour organizations: two for English and French nurses in Montreal, and one for all other regions across Quebec.

In 1972, many public services were affected by a strike of the Front commun (union collective) involving nurses who were members of the Alliance des infirmières et infirmiers de Montréal (AIM). These nurses were ordered to return to work when the National Assembly of Quebec passed legislation to end the interruption in public services. Between then and 1987, all three of the nurses' unions negotiated their members' agreements separately. To create stronger bargaining power, the three nursing unions merged in December 1987 to form La Fédération des infirmières et infirmiers du Québec (FIIQ).

The illegal walkout of members of the new organization in 1989, and the subsequent standoff between the nurses and the government in the midst of an election campaign, led to a 7-day strike that unified the nurses and gained them considerable public support for their cause. The nurses' gains in this situation were impressive, and their public image was improved. Quebec nurses and their labour organizations received significant financial penalties for this action, which included ending the deduction of union dues from nurses' pay, thus creating a financial burden for the union. During this time, the FIIQ received financial support from other nurses' labour organizations across Canada, which helped it to survive.

The FIIQ did not allow this battle to discourage it and went on to fight for its members' working conditions in 1999. This resulted in a 23-day strike, in the aftermath of which financial penalties were again imposed on the union. However, a new collective agreement was signed in 2000.

In the early 2000s, a Liberal government was elected and began promoting **neoliberalism** and austerity in public services. The beginning of the Liberals' 15 years in power signalled a turning point for the health and social services network and the unions that represented their workers. Two laws passed in 2003 triggered significant changes in the structure of the health network and the collective bargaining system. Bill 25 created local service networks in the form of health and social service centres; this legislation led nurses to start working just as much in hospitals as in local community service centres and long-term care centres (National Assembly, 2003a). These health institution mergers also led to union mergers. Bill 30 forced health care workers to be separated into four employee categories (National Assembly, 2003b); nurses were thus grouped with LPNs, respiratory therapists, and clinical perfusionists. The FIIQ was renamed the Fédération interprofessionnelle de la santé du Québec (FIQ), representing 57,000 members who work as nurses and cardiorespiratory therapists.

In 2015, just 10 years after the first reform, a new bill once again destabilized the health network and its unions. Bill 10 merged health institutions to form integrated health and social services centres (region-based megastructures) with only one public health institution per region. This law in turn led to more imposed union mergers (National Assembly, 2015). While the FIQ denounced the negative repercussions on its members' working conditions and their union life, the union emerged even stronger and now represents over 76,000 health care providers.

Since its formation, the FIIQ/FIQ has gone through three rounds of bargaining with the Quebec government. In 2006, the government abruptly ended negotiations by decree in order to implement reforms. The Quebec courts recognized that the government had negotiated in bad faith. In both 2010 and 2015, the union succeeded in negotiating collective agreements for its members. Gains that were achieved from those negotiations include a recognition that the shift overlap (passing on clinical information) counts as compensated work time; a 12% critical care premium for intensive care units; new mechanisms that promoted team stability; and a new salary structure. The negotiations also paved the way for a new job title in nursing (specialty NPs) and for implementing safe health care provider-to-patient ratios.

Using research evidence about safe provider-to-patient staffing ratios, the FIQ succeeded in obtaining two structural measures in its 2016–2020 collective agreement: care teams were stabilized by the addition of full-time positions, and a committee on safe health care provider-to-patient ratios was set up to study the pertinence and feasibility of such ratios through pilot projects (Fédération interprofessionnelle de la santé du Québec [FIQ], 2016).

At first, the union's work with the government on provider-to-patient ratios stalled, but ongoing lobbying helped to push the ratio pilot project forward. These actions included an international symposium on safe care; meetings with the political parties; the publication of *The Black Book of Care Safety* (FIQ, 2017), which brought together research and the personal stories of unsafe staffing ratios; and demonstrations held in the different regions of Quebec.

The pressure on the government was stepped up a notch in January 2018, when a nurse working in long-term care wrote to the minister of health through her Facebook account to inform him of her excessive workload and distress. This crisis was the subject of a media blitz in the days that followed (Marandolo, 2018). Health care providers mobilized and denounced the government's "rosy picture" of their practice conditions. At the same time, the FIQ met with the health minister to call for the stabilization of care teams, a stop to the use of mandatory overtime, and the implementing of the provider-to-patient ratio solution as soon as possible. These actions resulted in the commitment of 17 projects, as noted in Box 19.3.

New Brunswick

Originally, the New Brunswick Association of Registered Nurses (NBARN) provided the government with recommendations on salaries and working conditions on an annual basis. In the 1960s, nurses in New Brunswick became concerned about their socioeconomic status and

BOX 19.3 The Fight for Safe Health Care Provider-to-Patient Ratios in Quebec

Current management practices and successive reforms in Quebec's health care network have left health care providers facing difficult work and practice conditions: high workloads, mandatory overtime, substitutions, absences on work teams that are not replaced, and so on. These difficulties impact the quality of care; for example, health care providers reported that care was frequently left undone or not done to professional standards. A health care provider's workload, linked to inadequate care teams, was the reason most often cited to explain care rationing and omission.

Safe staffing has been linked to positive impacts for patients and health care providers. A solution backed by health care providers around the world to encourage adequate staffing is safe health care provider-to-patient ratios. Such ratios have been proven to increase the quality of care and staff satisfaction, notably in California and in some Australian states (FIQ, 2017).

The FIQ and its 76,000 members want to make safe health care provider-to-patient ratios a reality in Quebec. The nurses' current collective agreement includes a committee to study the pertinence and feasibility of such ratios through pilot projects. Seventeen projects are currently taking place in every region of the province in selected long-term care, acute care, and community care settings. Each project has three main components: a numerical chart of ratios based on the unit and shift, the enhancement of professional practice, and the possibility for the care team to upgrade the ratios as required by the patients' conditions or the care environment.

A joint analysis of the projects' results with the employer was expected later in 2020. However, general findings from the ratios pilot projects as observed and perceived by health care providers already include better clinical interventions, positive patient outcomes, and a better work environment.

The FIQ and its members believe that the best way to introduce and maintain safe ratios for the long term in Quebec is through legislation. The union will continue to mobilize to maintain the ratios pilot projects currently underway and obtain safe staffing legislation in Quebec.

Source: Fédération des interprofessionelle de la Santé du Québec. (2017). *The black book of care safety.* Montreal, QC: Author. Retrieved from http://www.fiqsante.qc.ca/wp-content/uploads/2017/12/FIQ-LivreNoir_ENG-Web.pdf.

disenchanted with the procedure for determining salaries. The first gain to achieve more power occurred when the NBARN Social and Economic Welfare Committee acquired standing committee status in 1967. With this status, the committee began helping nurses in health care agencies to organize staff associations throughout New Brunswick. In 1968, the NBARN Provincial Collective Bargaining Council was established as a separate entity from the NBARN.

The first serious collective bargaining in New Brunswick began in 1969, when employers agreed to negotiate with the NBARN Provincial Collective Bargaining Council (Kealey, 2008). When a stalemate occurred in the negotiations, most New Brunswick nurses resigned. These resignations were withdrawn when the employer group agreed to go back to the bargaining table to negotiate in a fair and equitable manner. An agreement was signed by both parties soon after. In the same year, provisions of the *Public Service Labour Relations Act* gave nurses in the public sector the right to bargain collectively. The right was extended to the private sector 2 years later, in 1971, through the *Industrial Relations Act.* The NBARN Provincial Collective Bargaining Council disassociated itself from the NBARN by becoming the New Brunswick Nurses' Provincial Collective Bargaining Council. The New Brunswick Civil Service Nurses' Provincial Collective Bargaining Council was also established because public- and private-sector bargaining were separated legislatively. The two organizations merged in 1978 to form the New Brunswick Nurses' Union (NBNU) (Botterill-Conroy, 1980).

In January 1975, after the wages of registered nursing assistants were negotiated to a level close to those of RNs, nurses attempted to reopen their contract by starting a campaign dubbed the "blue flu." Seven hundred nurses in 15 hospitals called in sick the first day. The media used this opportunity to scorn nurses for their actions but did agree there was an inequity. While the nurses' efforts did not result in their contracts being reopened, it did help to increase solidarity among New Brunswick nurses, as they started to see that both professional and union hats could be worn concurrently (Kealey, 2008).

In 1991, the provincial government imposed a wage freeze and rescinded a previously agreed-to salary adjustment for nurses. The NBNU threatened to strike, then reached a settlement with the provincial government. In 1994, nurses were able to prevent the government from removing "nursing" from job qualifications (McGee, 1994). In 2002, the *Nurses Act* was amended to enable the practice of NPs in New Brunswick, and the NBNU now represents them in the Regional Health Authorities.

Following the economic downturn of 2008, as with other provincial and territorial nursing organizations, the NBNU focused on recruiting and retaining the nursing workforce and improving the workplace for health care providers. The economic downturn also created difficulties for pension plan funds. The NBNU actively participated in provincial pension reform to ensure that full-time and part-time nurses would be assured of sustainable retirement pensions.

In 2009, the NBNU joined the New Brunswick Federation of Labour. Nurses recognized they could lend a credible, respected voice to issues that affected not only health but the broader labour movement and the province. In late 2009, the NBNU joined forces with other public-sector unions and led a successful provincial campaign to stop the sale of New Brunswick Power, a crown corporation.

Starting in the 2010, the Government of New Brunswick began making cuts to the provincial health care budget as part of austerity measures. These cuts contributed to lay-offs and skill-mix changes, which then led to staffing challenges and a deterioration in the quality of patient care. As a result, the NBNU spent considerable time in 2013 promoting the value of RNs through media campaigns, such as There is No Substitute for a Registered Nurse. To this day, the union continues to work on recruitment and retention strategies and improving the workplace, with a strong focus on reducing workplace violence.

Since the late 2000s, nurses have seen an increase in workplace violence and a deterioration in the general health status of nurses along with an increased prevalence of musculoskeletal injuries and mental illness. The NBNU continues to work with employers and the government on strategies to create healthier workplaces, including creating violence reduction programs with zero-tolerance policies. The union has lobbied for legislative changes to the provincial *Occupational Health and Safety Act* and is advocating for nurses to have a safe and secure workplace free from violence.

Nova Scotia

In 1966, the Registered Nurses' Association of Nova Scotia (RNANS) (predecessor of the College of Registered Nurses of Nova Scotia and later the Nova Scotia College of Nursing) organized the Committee on Social and Economic Welfare to press for higher wages and better working conditions. This pressure had built in response to nurses' feeling extremely undervalued.

In 1968, the RNANS was prepared to act as a bargaining agent for working nurses after the union's legislative mandate was changed. The union then sought to assist nurses with certification as bargaining agents under the *Trade Union Act*, starting with Highland View Hospital in Amherst on March 10, 1969 (*Health Authorities Act, 2014*, c. 32). In February 1970, bargaining broke down at Highland View. In October, after conciliation failed, nurses voted 43–1 in favour of a strike, which involved withdrawing non-nursing services. In May 1971, the RNANS formed a provincial bargaining committee with one member from each nurses' staff association.

In 1973, at a meeting of the Provincial Committee on Collective Bargaining, the Nurses' Staff Association of Nova Scotia was created as an independent representative of RNs in collective bargaining. At its formation, the association consisted of 18 certified staff associations and two associations that were in the midst of organizing. The Nurses' Staff Association of Nova Scotia had become an autonomous organization.

In 1975, nurses at 15 institutions withdrew their services because of a bargaining impasse. At that time, bargaining still occurred primarily at the local level. In 1976, the Nova Scotia Nurses' Union (NSNU) was formed, and in 1978, the provincial union gained certification rights and began to bargain collectively for its members. By the next year, most facilities were involved in the process (Botterill-Conroy, 1980). The NSNU has accomplished much in its history, including Supreme Court victories concerning workers' compensation and wage rollbacks, pension gains, improvements in workplace health and safety, sharps regulations, and influenza protections.

In the late 1970s, certified nurse assistants (now known as LPNs) began making requests to join the NSNU. In 1980, a motion was passed at the annual general meeting to accept certified nurse assistants into the union as full members in the then current RN bargaining units. On March 11, 1981, the labour board amended the NSNU's certification to include the first certified nurse assistants in the union.

In 2001, the collective bargaining process undertaken between the NSNU and the Province of Nova Scotia was particularly difficult (Cox & Mickleburgh, 2001). Although a tentative agreement was reached on May 26, 2001, the offer was rejected by the membership. On June 14, the Nova Scotia government introduced Bill 68, the *Health Care Continuation (2001) Act*. The measures in the proposed legislation stirred further anger and resentment toward the government because the amendment would suspend the right of employees to strike until March 31, 2004, and give cabinet the power to impose a collective agreement if one could not be reached through bargaining. On June 27, the Nova Scotia Government and General Employees Union (NSGEU), which represented former public-sector nurses in Halifax, submitted notices of resignation en masse. Through a contract provision, these resignations could be revoked without penalty to the nurses. In the meantime, on June 29, the NSNU received a strike mandate from its membership, and nurses prepared to walk off the job.

The government retreated from its original position, and on July 5 all parties agreed to invoke a final-offer selection process to settle the outstanding contract issues. The agreement provided that the legislation would not apply to nurses, that the final report of the selector should be issued in just over a month, and that a 3-year collective agreement would be agreed upon.

In 2014, the Government of Nova Scotia introduced legislation to merge the province's nine district health authorities into one provincial authority (*Health Authorities Act, 2014*). The IWK Children's Hospital would retain its separate governance structure. The legislation mandated that unionized workers be separated into four provincial bargaining units: nurses (RNs, LPNs, NPs), health care workers, support workers, and administrative professionals. The four existing unions representing health care workers in Nova Scotia (NSNU, NSGEU, CUPE, and Unifor) were each meant to represent one of these units, with workers being transferred between unions to accomplish this. Two of the unions represented RNs, all four unions represented LPNs, and the three unions other than the NSNU each represented health care, support workers, and administrative workers, respectively. Mr. James Dorsey was appointed mediator–arbitrator to guide the unions and employer through the process. The government finally introduced new legislation to allow the four unions to maintain their existing memberships and bargain collectively as councils of unions. The councils then successfully bargained their first contracts in 2018 and 2019.

In 2011, the NSNU became the first nurses' union in the country to introduce a standardized nurse uniform for its members, with funding provided in the collective agreement. The distinctive uniform of a white top and black bottom, with nursing designation identified, achieves several ends. It promotes a professional image of nursing and encourages respect; it helps patients to easily identify nurses in large institutions; and it helps the public to realize when there are decreasing numbers of nurses working in health care facilities. Nurse uniforms have since been introduced in several jurisdictions across the country, and research by the NSNU shows that the uniforms are popular with both nurses and patients (Corporate Research Associates, 2013).

In 2015, the NSNU released its publication *Broken Homes*, an examination of the province's long-term care sector from the perspective of working nurses (Curry, 2015). The report outlined the poor state of long term care in the province and ushered in several key reforms, such as the increased use of NPs in long-term care, an improved long-term care practicum for nursing students, leadership training for nurses in long-term care, specialized behavioural management units, and improved awareness of violence in long-term care. The report also increased the public's awareness of the staffing levels needed to provide quality care in nursing homes.

In 2017, the NSNU worked with employers and the government to improve safety in community hospital emergency departments. Together, they generated a report with 12 expansive recommendations designed to create safer working conditions for emergency care workers.

In 2019, the NSNU released *Nursing Potential—Optimizing Nursing and Primary Healthcare in Nova Scotia* (Curry, Hiltz, & Buckle, 2019), a report about improving primary health care in the province by expanding the role of nurses and removing barriers to their practice.

Newfoundland and Labrador

In 1971, represented by the Association of Registered Nurses of Newfoundland (ARNN), RNs signed their first collective agreement. The 2-year agreement attempted to improve compensation and conditions for RNs, but 3 years later it was apparent that little improvement had been made. Staff nurses continued to be poorly compensated, and a nurse's working life continued to consist of long days with little time off and few, if any, benefits.

In 1973, the *Public Service Collective Bargaining Act* was introduced, making it illegal for an employee organization to be influenced or dominated by management. As such, the ARNN Council, which consisted of both management and staff RNs, could no longer represent RNs in collective bargaining. In 1974, the Newfoundland Nurses' Union was founded to represent staff RNs. Today, this union is named the Registered Nurses' Union of Newfoundland and Labrador (RNUNL).

Throughout its history, the RNUNL has achieved significant gains for its members through collective bargaining and advocacy. The union has positively impacted nurses' wages, and the collective agreements now benefit RNs with competitive salaries, improved pension plans, health and disability benefits, family leave, maternity leave, and a 37.5-hour work week.

RNUNL has negotiated many collective agreements with only three strikes: a rotating strike in 1977, and two provincial strikes, in 1979 and 1999. In 1999, RNs were legislated back to work after 9 days on the picket line. But the fight for a respectful collective agreement did not end there. By putting constant pressure on employers and the government in the 12 months after the strike, the union achieved benefits for nurses that went far beyond what RNs had been looking for on the picket line. In 2009, the RNUNL was just 2 hours away from job action when a historic agreement was reached with the provincial government, proving that a strike mandate and a strike deadline can have a powerful influence on achieving membership priorities and moving government away from template bargaining.

Over the years, the RNUNL has become a recognized voice of the nursing profession, as well as an advocate for an improved health care system and the rights of patients, clients, and residents. One of the most significant campaigns for RNUNL is the Clarity Project. This multi-year, award-winning project focuses on promoting the value and identity of RNs. It captures the pride RNs have for their profession and the vital role they play in delivering quality health care. The project also encourages RNs to adopt the unique uniform colours of white and black, making them stand out in hospitals, health centres, and the community.

Prince Edward Island

Collective bargaining rights for nurses were included in the amended *PEI Nurses' Act* in 1972 because nurses had been excluded from the *PEI Labour Act*. Thus, the Provincial Collective Bargaining Committee of the Association of Nurses of Prince Edward Island (ANPEI) held legal responsibility for collective bargaining for nurses in the province. The first collective agreement was not negotiated until 1974 because the government and the ANPEI did not agree on the regulations to implement the act. Although nurses in PEI did not have the right to strike, a standoff between the nurses and the government was resolved when the government agreed to a compromise after the nurses threatened to resign.

For a time, it seemed that Prince Edward Island might be the only province that would not establish a separate organization for collective bargaining. Then, in 1987, the *PEI Nurses' Act* was amended to remove responsibility for collective bargaining from the ANPEI, and the *Labour Act* was amended to ensure that nurses would not be excluded from its provisions. As a result, the PEI Nurses' Union (PEINU) was established. Today, the union represents more than 1,200 RNs and NPs working in acute care, long-term care, community care, mental health, and addictions.

Following health care reform in the 1990s, nurses in PEI began facing staff shortages and difficult working conditions, problems similar to those in other provinces. Retention, recruitment, staffing, and occupational health and safety concerns remain on the forefront of PEINU's advocacy for their nurses.

Northwest Territories, Nunavut, and Yukon

The Registered Nurses Association of the Northwest Territories and Nunavut (RNANT/NU) was founded in 1975 and serves as both a regulatory body and a professional association. RNs and NPs are the only self-regulated health professionals in both territories. The RNANT/NU performs regulatory functions to ensure that nurses who are practicing in its jurisdiction protect the public through registration, professional conduct review, and approval of education programs. It does not advocate for the nursing profession as a union.

The Yukon Registered Nurses' Association is also a regulatory body and professional association. Nurses in these jurisdictions are employees of the federal and territorial governments and are represented by government employees' unions. For the most part, nurses are members of either

the Public Service Alliance of Canada or The Professional Institute of Public Service of Canada. These unions are multi-sectoral and represent more professions than the traditional nurses' unions in other provinces. These organizations work very closely with the professional nursing associations in these jurisdictions, as recruitment and retention of nurses are ongoing issues.

 APPLYING CONTENT KNOWLEDGE

Reflect on the development of a nursing union in one province or territory and explain the current issues the selected union is working on.

UNION OR MANAGEMENT: TWO SIDES OF THE SAME COIN?

Unions across Canada have many different recognition clauses that identify who is represented by what union. Staff nurses and NPs (in some provinces) are typically represented by their respective unions. The dilemma concerning union representation is most prevalent for first-line managers. Provincial differences exist with respect to whether certain employees can be included in the bargaining unit. In jurisdictions, the "hiring and firing" standard has been used, and managers who perform these functions are disqualified from being union members. In other instances, management has redefined functions to ensure that first-line managers are not included in the bargaining unit.

Many nurses do not wish to be removed from the bargaining unit because they will no longer have job security in the face of downsizing, replacement, or layoffs, nor the benefits afforded them under their collective agreements. Nurse managers have little protection in comparison to staff nurses and others covered by the collective agreement. Many provinces have therefore had difficulty enticing staff nurses to leave the bargaining unit to become "management" with no collective agreement rights.

The Quebec and New Brunswick nurses' unions represent nurses in management positions, but this is not the case in other provinces and territories. This dilemma was especially evident in the 1990s, when all middle-management positions were endangered as organizations aimed for lower-cost "flat" structures consisting of fewer managers. As a result, "nursing departments" have been dissolved, and some unit managers and directors who oversee nurses are not nurses themselves. Unions and nurse leaders claim that these factors are diminishing the potential power of nursing within health care organizations and silencing nursing leaders, who are in a unique position to evaluate the operational effectiveness of the system.

CASE STUDY
Professional Responsibility Clauses—Advocating for Quality Patient Care

A major concern for unions today is the work climate in which nurses are expected to function. The advent of professional responsibility clauses as part of collective agreements is tangible evidence of this trend. Emphasis on salaries and wages continues but working conditions for nurses have become a high priority in negotiations. One consequence of the deep cuts to health care system funding has been staff shortages, as fewer nurses are expected to carry heavier and heavier patient loads as well as work an unreasonable number of overtime hours.

Nurses are deeply concerned about the quality and safety of the care they provide. Structuring collective agreements to allow nurses to negotiate with their employer about certain resources that may be necessary for providing safe care is an integral part of the collective bargaining process. Examples of difficulty in providing adequate care can be documented using professional responsibility workload report forms (see Figure. 19.4). These records provide data to support concerns discussed at meetings with management on professional responsibility committees.

In 1976, RNs from the intensive care unit at Mount Sinai Hospital, Toronto, were disciplined for refusing to take on additional patients from emergency when appropriate staffing was not provided. The matter went to arbitration, and the arbitrator ruled against the union on the basis that the "obey and grieve" rule was appropriate in these circumstances. Outraged by this decision, the union took their workload concerns to the bargaining table. As a result, in 1977, ONA achieved the first "professional responsibility" clause in Canada at Mount Sinai Hospital through an arbitration award. The clause provided a forum for nurses to bring forward their concerns when assigned work that was inconsistent with proper patient care. If unresolved at the hospital level, an independent nurse tribunal known as an Independent Assessment Committee (IAC) would hold a hearing and then provide recommendations to address the nurses' concerns. By 1980, ONA had bargained for all hospitals to include this provision in their collective agreements.

The resolution of workload and professional practice concerns can have a positive impact on the health care setting and ensures safer patient care and better outcomes. As part of their leadership role in health care teams, RNs are mandated by their respective regulatory bodies to report their concerns about the health care system if it is not meeting patient care needs. RNs are also ethically obligated to make recommendations to address the concerns of quality and safe patient care.

A nurse's concerns and recommendations are documented on a professional responsibility workload report form that is presented and discussed with their manager. If a satisfactory resolution cannot be reached with an employer regarding the nurse's professional practice concerns, the matter is forwarded to an IAC panel composed of three RNs: one chosen by the union, one chosen by the employer, and a chair mutually agreed upon by the employer and the union. The panel is charged with evaluating whether the employer assigned a number of patients or a workload that is inconsistent with proper patient care. The IAC can make recommendations to alleviate issues it identifies as being a problem.

The recommendations arising from various IAC panels have been helpful to both the union and the employer in resolving professional practice issues. For example, at Humber River Hospital, a hearing was held from June 18 to 20, 2014, regarding the endoscopy units. The panel (chaired by Claire Mallette) released its decision on August 4, 2014, concluding that the RN staffing levels at Humber River Hospital's two endoscopy units were inadequate. The panel also made 32 recommendations to improve patient care by addressing RN staffing levels, fragmentation of patient care, improper staff support, and an incorrect skill mix that was putting patients at risk. The recommendations were grouped into nine categories: RN staffing; roles and responsibilities, including clarity regarding the role of RPNs; processes, including unit practices, calling in staff, and job descriptions; communication; collaborative working relationships; workplace conflict and violence resolution; leadership; education; and system change management (Mallette, Steed, & Gabrielli, 2014).

The Humber River panel made recommendations regarding the need to change the model of care, stating that "patient safety risks are even higher with the new practice model and introduction of the RPN role in the procedure room" (Mallette, Steed, & Gabrielli, 2014, p. 43). The panel also recommended that the endoscopy unit ensure that transfer of care of a sedated patient from the procedure room to the recovery room is from either an anesthetist to an RN or from one RN to another RN.

In the case of the 2014 Rouge Valley Hospital hearing about staffing issues in the post-acute care unit, the IAC panel concluded that the RNs were "unable to provide proper patient care" (Cardiff, Anderson, & Hubley, 2014).

(Continued)

CASE STUDY (*Cont.*)

The panel identified 50 recommendations, focusing on the areas of leadership and governance, nursing care delivery model and associated staffing, and clinical practice/unit processes.

The Rouge Valley IAC noted in its report that the hospital had cut 55% of its RN positions and that the unit had "suffered significantly" from a low number of full-time, unit-based RNs, RPNs, and other staff (Cardiff, Anderson, & Hubley, 2014). The panel called for an increase in the number of full-time RNs and other nurses to enable better coverage of the baseline schedule with full-time staff instead of a heavy reliance on the part-time pool and agency staff. The panel also recommended that Rouge Valley revise its model of care to better use the RN as a leader of the care team; that the hospital clarify the role of RNs, RPNs, and unregulated care providers; that evidence be used to achieve a safe staffing model; and that practices and voices of frontline nurses be valued and respected in order to improve patient care and patient outcomes.

More recently, in 2017, at the Southlake Regional Health Centre, the IAC conducted a 3-day hearing to investigate whether RNs were being asked to assume more work than is consistent with the provision of proper patient care. The issues were related to nurse-to-patient ratio, patient acuity/complexity of care requirements, and patient volumes in the emergency department. The RNs submitted over 120 professional responsibility workload report forms from January 2016 to the time of the hearing, documenting situations where patient care was at risk owing to significant professional responsibility and workload concerns.

Nurses across Canada continue to use the professional responsibility clause in their collective agreements to ensure that they meet their reporting obligations under their regulatory colleges. They also continue to advocate for safe and quality practice environments for the patients, residents, and clients they serve (Canadian Nurses Association, 2017).

Sources: Canadian Nurses Association. (2017). *Code of ethics for registered nurses*. Ottawa, ON: Author. Retrieved from https://www.cna-aiic.ca/-/media/cna/page-content/pdf-en/code-of-ethics-2017-edition-secure-interactive.pdf; Cardiff, J., Anderson, C., & Hubley, G. (2014). *Independent Assessment Committee report—Rouge Valley Health System and Ontario Nurses' Association.* Retrieved from https://www.ona.org/wp-content/uploads/ona_iacreport_rougevalleyhealthsystem_201402.pdf; Mallette, C., Steed, B., & Gabrielli, C. (2014, July). *Independent Assessment Committee report—Humber River Hospital and Ontario Nurses' Association.* Retrieved from https://www.ona.org/wp-content/uploads/ona_iacreport_humberriverhospital_20160612.pdf.

IMPACT OF LOSING THE RIGHT TO STRIKE

The denial of the right of any particular professional group to strike is unusual and represents legislative interference with the freedom to engage in the typical processes associated with collective bargaining (Anderson & Anderson, 1982). Most Ontario nurses lost the right to strike when the *Hospital Disputes Arbitration Act* of 1965 was passed. The right to strike was denied to nurses employed in hospitals in Alberta in 1983 after a period of acrimonious labour relations among Alberta nurses, the provincial government, and the Alberta Hospital Association. Three legal nurses' strikes between 1977 and 1982 motivated the Alberta government to enact legislation that denied hospital nurses and some other workers the right to strike because their services were deemed essential. This legislation imposed severe penalties on those who defied the law. As noted earlier, severe penalties under this legislation were imposed on the UNA because of an illegal strike in 1988. Quebec nurses also suffered penalties after their 23-day illegal strike in 1999. It is possible that events in Alberta convinced the government of British Columbia that legislation to prevent nurses' strikes was necessary. Nurses in Prince Edward Island also do not

have the right to strike; in several other provinces, the right of nurses to strike is severely limited by conditions that must be satisfied during a strike.

A question that is often asked is whether the presence or absence of the freedom to strike compromises a union's position at the bargaining table. In Ontario, nurses in hospitals and nursing homes have not had the right to strike for three decades, but salary levels appear to exceed those in most other provinces. Indeed, until Alberta nurses asserted themselves in the wake of a booming economy in the late 1970s and early 1980s, Ontario nurses had the highest salaries in Canada. Since then, nurses in Ontario, Alberta, and British Columbia have had very similar salaries, with minor shifts in position with ongoing contract settlements.

APPLYING CONTENT KNOWLEDGE

Explore the use of the right to strike in nursing, and discuss how you might respond if your bargaining unit voted to strike to support the members' bargaining objectives.

Activism and Professionalism go Hand-in-hand

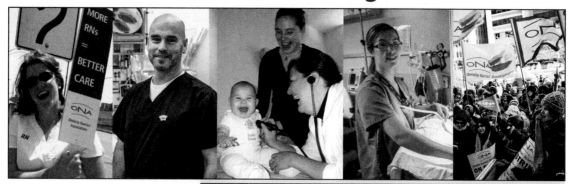

Are you concerned about the quality of care you can provide?

Most of ONA's collective agreements contain a process that lets you address concerns about your professional practice and workload issues.

The professional responsibility process has improved patient care including:

- Increased staffing levels.
- Developed safer workplaces.
- Improved communication between nurses.

ONA's Professional Responsibility Clause

✓ Gives you a say in the quality of care you provide.

✓ Provides a problem-solving approach that helps you meet your professional standards.

✓ Provides documented evidence.

✓ Provides you with union representation for practice concerns and as a venue for dispute resolution.

ONA is here to help you with your practice and workload concerns. Please visit the ONA Professional Practice website at www.ona.org/pp for important resources, information and tips that will help you to solve workplace issues.

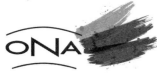

Ontario Nurses' Association

Reporting unsafe patient/client/resident care or practice to your employer is your professional responsibility.

How to report

- Obtain a *Professional Responsibility Workload Report Form* from your Bargaining Unit President.
- Fill out the form every time the employer creates an unsafe and/or unprofessional practice or setting.
- This form is the start of a paper trail to show there are problems that need a response from your employer.

When to use the form

Fill out a form when you encounter:

☐ Inadequate/inappropriate staff and/or skill mix for acuity/activity.

☐ Any delayed, incomplete or missed assessment, treatment or medication.

☐ Non-nursing duties and/or lack of support staff.

☐ Any workload, employer practice, policy or situation that is detrimental to patient/client/resident care and/or safety.

☐ New patients or overflow patients admitted to unit with inadequate staff.

☐ Lack of educational support including staff not given adequate orientation and/or mentorship in area assigned.

☐ Lack of leadership and/or leadership support.

☐ Lack of adequate equipment and/or supplies.

When completing the form

When completing the form, always contact your Bargaining Unit President for assistance.

Focus on:

- **Patient care factors** – for example, care requirements – acuity, complexity and predicatability, overcapacity/hallway patients, 1:1 patients, restraints, altered mental status, less than four hours post-op, etc.

- **Nurse** – ability to meet practice standards, category of nurse/care provider, new, experienced and familiar to the area/unit.

- **Environment** – practice supports, policies, time for consultation and collaboration, equipment.

- **Practice** – how was your practice affected?

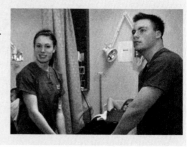

The Ontario Nurses' Association is the union representing 68,000 front-line registered nurses and allied health professionals as well as more than 18,000 nursing student affiliates providing care in Ontario hospitals, long-term care facilities, public health, the community, industry and clinics.

Fig. 19.4 An educational tool that assists nurses in meeting their professional obligations by reporting unsafe care to their employer. (Ontario Nurses' Association)

CHARACTERISTICS OF PROFESSIONAL ASSOCIATIONS AND UNIONS: WORKING TOGETHER

The development of both leadership and organizational culture and norms is an evolutionary process and thus takes time. Nurses have had to learn about the collective bargaining process and how to use collective power to their advantage. Professional nursing associations, dating formally from 1910 and informally for many years before that, have had a much longer history than nursing unions. The maturity that characterizes the relationship between professional associations and unions is extremely important, as it defines the nature of the interactions between them. The initial growth period of unions was characterized by both positive and negative relationships between these organizations. Because unions were organizational newcomers, their independence and determined challenges may have come as a surprise to professional associations that had not expected to be at odds over issues with their counterpart union groups.

Professional associations and unions have many common goals, including promoting the welfare of members and improving their working conditions. Since professional associations include many who are not members of nursing unions and whose economic interests are not served directly by unions, professional associations continue to play an important role in advising and assisting. Most nurses in management are included in this group, as Quebec and New Brunswick are the only provinces where the union represents nursing managers and supervisors. Professional associations are also interested in ensuring that salaries and benefits for staff nurses continue at sufficiently high levels to maintain the status of the profession and to encourage prospective candidates to pursue nursing as a career.

Unions and professional associations share a concern for professional ethics, supporting nursing students, improving social determinants of health, influencing health policy, promoting excellence in nursing practice, and increasing nurses' contributions to shaping the health care system. The major difference is that unions negotiate collective agreements for nonmanagerial nurses. However, the majority of their positions are aligned, and thus the joint work of unions and professional associations continues to evolve.

CANADIAN NURSING ADVOCACY TO SAVE MEDICARE

CFNU and the provincial nursing unions have long supported a universal publicly funded, administered, and delivered health care system. Canadian nursing unions, joined by other unions across Canada, have partnered with the Canadian Health Coalition (CHC) to advocate for and advance this ideal. When the CHC was formed in 1979, universal public health care in Canada was just over a decade old and was already being challenged. User fees and extra-billing, along with a change in transfer payments to the provinces, were chipping away at the health care system. This motivated unions, health care workers, churches, and concerned individuals to come together to advocate on a national scale for everyone to have access to the best possible health care. Since the beginning, nurses have made important contributions to the CHC's work.

The *Canada Health Act* was enacted in 1984; Chapter 1 details its particulars. This law banned extra-billing and placed conditions on the provinces and territories to access federal funding for health care. The CHC monitors the enforcement of the *Canada Health Act* to ensure that health care remains public and accessible to all.

The CHC has also been working to expand the public health care system to include pharmacare and senior care. As an example, the CHC has called for a National Seniors Care Strategy to ensure consistent funding, standards of care, and adequate staffing levels across the country so all seniors can access quality care, regardless of where they live in Canada.

SUMMARY OF LEARNING OBJECTIVES

- A Supreme Court ruling in 1973 determined that a professional association that represented both managers and staff posed a conflict of interest and therefore could not represent staff nurses in collective bargaining. As a result, nursing unions were formed to negotiate collective agreements on behalf of staff nurses.
- The gradual evolution of nursing unions is different for each province and territory in Canada. Several unions were formed when the professional associations were found to be in conflict by representing all levels of nurses (including managers). Therefore, unions in several provinces, including British Columbia, Alberta, Saskatchewan, Manitoba, Ontario, New Brunswick, Nova Scotia, and PEI, all began to address this issue by separating from their professional associations. Quebec did not, as it has had a nurses union since the 1940s, and nurses in the Northwest Territories, Yukon, and Nunavut are under federal jurisdiction for the most

part, and are members of either the Public Service Alliance of Canada or The Professional Institute of Public Service of Canada.

- The establishment of the CFNU in 1981 paralleled the formation of provincial nursing unions. The CFNU is the national voice for unionized nurses in Canada, representing nurses to governments, the public, and the national media. Some priorities championed by the CFNU include safe staffing, national pharmacare, and healthy and safe workplaces.
- Nurses' unions have helped to improve wages, health care benefits, pensions, and staffing. Unions have advocated for amending occupational health and safety legislation and for the rights of marginalized groups.
- Nursing unions in Canada have partnered with like-minded organizations, including the Canadian Health Coalition, to advocate for a publicly funded, administered, and delivered health care system. Unions are involved in provincial and federal committees that develop health care policy for the benefit of patients, clients, and residents, such as nurse-to-patient staffing ratios and coroner's inquest recommendations.
- Nurses' unions have helped to usher in improvements to health and safety legislation, including giving nurses added protection from infectious disease, workplace violence, PTSD, and needlestick injuries. Nurses' unions also helped to ensure that nurses were included as first responders in PTSD legislation in some provinces.
- The denial of the right to strike represents legislative interference with the freedom to engage in striking, a usual process associated with collective bargaining. After several acrimonious strikes took place, several provinces in Canada enacted legislation that replaced the right to strike with arbitration.
- When professional associations and unions created separate entities, their roles also changed. The professional associations addressed issues such as education, nursing policy, professional ethics, social determinants of health, health policy, and excellence in nursing practice. The unions were certified as the bargaining agents negotiating collective agreements for members. Now, the negotiation of collective agreements addresses social policies, professional ethics and responsibility, nursing policy, and government funding, resulting in unions working in tandem with their professional associations on common concerns.
- Provincial nurses' unions have worked together with their CFNU counterparts to advocate for a publicly funded, administered, and delivered health care system. Unions have partnered with and are members of the CHC. Together, they advocate for Medicare for all, so that regardless of race, income, religion, health, or gender, all individuals have access to the best possible health care. Unions also participate in advocacy efforts across Canada for a national pharmacare program.
- The professional responsibility clauses in collective agreements provide nurses with the opportunity to address concerns with their employers regarding workload, standards of practice, and professional responsibility. If their concerns are not addressed by their employer, nurses can request that an Independent Assessment Committee (made up of expert nurses) review these concerns and make recommendations to the employer and union to improve the working life of nurses and care and outcomes for patients.

CRITICAL THINKING QUESTIONS

1. Explain why nurses found it necessary to develop programs to bargain collectively for their salaries, wages, and benefits within various jurisdictions in Canada.
2. What impact has losing the right to strike had in provinces where this decision has been mandated by provincial governments?
3. In addition to fighting for better wages, explain other advocacy efforts by unions.
4. How does the use of the professional responsibility workload report form serve both patients and nurses?

REFERENCES

Aiken, L. H., Clarke, S. P., Sloane, D. M., et al. (2002). Hospital nurse staffing and patient mortality, nurse burnout and job dissatisfaction. *Journal of the American Medical Association, 288*(16), 1987–1993. https://doi.org/10.1001/jama.288.16.1987.

Anderson, J., & Anderson, M. (1982). *Union–management relations in Canada.* Toronto, ON: Addison-Wesley.

Archibald, T. (2004). Collective bargaining by nurses in Canadian health care: Assessing recent trends and emerging claims. *Health Law Journal, 11*, 77–198.

Ball, J. E., Bruyneel, L., Aiken, L. H., et al. (2017). Post-operative mortality, missed care and nurse staffing in nine countries: A cross-sectional study. *International Journal of Nursing Studies, 78*, 10–15. https://doi.org/10.1016/j.ijnurstu.2017.08.004.

Batt, S. (2019). *The big money club: Revealing the players and their campaign to stop pharmacare*. Ottawa, ON: The Canadian Federation of Nurses Unions. Retrieved from https://nursesunions.ca/research/big-money-club/.

Berry, L., & Curry, P. (2012). *Nursing workload and patient care*. Ottawa, ON: The Canadian Federation of Nurses Unions. Retrieved from https://nursesunions.ca/research/nursing-workload-and-patient-care/.

Botterill-Conroy, M. D. (1980). *Labour relations, collective bargaining and nursing*. Edmonton, AB: Unpublished manuscript. University of Alberta, Division of Health Services Administration and Community Medicine.

Canadian Federation of Nurses Unions. (2019a). *Our story*. Retrieved from www.nursesunions.ca/our-story.

Canadian Federation of Nurses Unions. (2019b). *Workplace violence toolkit*. Ottawa, ON: Author. Retrieved from https://nursesunions.ca/workplace-violence-toolkit-campaigns/.

Canadian Nurses Association & Canadian Federation of Nurses Unions. (2015). *Evidence-based safe nurse staffing toolkit*. Ottawa, ON: Author. Retrieved from https://www.cna-aiic.ca/-/media/cna/page-content/pdf-en/2019-evidencebasedsafenursestaffingtoolkitaccessiblecontent2.pdf.

Cimiotti, J. P., Aiken, L. H., Sloane, D. M., & Wu, E. S. (2012). Nurse staffing, burnout, and health care-associated infection. *American Journal of Infection Control, 40*(6), 486–490. https://doi.org/10.1016/j.ajic.2012.02.029.

Cohen, M., Village, J., Ostry, A. S., et al. (2004). Workload as a determinant of staff injury in intermediate care. *International Journal of Occupational and Environmental Health, 10*(4), 375–383. https://doi.org/10.1179/oeh.2004.10.4.375.

Corporate Research Associates. (2013). *Public opinion poll of 400 Nova Scotians*. Dartmouth, NS: Nova Scotia Nurses' Union.

Cox, K., & Mickleburgh, R. (2001, June 27). Nova Scotia girds for health strike. *Globe and Mail*. Retrieved from https://www.theglobeandmail.com/news/national/nova-scotia-girds-for-health-strike/article4150128/.

Curry, P. (2015). *Broken Homes – Nurses speak out on the state of long-term care in Nova Scotia and chart a course for a sustainable future*. Halifax, NS: Nova Scotia Nurses' Union. Retrieved from https://www.nsnu.ca/advocacy-campaigns/brokenhomes.

Curry, P., Hiltz, J., & Buckle, A. (2019). *Nursing potential — Optimizing nursing and primary healthcare in Nova Scotia*. Halifax, NS: Nova Scotia Nurses' Union. Retrieved from https://www.nsnu.ca/advocacy-campaigns/brokenhomes.

Duffield, C., Diers, D., O'Brien-Pallas, L., et al. (2011). Nurse staffing, nursing workload, the work environment and patient outcomes. *Applied Nursing Research, 24*(4), 244–255. https://doi.org/10.1016/j.apnr.2009.12.004.

Fédération interprofessionnelle de la santé du Québec. (2016). *Negotiated by us, for us. Collective Agreement July 2016 – March 2020*. Montreal, QC: Author. Retrieved from http://www.fiqsante.qc.ca/wp-content/uploads/2016/10/Convention_collective_Web_2016-2020_ANG.pdf?download=1.

Fédération interprofessionnelle de la santé du Québec. (2017). *The black book of care safety*. Montreal, QC: Author. Retrieved from http://www.fiqsante.qc.ca/wp-content/uploads/2017/12/FIQ-LivreNoir_ENG-Web.pdf?download=1.

Gagnon, M. A. (2014). *A roadmap to a rational pharmacare policy in Canada*. Ottawa, ON: Canadian Federation of Nurses Unions. Retrieved from https://nursesunions.ca/wp-content/uploads/2017/05/Pharmacare_FINAL.pdf.

Health Canada. (2019). *A prescription for Canada: Achieving pharmacare for all*. Advisory Council on the Implementation of National Pharmacare. Ottawa, ON: Author. Retrieved from https://www.canada.ca/en/health-canada/corporate/about-health-canada/public-engagement/external-advisory-bodies/implementation-national-pharmacare/final-report.html.

House of Commons Standing Committee on Health. (2018, April). *Pharmacare Now: Prescription Medicine Coverage for All Canadians*.14th Report. 42nd Parliament, 1st Session. Ottawa, ON: Parliament, House of Commons. Retrieved from https://www.ourcommons.ca/Content/Committee/421/HESA/Reports/RP9762464/hesarp14/hesarp14-e.pdf.

House of Commons. (2019). *Petitions: Petition E-1902. Healthcare workers*. Retrieved from https://petitions.ourcommons.ca/en/Petition/Details?Petition=e-1902.

Jacobson Consulting Inc. (2017). *Trends in own illness- or disability-related absenteeism and overtime among publicly employed registered nurses. Quick Facts 2017*. Retrieved from https://nursesunions.ca/wp-content/uploads/2017/05/Quick_Facts_Absenteeism-and-Overtime-2017-Final.pdf.

Kealey, L. (2008). No more 'Yes Girls': Labour activism among New Brunswick nurses, 1964–1981. *Acadiensis, 37*(2), 3. Retrieved from https://journals.lib.unb.ca/index.php/Acadiensis/article/view/11146.

Lopert, R., Docteur, E., & Morgan, S. (2018). *Body count: The human cost of financial barriers to prescription medications*. Ottawa, ON: Canadian Federation of Nurses Unions. Retrieved from https://nursesunions.ca/wp-content/uploads/2018/05/2018.04-Body-Count-Final-web.pdf.

MacDonald, L. (2014). UPN members vote to merge with BCNU. *British Columbia Nurses' Union Update, 33*(5). Retrieved from https://www.bcnu.org/news-and-events/news/upn-members-vote-merge-bcnu.

Mackenzie, H. (2016). *Down the drain: How Canada has wasted $62 billion health care dollars without pharmacare*. Ottawa, ON: Canadian Federation of Nurses Unions. Retrieved from https://nursesunions.ca/wp-content/uploads/2017/05/Down_The_Drain_Pharmacare_Report_December_2017.pdf.

MacPhee, M. (2014). *Valuing patient safety: Responsible workforce design*. Ottawa, ON: Canadian Federation of Nurses Unions. Retrieved from https://nursesunions.ca/research/valuing-patient-safety-responsible-workforce-design/.

Manitoba Nurses' Union. (2010). *MNU handbook*. Winnipeg, MB: Author.

Manitoba Nurses' Union. (2015). *Post-traumatic stress disorder (PTSD) in the nursing profession: Helping Manitoba's wounded healers*. Winnipeg, MB: Author. Retrieved from http://traumadoesntend.ca/wp-content/uploads/2015/04/75005-MNU-PTSD-BOOKLET-SCREEN.pdf.

Manitoba Nurses' Union. (2018). *The future of long-term care is now: Addressing nursing care needs in Manitoba's personal care homes*. Winnipeg, MB: Manitoba Nurses Union. Retrieved from https://manitobanurses.ca/system/files/MNU-Long%20Term%20Care%20Report%202018.pdf.

Manitoba Nurses' Union. (2019). *A history of caring*. Retrieved from https://manitobanurses.ca/system/files/81080-MNU-TImeline-History-Book-Digital-press.pdf.

Marandolo, S. (2018, January 31). Sherbrooke nurse's cry for help on social media prompts response from health minister. *CBC News*. Retrieved from https://www.cbc.ca/news/Sherbr/montreal/Sherbrooke-nurse-social-post-1.4513475.

McGee, A. H. (1994). *The strength of one: A history of the New Brunswick Nurses Union*. Fredericton, NB: New Brunswick Nurses Union.

National Assembly. (2003a). *Bill 25 (2003, chapter 21). An Act respecting local health and social services network development agencies*. Québec, QC: Québec Official Publisher. Retrieved from http://www2.publicationsduquebec.gouv.qc.ca/dynamicSearch/telecharge.php?type=5&file=2003C21A.PDF.

National Assembly. (2003b). *Bill 30 (2003, chapter 25). An Act respecting bargaining units in social affairs sector and amending the Act respecting the process of negotiation of the collective agreements in the public and parapublic sectors*. Québec, QC: Author. Retrieved from http://www2.publicationsduquebec.gouv.qc.ca/dynamicSearch/telecharge.php?type=5&file=2003C25A.PDF.

National Assembly. (2015). *Bill 30 (2015, chapter 1). An Act to modify the organization and governance of the health and social services network, in particular by abolishing the regional agencies*. Quebec, QC: Author. Retrieved from http://www2.publicationsduquebec.gouv.qc.ca/dynamicSearch/telecharge.php?type=5&file=2015C1A.PDF.

Needleman, J., Buerhaus, P., Mattke, S., et al. (2002). Nurse-staffing levels and the quality of care in hospitals. *New England Journal of Medicine., 346*(22), 1715–1722. https://doi.org/10.1056/NEJMsa012247.

Needleman, J., Buerhaus, P., Pankratz, S., et al. (2011). Nurse staffing and inpatient hospital mortality. *New England Journal of Medicine*(364), 1037–1045. https://doi.org/10.1056/NEJMsa1001025.

Rafferty, A. M., Clarke, S. P., Coles, J., et al. (2007). Outcomes of variation in hospital nurse staffing in English hospitals: Cross-sectional analysis of survey data and discharge records. *International Journal of Nursing Studies, 44*(2), 175–182. https://doi.org/10.1016/j.ijnurstu.2006.08.003.

Reichert, C. (2017). *Enough is enough: Putting a stop to violence in the health care sector. A discussion paper*. Ottawa, ON: Canadian Federation of Nurses Unions. Retrieved from https://nursesunions.ca/wp-content/uploads/2017/05/CFNU_Enough-is-Enough_June1_FINALlow.pdf.

Robinson, K. M., & Tappen, R. M. (2008). Policy recommendations on the prevention of violence in long-term care facilities. *Journal of Gerontological Nursing, 3*(34), 10–14. https://doi.org/10.3928/00989134-20080301-08.

Rowsell, G. (1982). Changing trends in labour relations: Effects on collective bargaining for nurses. *International Nursing Review, 29*(5), 141–145.

Schubert, M., Clarke, S. P., Aiken, L. H., & de Geest, S. (2012). Associations between rationing of nursing care and inpatient mortality in Swiss hospitals. *International Journal for Quality in Health Care, 24*(3), 230–238. https://doi.org/10.1093/intqhc/mzs009.

Sheward, L., Hunt, J., Hagen, S., et al. (2005). The relationship between UK hospital nurse staffing and emotional exhaustion and job dissatisfaction. *Journal of Nursing Management, 13*(1), 51–60. https://doi.org/10.1111/j.1365-2834.2004.00460.x.

Shindul-Rothschild, J., Flanagan, J., Stamp, K. D., & Read, C. Y. (2017). Beyond the pain scale: Provider communication and staffing predictive of patients' satisfaction with pain control. *Pain Management Nursing, 18*(6), 401–409. https://doi.org/10.1016/j.pmn.2017.05.003.

Silversides, A. (2019). *Taking our place: Stories from leaders of Canada's union movement*. Ottawa, ON: The Canadian Federation of Nurses Unions. Retrieved from https://nursesunions.ca/research/taking-our-place/.

Tatroff, D. (2006). Special twenty-fifth anniversary issue. *British Columbia Nurses' Union Update, 25*(2). Retrieved from https://www.bcnu.org/News-Events/UpdateMagazine/Documents/Update_Feb_Mar06.pdf.

Trinkoff, A. M., Johantgen, M., Muntaner, C., & Le, R. (2005). Staffing and worker injury in nursing homes. *American Journal of Public Health, 95*(7), 1220–1225. https://doi.org/10.2105/AJPH.2004.045070.

PART IV

Educating Nurses for the Future

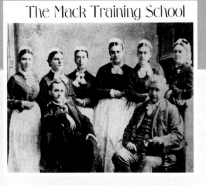
The Mack Training School

The Origins and Development of Nursing Education in Canada

Pauline Paul

LEARNING OBJECTIVES

After reading this chapter, you will be able to:
- Describe when women and nurses first had access to higher education and understand that women were discriminated against by that sector.
- Acknowledge the early preparation of nurses prior to Florence Nightingale.
- Understand how the Nightingale model of nursing education spread around the globe, including Canada.
- Describe the inception of the first hospital schools of nursing in Canada.
- Discuss how several key reports demonstrated the need for better standards in nursing education.

- Understand the movement to establish two-year schools of nursing and institutions and identify how it played out in various provinces.
- Discuss the emergence of university schools of nursing and the evolution of university nursing education overtime.
- Understand the meaning of the "entry-to-practice" position.
- Describe recent developments in nursing education that specifically prepare nurses who can better serve francophone official language minorities and Indigenous peoples.

OUTLINE

KEY TERMS

alumnae
Hall Commission Report
incidental instruction
normal school

private-duty nurses
royal commission
Weir Report

 PERSONAL PERSPECTIVES

What was the schedule of a nursing student in 1930? From November 1929 to July 1931, Dr. G. W. Weir, a professor of education at the University of British Columbia, conducted a national survey of nursing education. He had been appointed to conduct this survey by a joint committee of the Canadian Nurses Association and Canadian Medical Association (Weir, 1932). The extensive survey showed that the typical day of a nursing student was as follows: 9 hours of clinical practice, 1.5 hours of classes, 1.5 hours of study time, 2 hours for meals, 2 hours of recreation, and 8 hours of sleep. This type of schedule was followed 6 days a week. Dr. Weir was appalled at a schedule that required students to be "keyed up to a high pitch of tension for 12 hours a day . . . no other profession would tolerate such working conditions" (Weir, 1932, p. 171). At that time, hospitals hired very few registered nurses. Instead, most of the patient care was the responsibility of nursing students, who all had to live in nursing residences that had very strict rules.

WOMEN AND HIGHER EDUCATION

In the late 1700s in the United States, a crusade began to allow women entry into institutions of higher education. Feminist writer Mary Wollstonecraft (1787, 1792) presented an articulate case for the schooling of women. However, it was not until 1837 that women began to slowly enter higher education in the United States. The first university to admit women in Canada was Mount Allison University in New Brunswick in 1862. It was also the first university in the British Empire to confer a degree on a woman when, in 1875, Grace Annie Lockhart obtained a Bachelor of Science degree (Tunis, 1966; Mount Allison University, 2015).

Teaching was among the first professions to accept female students. One of the early schools to admit women into education programs was the New York College for the Training of Teachers. Founded in 1887 by philanthropist Grace Hoadley Dodge, the institution became Teachers College in 1892 and later a school of Columbia University

(The Editors of Encyclopaedia Britannica, 2018). In 1899, Teachers College established a course in nursing—the first time in the world that nursing was made a university subject area. Considering the concern that Hoadley Dodge had for working women, and that **normal schools** in general were the first to welcome large numbers of women, it is not surprising that the first department of nursing in a university was at Teachers College. Teachers College rapidly became the beacon of university education for women in North America. In 1906, Mary Adelaide Nutting, a Quebec-born American nursing leader, became the director of its nursing program at Columbia University and the first professor of nursing in the world. Columbia played a significant role in educating countless American and Canadian nursing leaders who shaped nursing education throughout the twentieth century.

However, in the beginning of the twentieth century, most nurses did not yet study in universities but rather at hospital schools (and later in colleges) to obtain their nursing diplomas. It is thus important to first consider how hospital nursing schools became the norm in the first half of the twentieth century in Canada.

EARLY PREPARATION FOR NURSING PRACTICE

Although lay nurses had some preparation for practice in the early days of the profession, the training was largely informal. Observation, passing knowledge from one person to another, and on-the-job training were the principal forms of educational preparation for lay nurses from the seventeenth through the nineteenth century. Members of religious nursing orders, including the Augustinians, who arrived at Québec in 1639, received their preparation within their order, which had dedicated itself to the care of the sick. For several centuries, women who joined religious orders were taught the skills of nursing by experienced members of the sisterhood. Lay nurses rarely received this type of education. Among the exceptions were Jeanne Mance and later, Florence Nightingale. Jeanne Mance, the founder of Hôtel-Dieu de Montréal and co-founder of the city, was the first lay nurse of New France. She designed her own course of nursing study, travelling to several centres in France to learn care methods before coming to New France in 1641. Similarly, Florence Nightingale sought nursing knowledge at the Institution for Nursing Deaconesses at Kaiserswerth in Germany and with the Sisters of St. Vincent de Paul in Paris. The genius of Florence Nightingale was that she transformed what she had seen and learned into a school of nursing for laywomen, which gave rise to modern nursing education.

THE NIGHTINGALE MODEL

In 1852, Florence Nightingale eloquently posed the question, "Why have women passion, intellect and moral activity—these three—and a place in society where no one of the three can be exercised?" (Nightingale, 1929, p. 396). In a way, Nightingale answered her own question in 1860, by founding the first school of nursing in conjunction with St. Thomas' Hospital in London. Evidently, this development was needed in Western society, for the idea swept the world, and many hospital nursing schools were established throughout Europe and North America. It can be argued that because Nightingale lived at a time when the British Empire was very strong, the Empire contributed to the propagation of her views about nursing education. However, the first hospital schools of North America lacked an important aspect of the original Nightingale school, namely financial autonomy. The term "the historical accident," coined by Esther Lucile Brown (1948, p. 164), referred to the failure to apply the fundamental philosophy of the Nightingale model to the new schools in North America. In many of these schools, the concept of autonomy was lost in the financial administration of the enterprise. Such schools became completely dependent on the financial stability of the hospital with which they were associated, and policies were dictated by a board of trustees. Nursing students became the workforce of hospitals. They were admitted to hospital schools of nursing to provide the patient care. Providing nursing students with a solid education was not the priority of hospital administrators. Thus, little attention was given to opportunities for instruction in the classroom or during clinical experience, and educational preparation was considered secondary to the needs of the hospital nursing service. It is important to understand that once they graduated, nurses predominantly worked in private homes as **private-duty nurses**. They did not work in hospitals, as hospitals relied on the next cohorts of nursing students to provide patient care.

Certain principles of the first Nightingale school were present in new schools: women who were as well prepared in nursing as possible were placed in charge of the schools, courses were spread over a period of 2 or 3 years, and **incidental instruction** was accompanied by extended periods of practice. It was an apprenticeship system that lacked the master craftsman. In North America, off-duty students attended 1 or 2 hours of lectures that were given each week by a physician or the superintendent of nurses. Those who could attend related the information to those who could not because they were assigned to care duties in the hospital.

One of the first schools in North America to advocate the principles of Florence Nightingale was the Bellevue Training School for Nurses, established in New York in 1873 by Sister Helen Bowden, an Anglican sister who had been educated at University College Hospital in England. Many Canadian women went to the United States to study during this period, and some, including Isabel Hampton Robb, Mary Adelaide Nutting, and Isabel Maitland Stewart, later became leaders in American nursing. Undoubtedly as a result of their influence, close contact was maintained between nurses in Canada and the United States through professional nursing organizations.

THE FIRST CANADIAN HOSPITAL SCHOOLS OF NURSING

The first hospital diploma school in Canada, the Mack Training School for Nurses in St. Catharines, Ontario, was initiated on June 10, 1874, by Dr. Theophilus Mack, an Irish-born physician who was convinced that "the prejudice held by many sick people against going into public hospitals could best be overcome by building up a profession of trained lay nurses" (Gibbon & Mathewson, 1947, p. 144). The picture on the first page of this chapter represents the first nurses to graduate from the school.

Healey (1990) noted that the date of the school's inception "so closely parallels the start of Bellevue that in later years there will be those who seek to prove it was the first on the Continent to incorporate Nightingale's ideas" (pp. 31–32). Healey (1990) also indicated that "Dr. Mack is credited with having the idea [for the establishment of the school] as early as 1864" (p. 43). Constraints were again imposed, as "nursing was considered an undesirable vocation for a refined lady, the only acceptable profession being teaching" (Healey, 1990, p. 44).

Admission standards were "plain English education, good character, and Christian motives" (*St. Catharines Annual Report*, cited in Healey, 1990). The philosophy of the school is reflected in a statement concerning instruction:

> *Every possible opportunity is seized to impart instruction of a practical nature in the art of nursing, while teachings will be given in Chemistry, Sanitary Science, Popular Physiology and Anatomy, hygiene and all such branches of the healing art as a nurse ought to be*

familiar with. . . The vocation of nursing goes hand in hand with that of physician and surgeon, and are absolutely indispensable one to the other. Incompetency on the part of a nurse renders nugatory the best effects of the doctor in the critical moments and has frequently resulted in loss of life. All the most brilliant achievements of modern surgery are dependent to a great extent upon careful and intelligent nursing. . . The skilled nurse, by minutely watching the temperature, conditions of skin, pulse, respirations, the various functions of all the organs and reporting faithfully to the attending physician, must increase the chances of recovery twofold. (Healey, 1990, pp. 45–46)

The School for Nurses associated with the Toronto General Hospital was established in 1881; 17 students enrolled, but eight resigned or were dismissed (Gibbon & Mathewson, 1947). When Mary Agnes Snively, a former schoolteacher from St. Catharines who had graduated from the Bellevue Hospital Training School of New York, was appointed superintendent of the school in 1884, there were no systems for work or study, no written orders, no history records, and no systems for obtaining ward supplies. The living conditions were distressing. The school was gradually reorganized and a modern plan developed (Gibbon & Mathewson, 1947). Snively worked hard to improve the educational component of the program as it developed, making it one of the most successful schools of nursing in the country (Kirkwood, 2005). Snively is also remembered for the roles she played in the International Council of Nurses (ICN) and the Canadian National Association of Trained Nurses (later the Canadian Nurses Association [CNA]).

At the Montreal General Hospital, founded in 1822, early interest in establishing a school of nursing led to the Committee of Management's correspondence in 1874 to secure assistance in developing "a system of trained hospital nurses such as approved of in England" (MacDermot, 1940, p. 17). Correspondence that ensued between Florence Nightingale and her brother-in-law, Henry Bonham Carter, the president of the Nightingale Fund, dealt primarily with plans for the new hospital building that had been promised by the Committee of Management. Miss Machin, a Quebec native who had been nursing at the Nightingale Home in London, set out for Montreal with four Nightingale nurses, but the mission failed. The difficulties that arose during Machin's tenure at the hospital included high staff turnover, and "there is reason to believe there was 'a lack of adaptability on the part of Miss Machin whose uncompromising purpose was to apply Nightingale principles of nursing care at whatever cost and without much thought for diplomacy'" (Redpath; cited in

Baly, 1986, p. 146). The problems she encountered and her failure to accomplish her initial objective—establishing a training school for nurses—led her to perceive that she had failed in her mission, and she returned to England in 1878. Baly (1986) notes that the Council of the Nightingale Fund did not make much of their efforts in Montreal or elsewhere because Cook (Nightingale's biographer) had given Montreal only a passing reference, and Carter clearly thought that the entire issue should be forgotten. Baly (1986) has taken issue with "nursing historians" who "have claimed that Nightingale missioners took reformed nursing to both Canada and Australia and have made much out of little evidence" (p. 147).

The School for Nurses at the Montreal General Hospital was finally initiated in 1890, under the direction of Nora Livingston, who was born to English parents in Sault Ste. Marie, Michigan, raised in Como, Quebec, and educated

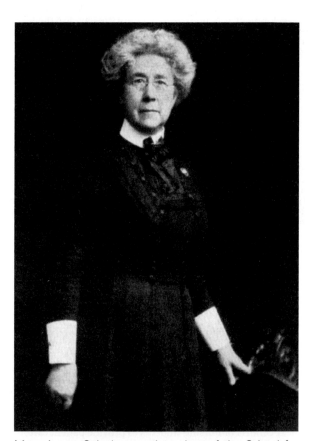

Mary Agnes Snively, superintendent of the School for Nurses at Toronto General Hospital and first president of the National Association of Trained Nurses (later the CNA). (With permission from National Library of Medicine)

at the New York Hospital's Training School for Nurses (MacDermot, 1940). When she arrived in Montreal, she found the conditions deplorable and undertook to improve them immediately to ensure that the hospital and its nurses were soon held in high regard: "By reorganizing the work, gradually encouraging the appointment of nurses to positions of responsibility, and establishing specific duties, Livingston helped to define the proper functions of a nurse" (Cohen, 2005, n.p.).

The popularity of the school increased rapidly. Livingston reported that there were 160 applications in the first year, 80 of which were accepted on probation. Of the 80 students accepted, 42 proved satisfactory (Gibbon & Mathewson, 1947). Recollections of Livingston's abilities are positive:

> What an extraordinary amount of tact and gumption this remarkable woman possessed. Not only had she to change the incredible conditions of nursing but above all she had to change the attitudes of the administrators, men animated by good intentions but more accustomed to conducting the affairs of business than those of a hospital. (Desjardins, 1971, p. 103)

The nursing education program gradually took shape, and one of the early graduates recalled, "Thinking of those days so long ago, I think I hear Miss Livingston say— 'Nurse—the patient—always the patient first!' I think that spirit still lives within these old walls" (Gibbon & Mathewson, 1947, p. 149).

The move to establish hospital schools of nursing swept the country. The Winnipeg General Hospital initiated the first Training School for Nurses in Western Canada in 1887. In Vancouver, the General Hospital began an educational program in 1891, and a school was initiated at Medicine Hat, Alberta, in 1894. In the Maritime provinces, the Saint John General Hospital in Saint John and the Victoria Public Hospital in Fredericton opened training schools for nurses in 1887, and the Victoria General in Halifax and the Prince Edward Island Hospital in Charlottetown followed suit in 1890. By 1930, there were approximately 330 schools of nursing in Canada (CNA, 1968).

 APPLYING CONTENT KNOWLEDGE

An older friend of your grandmother's asks you why nurses are no longer educated in hospital schools of nursing. She thinks nurses were better prepared when they were educated in hospitals. How will you respond to her question? How will you convince her that you are fortunate to be able to study toward a nursing degree and that your patients will benefit from your knowledge?

RECOGNIZING THE NEED FOR IMPROVEMENT IN STANDARDS

Because hospitals were staffed primarily by students in the late nineteenth and early twentieth centuries, there were few opportunities to secure a staff position after graduation. Graduates who practiced their profession usually did so as private-duty nurses in the homes of the sick. Therefore, one of nursing's first struggles after the hospital-based system of nursing education was established involved replacing students with graduate nurses as the primary providers of nursing care. Mabel Holt (1936) writes of an "experiment" in a Montreal hospital in which a nursing unit was totally staffed with graduate nurses and justified the endeavour as follows:

> There are, however, other and even more important benefits... which have come about as a direct result of this new policy. Instead of adding to the output of graduate nurses during these difficult years by increasing the enrolment of our school of nursing, we have created employment for those who otherwise would have been obliged to enter an overcrowded and highly competitive field. (p. 10)

The significance of the 1910 *Flexner Report* on medical education and its impact on nursing education have been noted by Allemang (1974). Funded by the Carnegie Foundation, the *Flexner Report* was commissioned because of concerns about the quality of medical practice and medical education and the concomitant inability of the American Medical Association and the Council on Medical Education to achieve reforms. As a result of the *Flexner Report*, the character of medical education changed quickly in both the United States and Canada; the proprietary schools that operated for profit were closed, and standards in medical education began to rise as the universities assumed major responsibility for the support and direction of the enterprise. According to Allemang (1974), "The Flexner report on medical education provided a model for the new approach to nursing reforms" (pp. 115–116). However, it has been argued that none of the reports on nursing education that were published in the twentieth century had an immediate impact equivalent to that of the *Flexner Report* (Gebbie, 2009). Thus, the call for improved standards of nursing education continued for decades. Increased awareness of deficiencies resulted in a number of surveys of nursing education in Canada and the United States. In 1923, the *Goldmark Report*, commissioned by the Rockefeller Foundation to investigate conditions in schools of nursing in the United States, described appalling conditions. The report advocated for more attention to be directed to the educational preparation of nurses, more stringent admission requirements for nursing schools, and the provision of federal grants to assist schools in raising their educational standards. Reports on schools of nursing made by of a joint committee of several professional nursing associations and professional organizations of related health fields restated the shortcomings of the system (Burgess 1928; Committee on the Grading of Nursing Schools 1934).

In Canada, similar unrest about hospital schools of nursing surfaced in the 1920s. In 1927, a joint committee of the Canadian Medical Association and the CNA was organized to study the problems. The committee appointed Dr. George Weir from the Department of Education at the University of British Columbia to conduct a survey to address these matters. The study documented the problems and drew attention to the changes needed to improve standards of education and service. The fact that small hospitals had established schools of nursing was a concern, as students' education could be compromised by the lack of variety in clinical experience offered at small institutions. The survey indicated that, in operating programs, schools associated with hospitals having fewer than 75 beds were more concerned with the financial needs of the hospital than with the educational needs of the nursing students (CNA, 1968; Gibbon & Mathewson, 1947; Weir, 1932). The health of students was also a concern raised in the **Weir Report**. It was common for schools to require students to work as many as 78 hours per week with just one half-day off-duty. This situation stood in sharp contrast to what was asked of tradespeople and skilled factory workers in 1936. Historical evidence indicates that tradespeople had a 40- to 50-hour work week, while unskilled workers in factories worked 25 to 60 hours a week (Statistics Canada, 2009). Nursing students often had to work overtime, and they were not given time off to compensate for it. Consequently, the grueling hours had an impact on the health of many students, and some did not complete their programs as a result. Classroom instruction was likewise lacking in planning and generally inadequate, with too few and ill-prepared instructors.

Suspicion about the motives of hospitals in offering educational programs led to the recommendation that authority and responsibility for schools of nursing be vested within the general provincial system of education, as stated in the *Weir Report*: "The development of training schools for nurses primarily as educational institutions functioning as an integral part of the general educational system of the province and financed on the same principle as are normal schools, should be made an immediate objective" (Weir, 1932, p. 116). This recommendation was repeated many times in the years before the basic diploma nursing education program began to move to be within the purview of the general postsecondary system of education.

The recommendations of the *Weir Report* led the CNA to organize a national curriculum committee with a mandate to develop a curriculum model (Letourneau, 1975, p. 6). The standard curriculum guide, published in 1936, was intended to serve as an interim measure that would help schools of nursing during their transfer to provincial educational systems (CNA, 1936).

GENDER CONSIDERATIONS

Modern nursing as conceived by Florence Nightingale was a feminine pursuit (Evans, 2004). In Canada, schools of nursing did not admit male students until the 1950s. Not all provincial legislation permitted the recruitment of male nurses. For example, it was not until 1969 that men in Quebec could join the profession. The provincial government was opposed to their becoming nurses, as society continued to view nursing as a woman's job. The first man to become a registered nurse (RN) in Quebec was Jean Robitaille. Six hundred men who had already graduated from Quebec nursing schools could finally become RNs (Anonymous, 1970).

Source: Anonymous. First male nurse licensed to practice in Quebec. *The Canadian Nurse, 66*(2), 10. Retrieved from https://archive.org/details/thecanadiannurse66cnanuoft/page/n65/mode/2up; Evans, J. (2004). Men nurses: A historical and feminist perspective. *Journal of Advanced Nursing, 47*(3), 321–328. https://doi.org/10.1111/j.1365-2648.2004.03096.x.

The Demonstration School

The minimal progress through the next decade led the CNA to secure Red Cross funding for a demonstration school that would ascertain the feasibility of preparing a nurse to practise in less than 3 years. The premise for such a plan was "that an autonomous academic institution run by nurses could attract better candidates to the field than existing hospital-controlled schools, provide superior training, and produce professional nurses in less time" (Palmer, 2013, p. 131). The school, known simply as the Demonstration School, was established in 1948 in conjunction with the Metropolitan Hospital in Windsor, Ontario. Red Cross funding enabled the Demonstration School to be financially independent from the hospital. The experiment continued until 1952, when the Demonstration School reverted to its former status of being financially dependent on the hospital. An extensive evaluation, conducted by a joint committee (chaired by A. R. Lord) of the CNA and the Canadian Education Association, indicated that the venture was a success; it was possible to prepare a nurse for practice in 2 years:

The conclusion is inescapable. When the school has complete control of students, nurses can be trained at least as satisfactorily in two years as in three, and under better conditions, but the training must be paid for in money instead of in services. Few students can afford substantial fees nor can the hospital pass on such additional costs to the "paying patient." Some new source of revenue is the only solution. (Lord, 1952, p. 54)

Although the program was discontinued in 1952, it served as a point of reference for the coming decades, when hospital schools of nursing would receive their own budgets and schools of nursing would be transferred to colleges (Palmer, 2013).

RESEARCH FOCUS

In his historical research using archival information, Palmer (2013) added new knowledge about why the Metropolitan Demonstration School in Windsor was discontinued in 1952. Issues surrounding the school budget and a "sex scandal" that occurred in 1949 seemed to have played a role. The scandal involved nurses, municipal politicians, and hospital administrators. Although none of the nursing school staff or nursing students were involved in the scandal, the community became skeptical. After the scandal came to light, the new, more conservative hospital administration that was appointed brought an end to the project. In his analysis, Palmer suggested that also at play were the views of the time about the place of women in society.

Source: Palmer, S. (2013). Windsor's Metropolitan Demonstration School and the reform on nursing education, 1944–1970. In P. D'Antonio, J. A. Fairman, and J. C. Whelan (Eds.), *Routledge handbook on the global history of nursing* (pp. 131–150). New York, NY: Routledge.

The Centralized Teaching Program

During the same era, in Saskatchewan, there was increasing concern about the lack of foundational courses in basic sciences for nursing students in diploma programs and the general shortage of suitably qualified faculty. The Saskatchewan Registered Nurses Association (SRNA) sought and secured financial support from the W. K. Kellogg Foundation to centralize the teaching of basic sciences for all schools of nursing in the Saskatoon and Regina areas. The program provided for

a duly authorized sixteen weeks' program of instruction in the basic sciences for nursing students. It is an integral part of the curriculum plan of the hospital school of nursing provided apart from the hospital school at a designated centre permitting centralization of effort and resources not immediately available in the local setting of the participating schools. (Schmitt, 1957, p. 6)

Although considerable effort was directed to organizing this model and it was declared a success, the model was not considered a panacea for the ills of basic nursing education. Although many areas of the country decided not to offer basic science instruction on a regional basis, this endeavour provided a solution to some problems in basic diploma nursing education.

Accreditation

The CNA next directed its attention to the quality of instruction in schools of nursing. A pilot project under the direction of Executive Director Helen K. Mussallem was designed to determine whether schools were ready for a national voluntary accreditation program. The findings were somewhat disappointing; only 16% of schools met the criteria for accreditation. It was also determined that little progress had been made in improving the quality of schools since Dr. Weir had made his report public some 30 years before. Dr. Mussallem thus recommended that rather than embark on an accreditation program, the CNA should first establish a school improvement program designed to lead to accreditation in the future (Mussallem, 1960). The CNA took this course of action, and accreditation was not seriously discussed again until the late 1970s. At that time, because of the associated costs, accreditation was not considered for diploma schools in the absence of an organization willing to provide the necessary funds.

In 1983, the Council of the Canadian Association of University Schools of Nursing (CAUSN, now the Canadian Association of Schools of Nursing [CASN]) adopted an accreditation program that had been designed by the organization. The first school of nursing to receive CAUSN Accreditation was the Faculté des sciences infirmières at the Université de Montréal in 1987 (Baker, Guest, Jorgenson et al., 2012). Accreditation and approval are discussed in more detail in Chapter 24.

The Royal Commission on Health Services

In its brief to the **Royal Commission** on Health Services, the CNA favoured "introducing diploma schools of nursing into the post-high school system of the country" (Mussallem, 1964, p. 137). The Royal Commission on Health Services, known as the Hall Commission, surveyed the entire range of health services (including nursing) and submitted its report in 1964 recommending that schools of nursing function independently from hospitals and offer programs shorter than 3 years:

The Commission believes this to be the right approach. The educational system for nursing should be organized and financed like other forms of professional education . . . not only [so] that we shall obtain equally, if not better, qualified personnel in shorter time, but that a substantial part of hospitalized patient care will no longer depend, as it does now, upon apprentices. (Hall, 1964, pp. 64–69)

A certain momentum created by the increased pace of change after the release of the **Hall Commission Report** may have led to the CNA's plan to press for change. Mussallem (1964) declared:

Whether nursing education should be placed within the general educational system can no longer be considered a point of debate. It is possible and it can be done. . . The Canadian Nurses' Association, in cooperation with its provincial counterparts, should take steps to implement the plan presented in the study . . .leading to the inclusion of all nursing education within the general educational system of each province. (pp. 183–185)

THE MOVEMENT TO ESTABLISH TWO-YEAR SCHOOLS

In its recommendations, the Hall Commission proposed that nursing programs could be shortened. Students were continuing to be used to various degrees as a hospital workforce. Eliminating this practice could lead to shorter programs that would be able to deliver the content in 2 years instead of 3 years. As will be seen in the following sections, not all regions of the country moved to shorter programs at the same time. Similarly, in some provinces, nursing education was rapidly relocated to colleges, while in others it took decades for hospital schools of nursing to close their doors. It is important to recall that education is a provincial responsibility. Canada is a vast country with multiple differences. Provincial governments do not always have the same priorities, as political, social, and cultural factors come into play.

Quebec

In Quebec, the Royal Commission of Inquiry on Education, also known as the Parent Commission, made its report in 1966 arguing against initiating 1- or 2-year schools, as suggested by the Association of Nurses of the Province of Quebec, and instead advocated for a total transfer of programs to the general system of education. The commission contended that the recommendations for nursing were totally consistent with findings in other fields. Campbell (1971) commented about the impact of the Parent Commission's report: "It would be difficult to name any royal commission in the history of Canadian education whose judgements more profoundly altered the structure

and process of the entire educational system of a province and with greater speed" (p. 54). One of the central foci of the Quebec government of the time was education. This attention to education meant that the province wanted nursing students to be like all other students enrolled in the newly created collèges d'enseignement général et professionnel (CEGEPs). In these institutions, diploma programs in all fields of study were to be 3 years in length. Besides learning their own field of study, all students were to receive an education that would focus on language (French or English), philosophy, and physical education. This context explains why the province did not agree with the implementation of 2-year programs.

In 1967, three programs were selected for transfer to CEGEPs to serve as pilot projects; 17 were selected in 1968, and others after that. "In 1972, the last Schools of Nursing attached to hospitals closed, ending three-quarters of a century of history. Now a network of 40 nursing options exists throughout 'la belle province'" (Association of Nurses of the Province of Quebec, 1972, p. 1). With the two English-language CEGEPs that already had diploma programs, the number of programs came to 42. Also, "a distinctively unique characteristic of education offered in a CEGEP is that it is tuition free for all full-time students" (Letourneau, 1975, p. 77). Thus, as nursing schools became part of the community college system in Quebec, nursing students began receiving the same educational benefits as students studying in other professions and vocations.

Ontario

The Nightingale School of Nursing in Toronto, established in 1960, was financed by the Ontario Hospital Services Commission. Situated near New Mount Sinai Hospital, where nursing clinical experience was obtained, the school was administered by an independent board of directors. The Quo Vadis School of Nursing was established in 1964 under the auspices of the Catholic Hospital Conference of Ontario with a mandate to attract mature students. Financial support was provided by the Ontario Hospital Services Commission, and the school was administered by an independent board of directors (McLean, 1964).

The School of Nursing established at Ryerson Polytechnical Institute in Toronto in 1964 had the distinction of being the first nursing diploma program in Canada to be initiated in an educational institution (Letourneau, 1975). The efforts of the Registered Nurses' Association of Ontario were influential in instigating this effort. Similar programs were developed in colleges across the country. Although Ryerson's program was initially structured as a 3-year program, it was later converted to a 2-year program. Dr. Moyra Allen of McGill University and Professor Mary Reidy of the Université de Montréal evaluated this program after 5 years and confirmed its soundness. The findings "point to the potential value of preparing a nurse in a college-level institution within the general system of education" (Allen & Reidy, 1971, p. 262).

In 1967, 20 colleges of applied arts and technology (CAATs) were created in the province by order of the Ontario government. In 1969, Humber College was the first of these institutions to develop a nursing program. Ontario moved ahead on another front before it began to develop schools of nursing within the CAAT system on a large scale—the province developed freestanding schools of nursing, or "regional schools," which were separate from the general education system. There were no regional schools in 1965, but "by the end of 1967 there were eight, and ten more . . . expected within the next five years" (Murray, 1970, p. 132). Some of the programs that opened in colleges were in fact the transfer of hospital schools into the mainstream education system. For example, in 1973, the Mack Centre of Nursing Education (its name by then) was relocated in the Niagara College of Applied Arts and Technology. This was a way to preserve a name that had been important. However, the program was now part of the education system and no longer part of the health system.

The government also decided, in spite of the reservations expressed by the College of Nurses of Ontario, to move to "two plus one" programs, initially in a "ten-year plan leading to a gradual shortening and regionalization of schools of nursing" (Letourneau, 1975, p. 144). This change occurred rapidly, but it was a passing phenomenon, as the move to establish 2-year schools under the aegis of the CAATs received overwhelming support, and "in 1972, policies with regard to free room and board were altered, the year of internship was discontinued, and nursing students were required to pay tuition fees" (Letourneau, 1975, p. 145). By 1973, 56 schools had been absorbed by 23 CAATs.

Western Canada

Saskatchewan was the first Canadian province to consider implementing 2-year diploma nursing schools. The Regina Grey Nuns Hospital School of Nursing received permission from the SRNA to develop a 2-year diploma program in nursing on an experimental basis, leading to the establishment of 2-year diploma programs in Saskatoon and Regina in 1967. Letourneau (1975) cites the difficulties that occurred because "Saskatchewan had forged ahead in legislating change without having an educational system fully established to absorb programs" (p. 25). To avoid the development of isolated institutions that would be for nursing only, the SRNA (1966) insisted "that diploma nursing for nurses be established in post-secondary institutions for higher education" (p. 1). In Saskatchewan, "the trend

was not for hospital schools of nursing to transmute to an educational institution, but rather to gradually phase out by ceasing to admit students" (Letourneau, 1975, p. 27). The two new 2-year programs in Saskatchewan were developed at the Kelsey Institute in Saskatoon and the Wascana Institute in Regina, respectively.

In British Columbia, the first diploma nursing program to be established within the general educational system was a jointly planned venture of the British Columbia Institute of Technology and the Registered Nurses Association of British Columbia (RNABC) in 1967. The RNABC's (1967) position was well known:

> Nursing can no longer be taught by apprenticeship methods; yet the students are part of the hospital service personnel . . . We believe that the method of financing nursing education partly through hospital operating costs and partly through service rendered by students is no longer an adequate or desirable one. (p. 20)

Funding for this program was obtained through an agreement between the federal and provincial governments for vocational–technical education. During the development of the program, the RNABC successfully lobbied for changes in existing legislation to allow for the development of new and innovative models of diploma nursing programs. Thus, community colleges throughout the province were able to develop nursing programs, and in 1965, Vancouver City College in Langara and Selkirk College in Castlegar initiated theirs. By 1974, four programs had been developed, and several others were in the planning stages, although four hospital diploma programs still remained in operation.

In Alberta, the transfer of diploma programs to the community colleges was a slow process. Mount Royal College in Calgary was the first college in the province to develop a diploma nursing program in 1967. Others included Red Deer College in 1968, Lethbridge Community College in 1969, Medicine Hat College in 1970, and Grant MacEwan Community College in 1972. Although seven hospitals had phased out their schools, six were still in operation in the province in 1974 (Letourneau, 1975). A report prepared by Dr. G. R. Fast in 1971 had recommended the transfer of remaining diploma programs to the Alberta college system, but lack of consultation and discussion prior to the report's release led to its shelving. The last hospital schools of nursing did not close their doors until the 1990s.

The first and only college diploma program established in Manitoba in the 1970s was at Red River Community College (in 1970) as a result of "action on the part of the Departments of Health and Education and the adjoining cooperative efforts of the MARN" (Letourneau, 1975, p. 253). The Manitoba Association of Registered Nurses

(MARN) was influential in establishing the program because it supported the inclusion of diploma nursing programs in the general system of education and the shortening of the programs to 2 years (Manitoba Association of Registered Nurses, 1968). Some diploma programs have been phased out in Manitoba, but Red River College continues to offer a diploma program in nursing.

Atlantic Canada

By the end of 1974, there had been some activity in the Atlantic provinces in relation to the movement that was sweeping other parts of the country, but this activity was limited. A study conducted by Katherine MacLaggan of nursing education in New Brunswick resulted in a recommendation that the general educational system be vested with responsibility for diploma nursing education (MacLaggan, 1965). According to Letourneau (1975), "Conflicting forces have rendered impossible the actual transfer of hospital programs to the system of education" (p. 275). In 1971, the *Abbis Report* recommended that four independent schools be established, similar to a pilot program at the Saint John School of Nursing, which had been converted to a 2-year program but financed through health dollars from the Department of Health (Study Committee on Nursing Education, 1971). Controversy over recommendations on registration and standards also contained in the document led the New Brunswick Association of Registered Nurses (1971) to say that it was "gravely alarmed at the import of these recommendations and quite surprised that they appear in the Report . . . [We] earnestly recommend that they be rejected" (p. 23).

Because there was no authority for establishing community colleges in New Brunswick until 1974, transfer of diploma nursing programs to the system of general education across the province was not possible. Thus, four independent schools and one hospital school were established in Bathurst, Edmundston, Moncton, and Saint John (Letourneau, 1975). These programs were autonomous in all respects except finance. However, as Letourneau observed, "Trends point to an eventual orderly transfer of independent programs to the provincial system of education, but first the community college system must develop sufficiently to absorb these programs" (p. 290).

The Registered Nurses' Association of Nova Scotia (RNANS) had a leading role in pressing for changes in the province's system of nursing education. RNANS' appointment of a curriculum council to determine each school's plan for change may have hastened and facilitated self-study by the schools so that "seven hospital schools of nursing were authorized, in the period extending from 1969 to 1970, to begin a two-year program or to effect a change in this direction" (Letourneau, 1975, p. 293). As with nurses

across the country, nurses in Nova Scotia had to stop an attempt in 1969 to remove the regulatory powers vested in their association. Like New Brunswick, Nova Scotia also faced the problem of having a community college system that needed to develop to accommodate the new programs.

The Association of Nurses of Prince Edward Island (ANPEI) requested that the three existing hospital schools of nursing in its province be phased out and replaced by one program to make the best use of staff and facilities and to provide the best possible education for students (Letourneau, 1975). The organization also sponsored a study that assessed the climate and readiness for change in the diploma nursing education system, reaching the conclusion that it was not the right time for major change (Rowe, 1967). In 1968, the ANPEI again pressed for change in the system, and this time the government responded by providing authority for developing one independent "two plus one" program for the province, replacing the three hospital schools (Letourneau, 1975). Efforts in 1974 to link the school with a community college, Holland College, were unsuccessful.

As for Newfoundland and Labrador, Letourneau (1975) stated that "The transfer of hospital schools of nursing to the system of education is, as in other Atlantic provinces, non-existent in Newfoundland" (p. 308). Four hospital schools of nursing continued to exist there, although the Association of Registered Nurses of Newfoundland (ARNN) tried to encourage change. Arpin (1972), a consultant hired by ARNN to help formulate goals, recommended that "the three schools of nursing in St. John's develop their curriculum plans so that the theory and experience essential for meeting the school objectives is included in the first two years of the program" (p. 1). By 1973, the three schools in St. John's had established "two plus one" programs, and the Corner Brook program had been reduced to 2 years.

EMERGENCE OF UNIVERSITY SCHOOLS OF NURSING

In view of the firm establishment and acceptance of the hospital-based educational system, the difficulty that the university-based system encountered in establishing its credibility in the eyes of patients, the public, and even nurses is easily understood. As Bonin (1976) commented, "So deeply time-honoured became this system of nursing education that it became difficult to imagine nursing, like other professions, as belonging to a university setting for the education of its practitioners" (pp. xii–xiii).

University education for nurses was the subject of an address by Dr. Malcolm T. MacEachern to the British Columbia Hospitals' Association in July 1919, after the Board of Governors' decision on May 26 to approve

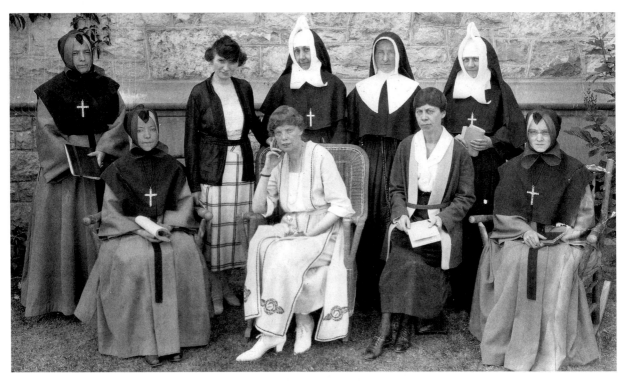

Ethel Johns, director of The University of British Columbia's Department of Nursing, the first university degree nursing program in Canada, with her students in the summer of 1922. (The University of British Columbia Archives)

the Senate's recommendation that a department of nursing be established at the University of British Columbia (Street, 1973). The founding of the department, a precedent in the history of Canadian nursing, occurred 4 years after the 1915 establishment of the university, largely through the efforts of Dr. MacEachern, the progressive medical superintendent of the Vancouver General Hospital. Universities were founded in the West as early as the second decade of the twentieth century, when agricultural and technical education were receiving attention from the federal government. The utilitarian philosophical orientation of the new Western universities explains the location of the first university school of nursing in the West—British Columbia.

The Department of Nursing at the University of British Columbia

When the decision was made to establish the University of British Columbia's Department of Nursing, the source of funding for the school was reviewed:

The Board was advised that the Department would not involve any additional expense to the University. The minutes of this meeting do not add a fact of which the

Board was aware: that the Vancouver General Hospital would pay the full salary of its director of nursing, who would also take charge of the University's Department of Nursing. (Street, 1973, pp. 118–119)

In subsequent communication to the Senate to inform members of the disposition of the recommendation, it was "emphasized that the action was taken on the understanding that the establishment of this Department would not involve any additional expense to the University" (Street, 1973, pp. 118–119). Under the terms of such a favourable arrangement, where the operating costs of the new department were to be borne by the hospital, the university was undoubtedly more easily persuaded by the persistent Dr. MacEachern that the entry of nursing into the academic world of the university was both possible and desirable.

The appointment of Ethel Johns as director of the new department was fortuitous; she was energetic, articulate, and of independent spirit. These qualities would be an asset, because in the beginning the way would not be easy for the first university school of nursing in the country. Street (1973) alluded to the "precarious early years" of the new program (p. 115). In an address to a joint session of the British Columbia Hospitals' Association and the Canadian Public Health Association in Vancouver in June 1920, Johns had an opportunity to make an appeal for positive attitudes, which had prevailed among physicians, toward the new development in nursing education:

> *To those who are in opposition or are in doubt, one last word, if there are any of such here: Will you not listen to the appeal of those upon whose shoulders you yourselves lay such heavy burdens? You see so many faults, so many blunders in our nursing service. So do we; they are not hidden from us. You cannot imagine why things should not run more smoothly, but we can; we know it is because of insufficient teaching and supervision. You do not realize how complex your own profession has become. How can we expect you to realize how difficult it is for us, with few of your educational advantages, to keep up with the advance shown in medicine?* (Street, 1973, p. 132)

The degree program thus established was based on the prevailing US model and "became the Canadian prototype of the pattern which came to be known as the non-integrated degree nursing course, or the 2 + 2 + 1 or 1 + 3 + 1 course, in which the university assumed no responsibility for the two or three years of nursing preparation in a hospital school of nursing" (Bonin, 1976, p. 7). The term "nonintegrated degree nursing course" referred to multiple variations of a 5-year nursing degree program, where students spent a number of years studying at the university and a number of years studying in hospital schools of nursing. These programs were sometimes referred to as a "sandwich program." For example, using a sandwich analogy, a 1 + 3 + 1 program was as follows: the first year (bottom slice of bread) was taught in a university; years 2, 3, and 4 (the sandwich filling) were taught in a hospital school of nursing and were in essence the diploma program; and year 5 (top slice of bread) was taught in a university. It was considered nonintegrated because the curricula of years 1 and 5 were the responsibility of the university, while the curricula of years 2, 3, and 4 were under the purview of the hospital school.

The new program gradually became established. After the program was approved for its fifth year, there was a request from the Library Committee

> *for a grant of two hundred fifty dollars with which to purchase books for the Department of Nursing. But the Board had a long memory. After some discussion, it was decided to direct the attention of the Library Committee to the undertaking of the Hospital authorities that the University would not be asked to*

> *assume any financial responsibility in respect to the Department of Nursing. It was decided that a sum not to exceed one hundred dollars should be granted for books.* (Street, 1973, p. 127)

The Impact of Red Cross Funding

After World War I, the Canadian Red Cross Society participated in the formation of the League of Red Cross Societies and the planning of an international program for peacetime activity in public health. "It was decided that there should be a great worldwide public health organization to help bring up the standards of physical and mental fitness of the world...the promotion of health, the prevention of disease and the mitigation of suffering throughout the world" (Gibbon & Mathewson, 1947, p. 342).

In Canada, the Red Cross Society first directed its efforts to providing funds for the provision of facilities for postgraduate instruction in public health nursing "by subsidizing special courses for three years at the Universities of Toronto, McGill, British Columbia, Alberta, and Dalhousie" (Gibbon & Mathewson, 1947, p. 342). The financial incentive provided by these grants contributed to the creation of departments for the study of nursing at four of the institutions and encouraged the extension of what had been initiated the previous year at the University of British Columbia:

> *In April 1920 the University of British Columbia accepted a proposal from the Provincial branch of the Canadian Red Cross Society to the effect that a Red Cross Chair of Public Health be established. For a period of three years from date of acceptance by the University, the Red Cross Society would pay five thousand dollars toward the salary of the professor. The expectation was that "the cause of Public Health, which everywhere is being regarded as of great importance, will be materially advanced throughout British Columbia." The Senate approved the proposal.* (Street, 1973, p. 128)

The Red Cross funds must have seemed like a windfall to the young institution, which had been founded during wartime and had received little tangible support from the government that was in power in the province at the time.

In addition to providing funds to institutions to stimulate the creation of new programs in public health nursing, the Canadian Red Cross Society provided financial aid to students who wanted to attend programs initiated under their sponsorship (King, 1970, p. 70). These actions were met with enthusiasm, and continued increases in enrollment ensured the survival of most of the universities after the 3-year period of institutional grants had ended. Not surprisingly, these certificate courses became the first in a series of such courses to be offered by the universities and also led to the development of degree programs in most of the institutions. However, these developments in 1920 were preceded by years of effort on the part of nurses to secure university education:

> The first documentation concerning efforts to establish a university nursing program in Canada appeared in 1905 when a memorandum was submitted by the Graduate Nurses' Association of Ontario to the University of Toronto requesting the university "to offer a course of training and education of nurses." (King, 1970, p. 70)

In 1918, Dr. Helen MacMurchy, a physician and the first editor of *The Canadian Nurse*, wrote to the presidents of the universities to urge them to encourage establishment of nursing programs at their institutions (MacMurchy, 1918). Although the influence of such communication remains a matter of speculation, it is reasonable to assume that it at least made administrators of higher education more aware of the needs and issues in nursing education. As one author concluded, "One of the most significant developments during the period from 1910 to 1930 was the growth of positive attitudes toward university education for nurses" (Allemang, 1974, p. 137).

The one exception to the lasting success of the stimulus provided by the Red Cross for the establishment of university nursing education was the public health nursing certificate program begun at Dalhousie University, which was also the first of its kind to be initiated (Tunis, 1966). The program at Dalhousie was short lived and, for financial and perhaps other reasons, did not survive after 1922. Although Dalhousie's program was the first to be initiated through Red Cross funds, the nature of the support differed in that it consisted of direct funding of students rather than institutional grants; it was therefore far less substantial than the funding given to other universities during those same years. It took until 1949 for Dalhousie University to establish a school of nursing (Twohig, 1998).

The 1920s and 1930s

During the 1920s, several new 5-year nonintegrated degree programs were initiated that were similar to the program at the University of British Columbia. The University of Western Ontario established a program in 1924, followed by one at the University of Alberta in 1925. At the request of the Grey Nuns, the Université de Montréal began offering courses to nurses in 1923. These beginnings led the Grey Nuns in 1934 to fund the Institut Marguerite d'Youville in Montreal as an affiliated school to the Université de Montréal. In 1962, the institute became the Faculté des sciences infirmières (Faculty of Nursing) of the Université

de Montréal. By establishing a nonintegrated degree program at their institute, the Grey Nuns became the leaders of nursing education in the French world. Indeed, they offered the first university nursing program available in French in the world. The sisters had clearly been influenced by the developments at the University of British Columbia, and because they owned and operated hospitals in Western Canada, they were well aware of continental trends in nursing education (Paul, 1994; Cohen, Pepin, Lamontagne et al., 2002). Finally, the University of Toronto experimented throughout the 1920s and 1930s with a new model of a diploma program that evolved into the integrated degree program. This model is discussed later in this chapter.

The 1920s were productive years during which adequate financial support had been available to support programs and expansion into new fields. During this period, nursing entered the university scene in Canada with the development of programs at six universities. However, growth and expansion in these institutions after 1929 was limited because of financial constraints. The early 1930s were difficult for Canadian universities. The struggles of the School for Graduate Nurses at McGill University best exemplify these hardships and are presented in the next section. There are frequent references to salary cuts that professors accepted rather than see colleagues lose their positions because of financial constraints. Evidence of the lack of growth in the decade after the stock market collapse was observed in all institutions, but particularly those in Western Canada. Nonetheless, by the end of the decade things began to improve—the University of Saskatchewan and the University of Ottawa introduced degree programs in 1938, followed by St. Francis Xavier University in 1939.

Crisis at McGill

The year 1929 spelled the end of a decade in which university nursing education in Canada had improved by leaps and bounds. According to Allemang (1974), the stock market crash in the fall of 1929 and the economic depression that followed "brought unemployment and hardship to nurses" (p. 172). Nurses had experienced difficulties in securing employment before 1929, and because of the worldwide economic depression, the situation rapidly worsened. People could no longer afford to employ private-duty nurses; this proved to be a major setback, as private duty had been the most promising area of employment for new nursing graduates (Gunn, 1933, p. 141).

For universities, the Great Depression meant a period of significant adjustment that included reduced revenues, staff layoffs, and difficult working conditions. However, despite this adverse environment, enrollments continued to show slow but steady growth throughout the decade; perhaps because no employment was available for people who had completed their high school educations, many chose to remain in school. The impact of the Great Depression on an institution in Canada was determined to a large extent by the amount of external support it received from government and private sources.

The Great Depression was hard on McGill University. A number of pages are devoted to this story because of its historical significance. As a private institution, McGill's mandate was to raise funds from private sources to operate its programs or else reduce the size of its enterprise. This mandate made financing difficult enough during prosperous times; during the lean years of the Great Depression, it became an onerous task. The School for Graduate Nurses at McGill was subjected to the impact of the financial crunch for more than a decade. Helen Reid, a member of the first class to graduate from McGill, was a strong proponent of the establishment of a school of nursing at McGill because she felt this would give women another means of entering the university. Although Reid had originally envisioned a 2-year degree course at McGill, advice that she received in 1920 from Isabel M. Stewart, the Canadian-born professor of nursing at Teachers College, Columbia University, suggested that "to attempt at present in any way to arrange for two-year courses would be a real injury to the undertaking" (Tunis, 1966, p. 22). The final announcement of the course reflected the intent to begin a degree program "in the near future" (Tunis, 1966, p. 22). After the nursing school appointed as its director the Canadian-born nurse educator, writer, and administrator Bertha Harmer, formerly of Yale University, the committee recommended "that a six-year undergraduate course leading to a degree be established at the School for Graduate Nurses" (Tunis, 1966, p. 42). The attitudes of the principal and vice-chancellor were said to be encouraging: "When we establish the degree course we can promise that Miss Harmer's rank will be that of professor" (Tunis, 1966, p. 42).

Because there was reason for optimism, work went forward under Harmer's direction to develop a framework for the curriculum that would facilitate the transition to the degree program when it was established. Students could select from five new areas of focus, each of which could lead to a university diploma rather than a certificate after 2 years of study. To implement the new programs, four new faculty members were appointed for the 1929–1930 academic year. Despite the optimism, however, the school's viability was threatened by the financial uncertainty brought about by the loss of Red Cross funding in 1923. To the new director, this uncertainty must have been a continuing source of anxiety:

I have just returned to the office after a repeated attack of illness and had hoped to find a favourable decision of the Finance Committee awaiting me. At the risk of seeming to trouble you unduly I am writing to

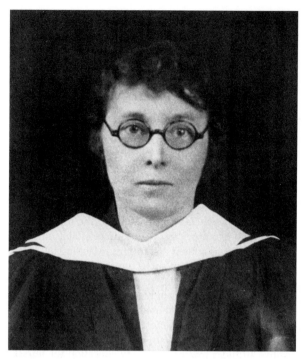

It was only through an unprecedented outpouring of financial support from alumni that Bertha Harmer, Director of the School for Graduate Nurses at McGill University, was able to maintain the school during the Great Depression. (McGill University Archives, PR039514)

ask the decision of the Finance Committee in regard to our budget. I should not trouble you if it were not that so many important matters are depending on it. (Harmer, 1929)

The undercurrent of suspicion toward nursing's place in the university environment surfaced again: "There are so many professors in the University who most cordially disapprove of schools of this kind. Their antagonism becomes more marked because of the necessity of reducing their salaries" (Currie, 1932).

A crisis was imminent, and the facts were given to Harmer by Sir Arthur Currie, the acting principal:

I quite agree with you that the School has had an increasing attendance, that it has done excellent work, and that the influence of its graduates on nursing and nursing education and administration has been most valuable. But there is the eternal question of finance. How are we to get the money to continue this School? (Currie, 1932)

In the face of the university's economic difficulties imposed by the Great Depression, the school would not be permitted to continue to drain McGill's financial resources. It was given only one alternative to being shut down: the school would have the opportunity to raise an endowment of $40,000 to provide for the annual operating expenses of $8,000, "which would keep it going for the next five years, in the hope that by that time financial conditions would be such that the expense of the School could be more readily provided for" (Currie, 1932).

The alumnae association and the advisory committee convened in a joint session to consider the crisis that had beset the school, and they offered their support for a national fundraising effort (Tunis, 1966). An appeal was sent to the presidents of all provincial nursing associations to assist with the campaign. In Harmer's words,

> The nursing profession has many interested and grateful friends who appreciate the service which it renders, and it is quite right and just that they, in addition to the provincial and city government boards, and boards of hospitals and public health and welfare associations, should now be asked as individuals to contribute to the support of nursing education. (Harmer, 1932)

Support was also to be solicited from foundations, businesses, and corporations; however, the appeals to these organizations failed, and the response was a great disappointment: "All was not lost, however, for the appeal to Canadian nurses did not go unheard and 'miraculously the money poured in. Within two months, more than $5,000 in cash was on hand and over $12,000 pledged'" (Tunis, 1966, p. 56).

The role of **alumnae** groups all over the country in ensuring the survival of the McGill School for Graduate Nurses was the critical factor in resolving the financial crisis that spanned more than a decade. In the process, the stature of nurses and nursing was raised, as nurses demonstrated a single-minded commitment to continuing the good work that had been started at McGill. It is clear from the documents that McGill administrators were surprised that nurse alumnae members and others would have sufficient interest or strength of purpose to donate funds so generously. Although the $20,000 that was raised by alumnae fell far short of the initial goal of $40,000, this money was applied to the school's annual operating costs and thus kept the School for Graduate Nurses open.

 APPLYING CONTENT KNOWLEDGE

The McGill nursing alumnae were very generous. Is it still important for nursing schools to have engaged alumnae? For example, are you aware of any scholarships at your school that have been funded by alumnae donations? Do you think nursing graduates today are as generous as nursing graduates of the past?

The fact that $20,000 was sufficient to see the school through 10 difficult years was attributed to strict control over spending by school administrators (Tunis, 1966). An example of the nature of the commitment and dedication to the school is found in Harmer's 1933 report to the principal on the results of the first, and possibly the most important, phase of the campaign:

> I am enclosing a statement showing results of the efforts of nurses to raise $40,000 to endow the School for the next five years. As it seemed hopeless, however, under present conditions, to raise this sum, efforts were concentrated on raising $8,000 in the hope that better times would enable us to raise an endowment later. Deducting my salary (my services were offered at the end of the year when it seemed the only hope of saving the School) left $5,000 as the objective. As the enclosed statement shows we have pledges for $5,597 for the next year, and $6,355.52 toward the next four years. (Harmer, 1933)

In addition, many special lecturers in the program accepted reduced fees for their services or waived them altogether. Operating costs were lowered further when faculty members bought books for the library and supplies out of their own pockets (Tunis, 1966). Sir Arthur Currie's announcement in 1933 that sufficient funds had been received in the first 5 months of the fundraising campaign to continue the school for one more year was a cause for rejoicing among faculty, alumnae, and friends of the school:

> On the understanding that the Budget for the next year does not exceed the year just closing, and relying on the pledges outlined in your letter of May first, 1933, I shall recommend to the Board of Governors that the School for Graduate Nurses be continued for another year, that is, until June 30, 1934. (Currie, 1933)

The struggle was to be long, however, and neither Harmer nor Currie lived to see its conclusion. After Harmer's resignation and death in 1934, the continuing struggle for existence was carried on under the direction of Marion Lindeburgh, who served as acting director until 1939 and as director thereafter until 1950. The stringent economies required that fewer courses be taught and that the 2-year diploma programs be dropped in favour of 1-year certificate programs (Tunis, 1966). The degree program had to be postponed until much later because program development priorities had to focus on retaining the programs that remained operational.

The Development of an Experimental School of Nursing at Toronto

It is ironic that at the very moment administrators served McGill's School for Graduate Nurses with notice of intent to terminate its programs, the University of Toronto's School of Nursing—started in 1926 thanks to the vision of the school's director, Edith Kathleen Russell—received financial support and explicit encouragement to continue its innovative experiment with basic curriculum design. This positive development had been preceded by many years of groundwork by Russell, and the grant was not the first the school had been awarded by the Rockefeller Foundation. The nursing program established in 1926 and the improved one in 1933 were diploma rather than degree programs. Their importance for Canadian nursing was that they were radical departures from the existing philosophy of university education for nurses.

Russell, who came to the university early in the national development of higher education in nursing, possessed the rare qualities of brilliant leaders. She had time to establish herself at the university and develop her ideas about the pursuit of knowledge and truth as applied to nursing in the university setting. The credibility of the work accomplished and Russell's unique capabilities for leadership were remarkable. Ultimately, these factors augured well for

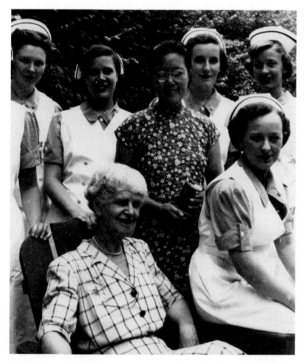

Edith Kathleen Russell with students of the University of Toronto's School of Nursing, class of 1949. Russell is credited with developing the integrated nursing program and obtaining Rockefeller Foundation grants to establish it. (University of Toronto Archives, University of Toronto. Faculty of Nursing Records, A1987-0024/001 (11))

the University of Toronto because, as Carpenter indicated about the Rockefeller Foundation, "in the 30-year period ending in 1953, the Foundation supported the development of nursing education in 48 countries. The University of Toronto was the only Canadian university to receive this support" (Carpenter, 1970, p. 94).

The proposal for the 1933 program—which also established the School of Nursing as an autonomous unit within the administrative framework of the university, allowing it to participate fully in university governance—was first submitted to the Rockefeller Foundation in 1929. The foundation agreed to support the project if support was also obtained from the university and the Ontario government, guarantees that were subsequently provided. The major feature of this 39-month program, which was unique from a developmental standpoint and made this curriculum model stand apart from the nonintegrated curriculum pattern, was the principle that the faculty of the school would assume total responsibility for students' education. Because the school was administratively independent from the hospital, new value was placed on clinical teaching. Student learning needs would no longer be put aside in favour of pressing hospital nursing service demands because students were not used in "staff" positions. They were viewed as learners, with the rights and responsibilities that accompany that role. The role of the faculty member in the clinical setting was one that was critical in facilitating the integration of theory and practice and fostering creative thinking and a questioning attitude (Carpenter, 1982). The function of the university school, as conceived by Russell (1956), was

> . . . to prepare professional women who, through studies in the humanities and social sciences, will grow in understanding and wisdom; with this education in the realm of human values they may approach with some degree of safety the work which is awaiting them. (p. 35)

NEW INITIATIVES AND INCENTIVES IN UNIVERSITY NURSING EDUCATION BETWEEN 1940 AND 1955

In 1940, as Canada became involved in World War II, the country's sluggish economy recovered as the demand for manufactured goods skyrocketed. The war also affected higher education. Education in the health sciences became a priority as Canada quickly recognized the need for health professionals to care for military personnel and the civilian population.

In the nursing profession, pressures arose from the conditions of returning prosperity in 1940, and as these mounted, the balance between supply and demand reversed abruptly from what it had been during the 1930s. Where at first there had been oversupply of nurses, there was now a distinct shortage. Increasing prosperity was partially responsible for this turn of events, as private-duty nurses were in demand again in both hospitals and homes, which put a tight squeeze on the nursing profession and health services in general. The economic conditions of the 1930s had forced many small hospitals to close their schools of nursing and hire from the large pool of unemployed nurses, who would work for low wages. By the end of the decade, general staff nursing in hospitals had become a major form of employment among nurses (Allemang, 1974). This trend contrasted sharply with that of the previous decade, when few staff nurse positions were available in hospitals and graduate nurses generally sought employment as independent practitioners whose services were retained by families to care for ill family members in hospitals and homes.

Other factors that contributed to the development of the shortage included the wartime demands on a profession with a contribution to make:

Nursing administrators, supervisors, head nurses, teachers and public health nurses left their civilian positions for those of military service. These were key people in providing quality in nursing services and nursing education. Since bedside nursing care accompanied by supervision and ward teaching was considered the core of the curriculum, their loss was deeply felt. (Allemang, 1974, p. 211)

Nurses were also needed in wartime industries, which generally offered better salaries and working conditions. For the most part, the shortages were most acute in rural areas for hospital and public health positions, as well as in specialized areas where nurses were badly needed, such as tuberculosis sanatoria, isolation hospitals, and psychiatric institutions. In fact, the needs became so great and the possibilities for meeting those needs were so limited that a new category of health care provider was created to fill the gap—the certified or registered nursing assistant or licensed practical nurse. Although some consideration was given to shortening nursing programs in Canada to meet specific needs related to the war, this development never occurred because enough nurses volunteered for the armed services (Lindeburgh, 1942).

University schools of nursing soon began to reap the benefits of federal interest in higher education. This support came in the form of government subsidy of university operations and a considerable response to the assistance requested by professional organizations. Federal funds for nursing education, distributed through the CNA to the schools, amounted to $150,000 in 1942 and $250,000

each in 1943 and 1944; the program was maintained until the end of the war. Funds were then awarded through the provincial nurses' associations to the diploma and university schools of the provinces. In addition, the W. K. Kellogg Foundation initiated a program of fellowships in nursing and, between 1941 and 1959, granted $11,680 to institutions and agencies to be awarded to Canadian nurses for additional study. The university schools of nursing received the greater part of these funds so that they could upgrade the academic qualifications of their faculties. The fellowships were tenable in the United States, as during that period there were no master's programs for nurses in Canada. The new funds, most of which were provided between 1941 and 1945, provided a stimulus to nursing education at a time when it was needed.

The W. K. Kellogg Foundation also made scholarship and loan funds available for students in programs at five universities between 1942 and 1944. Under this program, McGill University, Université de Montréal, the University of Toronto, and the University of Western Ontario each received $4,000, and Université Laval each received $6,000. For students seeking certificate or baccalaureate preparation, the Victorian Order of Nurses, a national agency that needed nurses with specific preparation in public health nursing, reactivated the bursary program that had been initiated during the 1920s and discontinued in 1933. The Canadian Red Cross Society also made scholarships in public health nursing available (Tunis, 1966).

An awakened interest in nursing and nursing education in the postwar period led to the founding of new programs in nursing at several universities. Programs were initiated by Queen's University and McMaster University in 1941, by the University of Manitoba in 1943, by Mount St. Vincent University in 1947, and by Dalhousie University in 1949. Federal funds made available for schools and fellowship and bursary programs under the auspices of private foundations and agencies played an important role in the new developments. As was the case in 1920, universities became aware of potential benefits from the sponsorship of nursing programs.

At McGill, the influx of additional funds was considerable and continuous. The courage and perseverance of those faculty, alumnae, and friends who had held out for the retention of the school through the long years of the Great Depression and the war were rewarded. Their steadfast conviction that the School for Graduate Nurses had a significant and critical function to fulfill at McGill was vindicated. The funds provided to McGill's School for Graduate Nurses from the federal grant program administered by the CNA included "$2100 [in 1942], an amount that was increased to $6000 in 1943, and which by 1945 totalled $27,750" (Tunis, 1966, p. 73).

Nursing faculty at McGill were again able to entertain the idea of a degree program. Preparations began in 1941 for a 5-year nonintegrated degree course, and the first students were accepted in 1944. In 1945, the alumnae of the school disbanded their Special Finance Committee, but simultaneously revitalized earlier efforts to establish an endowment fund for the Flora Madeline Chair in Nursing (Tunis, 1966).

DIPLOMA TO DEGREE: THE INCEPTION OF THE BASIC DEGREE PROGRAM AT THE UNIVERSITY OF TORONTO

The development of curricula for baccalaureate nursing education has not been without difficulties. These efforts have largely relied on contractual agreements between the university schools of nursing and hospitals and other agencies used for clinical experience. Brown (1948) cited two reasons to explain why major problems in curricula development arose: hospitals had a traditional outlook that viewed nursing education as service, and many university schools and students had meagre financial resources.

Probably the most influential event in the history of Canadian degree programs in nursing was the introduction of the basic degree program at the University of Toronto in 1942. This program provided an alternative to the existing pattern of baccalaureate nursing education. In the integrated program, studies in the arts and sciences were combined with the nursing component. Courses were carefully planned and sequenced so that individual student development would be enhanced: "For the first time in a nursing undergraduate degree programme full authority and responsibility for the teaching of nursing rested in the university. . . This simple fact, nonetheless, was a radical departure from existing degree programmes" (King, 1970, p. 72).

It is always difficult to break with tradition, and in nursing, the nonintegrated degree pattern had established its stepladder approach to nursing education well over 20 years before. In addition, the associated hospital programs had been entrenched for even longer. Effecting a change that made the basic degree program stand apart from its nonintegrated counterpart required a great leader. Edith Kathleen Russell was such an individual, as she exerted a profound influence on the thinking of her colleagues in nursing and was able to enlist the moral support of the Faculty of Medicine, the president of the University of Toronto, and the Rockefeller Foundation. In regard to her influence, Emory (1964) noted, "It has been said that greatness is attained through changing the course of events and changing them for always. If this be true, then in retrospect there

can be detected in Edith Kathleen Russell's professional life and work an element of true greatness" (p. 7).

A SECOND BASIC DEGREE PROGRAM BEGINS

In her study of basic degree programs in Canada, Bonin (1976) concluded, "The most salient driving forces which spurred the establishment of basic degree programs are key persons, especially Kathleen Russell and Gladys Sharpe, in two pioneering universities" (p. 178). Four years after the introduction of the University of Toronto basic degree program, a second such program was developed at McMaster University under the direction of Gladys Sharpe. Sharpe was largely responsible for phasing out its predecessor, a degree and diploma program at McMaster called Arts and Nursing, which had begun in 1941. At McMaster, the initiative of the Hamilton General Hospital had been important in developing the earlier affiliation between the hospital and the university, and the hospital continued to support the new program and its director. Similar support from an associated hospital had occurred in 1919 when the Vancouver General Hospital supported the establishment of the University of British Columbia School of Nursing. It was also evident that there was an extremely close working relationship between the Toronto General Hospital and the School of Nursing at the University of Toronto. In the early 1930s, consideration was given to combining the Toronto General nursing program with that of the University of Toronto (Carpenter, 1970).

 APPLYING CONTENT KNOWLEDGE

In your journal or notebook, reflect on the meaning of the evolution of university nursing education in Canada for the nursing profession.

REVISITING SURVEYS OF NURSING EDUCATION AND UNIVERSITY EDUCATION AND LOOKING TOWARD THE FUTURE

In the history of Canadian nursing education, periodic surveys have been undertaken by professional organizations and government to assess conditions and develop solutions to pressing problems. Kathleen Russell carried out one such survey in New Brunswick that addressed the whole gamut of issues in nursing education in the province. The survey had considerable impact on the thinking of nursing educators, as the establishment of the School of Nursing at the University of New Brunswick in 1959 was a direct result of her recommendations about higher education in nursing in New Brunswick (Russell, 1956). Soon afterward, the CNA launched its Pilot Project for Evaluation of Schools of Nursing to assess readiness for a system of accreditation and published its report in 1960.

One of Mussallem's (1960) recommendations, "that a re-examination and study of the whole field of nursing education be undertaken" (p. vii), was implemented within a short time. A royal commission was appointed by the federal government to investigate the problems and issues related to all aspects of the delivery of health care services in Canada. The report of that commission urged that 10 more university nursing programs, under administratively autonomous schools of nursing, be established in Canada as soon as possible (Hall, 1964). The report also recommended elimination of nonintegrated basic programs at a time when admissions were 22% higher than admissions to integrated programs. The impact of this report was impressive, as only 4 years later "admissions to integrated programmes constituted 97% of all admissions to baccalaureate programmes" (King, 1970, pp. 178–79). In addition, the number of candidates seeking postgraduate degrees after graduation from hospital or college diploma programs doubled during the same period. Schools of nursing made concerted efforts to increase maximum enrollment levels in response to the royal commission's recommendation despite limited space in clinical facilities:

> It is of the utmost importance that these schools be expanded in number to enable them to prepare approximately one-fourth of the total recruits to the nursing force. It is from this pool that the instructors, supervisors, administrators and other leaders in the profession must come. (Hall, 1964, p. 67)

All 10 of the new university schools recommended by the royal commission were established soon after the report's publication. Since 1965, the ratio of diploma- to baccalaureate-prepared nurses has increased considerably from nearly 1 in 10 nationally in 1988, to 1 in 16 in 1993, to 1 in 21 in 1998 (CNA, 2001). In 2007, 35.5% of Canadian nurses in the workforce held a baccalaureate degree as their highest level of education; 10 years later, the percentage had risen to 52.3% (CNA, 2017).

ENTRY TO PRACTICE AT THE BACCALAUREATE LEVEL

Since the 1980s, the endorsement of the baccalaureate entry-to-practice position by the CNA and most provincial/territorial professional nursing associations and colleges has exponentially increased the number of university colleges, departments, schools, and faculties of nursing.

By 2019, the CASN had 94 member schools and faculties, all of which are involved in the delivery of undergraduate nursing education.

The Alberta Task Force on Nursing Education made the first "official statement" recommending that the baccalaureate degree be the minimal requirement for new graduates planning to enter the profession (Government of Alberta, 1975). The Alberta Association of Registered Nurses, now the College and Association of Registered Nurses of Alberta, endorsed the position in 1976 (Alberta Association of Registered Nurses, 1976), while the CNA endorsed it in 1982 (CNA, 2013). The goal of entry-to-practice at the baccalaureate level was often misinterpreted as suggesting that diploma-prepared nurses would lose their ability to practice once regulators endorsed the entry-to-practice position. The goal of entry to practice was to prepare nurses who could provide increasingly complex nursing services.

New Brunswick was the first province to endorse the position in 1989. By 1998, all provinces in Atlantic Canada had adopted this position (CNA, 2019). However, as with anything else in nursing education, it took a long time to convince provincial governments that entry-to-practice requirements at the baccalaureate level were desirable. Consequently, it was not until the 2000s that most provinces had adopted the position. Saskatchewan adopted the position in 2000, Ontario in 2005, British Columbia in 2008, Alberta in 2010, the Northwest Territories and Nunavut in 2010, and Manitoba in 2012. The only provincial government that has not yet done so is the Quebec government, while in Yukon there are no entry-level nursing education programs (CNA, 2019).

The transition to baccalaureate-level entry to practice was greatly facilitated by the creation of collaborative programs. In these programs, collaboration occurs between schools of nursing located in colleges and their university partners, the degree-granting institutions that deliver the baccalaureate education. The first collaboration of this type was created in 1989 between the University of British Columbia School of Nursing and the Vancouver General Hospital School of Nursing (CNA, 1989). The first college–university collaboration began in 1990 between Red Deer College and the Faculty of Nursing at the University of Alberta. A year later, four more institutions joined the partnership—the University of Alberta Hospital School of Nursing, the Royal Alexandra Hospital School of Nursing, the Misericordia Hospital School of Nursing, and the Grant MacEwan College. In 1995, the hospital schools of nursing were closed by the province, and therefore the two colleges and the University of Alberta were left to deliver the program. In 1996, the colleges in Grande Prairie (Keyano) and Fort McMurray joined the collaboration. Initially, the college partners were obligated by the Government of Alberta to make available a diploma exit option; however, as the collaborative program developed, fewer and fewer students chose this option. In essence, by 2010, when the province finally endorsed the entry-to-practice position, students had already made it a reality because the great majority were choosing to complete their degrees.

Models similar to the one created at the University of Alberta rapidly spread in Western Canada, in Atlantic Canada, and eventually in Ontario. Although different in form, collaboration now also exists between colleges and universities in Quebec. Collaborative models also spread between provinces and territories. Since 2000, Aurora College in the Northwest Territories collaborates with the University of Victoria, while Nunavut Arctic College has been in a partnership with Dalhousie University since 1999. It can be argued that collaborative models generated momentum by offering a larger number of nursing students the more attractive option of pursuing their degrees without having to leave their communities. Once enrolled in these collaborative programs, students soon realized that completing their degrees was advantageous and they therefore opted to continue their education. Successful collaboration between institutions requires "an astute and visionary cadre of nursing education leaders" (Zawaduk, Duncan, Star Mahara et al., 2014, p. 586). Those who created the early collaborative programs because they shared a common goal exemplified this type of leadership. They did not wait for provincial governments to endorse the entry-to-practice requirement to take initiative—they took a chance and brought nursing closer to the goal of entry to practice at the baccalaureate level.

DESIGNING PROGRAMS FOR DIFFERENT LEARNERS

Since the 1990s, many programs have been designed for students wishing to enter nursing after the completion of a degree in another discipline. These programs are often referred to as "fast-track" or "after-degree" programs. Programs have also been developed to facilitate the entry into the profession of nurses from other countries. The threat of a shortage of nurses was the impetus behind the creation of both types of programs. These programs were also seen as being advantageous because they recognized prior education and were thus cost effective. In the case of internationally educated nurses (IEN), in 2010, Health Canada provided funding to the CASN to create a framework of guiding principles and essential components for IEN bridging programs (CASN, 2010) (see Chapter 26). The development of the framework was timely, as there were few bridging programs, especially in smaller provinces, and the cost to enroll in these programs could be prohibitive.

PREPARING NURSES TO SERVE FRANCOPHONE OFFICIAL LANGUAGE MINORITY POPULATIONS

In 1998, the Government of Ontario threatened to close Hôpital Montfort in Ottawa, the only francophone teaching hospital in Ontario. Francophone communities across Canada reacted to this threat and united. The province did not close the hospital, but the situation galvanized francophone communities (Centre national de formation en santé, 2019). The federal government became involved, and Heritage Canada began offering financial support to educate health care providers in French at the Hôpital Montfort and the University of Ottawa.

In 1999, the Centre national de formation en santé was created to support the education of health care providers in French outside of Quebec. The University of Moncton, the University of Ottawa, and Laurentian University already had French-language nursing programs, but the new consortium was beneficial because it provided new funding and an agreement to work together and share resources (Centre national de formation en santé, 2019). The creation of the consortium soon led to the development of a French-language nursing program at the Université de Saint-Boniface in Winnipeg, Manitoba, that was initially offered in collaboration with the University of Ottawa. It also led to the creation of the first bilingual nursing baccalaureate program in 2004 through a collaboration between the Faculty of Nursing and Campus Saint-Jean at the University of Alberta. Another bilingual program was initiated at the University of Regina in 2018. This program is a collaboration between the Faculty of Nursing, Saskatchewan Polytechnic, and la Cité universitaire francophone. Preparing nurses who can offer services in French to francophone minority populations is essential, as language barriers have a negative impact on the health of francophone minority populations (Fédération des communautés francophones et acadiennes, 2001; Bowen, 2001). Health Canada now provides funding to the Centre national de formation en santé.

INDIGENOUS NURSING STUDENTS AND THE RESPONSE OF SCHOOLS OF NURSING TO THE TRUTH AND RECONCILIATION CALLS TO ACTION

There is no evidence that Indigenous women were admitted into nursing education programs prior to 1917 (Toman, 2010). The Toronto Free Hospital for Consumptive Poor, also known as the Weston Sanatorium (now known as the West Park Health Centre), was the first institution to admit Indigenous women to its nursing program. In the 1930s, more programs began admitting Indigenous women, including the St. Boniface Hospital School in Winnipeg, Manitoba, and the Kootenay Lake Training School for Nurses in Nelson, British Columbia. However, the number of Indigenous graduates remained low. Even at times of nursing shortages, visible minorities found it difficult to gain entry into nursing programs. For example, it was not until the mid-1940s that Black women were admitted to Canadian nursing schools (Flynn, 2009).

The number of Indigenous students started to increase in the 1980s when some nursing programs began to create seats dedicated to this population. At that time, universities also began offering transition programs that assisted Indigenous students, who were often from remote areas, to transition into university education.

A major catalyst for change occurred with the publication of the Truth and Reconciliation Commission of Canada's (2015) Calls to Action. Between 2007 and 2015, the commission heard from more than 6,500 witnesses who shared their personal histories and experiences with the residential school system (Government of Canada, 2019). Call to Action 24 is directly related to the education of nurses:

> We call upon medical and nursing schools in Canada to require all students to take a course dealing with Aboriginal health issues, including the history and legacy of residential schools, the United Nations Declaration on the Rights of Indigenous peoples, Treaties and Aboriginal rights, and Indigenous teachings and practices. This will require skills-based training in intercultural competency, conflict resolution, human rights, and anti-racism. (Truth and Reconciliation Commission of Canada, 2015, p. 3)

This Call to Action has led nursing programs, colleges, and universities to design initiatives meant to address the issues raised. Courses that include the elements listed in Call to Action 24 have begun to be designed and offered. It is hoped that through these courses, nursing students of all origins will be better equipped to care for Indigenous populations and above all will be prepared to recognize and fight anti-Indigenous racism.

Although Indigenous peoples make up 4.9% of the population, only 3.0% of registered nurses have identified as being Indigenous (University of Saskatchewan College of Nursing and Canadian Indigenous Nurses Association, 2018). Enrollment and retention of Indigenous nursing students continues to be a priority in many institutions. The College of Nursing at the University of Saskatchewan provides an example of leadership in this area. The college developed a creative "learn where you live" model so that students can study in remote areas (Butler, Berry, & Exner-Pirot, 2018) and a strategic plan for engagement with Indigenous peoples (Butler, Exner-Pirot, & Berry, 2018).

🌐 CULTURAL CONSIDERATIONS

The College of Nursing at the University of Saskatchewan is a leader in the education of Indigenous nurses. In 1984, the college and its partners, the First Nations University of Canada and the University of Regina, established the National Native Access Program to Nursing with funding from Health Canada (Arnault-Pelletier, Brown, Desjarlais, & McBeth, 2006). In 1997, the program was restructured to become a provincial program, the Native Access Program to Nursing. The program has had a great impact on the recruitment and retention of Indigenous students. For example, before its inception, the College of Nursing at the University of Saskatchewan had admitted two to four Indigenous students a year out of a total of 320 students. By 2006, 12% of the students at the College of Nursing were Indigenous. By creating a welcoming and supportive climate and being engaged with the community, schools of nursing can become change agents and ensure that Indigenous students have the opportunity to become registered nurses.

Source: Arnault-Pelletier, V., Brown, S., Desjarlais, J., & McBeth, B. (2006). Circle of strength. *The Canadian Nurse, 120*(4), 22–26.

CONCLUSION

This cursory examination of important events and trends in the development of nursing education has revealed that changes occurred gradually and that nurses needed determination to establish the entry-to-practice requirement at the baccalaureate level. With the evolution of the discipline and the expansion of the knowledge base, concern about the appropriateness of the learning environment helped to drive the desire for change. Widespread recognition that nursing remains one of the last sex-segregated professions has underscored injustices caused by differential treatment of both nurses and the profession itself. Improvement in the status of women through attaining fundamental rights and privileges previously accorded only to men has led the profession to press for educational arrangements and advantages common in all other disciplines.

At the outset, nursing education was characterized by informal on-the-job training. Hospital schools of nursing began to develop in 1874, and university schools in 1919. Community college nursing education programs, which were established in the 1960s, also offered diploma preparation. Today, collaborations between colleges and universities give students the opportunity to study for a university degree in nursing across the country. Over time, there has been a progression in nurses' thinking about the means to educate members of the profession, a vision guided from the beginning by a concern for standards of education and practice leading to safe patient care. Shortages of nurses have contributed to the development of programs that better recognize students' prior learning. In the last two decades, more efforts have been devoted to preparing nurses who can better serve francophone official language minority populations and Indigenous peoples. It will be interesting to see what lies ahead for the future of nursing education.

SUMMARY OF LEARNING OBJECTIVES

- Women began entering Canadian universities in the 1860s; however, universities that accepted women were the exception, as women were seen as unsuited to higher education. Since most nurses were women, it took time to develop nursing programs in universities.
- Prior to Florence Nightingale, there was no formal education for lay nurses. Nurses who were members of religious nursing orders received nursing education from their order. Nightingale developed the first modern school of nursing where laywomen could be admitted. Her model, in whole or in part, spread throughout Europe, North America, and other parts of the globe. The fact that Nightingale lived during the territorial peak of the British Empire helped the model to spread.
- The first school of Nursing in Canada was the Mack School of Nursing in St. Catharines, Ontario. The founder of the school believed that opening a school of nursing would be beneficial to the hospital. Though it was patterned on the Nightingale model, the school had one important deviation: it did not have an independent budget and thus relied on the hospital for funding. This led to the use of nursing students as a workforce.
- As early as 1932 it was recognized that there were problems in nursing education. The *Weir Report* provided solid evidence indicating that change was needed. However, immediate changes did not transpire. In 1960, Helen Mussallem published *Spotlight on Nursing Education: The Report of a Pilot Project for the Evaluation of Schools of Nursing in Canada*. Although a few provinces adopted some of the reforms she proposed, others did not take action until the mid-1990s.

- Because hospitals had been using students as a workforce, it was believed that students spent a lot of time repeating tasks instead of learning. Proponents of the 2-year nursing programs argued that by removing repetition, students would be able to complete their education in 2 years instead of 3 years.
- The first baccalaureate in nursing programs opened in 1919 at the University of British Columbia, and soon after other university nursing programs developed across the country. The need for nurses with specialized knowledge in public health opened the doors of universities to nurses.
- Nursing education began in hospital schools of nursing but these were eventually replaced by college and university programs. The movement toward colleges and universities took decades. Nursing leaders eventually convinced governments that nurses should have the opportunity to learn like all other students, in institutions devoted to higher learning.
- The entry-to-practice position was proposed by nursing leaders who believed that a baccalaureate degree should be the required qualification to enter the profession of nursing as registered nurses.
- In the last two decades, there have been sustained efforts to increase opportunities for French speakers who live outside of Quebec to study nursing in French. At the same time, efforts have been made to increase the number of Indigenous nurses. Initiatives are being developed to address the Calls to Action of the Truth and Reconciliation Commission of Canada to decolonize nursing education.

CRITICAL THINKING QUESTIONS

1. What do you find most striking about the history of nursing education presented in this chapter? Why is this so?
2. If, following your graduation, your school of nursing were to experience serious financial difficulties similar to those encountered by McGill's School for Graduate Nurses in the 1930s, do you think you would be willing to help the way that graduates from McGill did? Please elaborate.
3. What was fundamentally different between the nursing education model developed by Nightingale and the model that emerged in North America?

4. Can you think of the reasons why it took so long for nursing education to be transferred from hospitals to mainstream educational institutions?

5. The last two decades have been marked by the development of programs and courses to serve different type of students and to better prepare students from particular populations. What do you think has contributed to the development of these programs and courses? Think broadly and beyond this chapter, considering Canadian society and political decisions.

REFERENCES

Alberta Association of Registered Nurses. (1976). *The response of the Alberta Association of Registered Nurses to the Government of Alberta's position paper on nursing education*. Edmonton, AB: Author.

Allemang, M. M. (1974). *Nursing education in the United States and Canada, 1873–1950: Leading figures, forces, views on education* [Unpublished doctoral dissertation]. University of Washington.

Allen, M., & Reidy, M. (1971). *Learning to nurse: The first five years of the Ryerson nursing program*. Toronto, ON: Registered Nurses, Association of Ontario.

Arpin, K. (1972). *Report of visit to the Association of Registered Nurses of Newfoundland*. St. John's, NL: AARN.

Association of Nurses of the Province of Quebec. (1972). *CEGEP nursing education after five years*. Montreal, QC: Author.

Baker, C., Guest, E., Jorgenson, L., et al. (2012). *Ties that bind: The evolution of education for professional nursing in Canada from the 17th to the 21st Century*. Ottawa, ON: Canadian Association of Schools of Nursing. Retrieved from https://www.casn.ca/wp-content/uploads/2016/12/History.pdf.

Baly, M. (1986). *Florence Nightingale and the nursing legacy*. London, UK: Croom Helm.

Bonin, M. A. (1976). *Trends in integrated basic degree nursing programs in Canada: 1942–1972* [Unpublished doctoral dissertation]. University of Ottawa.

Bowen, S. (2001). *Language barriers in access to health care*. Ottawa, ON: Health Canada.

Brown, E. L. (1948). *Nursing for the future*. New York, NY: Russell Sage Foundation.

Burgess, M. A. (1928). *Nurses, patients and pocketbooks*. New York, NY: Committee on the Grading of Nursing Schools.

Butler, L., Berry, L., & Exner-Pirot, H. (2018a). Conceptualizing the role of a strategic outreach and Indigenous engagement to lead recruitment and retention of Indigenous students. *Nursing Leadership, 31*(1), 8–17. https://doi.org/10.12927/cjnl.2018.25477.

Butler, L., Exner-Pirot, H., & Berry, L. (2018b). Reshaping policies to achieve a strategic plan for Indigenous engagement in nursing education. *Nursing Leadership, 31*(1), 18–27. https://doi.org/10.12927/cjnl.2018.25476.

Campbell, G. (1971). *Community colleges in Canada*. Toronto, ON: McGraw-Hill.

Canadian Association of Schools of Nursing. (2010). *Final report on the pan-Canadian framework of guiding principles and essential components for IEN bridging programs*. Ottawa, ON: Author. Retrieved from https://casn.ca/wp-content/uploads/2014/12/FinalReportPanCanadianFrameworkFinalVersion.pdf.

Canadian Nurses Association. (1936). *A proposed curriculum for schools of nursing in Canada*. Montreal, QC: Author.

Canadian Nurses Association. (1968). *The leaf and the lamp*. Ottawa, ON: Author.

Canadian Nurses Association. (1989). VGH School of Nursing joins UBC. *The Canadian Nurse, 85*(2), 12.

Canadian Nurses Association. (2001). *Education for registered nurses in a time of shortage*. Ottawa, ON: Author. Retrieved from http://www.cna-nurses.ca/pages.education/educationframe.htm.

Canadian Nurses Association. (2013). *One hundred years of service 1908–2008*. Ottawa, ON: Author.

Canadian Nurses Association. (2017). *Registered nurses profiles (including nurse practitioners) Canada, 2017*. Retrieved from https://www.cna-aiic.ca/en/nursing-practice/the-practice-of-nursing/health-human-resources/nursing-statistics/canada.

Canadian Nurses Association. (2019). *RN and baccalaureate education*. Ottawa, ON: Author. Retrieved from https://www.cna-aiic.ca/en/nursing-practice/the-practice-of-nursing/education/rn-baccalaureate-education.

Carpenter, H. M. (1970). The University of Toronto School of Nursing: An agent of change. In M. Q. Innis (Ed.), *Nursing education in a changing society* (pp. 86–108). Toronto, ON: University of Toronto Press.

Carpenter, H. M. (1982). *Divine discontent: Edith Kathleen Russell—Reforming educator*. Toronto, ON: University of Toronto Faculty of Nursing.

Centre national de formation en santé. (2019). *Historique*. Ottawa, ON: Author. Retrieved from http://cnfs.net/a-propos/historique/.

Cohen, Y. (2005). *Gertrude Elizabeth Livingston. Dictionary of Canadian Biography Online*. Toronto, ON/Québec, QC: University of Toronto/Université Laval. Retrieved from http://www.biographi.ca/en/bio/livingston_gertrude_elizabeth_15E.html.

Cohen, Y., Pepin, J., Lamontagne, E., et al. (2002). *Les sciences infirmières, genèse d'une discipline*. Montreal, QC: Les Presses de l'Université de Montréal.

Committee on the Grading of Nursing Schools. (1934). *Nursing schools today and tomorrow*. New York, NY: Author.

Currie, A. W. (1932, June 27). *Letter to Dr. Helen R. Y. Reid. Financial crisis: 1933 to 1943* [Acc. 2432, File]. Montreal, QC: McGill University Archives.

Currie, A. W. (1933, May 12). *Letter to Bertha Harmer. Financial crisis: 1933 to 1943* [Acc. 2432, File]. Montreal, QC: McGill University Archives.

Desjardins, E. (1971). *Heritage: History of the nursing profession in the province of Quebec*. Québec, QC: Association of Nurses of the Province of Quebec.

Emory, F. (1964, March 6). *Edith Kathleen Russell: An appreciation of her professional life and work* [Acc. A-73011, mimeographed]. Toronto, ON: University of Toronto Faculty of Nursing.

Fédération des communautés francophones et acadiennes. (2001). *Improving access to French-language health services.* Ottawa, ON: Author.

Flynn, K. (2009). Beyond the glass wall: Black Canadian nurses, 1940–1970. *Nursing History Review, 17*, 129–152. https://doi.org/10.1891/1062-8061.17.129.

Gebbie, K. M. (2009). 20th-century reports on nursing and nursing education: What difference did they make? *Nursing Outlook, 57*(2), 84–97. https://doi.org/10.1016/j.outlook.2009.01.006.

Gibbon, J. M., & Mathewson, M. S. (1947). *Three centuries of Canadian nursing.* Toronto, ON: Macmillan.

Government of Alberta. (1975). *Report of the Alberta Task Force on Nursing Education.* Edmonton, AB: Author.

Government of Canada. (2019). *Truth and Reconciliation Commission of Canada.* Ottawa, ON: Author. Retrieved from https://www.rcaanc-cirnac.gc.ca/eng/1450124405592/1529106060525.

Gunn, J. I. (1933). Educational adjustments recommended by the survey. *The Canadian Nurse, 29*(3), 139–145.

Hall, E. M. (1964). *Royal Commission on Health Services: 1964: Volume I.* Ottawa, ON: Government of Canada.

Harmer, B. (1929, May 6). *Letter to Dr. C. F. Martin. Financial crisis: 1933 to 1943* [Acc. 2432, File]. Montreal, QC: McGill University Archives.

Harmer, B. (1932, December 1). *Letter to presidents of provincial nursing associations. Financial crisis: 1933 to 1943* [Acc. 2432, File]. Montreal, QC: McGill University Archives.

Harmer, B. (1933, May 1). *Letter to Sir Arthur W. Currie. Financial crisis: 1933 to 1943* [Acc. 2432, File]. Montreal, QC: McGill University Archives.

Healey, P. (1990). *The Mack Training School for Nurses* [Unpublished doctoral dissertation]. University of Texas.

Holt, M. (1936). Staffing with graduate nurses. *The Canadian Nurse, 32*(1), 5–10.

King, M. K. (1970). The development of university nursing education. In M. Q. Innis (Ed.), *Nursing education in a changing society* (pp. 67–85). Toronto, ON: University of Toronto Press.

Kirkwood, R. (2005). Enough but not too much: Nursing education in English language Canada 1874–2000. In C. Bates, D. Dodd, & N. Rousseau (Eds.), *On all frontiers: Four centuries of Canadian nursing* (pp. 183–196). Ottawa, ON: University of Ottawa Press.

Letourneau, M. (1975). *Trends in basic diploma nursing programs within the provincial systems of education in Canada 1964–1974* [Unpublished doctoral dissertation]. University of Ottawa.

Lindeburgh, M. (1942). Important emergency measures. *The Canadian Nurse, 38*(12), 925–926.

Lord, A. R. (1952). *Report of the evaluation of the Metropolitan School of Nursing, Windsor, Ontario.* Ottawa, ON: Canadian Nurses Association.

MacDermot, H. E. (1940). *History of the School of Nursing of the Montreal General Hospital.* Montreal, QC: The Alumnae Association, Montreal General Hospital.

MacLaggan, K. (1965). *Portrait of nursing: A plan for the education of nurses in the province of New Brunswick.* Fredericton, NB: New Brunswick Association of Registered Nurses.

MacMurchy, H. (1918). University training for the nursing profession. *The Canadian Nurse, 14*(9), 1284–1285.

Manitoba Association of Registered Nurses. (1968). *A position paper on nursing in Manitoba.* Winnipeg, MB: Author.

McLean, C. D. (1964). *A report on the establishment of the Quo Vadis School of Nursing and the selection of the first class of students.* Toronto, ON: Quo Vadis School of Nursing.

Mount Allison University. (2015). History of Mount Allison. Retrieved from https://www.mta.ca/mtahistory/.

Murray, V. V. (1970). *Nursing in Ontario: A study for the committee on the healing arts.* Toronto, ON: Queen's Printer for Ontario.

Mussallem, H. K. (1960). *Spotlight on nursing education: The report of a pilot project for the evaluation of schools of nursing in Canada.* Ottawa, ON: Canadian Nurses Association.

Mussallem, H. K. (1964). *A path to quality: A plan for the development of nursing education programs within the general educational system of Canada.* Ottawa, ON: Canadian Nurses Association.

New Brunswick Association of Registered Nurses. (1971). *Position paper.* Fredericton, NB: Author.

Nightingale, F. (1929). *Cassandra: An essay.* Old Westbury, NY: Feminist Press.

Paul, P. (1994). *A history of the Edmonton General Hospital: 1895-1970 "Be faithful to the duties of your calling"* [Unpublished doctoral dissertation]. University of Alberta.

Palmer, S. (2013). Windsor's Metropolitan Demonstration School and the reform of nursing education in Canada, 1944-1970. In P. D'Antonio, J. A. Fairman, & J. C. Whelan (Eds.), *The Routledge handbook on the global history of nursing* (pp. 131–150). New York, NY: Routledge.

Registered Nurses Association of British Columbia. (1967). *A proposed plan for the orderly development of nursing education in British Columbia: Part one—Basic nursing education.* Vancouver, BC: Author.

Rowe, H. R. (1967). *A study of transition in nursing education in Prince Edward Island.* Charlottetown, PEI: Association of Nurses of Prince Edward Island.

Russell, E. K. (1956). *The report of the study of nursing education in New Brunswick.* Fredericton, NB: Government of New Brunswick.

Schmitt, L. M. (1957). *Basic nursing education study: Report of the status of basic nursing education programs in Saskatchewan.* Regina, SK: Saskatchewan Registered Nurses' Association.

Statistics Canada. (2009). *Rates of wages and hours of labour in various trades and for unskilled factory labour in certain cities of Canada, 1936.* Ottawa, ON: Author. Retrieved from https://www65.statcan.gc.ca/acyb02/1937/acyb02_19370782002a-eng.htm.

Street, M. (1973). *Watch-fires on the mountains: The life and writings of Ethel Johns.* Toronto, ON: University of Toronto Press.

Study Committee on Nursing Education. (1971). *A study committee on nursing education.* Fredericton, NB: New Brunswick Department of Health.

The Editors of Encyclopaedia Britannica. (2018). *Grace Hoadley Dodge.* Retrieved from https://www.britannica.com/biography/Grace-Hoadley-Dodge.

Toman, C. (2010). "My chance has come at last!": The Weston Hospital, the Women's Christian Temperance Union, and Indian Nurses in Canada, 1917–1929. *Native Studies Review, 19*(2), 95–119.

Tunis, B. L. (1966). *In caps and gowns.* Montreal, QC: McGill University Press.

Truth and Reconciliation Commission of Canada. (2015). *Truth and Reconciliation Commission of Canada: Calls to Action.* Winnipeg, MB: Author. Retrieved from http://trc.ca/assets/pdf/Calls_to_Action_English2.pdf.

Twohig, P. L. (1998). *Challenges and change—A history of the Dalhousie School of Nursing 1949–1989.* Halifax, NS: Fernwood Publishing and Dalhousie University.

University of Saskatchewan College of Nursing and Canadian Indigenous Nurses Association. (2018). *2018 University of Saskatchewan & CINA's Fact Sheet: Aboriginal Nursing in Canada.* Retrieved from http://indigenousnurses.ca/sites/default/files/inline-files/Nursing_AborigNursing_sheet_2018_3.pdf.

Weir, G. M. (1932). *Survey of nursing education in Canada.* Toronto, ON: University of Toronto Press.

Wollstonecraft, M. (1787). *Thoughts on the education of daughters.* Clifton, NJ: A. M. Kelley.

Wollstonecraft, M. (1792). *A vindication of the rights of woman.* London, UK: J. Johnson.

Zawaduk, C., Duncan, S., Star Mahara, M., et al. (2014). Mission possible: Twenty-five years of university and college collaboration in baccalaureate nursing education. *Journal of Nursing Education, 53*(10), 580–588. https://doi.org/10.3928/01484834-20140922-04.

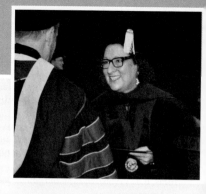

Licensure, Credentialling, and Entry to Practice in Nursing

Tammie R. McParland

(e) http://evolve.elsevier.com/Canada/Ross-Kerr/nursing

LEARNING OBJECTIVES

After reading this chapter, you will be able to:
- Describe what is meant by registration, licensure, and credentialling in the professional nursing context.
- Identify the current status of entry to practice for registered nurses in Canada.
- Describe the recent changes in the licensure exam for registered nurses in Canada.
- Understand the historical development of the current state of entry to practice for nursing in Canada.
- Describe the major credentialling mechanisms used in Canada for registered nurses, nurse practitioners, and advanced practice nurses.
- Discuss the issue of mandatory licensure in the nursing profession.
- Identify the reasons for specialization in nursing.
- Describe the programs available to credential nursing specialties in Canada.

OUTLINE

KEY TERMS

certification
credentialling
entry to practice
exam blueprint
licensure
licensure examination

mandatory licensure
Next Generation NCLEX
permissive licensure
registration
scope of practice
specialization

PERSONAL PERSPECTIVES

Upon graduation from his undergraduate program in nursing, Reed wrote and successfully passed his licensure exam to become a registered nurse in his province. Reed had the opportunity to experience working in the pediatric intensive care unit during his undergraduate education and decided that he wanted to specialize in pediatrics. Part of the unit's educational offerings included use of several types of simulation technologies to prepare new graduates for their role. Reed also found that he enjoyed this experience and wanted to know more about using simulation technologies. The nurse clinicians who used the simulation technologies were both certified simulation nurse educators and certified pediatric nurses. Reed now plans to learn more about how to become specialized in these two fields of nursing practice: simulation use in nursing education and pediatrics.

REGISTRATION, LICENSURE, AND CREDENTIALLING IN THE NURSING PROFESSION IN CANADA

All registered nurses (RNs) in Canada are licensed by their respective provincial or territorial regulatory body, but not all are graduates of a university baccalaureate program. **Entry to practice**, often confused for a baccalaureate degree, relates not to an educational achievement but to a **credentialling** requirement to qualify to practise as an RN. In Canada, for most provinces and territories, this requirement is satisfied by the graduation of a nurse from a university baccalaureate program. Quebec is the only jurisdiction that does not require a baccalaureate in nursing for entry to practice as an RN.

Entry to Practice

Historically, the baccalaureate degree as entry to practice was a hotly debated topic (see Chapter 20). The requirement for obtaining a baccalaureate degree to be able to practice as an RN was endorsed by the Canadian Nurses Association (CNA) and the provincial and territorial nursing associations in the latter decades of the twentieth century. In the late 1990s, "entry to practice 2000" (or EP2000) referred to the goal of attaining the baccalaureate standard for entry to practice by the year 2000. The rationale for this requirement was that the profession needed to prepare nurses who would be able to provide increasingly complex care. The only province in Canada to achieve this by 2000 was Newfoundland and Labrador. While the rest of the country was not able to achieve the goal of EP2000,

many provinces did eventually achieve it. Most legislatures quickly approved the request of professional nursing associations for baccalaureate entry to practice between 2001 and 2005. As of 2019, the only province that has not supported baccalaureate entry to practice is Quebec.

RNs who had graduated from a diploma program were grandfathered (to maintain their RN status) by the regulatory bodies across Canada and did not need to upgrade to a baccalaureate degree, although many did. Now, the demand for post-RN baccalaureate education from diploma-prepared nurses has declined, as there are few diploma-prepared nurses since the adoption of baccalaureate entry to practice. Currently, 44.7% of the Canadian RN workforce is diploma prepared (Canadian Nurses Association [CNA], 2019). As diploma-prepared nurses leave the workforce, and more baccalaureate-prepared nurses graduate and begin to practice, this percentage will decline even more. Of the many nurses who entered nursing practice with a diploma, some recognized both their personal need for additional education and the fact that additional study might improve their competitive position for promotions, particularly at a leadership level. As a result, many nurses chose to enroll in further education to become specialized or earn advanced degrees.

Interestingly, the initial leadership for the baccalaureate entry-to-practice initiative came neither from the profession nor from university faculties of nursing, but from the Alberta Task Force on Nursing Education, a government-appointed committee established to study needs in relation to nursing education in Alberta. The Alberta government subsequently issued a denunciation of the committee's recommendation, disagreeing with the recommendation to make a baccalaureate degree the requirement for practice (Government of Alberta, 2008).

Immediately after the government's refusal to accept the document, lively discussions ensued among all interested parties. The College and Association of Registered Nurses of Alberta (CARNA) (known as the Alberta Association of Registered Nurses [AARN] before November 2005) endorsed the task force's recommendations shortly after they were released. CARNA subsequently suggested the year 2000 as a more realistic target date for implementation of the entry-to-practice position than the 1995 goal suggested by the task force. At the 1980 Biennial Convention of the CNA, delegates debated a resolution to develop a statement on the minimum educational qualification needed to enter the profession. Following approval, the resolution became a priority for the 1980–1982 biennium. Momentum began to grow with the establishment of a committee to study the issue, and articles appeared in *The Canadian Nurse* debating both sides of the question (Rajabally, 1982). The decision to endorse the baccalaureate standard was taken by the CNA Board of Directors in February 1982. Support was high, and the motion was carried unanimously. Delegates to the 1982 Biennial Convention, in Newfoundland, added further strength to the position by adopting a motion of support. Support for the position grew within the profession as the issues were debated in provinces and territories that had not already adopted a position on the matter. Gradually, one jurisdiction at a time, positions in support of baccalaureate entry to practice were taken. With obvious enthusiasm and eagerness, nurses from one end of the country to the other identified and developed mechanisms to ensure that logical, well-articulated, and reasonable plans were made to achieve baccalaureate entry to practice.

CREDENTIALLING IN NURSING

Likewise, the way in which credentialling in nursing came about is illuminating, for it draws attention to the growth and development of nursing as a profession (see Chapter 3). Initially, nurses did not have to meet any credentialling expectations, as the profession did not have a set of professional standards or educational expectations. This began to change with the work of Florence Nightingale. The relation of credentialling to professionalization can be seen in what has been referred to as "the natural history of professionalization" a history that is both recognizable and sequential in nature:

> There is a typical process by which the established professions have arrived . . . [They] begin doing the work full time and stake out a jurisdiction; the early masters of the technique or adherents of the movement become concerned about standards of training and practice and set up a training school, which, if not lodged in universities at the start, makes academic connections within two or three decades; the teachers and activists then achieve success in promoting effective organization, first local, then national . . . Toward the end, legal protection appears; at the end, a formal code of ethics is adopted. (Wilensky, 1964, p. 144)

The presence of a specialized knowledge base is fundamental to the processes and mechanisms of credentialling in nursing. The perception of the defining characteristics of this knowledge determines identification and acceptance of any field as a profession, including the following elements: (1) the knowledge and skills are abstract and consist of principles considered relevant to everyday situations; (2) there is a belief that the specialized knowledge will produce positive results when applied to real problems; (3) those in the profession are involved in developing and applying the knowledge base and in providing expert opinion in difficult cases; and (4) the knowledge and skills are complex, and

only a few have the ability to acquire them (Goode, 1960). In a historical sense, Canadian nurses recognized early in the twentieth century that the knowledge and skills fundamental to the profession were important and that unqualified and unskilled practitioners could harm the clients for whom they cared. The profession needed to ensure that nurses graduated from recognized and high-quality schools of nursing and that professional standards were established to regulate nursing education and practice.

Hospitals in Canada did not need to be encouraged to establish schools of nursing in the late nineteenth and early twentieth centuries. They all sought to emulate the successful Nightingale model in Britain and to ensure an adequate number of staff members as well as a qualified and inexpensive staff. However, this design was the antithesis of what Nightingale intended, as her school was supported by the Nightingale endowment and was financially and administratively independent (see Chapter 20). Thus, evidence of graduation from a school of nursing was the earliest form of credentialling. This period of history was also characterized by a concerted drive by nursing leaders to secure legislation for **registration** of nurses to ensure that, for the protection of the public, the educated would be differentiated from the uneducated.

For the most part, credentialling issues are similar today, although the nature and extent of the knowledge and skills that must be acquired to practise nursing have changed. Important areas for discussion and study include the need for recognizing standards in programs, knowing the meaning of a certificate, securing qualified staff for many areas of **specialization**, establishing standards at the national level, and ensuring that practitioners update their knowledge and maintain competence throughout their careers. However, questions pertaining to protection of the public from unscrupulous, unqualified, and unskilled practitioners are as fundamental to credentialling processes and mechanisms today as they were in the past.

CREDENTIALLING MECHANISMS

Credentialling is a process used to indicate that an individual, program, institution, or product has met established standards set out by either a governmental or nongovernmental agency and can complete the tasks inherent in the standards (Styles & Affara, 1997). Thus, individuals who have knowledge and skills in a certain area are distinguished from those who do not have such skills. Describing credentialling as a mere system of checks and balances is appropriate. Nursing has two main credentialling mechanisms: professional and educational. On the professional side, registration and licensure are awarded to individuals for practise of the profession. Educational credentialling pertains to the requirements for acceptance into the profession. Nurses must satisfy the requirements for both educational (minimum required education) and professional credentialling (registration and licensure).

THE MOVEMENT TO SECURE LEGISLATION FOR REGISTRATION

The drive for the registration of nurses occurred early in the development of the profession in Canada. This was the issue that brought nurses together in professional organizations. The formation of the first national and international organization for nurses in 1893, the American Society of Superintendents of Training Schools for Nurses in the United States and Canada, was followed by the foundation of the Nurses' Associated Alumnae Association in the United States and Canada in 1896. The purpose of the latter organization was "to secure legislation to differentiate the trained from the untrained" (CNA, 1968, p. 35). Both organizations were initially headed by one of the most important nursing leaders of the time, Isabel Hampton Robb, a Canadian nurse from Ontario who was the first superintendent of nurses at the Johns Hopkins Hospital in Baltimore, Maryland. These groups inspired the formation, in both the United States and Canada, of many other local, regional, and national professional nursing organizations; in Canada, these organizations worked to complete the groundwork necessary for the passage of legislation to regulate nursing in the provinces and territories. The publication of the *American Journal of Nursing* in 1900 and *The Canadian Nurse* in 1905 helped the cause.

The US and Canadian groups separated as activity intensified, and it was evident that the battle for passage of legislation had to be fought regionally. In Canada, these efforts were spearheaded within the provinces because the *British North America Act, 1867* provided that the legislatures of each province be given exclusive right to make laws in relation to health and education. The Canadian Society of Superintendents of Training Schools for Nurses emerged in 1907, followed by the Provisional Society of the Canadian Nurses Association of Trained Nurses in 1908. The first president of both groups was Mary Agnes Snively, a graduate of Bellevue Hospital in New York who had headed the School of Nursing at Toronto General Hospital since 1884 (CNA, 1968).

From the beginning, there have been valid reasons for requiring registration. Professional registration and licensure make the benefits that accrue from the services of a highly skilled group available to society and protect society from those who are not highly skilled, as well as from those who might knowingly misuse their knowledge and skills to the disadvantage of the populace. In each province and territory in Canada, local graduate nurse groups joined forces to become provincial nurses' associations and sought legislation for the registration of nurses. These nurses believed that registration Acts that set standards for training schools would also improve the quality of care.

Two powerful social forces influenced the drive for legislation for the registration of nurses. The first was the consciousness-raising about women's rights, which was part of the movement for the enfranchisement of women. The second was that nurses' services were especially valued during World War I, when there was a tremendous need for nursing care on the battlefront and behind the lines. During this period of worldwide social upheaval, nursing and nurses became very much valued, as so many nurses volunteered for war service and served with dedication and valour. The worldwide influenza pandemic between 1916 and 1918 further drove home the need to recognize the qualifications of nurses as essential to protecting the health of the populace. The passage of legislation in every province and territory over a 12-year period may have been facilitated by these factors and represented general recognition of the need for a system that ensured nurses were qualified.

There was considerable activity for several years before legislation was first passed. In 1910, Nova Scotia was the first province to pass an Act that made registration

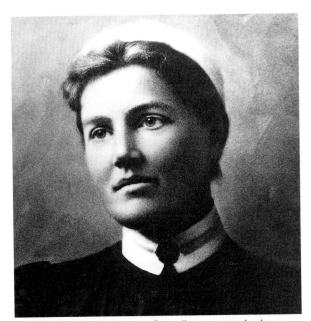

Isabel Hampton Robb, the Canadian nurse who became the first superintendent of nurses at Johns Hopkins Hospital in Baltimore, Maryland, in 1889. (From Wikipedia: Isabel Hampton)

TABLE 21.1	Chronology of Legislation Regulating Nursing in Canadian Jurisdictions		
Province/Territory	**Date Legislation First Enacted**	**Current status**	**Date of Change to Mandatory Legislation**
British Columbia	1918	Mandatory	1988
Alberta	1916	Mandatory	1983
Saskatchewan	1917	Mandatory	1988
Manitoba	1913	Mandatory	2001
Ontario	1922	Mandatory	1991
Quebec	1920	Mandatory	1973
New Brunswick	1916	Mandatory	1984
Nova Scotia	1910	Mandatory	1985
Prince Edward Island	1922	Mandatory	1972
Newfoundland	1931	Mandatory	1953
Northwest Territories and Nunavut	1976	Mandatory	1975
Yukon	1994	Mandatory	2004

Sources: Good, S. R., & Kerr, J. C. (Eds.). (1973). *Contemporary issues in Canadian law for nurses* (p. 189). Toronto, ON: Holt, Rinehart & Winston; Prowse, A. J. (1983). *Nursing legislation in Canada: An overview for health services administrators* (pp. 10–28, 36–41) [Unpublished master's thesis]. University of Alberta; College of Nurses of Ontario. (2005). *The Regulated Health Professions Act.* Retrieved from http://www.cno.org/docs/policy/41052_RHPAscope.pdf; Registered Nurses Association of the Northwest Territories and Nunavut. (2019). *Legislation.* Retrieved from http://www.rnantnu.ca/documents/acts-legislation; Yukon Registered Nurses Association. (2019). *Nursing practice—registration.* Retrieved from https://yukonnurses.ca/.

voluntary and allowed nongraduate nurses to register. Subsequent legislation in other provinces incorporated more restrictive standards. Minimum standards for admission and curricula in schools of nursing were set, as were rules governing registration and discipline of practising nurses. Ontario was the last province to approve legislation for nursing because of a lobby against the legislation, led by hospitals whose administrators feared that the educational standards for nursing schools could not be met or maintained. Opposition also arose from nurses who thought they could not meet the qualifications. These objections were overcome or overruled, and legislation was passed in Ontario in 1922 (Sabin, Price, & Sellers, 1973).

In all provinces except Alberta, the initial legislation gave provincial nursing associations the responsibility for administering the legislation. In Alberta, the *Registered Nurses Act* was passed in 1916, and uniform registration examinations were instituted in 1919. This statute was unusual because it placed nursing education under the aegis of the senate of the University of Alberta. A chronology documenting the process of securing registration in each of the provinces is presented in Table 21.1.

Registration and Licensure Requirements

Registration allows the profession to maintain an official roster of member nurses. To be named on a register, a nurse must be a member in good standing of the organization incorporating the statutory responsibility for registration. There are two types of registration: permissive and mandatory. Under permissive registration, the legislation protects only the title of "registered nurse"; that is, a person may practise nursing without being registered, but may not use the initials "R.N." Permissive registration does not exist in Canada. In Acts that provide for mandatory registration, the nature of the service provided by the profession is defined. This means that those who do not meet the requirements of the legislation may not practise nursing. The title is protected, as in permissive Acts, but the definition of nursing and the restriction of practice as it applies to RNs are the critical features that differentiate the two types of registration.

As noted, registration is the term that identifies who is on the official roster of a professional discipline, while licensure relates to professional credentialling expectations. Licensure and registration are often used interchangeably but they are not the same. Mandatory licensure was the result of a desire for the nursing profession to be accountable to the public, while **permissive licensure** did not expect accountability to the public, such that practitioners could engage in practice known to the discipline as long as they did not use any protected title. The title "nurse" has been protected since 1922, when Ontario approved mandatory registration. Therefore, permissive licensure no longer exists in Canada.

Mandatory registration is the requirement for licensure and is similar in all provinces. An applicant must be a graduate of an approved school of nursing and must pass a credentialling examination. Minimum standards for nursing education were established by a governmental body. In all provinces except Ontario and Quebec, the approval body was the professional association; this responsibility has since been taken under the auspices of the regulatory body of the province. In Ontario, the *Health Disciplines Act, 1980* and the *Regulated Health Professions Act, 1991* granted authority for the approval and monitoring of diploma programs to the Ministry of Training, Colleges and Universities, the Council of Ontario University Programs in Nursing (COUPN), and the university senate or governing council (for university programs).

Subsequently, COUPN delegated its authority to approve university nursing programs to the Canadian Association of Schools of Nursing (CASN). COUPN still has requirements for development and review of nursing programs at the provincial level, with CASN continuing to review educational programs through an accreditation process (Council of Ontario University Programs in Nursing [COUPN], 2019). Before 2018, accreditation of the university nursing program denoted governmental approval; however, after 2018, the regulatory members of the Canadian Council of Registered Nurse Regulators (CCRNR) indicated they would be approving nurse education programs. Approval of educational programs would grant the students who successfully passed the individual program the ability to write the **licensure examination** approved by the regulatory body. This exam is now the NCLEX-RN (National Council Licensing Exam for Registered Nurses), except in Quebec. In Quebec, the Ministère de l'Éducation et de l'Enseignement supérieur holds the responsibility for monitoring diploma programs in the Collèges d'enseignement général et professionnel (CEGEP). University programs in nursing are monitored by the individual universities through their respective provincial ministry of education–mandated quality assurance programs.

In Ontario, the College of Nurses began the process by approving nurse practitioner (NP) programs in 2018, followed by baccalaureate programs in 2019, and registered practical nurse programs in 2020. Program approval for RNs, NPs, licensed practical nurses, and registered psychiatric nurses in British Columbia was announced when the three regulatory bodies in British Columbia amalgamated into one regulatory college in 2018 (British Columbia College of Nursing Professionals, 2018).

The terms **registration** and **licensure** have different meanings, although they are used interchangeably in some situations. As previously noted, registration refers to the listing of a member in good standing of an organization on the roster of members, with the use of a specific protected title such as "nurse." Licensure refers to the granting by a government body to a member in good standing of the exclusive right to practise a profession as well as use of the protected title. In provinces where registration is mandatory, the same process may also be described as licensure. Practice of the profession by any person who has not been granted such a right is prohibited and punishable by law.

NCLEX-RN Licensure

The adoption of the American-based NCLEX-RN licensure exam in 2015 ushered in a change for all Canadian nurse educators and nursing students. The NCLEX-RN exam is based on an **exam blueprint** developed through a practice analysis of the work done by American nurses in their first year of practice in acute care settings. While opposition to the exam has lessened (except from francophone students—please see the Cultural Consideration box in this chapter), some criticism of the NCLEX continues; one deficit cited is the lack of focus on Canadian entry-to-practice requirements. In an attempt to address the criticism, the National Council of State Boards of Nursing (NCSBN), the creator of the exam, includes Canadian nurses as writers and reviewers.

In 2023, a new RN licensure exam will be released: the **Next Generation NCLEX** (NGN) exam. This exam will be focused on critical thinking and clinical judgement of RNs and follows a framework called the NCSBN Clinical Judgment Measurement Model. This model, which complements the nursing process and other evidence-informed theories of practice, details the layers involved between a client's needs and a nurse's decisions based on these needs. Research and surveys conducted by the NCSBN found that novice nurses were not readily prepared to make the complex clinical decisions required nowadays, and employers rated clinical judgement from "important" to "critically important" (National Council of State Boards of Nursing [NCSBN], 2020). The NGN exam will include questions that focus on interactions between nurses and clients, the needs of clients, and the expected outcomes of the care given by the nurses based on their clinical judgement. The new questions will reflect real-world nursing care. Since 2017, the NCSBN has been testing items for the new exam through a special research section of the NCLEX licensure exams. All writers are asked to complete this section after completing their NCLEX exam; participation is voluntary and will not affect the writers' scores (NCSBN, 2020).

THE CASE FOR MANDATORY LICENSURE

Licensure laws were designed to protect the public from unethical and incompetent practitioners, not to protect the nursing profession from competition. The only justifiable reason for adopting legislation to guarantee professionals exclusive right to practise is to protect the public from unqualified and incompetent practitioners. The legislation cannot and must not bestow a special benefit on people who have completed a certain educational program and demonstrated designated qualifications where there is no public protective component.

In recent years, there has been public concern about self-rule by professional groups, the fear being that power may be exercised in the interest of the profession. The thrust of the consumer movement is to present challenges in areas in which the consumer interest may not be protected. The health care field is no exception in such efforts. This phenomenon, and the fact that it is not easy to change existing legislation that governs professional groups, explains why it was difficult for provinces and territories to replace their original permissive legislation with mandatory statutes. **Mandatory licensure** has been achieved by emphasizing the need to assure the public that licensed nurses have met an appropriate standard of practice as determined by the profession.

All Canadian nursing jurisdictions have now achieved legislative provision for mandatory registration of nurses. The presence of a statutory definition of the scope of nursing practice is an important feature of legislature in jurisdictions with mandatory licensure. Nurses' functions are delineated more explicitly when a definition of nursing practice is incorporated into the statute. The potential for overlap with functions performed by other health care providers that exists in mandatory jurisdictions may be addressed through specific exemptions or by extending rights only to health care providers practising by virtue of other statutes.

In 1991, Ontario enacted legislation affecting all health care providers. This legislation, the *Regulated Health Professions Act*, provides for the regulation of 23 professional groups under 21 individual professional Acts. Each individual Act describes a **scope of practice** and allows for restrictive use of a title. To ensure public protection, however, the *Regulated Health Professions Act* identifies 13 controlled acts that may be performed only by specific registered members as identified in the individual legislation. In this manner, it is the activity that is licensed, not the individual provider (College of Nurses of Ontario, 2019). Alberta also passed omnibus legislation for the health professions and proclaimed the schedule for RNs in 2005. The scope of nursing practice is incorporated into the statute as previously described. The legislation also provides for the practice of restricted activities as authorized in the regulations (Government of Alberta, 2008).

Registration and licensure ensure a minimum level of safe practice at the time of initial registration. Those registered are eligible for re-registration annually if practice requirements are met and there is no evidence of unsafe practice. New knowledge is continually introduced to the field, and the individual must maintain and extend competence to meet the changing requirements. The nursing profession has wrestled with the problem of maintaining competence in an effort to demonstrate public accountability. The merits of mandatory versus permissive continuing education programs have been debated at length. In most provinces, mandatory continuing education has been rejected in favour of requiring a certain number of days of employment within a specified time and a record of satisfactory practice as evidence of current knowledge and skills. Quality assurance is the banner under which several provinces and territories assure the public that members are maintaining competency. While some similarities exist across provinces and territories, such as the setting of learning goals to meet an identified need, there is also some variability—for example, some provinces/territories require peer review and feedback, while others do not. For instance, Alberta calls the program a "continuing competency" program. Some provinces, like British Columbia, also expect nurses to engage in peer review. Failure to meet quality assurance expectations can lead to disciplinary action by the regulatory body against the nurse.

The move toward offering refresher courses for those who have been out of practice, upgrading programs, and opportunities for continuing education has become an integral and essential part of the nursing education system, as those who practise a profession must incorporate a commitment to lifelong learning. Nurses have a legal and ethical duty to maintain competence. In the event that a nurse's conduct is questioned by a patient, the practitioner may be called upon in a hearing of peers or in a court of law to provide evidence that reasonable effort has been expended to attend continuing education seminars and workshops to maintain competence in practice. Recently, some provinces have moved to incorporate mandatory continuing education as part of the continuing registration process. The intent here is protection of the public interest by ensuring that nurses maintain their knowledge and skills throughout their careers.

APPLYING CONTENT KNOWLEDGE

In your journal or notebook, explore the importance to public health and safety of legislation to regulate the practice of nursing.

NURSE PRACTITIONERS

The NP movement began in Canada in the 1960s, spurred on by advances in health care that led to evolving nursing roles, increasing specialization in nursing, and a developing

CASE STUDY

The Implementation of an American-Based Exam to License Canadian Registered Nurses

In 2011, RNs were informed by their respective regulatory bodies that a new licensure exam was being introduced to Canada as of January 1, 2015. This exam was developed in the United States by the National Council of the State Boards of Nursing (NCSBN) and was called the NCLEX-RN (National Council Licensing Exam for Registered Nurses). The choice to move to the NCLEX-RN was made by the Canadian Council of Registered Nurse Regulators (CCRNR), a group of representatives from regulatory bodies across Canada that is responsible for the licensure and regulation of RNs in Canada.

Efforts to bring a new exam to Canada began in 2009, when Ontario and British Columbia asked a sample group of RNs to provide their perceptions of the 142 nursing activities that US nurses undertake (NCSBN, 2010a, 2010b). The 145 national competencies for entry-level practice from the College of Nurses of Ontario were also compared with the 142 activities in the 2008 NCSBN test plan (NCSBN, n.d.). The NSCBN found that nurses in both provinces had similar perceptions of the activities of nurses for entry-level practice (McGillis Hall, Lalonde, Kashin et al., 2018). At this point, a suggestion was made that the provinces consider joint licensure discussions with the NCSBN to enhance licensure portability, a move that would benefit the two provinces, the United States, and ultimately the public (McGillis Hall, Lalonde, Kashin et al., 2018). This report was released 1.5 years before the selection of the NCLEX-RN by the Canadian regulatory body committee—the CCRNR.

In December 2011, the upcoming switch was communicated by the regulators, and preparatory work was done by nurse educators, especially the educational associations such as the Canadian Association of Schools of Nursing (CASN). The CASN held webinars to highlight the differences between the previous exam (the Canadian Registered Nurse Exam) and the new NCLEX-RN; developed fact sheets and resources; and liaised with stakeholders such as the Canadian Nursing Students' Association (CNSA) to engage them in preparatory work

for the new exam. Despite these efforts, the examination results in the first three-quarters of the year for first-time writers of the new NCLEX exam indicated a pass rate of around 70%, while in previous years, with the CRNE, the pass rate was 87%. Francophone writers, such as those in New Brunswick, fared even worse, with only 27% passing. These poor results led to concerns about the exam and its applicability to Canadian contexts and education. McGillis Hall and colleagues (2018) identified problems with the exam: its applicability to Canadian health care; curriculum alignment; examination translation for francophone students; lack of stakeholder engagement by the CCRNR; and a dearth of communication about the changes to the exam or addressing concerns about it. Students identified problems such as questions that included trade names for drugs not used in Canada; different lab results (US imperial measurements and not the metric units used in Canada); as well as policy statements about American health care (e.g., "Obamacare").

The CNSA submitted a letter to the NCSBN identifying the concerns of those who would be required to write the new exam in French and highlighting the lack of francophone preparatory resources, despite receiving assurance from the NCSBN that translation and resources would be available, and based upon earlier communication with the NCSBN (NCSBN, n.d.). Nurse educators were upset that they would have to revise curricula; in essence, they were "teaching to a test" and not to a set of professional competencies or Canadian-based framework. Several professional nursing associations expressed dismay about the results; they then initiated research to investigate why the pass rate was that much lower and implemented strategies to address the concerns expressed by nursing students and educators alike. The CNA voiced concerns that the exam result could impact the sustainability of the nursing workforce (CNA, 2015). There was a corresponding dip in the number of RNs for the year in which the exam was introduced (Canadian Association of Schools of Nursing, 2017).

Sources: Canadian Association of Schools of Nursing. (2017). *Registered nurse education statistics in Canada*. Retrieved from https://www.casn.ca/wp-content/uploads/2017/12/2015-2016-EN-SFS-FINAL-REPORT-supressed-for-web.pdf; Canadian Nurses Association. (2015). *Framework for registered nurse prescribing in Canada*. Retrieved from https://www.cna-aiic.ca/-/media/cna/page-content/pdf-en/cna-rn-prescribing-framework_e.pdf; McGillis Hall, L., Lalonde, M., Kashin, J., et al. (2018). Changing nurse licensing examinations: Media analysis and implications of the Canadian experience. *International Nursing Review, 65*, 13–23. https://doi.org/10.1111/inr.12367; National Council of State Boards of Nursing. (n.d.). *Test plans*. Retrieved from https://www.ncsbn.org/testplans.htm.

CULTURAL CONSIDERATIONS

Is the Licensure Requirement of the NCLEX-RN Fair to Francophone Canadian Nurses?

When the NCLEX-RN was written by students for the first time in 2015, it became evident that the average passing rate had dropped. The pass rate was 69.7% in the first year and rose to 82% in 2017 (first attempts). However, francophone students had a pass rate of only 27% in 2015, a number that barely increased (29%) in 2017. McGillis Hall, Lalonde, & Kashin (2016) interviewed 202 graduate Canadian nursing students who were the first to write the NCLEX-RN exam in 2015 and 2016. One of the major concerns identified by the students was the lack of French-language resources as well as the translation of the exam, which was done by American and not Canadian translators. Also identified was the inability of the NCSBN corporation to respond to students' queries in their mother tongue. As one student recounted to the researchers, "One of my colleagues wrote an email to the NCSBN in French and they came back to her stating 'sorry, please write to us in English—we have no idea what you are saying'" (McGillis Hall, Lalonde, & Kashin, 2016, p. 46).

The CNA expressed its concerns in 2015 and again in 2016 that the first-time results of the 2015 NCLEX-RN signalled that the exam was fraught with issues; the CAN also noted the difficulties experienced by francophone nurses as a major issue (CNA, 2015, 2016; St-Denis, 2017). The CNSA addressed the inequity in 2017 with a letter-writing campaign. In May 2018, the Société de l'Acadie du Nouveau-Brunswick, along with the student federation at the University of Moncton, brought a lawsuit against the regulatory body in New Brunswick (Fahmy, 2018). The groups indicated that the regulatory body did not adequately ensure that the test was properly translated, nor did they provide appropriate French-language study resources for francophone students (Lund, 2018). A parliamentary finding in November 2018 agreed that the "decision to adopt the NCLEX-RN without coordinating its translation with certified Canadian translators or developing French study resources of equal quality to those available in English did significant harm to minority francophone registered nurses" (Parliament of Canada, 2018). Four recommendations were made to address the inequity in language parity in the NCLEX-RN and ensure that the NCLEX-RN reflected the bilingual reality that exists in Canada.

Sources: Canadian Nurses Association. (2015, April). *Framework for registered nurse prescribing in Canada.* Retrieved from https://www.cna-aiic.ca/-/media/cna/page-content/pdf-en/cna-rn-prescribing-framework_e.pdf; Canadian Nurses Association. (2016, March 7). *2015 NCLEX-RN results signal several major issues with nurse licensing exam.* Retrieved from https://cna-aiic.ca/en/news-room/news-releases/2016/2015-nclex-rn-results-signal-several-major-issues-with-nurse-licensing-exam; Fahmy, G. (2018, May 14). *Nurses association faces lawsuit over "atrocious" failure rate by francophones.* CBC News. Retrieved from https://www.cbc.ca/news/canada/new-brunswick/nursing-association-lawsuit-exam-francophones-1.4661749; Lund, S. (2018, May 11). *Watchdog says nursing exam puts francophone students at a disadvantage.* CBC News. Retrieved from https://www.cbc.ca/news/politics/nursing-exams-translation-francophones-1.4657119; McGillis Hall, L., Lalonde, M., Kashin, J. (2016). People are failing! Something needs to be done: Canadian students' experience with the NCLEX-RN. *Nurse Education Today, 46,* 43–49. https://doi.org/10.1016/j.nedt.2016.08.022; Parliament of Canada. (2018). *House of Commons Standing Committee on Official Languages. Presentation of report on the success rate of francophone registered nurses who take the National Council Licensure Examination (NCLEX-RN)* [Press release]. Retrieved from https://www.ourcommons.ca/DocumentViewer/en/42-1/LANG/news-release/10184635; St. Denis, V. (2017, September 5). *The NCLEX-RN and the future of French-language health-care services.* Canadian Nurse. Retrieved from https://www.canadian-nurse.com/en/articles/issues/2017/september-october-2017/the-nclex-rn-and-the-future-of-french-language-health-care-services.

shortage of family physicians. The first program for outpost nurses at Dalhousie University began in 1967. It led to similar programs at other Canadian universities that were jointly sponsored by faculties of nursing and medicine but operated separately from ongoing degree programs in nursing. However, the graduates of the programs found themselves working in a legislative vacuum and, for the most part, were employed in northern and remote areas. Those who worked in cities were employed under physician supervision. Articles written in the 1970s began to advocate for the expanded role of nurses as a priority

(Hastings, 1972; Resnick, 1972). Responding to the perceived need for programs, in the 1980s, university nursing programs began to develop undergraduate and graduate courses in health assessment and to discuss developing advanced nursing practice programs at the master's level. Gradually, more of these programs became available and began to replace existing programs as student demand for them increased.

In the late 1990s, a movement gained momentum to develop legislation to allow NPs to become credentialed and work under legislative and legal authority. For the most part, the legislation has taken the form of amendments to the legislation for RNs in each jurisdiction. The expanded scope of practice allowed under each piece of legislation varies somewhat from jurisdiction to jurisdiction, but generally allows NPs to perform an assessment of health status leading to diagnosis of disease, order diagnostic and screening tests, and prescribe medications (CNA & Canadian Institute for Health Information, 2006). The scope of practice for NPs in Ontario recently expanded to included prescribing opiates. This expansion in scope of practice was moved forward in preparation for RN prescribing on Ontario, and while other provinces have already included prescribing medications as a part of the scope of practice of NPs, most do not include opiate ordering.

Credentialling for NPs now includes an exam after completion of advanced education. Passing the exam entitles the NP to practice with the initials "E.C.," meaning extended class, after their regulated title of RN. NPs must also complete required hours and assessments as part of remaining credentialed and entitled to use E.C.

🔍 RESEARCH FOCUS

Prescriptive Authority for Nurses: The Canadian Perspective

In Forchuk and Kohn's (2009) unique discussion of the evolution and status of prescriptive authority for nurses in Canada, the linkage to the development of advanced nursing practice was underscored. The authors noted that prescriptive authority is a "work in progress," because legislation to enact it is not yet universal across the country. However, the initial form of legislation according prescriptive authority to nurses with specialized preparation hinged on the availability of medical practitioners, while more recent legislation tends not to make it a requirement. The authors further outlined facilitators and barriers to putting prescriptive authority into place in any jurisdiction.

Source: Forchuk, C., & Kohn, R. (2009). Prescriptive authority for nurses: The Canadian perspective. *Perspectives in Psychiatric Care, 45*(1), 3–8. https://doi.org/10.1111/j.1744-6163.2009.00194.x.

CHANGES TO NURSES' SCOPE OF PRACTICE AND CREDENTIALLING

Nursing, as a self-reflective profession, is constantly assessing and responding to the needs of the public to whom it is accountable. Nursing education itself was transferred from hospital to college or technical school diploma to university because of the complexity of knowledge and skills required

and because it is through the educational process that nursing students acquire the essential foundation for practice.

Recently, there has been a movement across the country to allow RN prescribing outside of the NP role. RNs in other countries, such as Ireland and England, have had the skill of drug prescribing included in their scope. Historically, only NPs were allowed to prescribe, communicate a diagnosis for the purpose of prescribing, and perform certain medical procedures usually performed by physicians.

In addition, the scope of practice of registered practical nurses in Ontario is being opened to include several skills previously designated only to RNs, allowing this group of health care providers to be added to specialty **certification** groups such as gerontology (CNA, 2019). In addition, the NP role is expanding to allow the prescribing of opioids and the ordering of more diagnostic tests to address the needs of clients in rural, northern, and remote areas (Government of Ontario, 2017). See the previous discussion regarding the expansion of NP scope of practice, especially in Ontario.

SPECIALIZATION IN NURSING

The tremendous change in the nature and scope of nurses' practice in Canada in the past 40 years has been almost imperceptible, but this evolution has nonetheless had a profound effect on health care and society. It has become increasingly difficult for nurses to master the knowledge required for practice in every area in which nurses function. The rapid growth of knowledge in the health care field has led to specialization in just about every area of nursing,

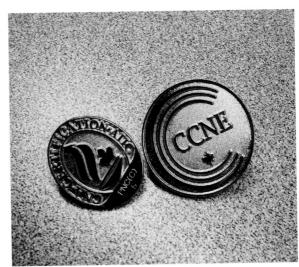

Certification pins from the Canadian Nurses Association and the Canadian Association of Schools of Nursing. (Courtesy Tammie R. McParland)

a change that has prompted questions about how to ensure the competence of those practising in specialized areas. The regulatory bodies for nursing require that nurses meet broad entry-to-practice competencies. As nurses practise, they become more knowledgeable in their particular area of practice—be it medical, surgical, maternal, pediatric, emergency, or critical care; rural or remote; and any other place a nurse works—and their generalized knowledge narrows.

The medical profession is highly specialized. The movement toward specialization in medicine has been strong and has, to a certain extent, influenced nursing. Although medicine has attempted to place greater value on the role of the general practitioner, more physicians are specializing. Given the tremendous growth in medical knowledge, this trend is not surprising. Nursing has also been influenced by tremendous knowledge growth in every area of practice, resulting in the development of discrete and increasingly complex nursing specialties.

The transfer of functions from medicine to nursing is also relevant. Many functions that were previously restricted exclusively to medical practice have been redefined as nursing responsibilities. Although this is primarily a task-oriented approach to practice in an area in which functions overlap, it is important because the changes in medical practice that produce the changes in nursing practice are immediately apparent. It is also important to recognize that (1) the transfer of functions among the health professions is an ongoing process and (2) there will always be an overlap of functions among professions. With increases in knowledge, skills, and functions, the nurse is in a pivotal position in the delivery of health care. The nurse of today assumes roles and functions that were expected of the general medical practitioner of yesterday. In fact, the general practitioner of yesterday might be overwhelmed at the complexity of the nursing roles of today. Three decades ago, there were five or six distinct areas of hospital- and community-based practice. Today, there are upward of 30 different clinical nursing areas, each requiring mastery of a unique and specialized knowledge base. Several of these require that nurses complete formal specialization processes before they can work in the specialty.

The trend toward specialization in the nursing profession is due to the increase in knowledge and the corresponding increase in skill needed for sound judgement and decision making. There is an almost constant demand for nurses who have expertise in highly specialized areas, so nurses must recognize their specialized skills and value the knowledge they require.

Recognition of Specialization

Specialized practice refers to a focus on a certain feature of nursing, be it age, health problem, medical diagnosis, environment of care, or type of care (CNA, 2019). Specialization has become an important phenomenon in nursing practice. Canadian nurses initially sought certification from programs in the United States to demonstrate knowledge in their areas of practice. At the 1980 Canadian Nurses Association Biennial Convention, the CNA Board of Directors passed a resolution to study the feasibility of developing certification examinations in major nursing specialties. Consideration of the issues involved led the CNA to develop a policy statement on credentialling in nursing and to make a commitment to facilitate the development of certification in nursing specialties (CNA, 1982).

Guidelines for a certification mechanism were adopted, and a certification program was designed (CNA, 1986a). The process involved designation of a specialty for certification, development of a certification examination by the Canadian Nurses Association Testing Services (CNATS), and certification of individuals. The CNA differentiated those acquiring certification in this manner from the clinical nurse specialist, who is designated as a nurse with advanced preparation in a clinical area at the master's level (CNA, 1986b).

The issues presented by specialization and certification seem to be those in which the national association is best suited to provide leadership. Since membership in specialty groups tends to be reasonably small, it is unlikely that the cost of developing a quality program could be borne by a province. Also, reciprocity would be an issue if different programs were developed in each province. Because specialization and certification are not part of basic preparation for practice (regulated by provincial or territorial legislation pursuant to the jurisdiction of provinces and territories as designated in the *Constitution Act*), development of programs at the national level appears to be the most appropriate and reasonable course of action.

The development of the CNA Advisory Council "to provide a forum for discussions between the Council and the CNA board of directors on health and nursing issues" (CNA, 1989b, p. 10) enabled special-interest groups to address the CNA. The approach to the certification process taken by the CNA is broad: "The designation process applies to an area of nursing rather than to a group or an association, and the process may be initiated by any group of nurses that is able to provide evidence that a specific nursing area meets the required criteria" (CNA, 1989b, p. 10).

In addition to national certification and specialization programs delivered by the CNA and CASN, there are several professional development programs throughout Canada that complement certification and specialization. These programs are delivered by educational institutions such as universities through their continuing education departments or are specific to working in a specialized area such as emergency or critical care. For example, professional development includes the certificates offered at the University of Toronto's Bloomberg School of Nursing (Certificate in Hospital & Acute Care for Nurse Practitioners, Certificate in Nursing Education for the Practice Setting) and several critical care nursing certificates at community colleges across Canada such as Humber, George Brown, Mohawk in Ontario, and BCIT in British Columbia. Examples of specific institutional certifications include such topics as PICC line care, defibrillation,

or specialty equipment use in the neonatal intensive care unit in the hospital.

 APPLYING CONTENT KNOWLEDGE

Discuss the advantages of the following to nurses who practise in specialty areas: one, the CNA or CASN certification mechanism, and two, specialty programs offered by Canadian universities at the master's level.

TABLE 21.2   Certification Programs in Nursing Specialties Offered by the Canadian Nurses Association

Name of Specialty	National Nursing Specialty Association	Designation	Program Established
Cardiovascular Nursing	Canadian Council of Cardiovascular Nurses	CCN(C)	2001
Community Health Nursing	Community Health Nurses Association of Canada	CCHN(C)	2006
Critical Care Nursing	Canadian Association of Critical Care Nurses	CNCC(C)	1995
Critical Care–Pediatric Nursing	Canadian Association of Critical Care Nurses	CNCCP(C)	2003
Emergency Nursing	National Emergency Nurses' Affiliation Inc.	ENC(C)	1994
Enterostomal Therapy Nursing (as of 2018, referred to as Nurses Specialized in Wound, Ostomy and Continence)	Nurses Specialized in Wound, Ostomy and Continence Care Canada	WOCC(C)	2008
Gastroenterology Nursing	Canadian Society of Gastroenterology Nurses and Associates	CGN(C)	2004*
Gerontology Nursing for RNs and NPs	Canadian Gerontological Nurses Association	GNC(C)	1999 for RNs
Gerontology Nursing for RPNs/LPNs	Canadian Gerontological Nurses Association	GPNC(C)	2019
Hospice Palliative Care Nursing	Canadian Hospice Palliative Care Association	CHPCN(C)	2004
Medical-Surgical Nursing	Canadian Association of Medical and Surgical Nurses	CMSN(C)	2009
Nephrology Nursing	Canadian Association of Nephrology Nurses and Technologists	CNeph(C)	1993
Neuroscience Nursing	Canadian Association of Neuroscience Nurses	CNN(C)	1991*
Occupational Health Nursing	Canadian Occupational Health Nurses Association	COHN(C)	1992
Oncology Nursing	Canadian Association of Nurses in Oncology	CON(C)	1997
Orthopedic Nursing	Canadian Orthopedic Nurses Association	ONC(C)	2006*
Perinatal Nursing	Association of Women's Health, Obstetric and Neonatal Nurses Canada	PNC(C)	2000
Pediatric	Canadian Association of Pediatric Nurses	CpedN(C)	2019
PeriAnesthesia	National Association of PeriAnesthesia Nurses of Canada	PANC(C)	2012*
Perioperative Nursing	Operating Room Nurses Association of Canada	CPN(C)	1995
Psychiatric/Mental Health Nursing	Canadian Federation of Mental Health Nurses	CPMHN(C)	1995
Rehabilitation Nursing	Canadian Association of Rehabilitation Nurses	CRN(C)	2006*

*Exam being retired in 2019, but nurses with existing certification can renew via continuous learning opportunities.
Source: Canadian Nurses Association. (2019). *CNA certification program.* Retrieved from https://www.cna-aiic.ca/en/certification.

TABLE 21.3   Certifications* Available From the Canadian Nurse Educator Institute (CNEI) of the Canadian Association of Schools of Nursing

Certification	Designation	Components
Canadian Certified Clinical Instructor	CCCI	6-week online course with final exam
Canadian Certified Nurse Educator	CCNE	3 × 6-week online modules with final exam plus professional portfolio
Canadian Certified Simulation Nurse Educator	CCSNE	4 × 6-week online modules with final exam

*The CNEI also provides continuing education, retreats, and webinars as part of their mission.
Source: Certified Nurse Educator Institute. (2019). *Certification programs.* Retrieved from http://cnei-icie.casn.ca/our-programs/certification-programs.

In 1981, the CNA agreed to develop a certification examination for the Canadian Council of Occupational Health Nurses, which had received a grant to develop this program. They hired the CNATS to create the examination. Consultation services for the development of the examination were offered "on the understanding they would join the CNA certification program when it became a reality" (CNA, 1989a, p. 7). However, the disappointing announcement was made that "following discussion and correspondence between CNA and the Canadian Council of Occupational Health Nurses Inc., the process of integrating the occupational health nursing examination into the CNA certification program has been suspended" because the occupational health nurses "would like more time to consider integration criteria, and [have] suggested waiting until at least 1991 to begin the process" (CNA, 1990, p. 14).

At that point, the CNA decided that groups that had been scheduled to enter the certification program after the Canadian Council of Occupational Health Nurses would be accommodated first (CNA, 1990). Thus, the first specialty groups to complete a certification program were nephrology nursing and neuroscience nursing. However, in March 1992, occupational health nursing was integrated into the CNA certification program, bringing the total number of specialty areas available for certification to three. Other specialty groups quickly followed suit, and by 2010 there were 19 such groups involved with and endorsing the CNA certification program. (See Table 21.2 for information about certification programs offered by the CNA.)

Meanwhile, demand for still other certification programs continued to grow, and the CNA recognized the need to expand the existing program. Based on recommendations of an ad hoc committee, the CNA Board of Directors reaffirmed its commitment to certification by adopting a plan for the accelerated expansion of the program. The expanded certification program offers certification to any specialty area with 10,000 or more nurses employed in that area in Canada, an approach that would provide the CNA

with enough financial support to continue expanding the program. The certification programs have grown exponentially; as of January 29, 2020, there were over 15,000 nurses certified across 23 nursing specialties (CNA, 2020). Effective November 2019, five speciality exams were retired by the CNA owing to sustainability issues, but nurses who hold this certification can renew every 5 years thorough continuous learning (CNA, 2019).

Although the development of its certification program has taken time and had its share of challenges, the CNA has successfully brought special-interest groups into the mainstream of professional association activities by establishing the process, developing an advisory council of representatives from specialty associations, and creating a position on the CNA Board of Directors for a representative from this group. The profession has been strengthened by these initiatives, and it is likely that such efforts will continue as more specialty groups become part of the certification program.

Canadian Association of Schools of Nursing and Certification for Nurse Educators

The CNA specialization focuses on practice specialities. In 2013, the CASN developed a Clinical Instructor course for nurse educators. From there, the CASN went on to create the Canadian Nurse Educator Institute (CNEI). The CNEI "contributes to the strength and growth of Canadian Nurse Educators through high-caliber professional development opportunities" (Canadian Association of Schools of Nursing, 2020). See Table 21.3 for the certifications available through the CASN and the components of each.

CONCLUSION

Nursing is a complex, comprehensive profession. As knowledge and complexity increase in health care, nurses are ideally placed to shape the benefits of such changes for the public. Because of the complexity of health care, and the role nurses play, basic entry-to-practice knowledge is not enough. Nurses will need to develop expertise wherever they work. Their scope of practice will adapt to address health care changes—policy will legitimize it, and the public will demand it. Whether or not nurses formalize the mastery of their specialization through a certification process, all nurses must develop expertise in their area of practice. It is a moral as well as professional imperative.

SUMMARY OF LEARNING OBJECTIVES

- While the terms registration, licensure, and credentialling are at times used interchangeably, they are in fact different mechanisms for creating accountability of professional nurses to the public through different requirements, such as education, final assessment, or specialized skills.
- Entry to practice for most registered nurses in Canada, except in Quebec, means the successful completion of a baccalaureate in nursing from an approved school of nursing. Program approval was nationally done by the CASN, but now each provincial/territorial regulatory body has taken over program approval. In several provinces, competencies set out by the regulatory body are required to meet entry-to-practice requirements.
- Entry to practice in Canada developed from an apprenticeship model, as nurses early in the twentieth century first followed the Nightingale model of nurse education. This model saw graduation as credentialling, to the point where nurse leaders wanted nurses licensed to differentiate between educated and uneducated practitioners.
- There are two credentialling types in nursing: professional and educational. Professional credentialling in Canada is accomplished through the successful completion of required education at the entry-to-practice level and successful passing of the licensure exam. Credentialling is undertaken by regulatory bodies in each province. Educational credentialling is concerned with the educational requirements to achieve the minimum entry-to-practice requirements, which in Canada (except Quebec) is a baccalaureate from a degree-granting institution (usually a university).
- Mandatory licensure in Canada came about as a result of the nursing profession's desire to be accountable to the public and to show that its members are well educated. Permissible licensure was present where practitioners did not have to pass any examinations but could still practice in the profession, so long as they did not use any protected title. The title "nurse" became protected in 1922 when Ontario was the last province to approve licensure. Permissive licensure no longer exists in nursing, as "nurse" is a protected title.
- Specialization refers to a focus on a certain feature of nursing, be it age, health problem, medical diagnosis, environment of care, or type of care. Specialization came about as the increasing complexity of care required by the public led to problems for nurses trying to maintain competence as general practitioners. It became apparent that nurses were generalists only when they first graduated; as they worked, nurses began to either formally or informally develop expertise in their area of practice. Specialization in nursing was driven at the national level and remains the focus of the CNA.
- There are several credentialling programs in Canada that allow nurses to specialize. The majority are developed and maintained by the CAN as a national recognition of expertise in a specific practice topic, practice area, or age. The CNA specialty designations have grown to 44 and focus mostly on practice or clinical specialties. The CASN also credentials specialization in nursing education with three certificate programs: Certified Canadian Clinical Instructor, Canadian Certified Nurse Educator, and Canadian Certified Simulation Nurse Educator. Several universities and colleges also offer education that may lead to the ability to become credentialed in a specific area.

CRITICAL THINKING QUESTIONS

1. How did early Canadian schools of nursing established by hospitals in the late nineteenth and early twentieth centuries differ from schools that followed the Nightingale model?
2. Describe the forces that drove the development of legislation to regulate nursing.
3. Describe the impact of specialization and certification on the profession of nursing today.
4. Describe the way in which nurse practitioner specialties are recognized. Does this differ from other specialties? If so, in what way?
5. What might be the implications for (i) the profession and (ii) the public of a decline in the number of successful passes of the NCLEX-RN test?

REFERENCES

British Columbia College of Nursing Professionals. (2018). *Becoming a nurse. Types of nurses.* Retrieved from https://www.bccnp.ca/becoming_a_nurse/Pages/Types_of_nurses.aspx.

Canadian Association of Schools of Nursing. (2020). *About CNEI.* Retrieved from http://cnei-icie.casn.ca/about/.

Canadian Nurses Association. (1968). *The leaf and the lamp: The Canadian Nurses' Association and the influences which shaped its origins and outlook during its first sixty years.* Ottawa, ON: Author. Retrieved from https://www.cna-aiic.ca/-/media/cna/page-content/pdf-fr/the_leaf_and_the_lamp_e.pdf.

Canadian Nurses Association. (1982). *Credentialling in nursing: Policy statement and background paper.* Ottawa, Canada: Author.

Canadian Nurses Association. (1986a). *CNA's certification program: An information booklet.* Ottawa, ON: Author.

Canadian Nurses Association. (1986b). *Statement on the clinical nurse specialist.* Ottawa, ON: Author.

Canadian Nurses Association. (1989a). Review of competencies and blueprint. *Canadian Nurse, 85*(1), 14.

Canadian Nurses Association. (1989b). Specialization stimulates debate. *Canadian Nurse, 85*(9), 10.

Canadian Nurses Association. (1990). Broad agenda highlights November board meeting. *Canadian Nurse, 86*(1), 14.

Canadian Nurses Association. (2019). *CNA certification programs.* Retrieved from https://www.cna-aiic.ca/en/certification.

Canadian Nurses Association. (2020). *Number of valid CNA certifications by specialty/area of nursing practice and province or territory.* Retrieved from https://www.cna-aiic.ca/-/media/cna/page-content/pdf-en/certification-statistics-2020-by-specialty-area-and-province_territory-en.pdf.

Canadian Nurses Association & Canadian Institute for Health Information. (2006). *The regulation and supply of nurse practitioners in Canada: 2006 update.* Retrieved from https://secure.cihi.ca/free_products/The_Nurse_Practitioner_Workforce_in_Canada_2006_Update_final.pdf.

College of Nurses of Ontario. (2019). *Legislation and regulation. RHPA: Scope of practice, controlled acts model.* Retrieved from http://www.cno.org/docs/policy/41052_RHPAscope.pdf.

Council of Ontario University Programs in Nursing. (2019). *Process of program approvals.* Retrieved from https://oucqa.ca/program-approvals-menu/program-approval-process/.

Fahmy, G. (2018, May 14). *Nurses association faces lawsuit over "atrocious" failure rate by francophones.* CBC News. Retrieved from https://www.cbc.ca/news/canada/new-brunswick/nursing-association-lawsuit-exam-francophones-1.4661749.

Goode, W. J. (1960). Encroachment, charlatanism, and the emerging professions: Psychology, sociology and medicine. *American Sociological Review, 25,* 903.

Government of Alberta. (2008). *Health Professions Act.* Retrieved from https://www.qp.alberta.ca/.

Government of Ontario. (2017, April 19). *Health bulletin: Ontario providing new prescribing authority for nurse practitioners.* Retrieved from http://www.health.gov.on.ca/en/news/bulletin/2017/hb_20170419.aspx.

Hastings, J. E. G. (1972). *Community health centres in Canada: Report of the Hastings Committee.* Ottawa, ON: Canadian Public Health Association.

National Council of State Boards of Nursing. (n.d.). *Test plans.* Retrieved from https://www.ncsbn.org/testplans.htm.

National Council of State Boards of Nursing. (2020). *NCLEX and other exams. NGN facts for educators.* Retrieved from https://www.ncsbn.org/11447.htm.

National Council of State Boards of Nursing. (2010a). *NCSBN Research Brief. Vol. 47. Report of Findings from the Comparison of Entry level Registered Nurses in the U.S. and Ontario, Canada.* Retrieved from https://www.ncsbn.org/10_Ontario_Vol47_web.pdf.

National Council of State Boards of Nursing. (2010b). *NCSBN Research Brief. Vol. 48. Report of Findings from the Comparison of Entry level Registered Nurses in the U.S. and British Columbia, Canada.* Retrieved from https://www.ncsbn.org/10_BC_Vol48_web.pdf.

Rajabally, M. H. (1982). Point of view: the entry to practice issue. We have seen the enemy. *Canadian Nurse, 78*(2.), 40–42.

Sabin, H., Price, D., & Sellers, B. (1973). Nursing: What it is and what it is not. In S. Good & J. C. Kerr (Eds.), *Contemporary issues in Canadian law for nurses* (pp. 63–82). Toronto, ON: Holt, Rinehart & Winston.

Styles, M. M., & Affara, F. A. (1997). *ICN on regulation: Towards 21st century models.* Geneva, Switzerland: International Council of Nurses.

Wilensky, H. L. (1964). The professionalization of everyone. *American Journal of Sociology, 70*(2), 143–144.

Yukon Registered Nurses Association. (2019). *Nursing practice—registration.* Retrieved from https://yukonnurses.ca/.

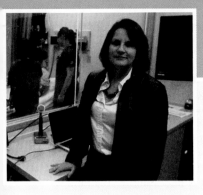

The Growth of Graduate Education in Nursing in Canada

Linda J. Patrick and Amanda E. McEwen

e http://evolve.elsevier.com/Canada/Ross-Kerr/nursing

LEARNING OBJECTIVES

After reading this chapter, you will be able to:
- Discuss the development and advancement of graduate nursing education in Canada.
- Explore variations in course and program delivery that facilitate student access to graduate education in nursing in Canada.
- Analyze enrollment trends in master's programs at Canadian nursing schools since the 1990s.

- Explain the process of developing faculty resources for graduate programs.
- Identify the challenges of sustaining graduate education in Canada.
- Appreciate the growth of doctoral programs in nursing at Canadian universities.
- Understand the need for postdoctoral programs to facilitate research development.

OUTLINE

KEY TERMS

advanced practice nursing
Doctor of Nursing
Doctor of Philosophy

Doctorate of Nursing Practice
nurse practitioner
tenure track

PERSONAL PERSPECTIVES

Rashad has just completed a Bachelor of Science degree in Honours Biology. He was recently accepted into a second-entry undergraduate nursing degree program with an expected completion date in 18 months. Rashad's career goal is to complete a master's degree in the **advanced practice nursing** stream with eligibility to write the nurse practitioner entry-to-practice exam. He is disappointed to learn that there is a minimum practice requirement for admission to the program. Rashad is seeking guidance and mentorship with his career goals and advice on options for employment in an advanced nursing practice role while he gains critical clinical experience.

Nurse practitioner programs build on undergraduate nursing education at the baccalaureate level. Programs in some provinces began as a postbaccalaureate certificate, but with the expansion of the scope of practice for nurse practitioners, it has become essential to move the education to a graduate degree with prior clinical experience. Clinical experience is essential to enhance the critical thinking required to make complex decisions and meet the competencies for safe practice.

INTRODUCTION

The development of graduate nursing education in Canada has achieved significant momentum in recent years, with improved access to both master's and doctoral programs. Improved access has been achieved not only through program growth at universities across Canada, but also through online and other innovative delivery approaches. The number of doctoral nursing programs in Canada has grown from only six in 1998 to 19 two decades later in 2018. Increased research activity in nursing has occurred as a result of a rapidly growing pool of nurses with preparation in research and the wider availability of funding for nursing research and interprofessional team investigations. This development goes hand in hand with, and is a necessary condition for, establishment of graduate education in nursing. Most of the research in any field takes place in university settings, and teaching research methods is an important facet of graduate education. Approval of new programs by universities is unlikely to occur without evidence of substantial research activity and the **Doctor of Philosophy** (PhD) as a standard qualification for faculty appointments.

A graduate degree in nursing is the educational preparation required to be an advanced practice nurse in Canada (Canadian Nurses Association [CNA], 2019). It is also essential that educational preparation is further combined with clinical experience and focused specialty expertise to practice. Universities offering master's-level education in nursing have grown significantly across Canada in recent decades. Access to graduate education in nursing has been further facilitated by the ability of students to access totally online degrees or programs with flexible delivery through a combination of online classes and short residency experiences on campus.

Graduate education is increasing in "the number and types of specialization streams" (Canadian Association of Schools of Nursing [CASN], 2015, p. 5). In response to this growth, the Canadian Association of Schools of Nursing (CASN) developed the National Nursing Education Framework to identify the fundamental expectations for all master's programs, "regardless of stream or specialization, as well as to clarify how a master's degree adds value and builds on baccalaureate education in nursing" (CASN, 2015, p. 5). While a master's degree may be the minimum requirement for admission to doctoral programs in nursing, individual schools have their own admission requirements for graduate study at both the master's and doctoral levels; therefore, anyone contemplating educational preparation beyond the baccalaureate in nursing should speak with an academic advisor.

THE ROOTS OF GRADUATE EDUCATION IN NURSING

Although the primary educational problems confronting the nursing profession in the 1940s and 1950s centred on issues of quality in baccalaureate and diploma nursing education, nurses recognized the critical need for nursing leaders who were prepared at the master's and doctoral levels. In her study of the needs and resources for graduate nursing education in Canada, Hart (1962) observed that

> *an increasing number of Canadian nurses recognized that graduate education was necessary to qualify for other specialized functions besides teaching. Canadian nurses had enrolled in programs leading to the master's degree to prepare for positions such as administration, supervision and consultation. Canadian nurses secured preparation for the specialized functions in nursing education as well as in nursing service in hospitals and health agencies. In spite of increasing demands for graduate education, by the time the study was undertaken there was still no provision for graduate study in nursing in Canada.* (p. 51)

Hart (1962) noted that the pursuit of graduate education often required study outside of Canada owing to limited opportunities geographically and a small number of program offerings. This was problematic given the increasing demand for nurses to have graduate preparation for leadership positions.

The Canadian Nurses Association (CNA) was in the forefront of developments and strongly supported the call for graduate programs in nursing. The CNA's Committee on Nursing Affairs (CNA, 1962) reported to the 31st Biennial Convention in 1962:

> We should promote immediately an assessment of present facilities, both university and clinical, in order to ascertain what is needed by way of the expansion of university nursing education . . . On the principle that one can never go wrong with an investment in human beings, a crash program for the development of qualified faculty for Canadian schools of nursing should be undertaken by CNA . . . CNA might also interest itself in giving some leadership to the development of graduate programs in nursing education, especially in terms of the pooling of university resources in particular specialties. (pp. 23–25)

The Committee on Nursing Education also made the following recommendations:

- Programs in nursing at the baccalaureate level should be expanded;
- The director of the school of nursing should be a nurse with preparation at a master's level with the necessary qualifications to assume the responsibility for administration of the school;
- All nurses responsible for teaching nursing students should have professional and academic preparation at least at the baccalaureate level and have demonstrated professional competence; and
- Programs should be developed at the master's and doctoral level to prepare nurses who will be qualified as nursing specialists and for administration, consultation, research, and teaching. (CNA, 1962, p. 46)

Thus, the focus of the profession was broadened to include graduate education as a necessary adjunct in the quest for quality in basic professional education. As was the case when baccalaureate programs were in their incipient stages, the first stage involved developing fellowship programs to prepare nurse faculty to take on the responsibilities associated with graduate education. Hart (1962) reported that in 1957

> a few unrestricted scholarships and fellowships were found to be available for graduate study in Canadian colleges and universities. Some scholarships were available specifically for nurses and other members of the health professions . . . If programs for graduate study

> were available in Canada, it is likely that students in the nursing field would utilize such scholarship and fellowship aid. (p. 47)

However, the W.K. Kellogg Foundation fellowship program, which spanned two decades, provided a much-needed source of funds for graduate students who had to incur the cost of taking up residence in a foreign country to find appropriate graduate-level educational opportunities (Table 22.1). In 1962, the Canadian Nurses Foundation (CNF) was formed with the assistance of a $136,639 grant from the W.K. Kellogg Foundation. The grant helped to establish a fellowship program for nurses to study at the master's and doctoral levels and work as research assistants. The grant has completed its first mandate admirably. Between 1962 and 2002, a total of 755 graduate fellowships were awarded, 494 for study at the master's level and 261 for doctoral work. The total amount given for fellowship awards over this 40-year period of the fund was $3,004,109.

It is noteworthy that the CNF has been actively fundraising and that provincial and territorial professional associations have been regular and substantial donors. In addition, many individuals, institutions, and businesses have contributed funds. However, owing to problems in maintaining the size of the fund in the first decade of its existence, the Research Committee of the CNF "formulated plans for developing nursing research in Canada but unfortunately, due to lack of funds, these could not be implemented" (Imai, 1971, p. 90). The CNF later initiated a program of research grants. The first such grant was one given to the Canadian Association of University Schools of Nursing for a research project on accreditation of university schools of nursing. With the establishment of the Ad Hoc Research Committee in 1983, the CNF Board of Directors initiated a program of research grants, which, although small, has been important in encouraging nurses to undertake research. As of 2019, the CNF has awarded nearly $15 million in scholarships and research grants, and opportunities for funding continue to grow. Annually, a total of $275,000 is awarded to both nurses and nursing students across Canada (Canadian Nurses Foundation, 2019).

THE ESTABLISHMENT OF MASTER'S PROGRAMS IN NURSING

The efforts of the University of Western Ontario to develop a 1-year diploma program in nursing service administration led to the establishment of a master's program in that area, one that became the first graduate program in nursing in Canada (Overduin, 1970). In 1957, the president of the university, Dr. G.E. Hall, applied for W.K. Kellogg funding

TABLE 22.1   W.K. Kellogg Foundation Grants to Canadian University Schools of Nursing and Selected Other Agencies, 1940–1981

Organization	Type of Grant	Date	Grant Amount
Alberta			
University of Alberta	Fellowships in nursing	1949–1954	$10,862
British Columbia			
The University of British Columbia	To help establish nursing education curricula leading to RN licensure and baccalaureate, master's, and doctoral degrees		$333,225
	Fellowships in nursing	1974–1977	$18,032
Vancouver Metropolitan Health Department	Fellowships in nursing	1946	$675
Manitoba			
University of Manitoba	Fellowships in nursing	1941–1949	$2,815
New Brunswick			
New Brunswick Association for Registered Nurses	Fellowships in nursing	1953	$715
University of New Brunswick	To help establish a degree program in basic nursing	1958–1965	$198,857
	To help establish a program of continuing education in nursing	1958–1961	$17,504
Ontario			
Canadian Nurses Association (for Province of Ontario)	Fellowships in nursing	1950	$1,493
McMaster University	Fellowships in nursing	1948–1954	$19,787
	To help establish a graduate education curriculum in nursing	1973–1978	$290,935
Quebec			
McGill University	To develop a master's degree program for non-nurse graduates	1981	$86,279

Sources: W. K. Kellogg Foundation. (1966). *Annual report.* Battle Creek, MI: Author; W. K. Kellogg Foundation. (1970). *Annual report.* Battle Creek, MI: Author; W. K. Kellogg Foundation. (1971). *Annual report.* Battle Creek, MI: Author; W. K. Kellogg Foundation. (1974). *Annual report.* Battle Creek, MI: Author; W. K. Kellogg Foundation. (1975). *Annual report.* Battle Creek, MI: Author.

to implement the diploma program, which had received the approval of the university senate as early as 1956:

> [He] requested $100,000 from the Foundation . . . $50,000 of which was slated for the "intensive development" of the new DNSA program—the Foundation indicated its willingness to support the school of nursing in its educational efforts in nursing administration. It supported the development of a master's program in Canada, to be supported by the Foundation over a five-year period just as it had done earlier in American universities. (Overduin, 1970, p. 84)

A brief was prepared and submitted to the W.K. Kellogg Foundation:

> [It] showed that Western met all the requirements set by the Foundation, described in detail the programs and courses offered by the school of nursing, and a

> projected budget for a five-year period indicating the cost of five major areas which would be supported by the Foundation: the master's program, and project of case-writing in administration, two fellowships per year to be granted during each year of the grant—each fellow to receive $2000 per year for each year of her two-year program, an annual seminar for senior nursing executives, and continuing education for faculty. (Overduin, 1970, p. 84)

Although $142,000 was said to have been awarded by the foundation for the establishment of this program (Overduin, 1970; University of Western Ontario School of Nursing, 1967), Kellogg records indicate that $128,618 was in fact expended between 1959 and 1965 "to help establish a program of graduate education in nursing service administration" (W.K. Kellogg Foundation, as cited in Kerr, 1978, p. 261) (see Table 22.1). Planning for the implementation of the new program began in March 1959, and "on October 30, 1959, the Senate approved the first year of the program, and the entrance requirements" (Overduin, 1970, p. 85). Of note was the recognition that "the great need for research, especially research in appraising nursing care and service, was instrumental in the decision that a student would be required to produce a thesis" (Overduin, 1970, p. 85).

At McGill University, much progress had occurred since 1944, when the baccalaureate degree program was established. The transition to the integrated program occurred in 1957. However, planning for a master's program began even earlier:

> Research in nursing at McGill had been urged in Miss Green's report of 1953. The following year students in the second-year degree programme undertook small research projects under the direction of staff members. Miss Chittick began to press for the creation of a Master's programme in nursing at the School for Graduate Nurses. (Tunis, 1966, p. 11)

After a resolution was passed at the 1958 CNA convention expressing the need for opportunities for graduate study in nursing at Canadian universities, "at McGill a two-year program leading to a degree of MSc (Applied) was drawn up for approval by the Faculty of Graduate Studies and Research" (Tunis, 1966, p. 112). Senate approval, in principle, was received in September 1959, and again the W.K. Kellogg Foundation provided financial support through a grant of $195,000 over 5 years to make the program plans operational (Tunis, 1966). This brought the total amount of W.K. Kellogg Foundation assistance received by McGill for the development of curricula to $221,252 between 1946 and 1967. Once again in the vanguard of developments in university nursing education in Canada, the W.K. Kellogg Foundation expressed its rationale for the assistance: "Graduate programs in Canadian universities are greatly needed. Better teachers of nursing produce better practitioners and, hence, improve patient care" (W. K. Kellogg Foundation, 1966, p. 56).

Considerable time lapsed following the early activity to establish master's programs at Western and McGill. However, program demonstrations made possible by the grants from the W.K. Kellogg Foundation had already begun, and it was up to the institutions to obtain their own resources if they wished to initiate graduate programs in nursing. Given the historical reluctance of universities to approve the development of new and costly graduate programs requiring ongoing and increasing operating expenditures, it is not surprising, particularly in the absence of financial inducements, that 5 years passed before another program was established. In 1966, a graduate program was initiated at the Université de Montréal, the first

French-language master's program in the world, and in 1968 a program was developed at The University of British Columbia (Good, 1971).

The W.K. Kellogg Foundation again offered support for the development of master's programs with an award of $178,000 to the Faculty of Nursing at the University of Toronto "to establish a graduate program to prepare clinical nurse specialists" (W. K. Kellogg Foundation, 1971, p. 28). In her annual report to the president, Dean Helen Carpenter (1970) describes the nature of the program in its first year of operation:

> The Master's Degree programme embodies specialization, mastery in depth of a specific area of knowledge, independent and critical study, and research. The purposes of the course are to make available advanced preparation for leadership roles in selected areas of nursing, and to advance nursing knowledge and skills through analytical study and investigation. Opportunity is provided for the students to acquire knowledge from nursing and the related sciences to provide the rationale for the management of complex health problems. (p. 74)

Another indication of the interest in developing innovative nursing curricula in Canada was W.K. Kellogg Foundation support, granted in 1973 for a 5-year period, to the School of Nursing at McMaster University for an "interdisciplinary graduate program to prepare clinical nurse specialists in primary and ambulatory care" (W. K. Kellogg Foundation, 1975, p. 19). This program award was in the amount of $290,196. An excerpt from the foundation's annual report (W. K. Kellogg Foundation, 1974) discusses the nature of this unique program:

> Foundation funds are helping the Division of Health Sciences of McMaster University, Hamilton, Ontario, develop an interdisciplinary graduate program to prepare nurses for advanced clinical practice in primary and ambulatory care. Students may choose clinical practice in maternal child health, family practice, or rehabilitation. Every attempt is made to include a true interdisciplinary experience, with members of several health professions learning together about issues in the delivery and management of health care. Nursing students will work with a physician preceptor during their clinical experience. The physician preceptor will also work with medical residents and will relate to both groups toward effective interdisciplinary clinical practice. (pp. 10–11)

Although the master's program at the University of Alberta, established in 1975, did not receive external funding, it derived substantial benefit from the development of the Master of Health Services Administration program in 1968.

This program was initiated under the auspices of the Western Canadian Council on Education of Health Personnel with the help of a W.K. Kellogg Foundation grant of $212,250 for a 5-year period (W. K. Kellogg Foundation, 1970). This program incorporated a stream for nursing administrators, paving the way for the 1975 development of the Master of Nursing program by providing for a joint appointment between the Division of Health Services Administration and the Faculty of Nursing and by developing a program with a strong research component. Both developments were assets to the Faculty of Nursing and facilitated the development of its master's program in 1975.

The University of British Columbia's first master's program was initiated without any external funding. However, 5 years later, a large W.K. Kellogg Foundation grant was awarded to the School of Nursing "to aid in establishing nursing education curricula leading to registered nurse licensure, baccalaureate, master's and doctoral degrees" (W.K. Kellogg Foundation; cited in Kerr, 1978, p. 259). Although the basic elements of such a ladder-system approach were developed before the termination of the grant in 1977, the doctoral part of the program was not established during the 5-year time frame. Noteworthy, too, is the fact that The University of British Columbia dropped the ladder concept before the end of the decade to concentrate on its basic baccalaureate, post-basic registered nurse (RN) baccalaureate and master's programs. Another development in the availability of master's programs was the establishment of the first program in the Atlantic Provinces at Dalhousie University in 1975.

Documentation of the W.K. Kellogg Foundation's annual expenditures between 1959 and 1982 paints a clear picture of how the foundation supported the first phase of development of graduate nursing education in Canada (see Table 22.1). The funds, which were awarded to the CNA for the establishment of the CNF and were also included as CNF awards for graduate study, were a critical factor in the development of the faculty resources needed to offer graduate nursing programs in Canada.

EXPANSION OF MASTER'S PROGRAMS IN NURSING

Since the first master's programs in nursing were developed at the University of Western Ontario in 1959 and at McGill University in 1961, master's offerings in Canada have expanded considerably (Table 22.2). The first programs offering study in clinical content areas were developed, beginning with the program at the Université de Montréal in 1966. The number and the focus of master's programs in nursing has also grown significantly since 2006. According to the 2017–2018 report *Registered Nurses*

TABLE 22.2 Establishment of Master's Degree Programs in Nursing	
Institution	**Date Program Established**
Faculty of Nursing, University of Western Ontario	1959
School of Nursing, McGill University	1961
Faculté des sciences infirmières, Université de Montréal	1966
School of Nursing, The University of British Columbia	1968
Faculty of Nursing, University of Toronto	1975
Faculty of Nursing, University of Alberta	1975
School of Nursing, Dalhousie University	1975
Faculty of Nursing, University of Manitoba	1979
Faculty of Nursing, University of Calgary	1981
School of Nursing, Memorial University of Newfoundland	1982
College of Nursing, University of Saskatchewan	1986
École des sciences infirmières, Université Laval	1991
School of Nursing, University of Ottawa	1993
School of Nursing, Queen's University	1994
School of Nursing, University of Windsor	1994
School of Nursing, McMaster University	1994
Faculty of Nursing, University of New Brunswick	1995
École des sciences infirmières, Université de Moncton	1998
Centre for Nursing and Health Studies, Athabasca University	2000
School of Nursing, Laurentian University	2003
Faculty of Health, York University	2004
Faculty of Community Services, Ryerson University	2004
Faculté de médecine et des sciences de la santé, Université de Sherbrooke	2005
Université du Québec à Chicoutimi, Outaouais, Rimouski et Trois-Rivières	2006

Note: As of 2020, graduate programs were not available in Nunavut, the Northwest Territories, or Yukon.

Education in Canada Statistics (CASN, 2019), 33% of schools (32 of 97 schools surveyed) offered one or more master's programs. During this same time period, **nurse practitioner** (NP) programs were offered by 28 schools nationally at three educational levels (post-RN, master's, and post-master's). Note that these statistics do not include interdisciplinary programs in which nursing may be one of several disciplines that offer a master's degree program. Such programs have existed for some time and include the University of Alberta's Master of Health Services Administration program and McMaster University's interdisciplinary Master of Health Sciences program.

🌐 CULTURAL CONSIDERATIONS

Truth and Reconciliation Commission of Canada's Calls to Action: Graduate Nursing Education

At a council meeting of the CASN (2017), a motion was adopted to formally respond to the Truth and Reconciliation Commission of Canada's (TRC) Calls to Action (2015) in partnership with the Canadian Nursing Students' Association and the Canadian Indigenous Nurses Association (CASN, 2018). Call to Action 24 specifically pertains to graduate education in nursing by requiring a course on Indigenous health issues. Graduate programs nationally will need to prioritize the inclusion of skills-based training in "intercultural competency, conflict resolution, human rights and anti-racism (Truth and Reconciliation Commission of Canada, 2015, p. 3). Universities are at different stages of development of graduate courses to meet the TRC recommendations with further information available on school websites.

Source: Canadian Association of Schools of Nursing. (2018). Minutes. *CASN Council meeting.* Retrieved from https://www.casn.ca/wp-content/uploads/2018/11/COUNCIL-Minutes-Nov-2017_FINAL-DRAFT-EN.pdf; Truth and Reconciliation Commission of Canada. (2015). *Truth and Reconciliation Commission of Canada: Calls to Action.* Winnipeg, MB: Author. Retrieved from http://trc.ca/assets/pdf/Calls_to_Action_English2.pdf.

ANALYSIS OF ENROLLMENT TRENDS IN MASTER'S PROGRAMS

Enrollment in master's programs has changed dramatically over the years. In 1959, the total enrollment at the University of Western Ontario was only two students (Overduin, 1970); in the 1960–1961 academic year, the combined enrollment at Western and McGill was 16 students. Over the next 5 years, total enrollment grew by 56%. In the next 5-year interval, three more programs were established, increasing the total enrollment to 675 students. During this time, programs that offered study in a clinical area were developed, beginning with the program at the Université de Montréal in 1966. An analysis of early trends in the development of graduate education in nursing prompted one author to speculate on the reasons why Canadian nurses were still travelling to the United States for graduate study instead of enrolling in the new Canadian programs. The reasons included historical precedent, more and better-qualified nurse faculty, and greater variety in programming. At that time, US universities offered advanced study in five to eight clinical content areas, as well as in the functional specialties, whereas only one Canadian master's program offered study in a clinical content area; the majority offered functional specialization (Good, 1969, p. 7).

Also interesting are enrollment trends since 1965. Erratic changes characterize the first 5-year period after 1965, probably because of the smaller aggregate numbers on which the calculations are based and because of the beginnings of retrenchment, as growth was replaced by shortfalls in enrollments nationally. The academic year 1969–1970, when four programs were operational, was the only one of the decade in which there was a decrease in enrollment over the previous year. The next academic year saw a 35% increase, and a 26% increase occurred in 1971–1972. In the period between 1970 and 1976, three more new master's programs were initiated, and total enrollment grew by 47%. For the academic years from 1971 through 1975, enrollment increases were lower, ranging from 3% to 8%, representing a slow but steady increase in student numbers and increased access to programs made possible by the addition of two programs after 1969–1970. In 1975–1976, there was a larger overall increase—about 13%—in the total enrollment figures. The new programs accounted for the larger percent increase. Exponential increases occurred over the next decade with the addition of new programs and increases in the size of existing ones. By 1993, total enrollment in master's programs had reached 904 students, and by 1999–2000 there were 1,491 students enrolled in master's programs in Canada. Demand was apparent, as more students applied for admission than could be accommodated in programs.

NURSE PRACTITIONER EDUCATION IN CANADA

Many master's programs in nursing also include an NP option that prepares graduates to perform advanced medical care. Athabasca University was one of the first to offer this option. Their program began as an Advanced Graduate Diploma in 1996 and evolved into the Master of Nursing program with an NP option in 2002. Ontario has taken the unique approach of offering postbaccalaureate education for nurses seeking entry to practice as NPs. The Ontario Ministry of Health and Long-Term Care tasked the Council of Ontario University Programs in Nursing with developing an accessible NP program following a 1994 report that documented how NPs were being used in Ontario (Mitchell, Pinelli, Patterson, & Southwell, 1993). The findings of the report led to the creation of the Ontario Primary Health Care Nurse Practitioner (PHCNP) program in 1995, a consortium of Ontario universities that offer programs in both English and French. The master's-level NP program can be taken either in conjunction with a larger master's in nursing or as a post-master's certificate. In 2019, nine universities were a part of the PHCNP Consortium with an annual enrollment of 200 students. The University of Toronto offers NP programs with an adult, pediatric, or global health focus.

The College of Nurses of Ontario (2017, 2020) reported that the number of RNs working in Ontario in the extended class is 3,938, up from the 938 RNs reported in 2008. According to the Canadian Institute for Health Information (2020), the total number of NPs in Canada is 6,159, with the highest rate of growth occurring between 2017 and 2018.

ISSUES IMPACTING NURSE PRACTITIONER EDUCATION IN CANADA

Insufficient access to primary care in many provinces is influencing investment in NP growth. Increased employment opportunities for NPs will drive student enrollments at universities across Canada wherever NP programs are offered. This will require schools of nursing to seek additional faculty, preceptors, and clinical placements to support the influx of students. The media in New Brunswick (Fraser, 2017) drew attention to a reported 20,000 residents who were without a health care provider, identifying that a barrier to care was that NPs were not able to access payment through direct funding. This is a contentious issue, as NPs earn an average salary of about $88,999 (PayScale, Inc., 2019). In British Columbia, inadequate access to primary care providers led the province to create a team-based system of care that will fund 200 new NP positions (British Columbia Ministry of Health, 2018). Similar investment in NPs is occurring across the country as provincial governments grapple with providing efficient access to primary care in response to hallway medicine and the aging demographic. In 2019, the Quebec government announced its goal of reaching 2,000 NPs by 2024, but as of 2019 growth was falling behind with only 600 NPs practicing (La Presse Canadienne, 2019).

> ### 👤 APPLYING CONTENT KNOWLEDGE
>
> The majority of nurses working as NPs are paid a salary with benefits. Considering the growth of the number of NPs working independently with an autonomous scope of practice, what method of payment would most benefit the profession and/or patients?

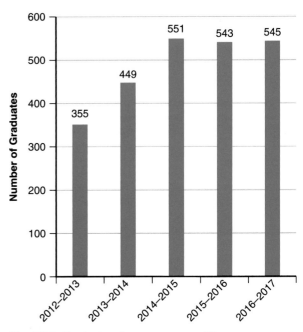

Fig. 22.1 Graduates from nurse practitioner programs, 2013–2017. (**Source:** National Student and Faculty Survey of Canadian Schools of Nursing)

The Canadian Association of Schools of Nursing (CASN) national survey reported that NP programs are offered in all provinces and territories except the Northwest Territories, Nunavut, and Yukon. National statistics indicated that 1,764 students were enrolled in NP programs and 564 students graduated in 2017 (CASN, 2019) (Figure 22.1).

ANALYSIS OF ENROLLMENT TRENDS IN DOCTORAL PROGRAMS

With the establishment of the first doctoral program in nursing at the University of Alberta on January 1, 1991, followed in September 1991 by the implementation of a second program at The University of British Columbia, nursing students no longer had to study in other disciplines or be admitted as special-case doctoral students in nursing. Programs at the University of Toronto and a joint program between McGill University and the Université de Montréal were initiated in the fall of 1993, and a fifth program commenced at McMaster University in September 1994. The University of Calgary initiated a doctoral program in nursing in 1999, and Dalhousie University planned to begin a program in 2003.

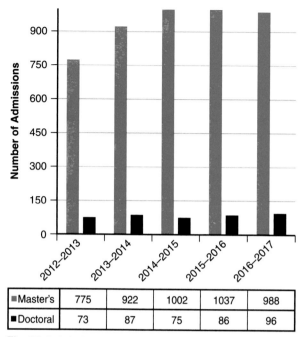

	2012–2013	2013–2014	2014–2015	2015–2016	2016–2017
Master's	775	922	1002	1037	988
Doctoral	73	87	75	86	96

Fig. 22.2 Admissions to master's and doctoral programs, 2012–2013 to 2016–2017. (**Source:** National Student and Faculty Survey of Canadian Schools of Nursing)

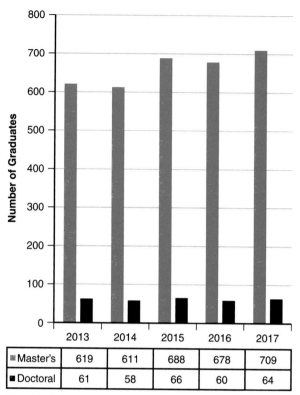

	2013	2014	2015	2016	2017
Master's	619	611	688	678	709
Doctoral	61	58	66	60	64

Fig. 22.3 Graduates from master's and doctoral programs, 2013–2017. (**Source:** National Student and Faculty Survey of Canadian Schools of Nursing)

As doctoral programs have become established, enrollments have climbed. The first students in doctoral programs in nursing enrolled between 1976 and 1988, and by 2000 enrollment across the country had reached 151. Enrollment in doctoral programs more than doubled from 2000 to 2005, and grew about 1.5 times from 2005 to 2017 (Figures 22.2 and 22.3).

The number of PhD programs across Canada has grown substantially over the past decade. Yet even with so many programs, they far from being able to meet the need for faculty members across the country and the need to strengthen the research base in nursing. According to the 2017–2018 report *Registered Nurses Education in Canada Statistics* (CASN, 2019), admissions to graduate programs for both master's and doctoral degrees have increased, but gains in graduates are relatively small compared with the number of faculty retiring. An increased number of nursing programs and ongoing retirements are creating a shortage of qualified faculty. The CASN report also indicated a 2.0% vacancy rate, with schools unable to fill 46 full-time faculty positions in 2016–2017 (CASN, 2019). This situation will escalate quickly, with 21.4% of permanent RN faculty eligible to retire and others choosing to retire early (2.3%) (CASN, 2019).

APPLYING CONTENT KNOWLEDGE

What would the outcome be for nursing if graduate education were not available in nursing and nurses continued to switch to other disciplines (education, sociology, etc.), as they did in the past, for advanced degrees?

DEVELOPING THE FACULTY RESOURCES FOR GRADUATE PROGRAMS

The element that constitutes the most essential resource in successfully operating a graduate program is its faculty. Securing faculty members with the requisite skills to offer quality graduate nursing programs is the most critical and difficult task. This was recognized earlier by Kathleen Russell (cited in Carpenter, 1970) as she laid the foundations of the basic baccalaureate degree program at the University of Toronto:

> Among the criteria established for faculty positions were: the capacity for independent and creative thought and critical analysis, a broad concept of nursing, a university degree representing sound, general education in the humanities, and preparation for teaching. As nurses with these qualifications were difficult to find, fellowships were secured to assist those selected to undertake additional study and to broaden their understanding of nursing through travel and observation in other countries. (p. 93)

Although skills such as creative thinking and critical analysis—complemented by research skills and a broad knowledge of nursing—can be learned in settings other than the formal university environment, Stinson (1977) observed that when it came to the development of research skills, "One must consider the point that a great deal about research can be learned from participating in increasingly more complex projects" (p. 29). However, she also noted that "it is only in the rare instance that sound research preparation and high research productivity can occur in the absence of substantial amounts and kinds of formalized instruction" (Stinson, 1977, p. 29).

University nursing administrators have experienced difficulty in securing suitably qualified teaching faculty for university programs. This was a major concern during the formative years of baccalaureate programs, and there were times when schools were forced to operate with fewer staff than was desirable because of unfilled faculty positions. Supply and demand questions aside, there is still the leadership connection—that is, whether administrators of university schools were sufficiently perceptive and aggressive in recognizing the necessary skills and in encouraging the development of such skills in faculty members who showed promise.

Fellowship programs for faculty development have been available since the 1920s. In the early years, these were, for the most part, under the sponsorship of private foundations and earmarked for faculty development. Fellowships were also often awarded directly to the institutions to offer to suitable candidates. However, in the late 1950s, public funds became available from federal sources administered through the provinces. With the establishment of the CNF, fellowship funds for graduate study also became available from that source. Although they have been used primarily for faculty development, the new funds were not specifically earmarked for this purpose and have also been directed to graduate preparation of nurses for practice, educational, and administrative settings.

The dearth of graduate-prepared faculty prompted Good (1969) to conclude that "the void in qualified nurse faculty in Canada has deterred development of Canadian graduate nurse education, and subsequent nursing research" (p. 8). In 1960–1961, shortly after master's programs in nursing were first initiated, 58% of teaching faculty in university schools of nursing held baccalaureate degrees and 38% held master's degrees, a level of preparation that Mussallem (1965) considered inadequate:

> Although the academic qualifications of faculty in university schools of nursing are higher than those for hospital schools, it should be recognized that university instructors are teaching at the baccalaureate level and their preparation should be beyond that of their students. (p. 84)

The situation changed slowly during the next decade as more master's programs became available; by 1970–1971, 1.43% of faculty in university programs held doctoral degrees, 44% held master's degrees, and 49% held baccalaureate degrees. In the 5-year period ending in 1975–1976, there was evidence of additional progress, as 3.74% of faculty held doctoral degrees, 31.28% held master's degrees, and 58.02% held baccalaureate degrees (Statistics Canada, 1976).

In 1980, Larsen and Stinson (1980) conducted a national survey to determine how many nurses held doctoral degrees. Of the 81 nurses qualified at the doctoral level, 69% were employed by universities. By 1989, 257 nurses held doctoral degrees, and of these, 79% were employed by universities (Lamb & Stinson, 1990, p. 9). By 2000, the majority of faculty teaching in graduate nursing programs held doctoral degrees, a trend that has continued into 2020. There are many more faculty who hold doctoral degrees in nursing, coinciding with the growth of doctoral programs in nursing across Canada.

PREPARATION TO ESTABLISH DOCTORAL PROGRAMS IN NURSING

In 1975, at the Fourth National Nursing Research Conference held in Edmonton, Alberta, a group of participants interested in facilitating the establishment of doctoral programs in the country held an informal meeting to discuss how this might be accomplished. Other discussions were held at national nursing meetings, and in 1976, a resolution was passed at the CNA Biennial Convention directing the association to provide leadership in the quest to establish doctoral education in Canada. Through a joint initiative of the CNA, CNF, and Canadian Association of University Schools of Nursing, a national seminar on doctoral education in nursing was convened in 1978. The W.K.

Kellogg Foundation funded the seminar, which brought together the deans and directors of university schools of nursing and the deans of graduate studies at those same institutions to begin planning the establishment of doctoral education in Canada. The meeting produced a commitment to establish at least one PhD program in nursing (Zilm, Larose, & Stinson, 1979). This was the first public recognition of the need to develop doctoral programs in nursing in this country. As was the case when access to baccalaureate and later master's programs was limited, Canadian nurses emigrated to the United States to take advantage of the doctoral educational programs there. Some never returned to Canada, as they were offered attractive positions in the United States.

Another federal initiative, this one led by the Medical Research Council of Canada (MRC), resulted in the establishment of the Working Group on Nursing Research in 1982. This group came about thanks to the CNA's efforts to document how very little nursing research was being funded by the national granting councils. As the smallest funding body, the National Health Research and Development Program (NHRDP) provided limited funding, and the funds that were available were not specifically earmarked for nursing. In addition, many other disciplines depended on the NHRDP for the majority of their funding. Although both the MRC and the Social Sciences and Humanities Research Council of Canada (SSHRC) stated that nursing was included among the disciplines that could be funded, nurses had difficulty getting either council to review their nursing proposals. Consequently, few nursing proposals were funded by either research funding body. In 1985, in response to these funding problems, the Working Group issued a report recommending, among other things, that funding bodies assist with creating opportunities to establish doctoral nursing programs. Also addressed was the need to designate nursing research for funding within the MRC (1985).

A special initiative to develop nursing research was jointly established in 1988 by the MRC and NHRDP using the model developed for medicine and science, in which career funding is provided to outstanding candidates with proven track records. These funded scientists are then expected to develop others within their research programs. Unfortunately, there were too few outstanding candidates who could be funded under this system; in many of the smaller universities, there were none. Nursing faculty members, apart from a few unique individuals, had not developed the necessary track records to qualify. There are many reasons that nursing faculty found themselves in this situation, including heavy teaching loads, lack of access to research funding, and an emphasis on service and teaching within faculties across the country. The first round of this joint program funded six nursing faculty from across the country. Members of the nursing profession were outraged at this outcome, believing that the limited funding was merely a token effort toward increasing the development of research capacity in nursing.

A second round of this competition was held in 1989, but the result was even more meagre than the first, with only three institutions receiving funding. The NHRDP–MRC program was then suspended for an evaluation, which took nearly 3 years to complete. After reviewing the results, the MRC and NHRDP decided to hold one final competition. According to members of the review committee, this last round received significantly better proposals than previous rounds did. It appears that the funding of those first nurse scientists and scholars had launched a new era of nursing research in Canada. Looking back from the vantage point of 2020, this effort by the major funding agencies to build research capacity in nursing proved to be successful.

The MRC spent many years struggling to broaden its mandate to include health research, which it finally did in 1994. The exclusive focus of the MRC on biomedical research had excluded many disciplines conducting health research, including nursing. Nursing research was clearly included as being eligible for funding under this broadened mandate. This new mandate followed by the transformation of the MRC into the Canadian Institutes of Health Research in 2000 completely changed the picture for nursing research in Canada (see Chapter 8 for details).

Today, the prospects for nursing research are vastly different than they were 30 years ago. Although nursing competes on a level field with other disciplines for funds, it is often difficult to secure grants for a single project. There is now greater emphasis on funding interdisciplinary teams of researchers who have varied experiences, education, specialties, and skill sets, and nurses have proven themselves to be highly valued members of these research teams.

THE ESTABLISHMENT OF DOCTORAL PROGRAMS IN NURSING

After the Kellogg National Seminar in 1978, McGill University and the Université de Montréal prepared a joint submission for a cooperative bilingual PhD program but it failed to receive approval when it was first proposed in 1980 (it would be approved over a decade later; see later in this section).

The University of Toronto Faculty of Nursing developed an arrangement with the university's Institute of Medical Science whereby nurses could be admitted to the PhD program offered by that unit to pursue doctoral studies in nursing. This arrangement included some Faculty of Nursing input into the program and allowed nurses to enroll in a doctoral program that was more closely related to their own discipline.

TABLE 22.3 Historical Overview of the First Doctoral Programs in Nursing in Canada		
Institution	Date First Students Accepted	Preceded by a Special Case Arrangement
Faculty of Nursing, University of Alberta	January 1, 1991	Yes
School of Nursing, Faculty of Applied Sciences, The University of British Columbia	September 1, 1991	No
Faculty of Nursing, University of Toronto*	September 1, 1993	No
School of Nursing, Faculty of Medicine, McGill University/Faculté des sciences infirmières, Université de Montréal	September 1, 1993	Yes
School of Nursing, Faculty of Health Sciences, McMaster University	September 1, 1994	No
Faculty of Nursing, University of Calgary	September 1, 1998	No

*The Faculty of Nursing at the University of Toronto had some involvement in a doctoral program established at the Institute of Medical Science. Prior to the establishment of their own nursing program, a number of University of Toronto nurses enrolled in and graduated from the institute's program.

In 1980, the Council of the Faculty of Nursing at the University of Alberta approved the development of a proposal for a PhD program. Once the proposal was developed and approved by the council in 1985, it received approval from the university's Board of Governors in 1986. The program was funded by the Alberta government on January 1, 1991, allowing students to be admitted to the first PhD program in nursing in Canada (Table 22.3).

A second doctoral program in nursing was implemented shortly thereafter at The University of British Columbia in September 1991. Two additional programs began in the fall of 1993: a PhD program at the University of Toronto and a joint PhD program at McGill University and the Université de Montréal. In the fall of 1994, a fifth PhD program got underway at McMaster University, and in 1998 a PhD program was implemented at the University of Calgary. Dalhousie University began a doctoral program in 2003, which brought the total number of PhD programs in nursing to seven.

In the late 1990s, prior to the funding of bona fide PhD programs, a number of special-case students were admitted to McGill University and the University of Alberta. The first graduate to receive a PhD in nursing from a Canadian university was a special-case student, Francine Ducharme, who graduated from McGill University in the fall of 1990.

In the early 2000s, the School of Nursing at the University of Victoria offered a "PhD by special arrangement," an individualized PhD program of studies similar to the special-case arrangements developed at other universities, including McGill and Alberta, prior to the establishment of their PhD programs (University of Victoria School of Nursing, 1995). This program has now been implemented by the University of Victoria as a PhD in nursing program.

Doctoral education has become much more accessible to nurses in Canada since the inception of the first program at the University of Alberta in 1991. Research in nursing is likely to continue to grow with the preparation of doctoral candidates who have expertise in research. The purpose of doctoral education is to prepare scholars and scientists who will develop knowledge for their discipline. In nursing, this knowledge provides the basis for practice and is therefore inextricably entwined with practice. It also informs health policy and provides the basis for educating future nurses. To be able to contribute at this level, students must have a good grasp of the discipline of nursing: its history, philosophy, research, and practice.

Doctoral programs in the United States have been around for about 100 years and underwent enormous expansion in the 1970s and 1980s. There are currently more than 80 universities with doctoral nursing programs in the United States. Programs typically follow a model that requires a minimum of 30 credits of course work and the completion of a supervised research project. Most courses are compulsory for all students, with some flexibility allowed in elective courses to meet students' individual interests and needs. Students typically do not require a faculty supervisor until their course work is finished and they are ready to begin the research. This model has the advantage of being able to accommodate large numbers of students who are taking course work and the disadvantage of postponing socialization of students into research roles until they are well into their course of study.

In contrast to the US approach, there was a deliberate effort in Canada to provide a more research-intensive experience for doctoral students. Canadian doctoral programs are remarkably similar in their goals, and all provide a major emphasis on research training, using, at least to some extent, the apprenticeship model. There is a continuum of flexibility in course requirements, varying from no credits to 18 credits. In most programs, students are assigned to a faculty supervisor upon admission, and a program of study is approved by the supervisor or, in some cases, a supervisory committee. The intent is for the course requirements to be individualized to meet a student's needs and to support the research the student will be doing.

From the standpoint of research training, the apprenticeship model is still unsurpassed. Students should expect to be involved in their faculty supervisor's research program. The more deeply students are involved with ongoing research, the better their socialization into research and scholarship will be, and the better prepared they will be to launch an academic career upon graduation.

In Canada, the Doctor of Philosophy (PhD) is considered the "terminal degree," or highest level of academic achievement. RNs who study for a PhD prepare for a career that includes leading a program of original research. The PhD is required for tenure-track academic positions in Canadian universities. The **Doctorate of Nursing Practice** (DNP) focuses on the preparation of leaders for clinical practice, health policy, and clinical or applied research. Acorn, Lamarche, and Edwards (2009) advocated for the development of both PhD and DNP degrees in Canada to advance nursing knowledge and to provide leadership in health care. They argued that individuals whose goals are to be educated in providing leadership in nursing and health care must currently take positions in PhD programs whose primary focus is research training.

Opponents to the DNP are concerned that practice doctorates will reduce enrollments in PhD programs and weaken the research mandate of the profession because of limited resources available to support graduate education in nursing. The CASN (2011) published a position statement on doctoral education in nursing in Canada that identified doctoral education as a critical priority to increase the number of PhD graduates in Canada for the next 5 years. Unfortunately, even with the expansion of doctoral programs and the growing number of graduates nationally, the vacancies for faculty continue to increase with the large number of retirements of the professoriate. Whether to promote the PhD or DNP (or both) is an ongoing debate that requires national dialogue. There were proposed nonresearch-focused **Doctor of Nursing** (DN) and DNP programs at Canadian universities in the planning and approval stages at the end of 2019. For instance, the University of Toronto's Faculty of Nursing had proposed a Doctor of Nursing program that was expected to begin accepting students in September 2020; the program is currently on hold until 2021 because of the COVID-19 pandemic.

🛈 RESEARCH FOCUS

Perspectives from Academic Leaders on the Nursing Faculty Shortage in Canada

The growing shortage of nursing faculty in Canada is a complicated issue that, left unresolved, threatens the viability of nursing education across the country. Contributing to this shortage is the insufficient number of graduates from PhD programs at a time when there is an increasing number of retirees and vacant **tenure-track** positions. Vandyk and colleagues (2017) used a descriptive design with a postpositivist lens to explore "how Deans and Directors of Canadian Schools of Nursing (SON) describe and work within the context of a faculty shortage." All 12 participant schools had an undergraduate nursing program, 11 of the 12 offered at least one graduate program at the master's level and seven offered a doctoral degree in nursing (PhD). At the time the study was conducted, there were 44 vacant tenure-track positions needing to be filled across the country, and 15 of these positions were at the schools participating in the study. Data collection involved semi-structured interviews with 12 deans and directors of Canadian schools of nursing. Data analysis used the constant comparison method of Glaser & Strauss (1967).

Participants spoke about their experiences with the faculty shortage in terms of demand, supply, and the strategies used to continue the viability of programs offered at their schools. The strategies used included targeted recruitment, casting a wide net, growing your own, adjusting workload and program delivery to meet needs, and fostering competition and collaboration (Vandyk, Chartrand, Beké et al., 2017, p. 1). Other strategies that did not have consensus among the group were identified as requiring more discussion. This includes the contentious issue of using nurses who have earned a Doctorate of Nursing Practice (DNP) to teach undergraduate students, as schools of nursing do in the United States.

The authors of this study explain the impact of the nursing shortage on academe and offer insight into the need to find strategies to navigate the growing shortage. The academic leaders who participated in this study expressed their commitment to protecting the integrity of the profession of nursing, underpinned by sound research to drive future decisions.

Sources: Vandyk, A., Chartrand, J., Beké, É., et al. (2017). Perspectives from academic leaders of the nursing faculty shortage in Canada. *International Journal of Nursing Education Scholarship, 14*(1), 286–297. https://doi.org/10.1515/ijnes-2017-0049; Glaser, B., & Strauss, A. (1967). *The discovery of grounded theory: Strategies for qualitative research.* Mill Valley, CA: Sociology Press.

POSTDOCTORAL EDUCATION IN NURSING

Postdoctoral education provides a form of socialization to the academic world that has been common in other disciplines for decades. Graduates with doctoral degrees in nursing have access to growing opportunities to pursue postdoctoral education, but the uptake of such an opportunity is dependent on the career goals of the graduate. Often, nurses obtain a doctoral degree while they are already employed in a teaching role at a college or university with the expectation that they will return to continue their employment after completion of their degree.

Postdoctoral study is facilitated by access to funding, and postdoctoral fellowships provide PhD graduates with the opportunity to develop their research programs beyond the completion of their dissertation research. Typically, a new PhD graduate will submit an application outlining a proposed research program of 1 to 3 years that will be supervised by an established researcher. Candidates are encouraged to seek opportunities in settings other than the one in which they earned their PhD to expand their opportunities into a new intellectual environment. Postdoctoral funding allows a new graduate to continue research development activities prior to assuming the full responsibilities of an academic appointment. Although postdoctoral funding covers research activities, no regular teaching activities are allowed during this time.

Those who aspire to work as career scientists in research will find that postdoctoral funding is essential. These individuals will use their fellowship time to present and publish the results of their doctoral dissertations and to undertake new research activities, as well as to acquire grants for the next phase of their research. Doing research and securing funding are the essential components of a career scientist application, the next step of the process.

Postdoctoral educational opportunities in nursing are essential if graduates of the new doctoral nursing programs are to have an opportunity to develop ongoing research programs as they take up academic appointments in universities. Experience has shown that new PhD graduates require support from more experienced researchers, as well as the time to plan their research and submit research proposals to funding agencies. If new PhD graduates have the opportunity to work on a collegial basis with established researchers, they are far more likely to be successful when they take up their appointments in faculties and schools of nursing. Given the significant time and resources that have been invested in the brightest and best academics, it is worthwhile to create the conditions for new researchers to succeed.

SUMMARY OF LEARNING OBJECTIVES

- Graduate education in nursing is a relatively new phenomenon in Canada. The first master's program began in 1959, and the first doctoral program in 1991.
- Graduate programs are offered across Canada in a variety of delivery formats, including fully online, face to face, and combinations of short residencies and online study. Students can study at the university of their choice without relocating.
- Graduate enrollments have grown across Canada with the establishment of more schools offering graduate programs. Despite increased access, graduate completion numbers are not sufficient to address the faculty shortage in Canadian nursing schools.

- A Master of Nursing can be course or thesis based, or it can be combined with another specialty focus. The nurse practitioner graduate degree is an example of the specialty focus combined with a master's degree of nursing.
- Sufficient faculty resources include faculty who are prepared at the doctoral level with established programs of research to support both the growth and sustainability of graduate education.
- Postdoctoral opportunities assist PhD graduates with establishing strong programs of research after completing their doctorates.

CRITICAL THINKING QUESTIONS

1. Why do you think graduate education is important to nursing?
2. The difficulty encountered by university schools of nursing in establishing and sustaining doctoral programs in nursing might be similar to the difficulties encountered by pioneers in other professions. What might these be, and how were they similar to or different from those in other professions?
3. What is the main argument against hiring nurses with Doctorate of Nursing Practice degrees as tenure-track faculty in Canadian universities?

REFERENCES

Acorn, S., Lamarche, K., & Edwards, M. (2009). Practice doctorates in nursing: Developing nursing leaders. *Nursing Leadership, 22,* 85–91. https://doi.org/10.12927/cjnl.2009.20801.

British Columbia Ministry of Health. (2018, May 23). *Creating new opportunities for nurse practitioners as part of team-based care system.* Retrieved from https://news.gov.bc.ca/releases/20 18HLTH0034-000995.

Canadian Association of Schools of Nursing. (2011). *Doctoral education in nursing in Canada.* Retrieved from https://casn.ca/wp-content/uploads/2014/10/DoctoralEducation2011.pdf.

Canadian Association of Schools of Nursing. (2015). *National nursing education framework: Final report.* Ottawa, ON: Author.

Canadian Association of Schools of Nursing. (2019, December). *Registered nurses education in Canada statistics. 2017–2018. Registered nurse workforce, Canadian production: Potential new supply.* Ottawa, ON: Author. Retrieved from https://www.casn.ca/wp-content/uploads/2019/12/2017-2018-EN-SFS-DRAFT-REPORT-for-web.pdf.

Canadian Institute for Health Information. (2020). *Nursing in Canada, 2019.* Retrieved from https://www.cihi.ca/en/nursing-in-canada-2019.

Canadian Nurses Association. (1962). *Folio of reports 1962.* Ottawa, ON: Author.

Canadian Nurses Association. (2019). *Advanced practice nursing: A pan-Canadian framework.* Ottawa, ON: Author.

Canadian Nurses Foundation. (2019). *Scholarships and research grants.* Retrieved from https://-fiic.ca/what-we-do/scholarships-and-bursaries/.

Carpenter, II. M. (1970). The University of Toronto School of Nursing: An agent of change. In M. Q. Innes (Ed.), *Nursing education in a changing society* (pp. 86–108). Toronto, ON: University of Toronto Press.

College of Nurses of Ontario. (2017). *Membership statistics report 2017.* Retrieved from http://www.cno.org/globalassets/docs/general/43069_stats/2017-membership-statistics-report.pdf.

College of Nurses of Ontario. (2020, July 2). *Membership totals at a glance.* Retrieved from http://www.cno.org/en/what-is-cno/nursing-demographics/membership-totals-at-a-glance/.

Fraser, E. (2017, November 16). *Province doesn't let nurse practitioners fill health-care gaps, group says.* CBC News. Retrieved from https://www.cbc.ca/news/canada/new-brunswick/nurse-practitioners-doctors-1.4404747.

Good, S. R. (1969). *Submission to the study of support of research in universities for the Science Secretariat of the Privy Council.* Ottawa, ON: Canadian Nurses Association and Canadian Nurses Foundation.

Good, S. R. (1971). *Submission to the Association of Universities and Colleges of Canada.* Calgary, AB: University of Calgary.

Hart, M. E. (1962). *Needs and resources for graduate education in nursing in Canada* [Unpublished doctoral dissertation]. Columbia University.

Imai, H. R. (1971). Professional associations and research activities in nursing in Canada. *National Conference on Research in Nursing Practice.* Vancouver, BC: The University of British Columbia School of Nursing.

Kerr, J. C. (1978). *Financing university nursing education in Canada: 1919–1976* [Unpublished doctoral dissertation]. University of Michigan.

La Presse Canadienne. (2019, October 9). *Quebec's super nurses set to get new powers as Bill 43 in introduced.* CTV News. Retrieved from https://montreal.ctvnews.ca/quebec-s-super-nurses-set-to-get-new-powers-as-bill-43-in-introduced-1.4631533.

Lamb, M., & Stinson, S. M. (1990). *Canadian nursing doctoral statistics: 1989 update.* Ottawa, ON: Canadian Nurses Association.

Larsen, J., & Stinson, S. M. (1980). *Canadian nursing doctoral statistics.* Ottawa, ON: Canadian Nurses Association.

Medical Research Council of Canada. (1985). *Report to the Medical Research Council of Canada by the Working Group on Nursing Research.* Ottawa, ON: Author.

Mitchell, A., Pinelli, J., Patterson, C., & Southwell, D. (1993). *Utilization of nurse practitioners in Ontario. A discussion paper.* Working Paper Series, Paper 93-4. Hamilton, ON: The Quality of Nursing Worklife Research Unit, University of Toronto/McMaster University.

Mussallem, H. K. (1965). *Nursing education in Canada.* Ottawa, ON: Queen's Printer.

Overduin, H. (1970). *People and ideas: Nursing at Western 1920-1970.* London, ON: University of Western Ontario.

PayScale. (2019). *Average nurse practitioner (NP) salary in Canada.* Retrieved from https://www.payscale.com/.

Statistics Canada. (1976). *Nursing in Canada. Canadian nursing statistics. 1976.* Ottawa, ON: Author.

Stinson, S. M. (1977). Central issues in Canadian nursing research. In B. LaSor & M. R. Elliott (Eds.), *Issues in Canadian nursing* (pp. 3–42). Toronto, ON: Prentice-Hall.

Tunis, B. (1966). *In caps and gowns.* Montreal, QC: McGill University Press.

University of Western Ontario School of Nursing. (1967). *Calendar.* London, ON: Author.

University of Victoria School of Nursing. (1995). *PhD by special arrangement: Brochure* (pp. 1–5). Victoria, BC: Author.

W. K. Kellogg Foundation. (1966). *Annual report.* Battle Creek, MI: Author.

W. K. Kellogg Foundation. (1970). *Annual report.* Battle Creek, MI: Author.

W. K. Kellogg Foundation. (1971). *Annual report.* Battle Creek, MI: Author.

W. K. Kellogg Foundation. (1974). *Annual report.* Battle Creek, MI: Author.

W. K. Kellogg Foundation. (1975). *Annual report.* Battle Creek, MI: Author.

Zilm, G., Larose, O., & Stinson, S. (1979). *PhD (nursing).* Ottawa, ON: Canadian Nurses Association.

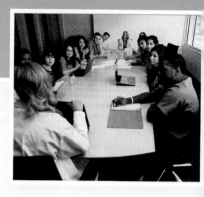

23

Career Development in Nursing

Noeman A. Mirza

 http://evolve.elsevier.com/Canada/Ross-Kerr/nursing

LEARNING OBJECTIVES

After reading this chapter, you will be able to:
- Describe advanced nursing practice roles in Canada.
- Identify how baccalaureate- and postgraduate-prepared nurses can develop their careers and become employable.
- Delineate the various types of research opportunities for nurses at different levels of education.
- Describe the activities that aspiring nurse researchers need to undertake to succeed in building a research record of accomplishment.
- Explain how an individual interested in postgraduate education would go about selecting a graduate program in nursing.

KEY TERMS

advanced practice nursing
employability
practice readiness

self-efficacy
self-regulated learning

As a faculty member in my mid-30s, I have been in an academic position for 5 years and have cherished every moment of my role as a university professor. My interest in research began when I was a teenager. In high school, I worked in a cancer biology research lab at Toronto's Sunnybrook Hospital and became a research assistant to a doctoral student at the University of Toronto during the summers. As a nursing student at McMaster University, I took on leadership roles as a student, securing council positions at school and nationally with the Canadian Nursing Students' Association. In my late teenage years, my time management skills were still developing, and I finally realized that my extraordinary commitment to extracurricular activities had to be cut significantly if I was to do well in my studies. In my final two years of study, I became more focused and secured a CIHR Undergraduate Summer Student Health Research Award. I also assisted a professor with a study on nurse practitioner education, which became my first publication in 2010. After working as an RN for 2 years, I rejoined McMaster for graduate studies. I fast-tracked into the PhD program after a year. I continued working part-time as a staff RN to maintain my clinical skills. I also accepted a sessional teaching position with the University of Toronto and went on to complete an RNAO clinical fellowship to develop clinical leadership skills. After completing my PhD, I applied for academic positions and accepted a tenure-track appointment at Thompson Rivers University in British Columbia. This was an exciting move. I was involved in developing the new Master of Nursing program and served as the program's coordinator a year after its inception. With my background in educational research, I founded the Collaboratory for Educational Research and Development, a centre for excellence in nursing education research. To develop skills in community-based research, I reached out to an experienced researcher in social work to act as my mentor based on our mutual interests in gerontology. Together we successfully secured several external grants, supervised graduate and undergraduate students, and presented and published in peer-reviewed conferences and journals. Today, I continue to grow as a teacher and researcher while giving back to academia through mentorship of students and early-career faculty members.

INTRODUCTION

Nursing is a desirable career that has attracted not only women but also an increasing number of men to its ranks. Today, nurses are a culturally diverse group of professionals who are equipped to provide high-quality care to individuals, families, and groups with diverse culturally specific care needs. Registered nurses (RNs) play a variety of professional roles and have the responsibility to advance the discipline of nursing (i.e., nursing's body of knowledge) and to uphold it as a profession (i.e., the operationalization of nursing's body of knowledge). There are unlimited opportunities for nurses who have the right competencies and are eager to learn and explore new roles within the profession. While most nurses work in staff positions to promote the health and well-being of the public in organizational and community settings, some take on leadership responsibilities as advance practice nurses, educators, consultants, legal advisers, researchers, managers, directors, vice presidents, chief nursing officers, and presidents of health care organizations. These nurse leaders often possess higher education, years of practice experience, and a strong history of ongoing career development that assists them in securing influential positions.

Most nurses enter the profession because they want to provide nursing services to the public. With an increasingly complex health care system, current practice environments have fostered the expansion of nursing roles and restructured traditional roles and responsibilities of all health care professions. While many nurses are satisfied with staff nursing positions in a health care organization for the duration of their careers, others may look for advancement. Whether or not one seeks career advancement, maintaining one's skills and furthering one's knowledge are essential to every nurse's success and should be part of a **self-regulated learning** career plan. Self-regulation allows individuals to engage in lifelong learning by setting goals and monitoring their progress toward achieving those goals (Zimmerman, 2002). Opportunities for advancement in clinical practice include the positions of advanced practice nurse, nurse practitioner, clinical nurse specialist, and clinical nurse educator. All involve graduate education and a specific area of specialization. An awareness of the issues involved in career advancement, including selecting a graduate program and searching for a suitable position, can help nurses take the risks and make the professional transitions necessary to a successful career. Aside from an individual's aspirations, it is important to understand the processes involved in making sound decisions about one's career. This chapter provides an overview of career development in nursing with an emphasis on how nursing students and new nursing graduates could plan their careers and what paths might be available to nurses who are seeking to advance their nursing education and career trajectory.

BUILDING A CLINICAL PRACTICE CAREER: PATHWAY TO SUCCESS

A nursing career in clinical practice is one of the most rewarding paths a new nursing graduate can take. Opportunities are endless as new nursing roles continue to emerge. Nurses who elect to build their careers in the practice arena must narrow their focus away from general practice and become experts in a specialized practice area (e.g., gerontology). The acquisition of higher education often accompanies this specialization. For example, one nurse might decide to become a Certified Diabetes Educator by completing the Diabetes Educator Certificate; another might consider a Master of Health Management to become a patient care manager; yet another might complete a Master of Nursing to become an Advanced Practice Geriatric Outreach Nurse. Regardless of the educational program, a nurse's choices to develop their career often rests on deep reflection that takes into consideration their interests, future goals, and advice from colleagues and field mentors.

Clinical nurse specialists (CNSs) and nurse practitioners (NPs) are two types of advanced practice nurses in Canada. CNSs are currently regulated as registered nurses (RNs), while legislation and regulations for NPs exists in all provinces and territories (Canadian Nurses Association [CNA], 2019). In their latest advanced nursing practice framework, the CNA (2019) states that **advanced practice nursing** is "an umbrella term for registered nurses (RNs) and nurse practitioners (NPs) who integrate graduate nursing educational preparation with in-depth, specialized clinical nursing knowledge and expertise in complex decision-making to meet the health needs of individuals, families, groups, communities and populations" (p. 13). The role of advanced practice nurses (CNSs and NPs) is to:

- Analyze and synthesize knowledge;
- Critique, interpret, and apply theory;
- Participate in and lead research from nursing and other disciplines;
- Use their advanced clinical competencies; and
- Develop and accelerate nursing knowledge and the profession as a whole. (CNA, 2019, p. 13)

In their seminal book on Canadian perspectives on advanced practice nursing, Staples, Ray, and Hannon (2016) provided a comprehensive overview of what advanced practice nursing entails in Canada. The two advanced practice nursing roles that are currently recognized in Canada are the CNS and NP.

Both the CNS and NP roles enable nurses to engage directly with clients to promote health and quality of life as well as to assist clients in dealing with and managing changes in their health (Staples & Ray, 2016). Despite their commonalities, "NPs possess the legislative authority, knowledge and skills to autonomously diagnose, order and interpret diagnostic tests, prescribe treatment (including drugs) and perform specific procedures (within their legislated scope of practice)" (CNA, 2019, p. 19). CNSs, on the other hand, possess "expert specialty knowledge, skills and abilities [that] enable them to autonomously provide consultation on highly complex clients with primary care providers that impacts diagnosis and prescribed treatments (including medications) and to assist in the performance of specific treatments within their legislated scope of practice" (CNA, 2019, p. 19).

The CNS role arose to meet institutional needs for the support of nurses involved in managing complex patients and improving quality of care. Nevertheless, the NP role came out of the need for nurses to assume expanded roles in areas where medical care was lacking, that is, in rural and northern areas. The NP role was extended to meet the needs of patients and families in tertiary care hospitals because of the reduction of doctors, particularly in Ontario, during the 1980s and 1990s (Staples & Ray, 2016). Nurse educators (clinical or academic), researchers, and health care administrators with graduate education who demonstrate advanced nursing practice in their positions are not, however, considered advanced practice nurses because they do not engage in direct clinical, comprehensive care as part of their roles (CNA, 2019).

Regardless of the professional direction taken, every nurse will apply for a job at some point. Therefore, it is vital for nurses with baccalaureate or graduate degrees to understand the type of work for which they are qualified, engage in honest self-appraisal, and present themselves in the best possible way to a prospective employer. Following a job interview, it is essential for nurses to think critically about the employer's expectations and the context of the prospective work environment. The "right" decision is based on the suitability of the position to their abilities and the likelihood of personal satisfaction in carrying out the responsibilities of the job. Baccalaureate-prepared nurses entering the job market must bear in mind that every position provides basic experience that will increase knowledge and understanding in a particular clinical area. Since every position is by nature career building, nurses must select employment opportunities that can enhance their experience as well as their ability to advance within the profession. Various nursing roles require different

TABLE 23.1 Employment Options with Different Levels of Nursing Education

Degree	Degree Examples	Employment Options
Baccalaureate	Bachelor of Nursing (BN) Bachelor of Science in Nursing (BScN, BSN)	Staff nurse, research nurse, or research assistant
Postgraduate certificate/ diploma	Occupational Health Nursing Certificate Diabetes Educator Certificate Clinical Research Graduate Certificate	Occupational health and safety nurse, Certified Diabetes Educator, research associate
Master's	Master of Nursing (MN) Master of Science in Nursing (MScN, MSN)	Advanced practice nurse, clinical nurse specialist, nurse administrator (manager, director, vice president), nurse educator, instructor/lecturer
Master's (nurse practitioner stream)	Master of Nursing – Nurse Practitioner (MN-NP)	Nurse practitioner or instructor/lecturer
Doctorate	Doctor of Philosophy (PhD)	Professor, postdoctoral fellow, researcher/ scientist

types of education. Table 23.1 provides an overview of the types of roles nurses can undertake with the nursing education options currently offered in Canada.

RESEARCH FOCUS

Succession Planning During a Nursing Shortage

With the current nursing shortage in Canada, health systems are also seeing a shortage in nurse leaders. In the Central Interior of British Columbia, new nursing graduates often have to take on leadership roles (e.g., charge nurse), sometimes within the first year after graduation. While new nursing graduates are perceived as novices or advanced beginners, they are occasionally expected to fill the roles of nurse leaders who are typically viewed as experts. More and more research is advocating for the need to engage in nurse manager succession planning. While some scholars have explored the various aspects of succession planning (Titzer, Phillips, Tooley et al., 2013), others are testing programs to improve self-perceived readiness of frontline nurses for leadership roles (LaCross, Hall, & Boerger, 2019). However, more research is needed on new nursing graduates who are taking on leadership roles so early in their nursing careers.

Sources: Titzer, J., Phillips, T., Tooley, S., et al. (2013). Nurse manager succession planning: Synthesis of the evidence. *Journal of Nursing Management, 21*, 971–979. https://doi.org/10.1111/jonm.12179; LaCross, E., Hall, N., & Boerger, J. A. (2019). Nurse manager succession planning: Evaluating a pilot program's effect on self-perception of readiness. *Journal of Nursing Administration, 49*(6), 331–335. https://doi.org/10.1097/NNA.0000000000000761.

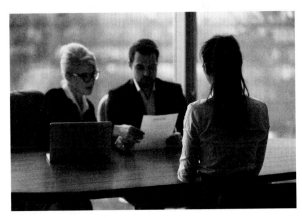

(istock.com/fizkes)

Employability and Readiness for Practice

Many nursing students in baccalaureate programs are often so immersed in their studies that they do not give much thought to **employability**. Employability is the process that an individual undertakes to prepare themselves to fulfill the specifications of a job (Taylor, 2016). Employment is the successful outcome of this process, and schools of nursing must ensure that undergraduate and graduate nursing curricula foster the development of employability among graduates. In their important and well-referenced paper on employability, Fugate, Kinicki, and Ashforth (2004) pointed out three dimensions of employability:

1. Career identity—One's sense of being a nurse;
2. Personal adaptability—Remaining productive, optimistic, self-efficacious, and open to change in a dynamic health care system; and
3. Social and human capital—Formal and informal networks and relationships; age, education, and experience.

While Fugate, Kinicki, and Ashforth (2004) proposed dimensions that are broad and not initially intended for nurses, these can guide new nursing graduates to become employable. For example, studying to become a nurse or an advanced practitioner requires more than just a passing grade in nursing courses; it also requires the learner to master undergraduate or graduate competencies depending on their level of study. A high level of mastery in nursing competencies shows a learner's motivation and desire to learn and become a professional at the level for which they are trained. This personal undertaking helps to form the identity of the nurse or advanced practitioner. Graduates of undergraduate and graduate programs who are adaptable are often productive, optimistic, self-efficacious, and open to change in the dynamic health care system. Their adaptability may often be reflected in their maturity and educational, practice, and life experiences (Fugate, Kinicki, and Ashforth, 2004).

In addition to the dimensions of employability, graduates must also be practice ready; that is, they must exhibit performance attributes that indicate competence at the level for which their current education prepares them. Graduates of advanced practice nursing programs must meet specific competencies that are outlined by the CNA (2019)'s framework (pp. 29–35). Similarly, graduates of baccalaureate programs must meet national and provincial competencies of entry-level nursing practice. However, successfully passing the licensing exam does not guarantee employment—graduates must also ensure that they are practice ready. Given today's complex health care systems, employers are increasingly demanding that new graduates be practice ready. According to Mirza, Manankil-Rankin, Prentice et al. (2019), **practice readiness** currently consists of three capabilities:

1. Cognitive capability—Competence, clinical reasoning, and situational awareness;
2. Clinical capability—Psychomotor skills, clinical assessment, care delivery and coordination; and
3. Professional capability—Professional identity, ethical practice, and self-esteem and self-worth.

The integrative nature of these three capabilities contributes to a new graduate's sense of **self-efficacy**, which is the belief in one's capabilities to respond appropriately to a situation (Bandura, 1995). Fugate, Kinicki, and Ashforth's (2004) dimensions of employability not only cover identity (analogous to professional capability) but self-efficacy as well. They also discuss age, experience, and education as part of social and human capital. Mirza, Manankil-Rankin, and Prentice (2019) discuss similar descriptors (age, experience, maturity, and educational socialization) as antecedents to becoming practice ready. To be employable, new nursing graduates must be able to demonstrate mastery of entry-level cognitive, clinical, and professional capabilities. Graduates' strengths in these capabilities may become noticeable through the self-efficacy that display when responding to an employer's questions during an interview.

The Work Search

In approaching the search for suitable employment, baccalaureate and advanced practice nursing students must be able to recognize positions that will be a good fit with their interests, values, and skills. Beginning the job search well in advance enables students to build some knowledge of the range of positions available. This preparation will allow graduates to apply for positions that offer the best opportunities to use their knowledge and skills, and will consequently result in a high level of job satisfaction. Students looking for an entry-level position following graduation from a baccalaureate nursing program should begin their search many months before they expect to be available for work. Those graduating from advanced practice nursing programs may first want to use their informal networks within the organization where they are currently employed. This might include looking at internal job postings or speaking to administrators, such as the manager or the director of nursing, to obtain an idea of the potential jobs they might be eligible for as a graduate.

Plan of Action

Organization is often the key to success in looking for a position (Haroun, 2016). At the outset, it is helpful to develop an outline of what needs to be done and then proceed through this plan in a stepwise manner. The first step is to identify what is being sought in a work situation, and then to specify the skills and aptitudes needed for such work. The work search should then focus on a particular type of position that will be congruent with the applicant's abilities and interests, sufficiently remunerative, and conveniently located. A good strategy is to look for potential jobs ahead of time, even a year in advance. By examining job postings, graduates-to-be may realize that they have some gaps they need to work on over the next year to fulfill employer requirements. For example, on realizing that they need to strengthen their research skills, an advanced practice nursing student may decide to become a research assistant or a collaborator on a research study being carried out by one of their professors or mentors.

Self-appraisal is a central part of the process of finding a career that fits one's values and passions. Those looking for challenging and satisfying positions should be honest with themselves in acknowledging what they like, and want, to do. Self-appraisal also includes honest and critical evaluation of one's level of knowledge and skills, such as technical skills and knowledge in a particular area; problem-solving, organizational, and communication skills; leadership skills; creativity; and personal qualities such as capacity for responsibility, attitude toward work, intrinsic motivation, flexibility, and so on. Student organizations offer an opportunity to learn through dialogue with other students at various levels throughout the local educational program as well as regionally and nationally.

Since nursing builds on humanistic values, individuals completing baccalaureate or graduate programs must ensure that their knowledge and skills will enable them to work respectfully with people from diverse backgrounds (including equity-seeking groups). Thus, skill in communicating with others and establishing rapport with patients, their families, and the interprofessional team will be of particular interest to prospective employers (Casey, Fink, Jaynes et al., 2011; Pillai, 2014). In contemporary Canadian society, there is an expectation that current and future nurses are able to skillfully provide culturally safe care to individuals, families, and communities. Canadian schools of nursing are in the process of integrating the Truth and Reconciliation Commission of Canada's (TRC, 2015) recommendations into nursing curricula. It is of the utmost importance that new graduates from any nursing program, completing any educational degree, familiarize themselves with the Calls to Action (TRC, 2015).

 APPLYING CONTENT KNOWLEDGE

Identify one career goal of your own and outline a strategy for achieving it. Think about the challenges you might face and how you would overcome them.

The Résumé or Curriculum Vitae

Depending on the type of job one is looking for, a nurse will need to develop either a résumé or curriculum vitae (CV) that speaks to their qualifications, attributes, and experience. Practice-based positions in health care organizations (e.g., hospitals) often require résumés, while academic institutions (colleges and universities) may request a CV. A résumé often includes personal data, educational achievements, skills and attributes, previous employment and volunteer experience, and references. Nurses often use CVs when applying for academic positions such as instructors, lecturers, or professors in colleges and universities. Compared with a résumé, a CV is slightly longer and may consist of teaching and research experience, publications and presentations, and any academic achievements such as teaching awards.

In a résumé or CV, it might be useful to consider including one's nursing philosophy to show employers one's commitment to and vision of professional caring. Some

applicants might also include evidence of ongoing development, such as leadership roles, attendance at conferences and workshops, and completion of informal courses and self-directed learning. Baccalaureate nursing students can mention extracurricular activities. Advanced practice nursing students can discuss their participation in workplace initiatives such as the journal club or the nursing advisory committee, or their experience of having been a charge nurse or the unit's "practice coach" on fall prevention. These additions to one's résumé or CV are useful when switching jobs or applying for highly competitive positions. A personal philosophy and information on ongoing professional development speak highly of an individual's passion for nursing and their potential as a lifelong learner and professional. Table 23.2 outlines some of the important components to include in one's résumé or CV.

The résumé or CV should be straightforward and clear. Applicants should include a cover letter to highlight the skills, attributes, experience, and education relevant to the position. The covering letter should reflect an applicant's personality as well as their qualifications for a position. A thoughtfully composed cover and well-written résumé can go a long way toward impressing an employer. It is a good

TABLE 23.2 Key Components of a Résumé or Curriculum Vitae

Section	Résumé	Curriculum Vitae
Personal data	•	•
Skills and attributes	•	
Educational achievements	•	•
Previous employment	•	•
Volunteer experience or service	•	•
Clinical leadership roles	•	
Teaching experience		•
Research experience		•
Student supervision		•
Practice-related training (fellowships)	•	
Research-based training (fellowships)		•
Publications		•
Presentations		•
Grants received		•
Teaching awards		•
Practice awards	•	•
Teaching philosophy		•
Scholarship philosophy		•
References	•	•

idea to ask one or two other individuals with excellent writing and editing skills to provide feedback on the résumé or CV. Avoiding spelling and grammatical errors is essential when presenting a résumé to a prospective employer. Applicants should also explain in their résumé or CV any career interruptions or breaks in work history due to family responsibilities (e.g., parental leave or leave to care for an ill family member).

Initial Contact and Use of Social Media

Job searches involve extensive research on positions available in a nurse's area of interest. Many people send out résumés in large numbers to prospective employers. However, it is better to make personal contact with a prospective employer and then send them a résumé or CV if invited to do so. One way to make personal contact is by using informal networks—such as asking a placement preceptor or the manager where one may have completed their consolidation or internship—or by attending career fairs to meet potential employers. If an employer invites an individual to send them a résumé or CV, it is best to remind the employer—in the cover letter—that they requested the résumé or CV. The objective of sending a résumé or CV is to gain an interview. A polite follow-up call a few days after sending the résumé is a good practice, especially if the employer invited the individual to apply.

As the labour market has become technologically advanced, employers now direct applicants to submit their résumés and CVs online. There are also job search websites that re-advertise most jobs posted by organizations. This online, "no cost" method of application submission might encourage applicants to submit tens of résumés in a matter of hours. The risk of online submission is that one's résumé could get lost in the pile of hundreds of applicants' résumés. One way to tackle this problem is by using social media (e.g., Twitter) to interact with prospective employers, learn about what their organization is doing, comment on their posts, tweet questions to them, and demonstrate ongoing interest in an organization and their mission. Some people also create blogs or websites on which they highlight their credentials, mention what type of job they are seeking, and include a link to their résumé or CV. This approach allows prospective employers to access an applicant's blog through their Twitter posts and get in touch with them.

Undergraduate or graduate students could make use of two other ways to secure work. First, they could join formal networks or organizations (e.g., interest groups of their provincial nursing organization, such as the Registered Nurses' Association of Ontario [RNAO]). By attending the organization's events or meetings, students can connect with managers and administrators that represent prospective employers. Student can also meet other nurses who might

be able to point them in the right direction or offer to pass on résumés to managers in their organization. Since organizations have relegated application submissions to online forms without a human component, increasing one's personal network may be a potential way to navigate toward that ideal job without having to compete with so many other applicants. Another way to find work, which might be more useful for graduate students, might be to secure entry-level jobs in bigger organizations while completing one's graduate education. This way, upon graduation, candidates can apply for their ideal position (e.g., CNS, nurse educator) internally, giving them first priority, and relieving the organization of the need to hire an external applicant.

The Interview

An interview is an opportunity for applicants to present themselves favourably to a prospective employer. Since applying for a position is competitive, arriving well prepared gives candidates a huge advantage. It is wise to find out in advance the names and positions of those who will be conducting the interview. If an applicant has applied for hundreds of jobs, it might be a good idea to ask for a copy of the job description beforehand. Information on the organization may be gathered (via the Internet or other sources) to gain some understanding of the organization's core values and mission, as well as what its key service area or population might be. Employers are often impressed with applicants who have done some work to learn about the organization for which they hope to work. It is also important to explain any breaks in work history if these were the result of family responsibilities. If the interview is conducted by telephone or video conferencing, steps should be taken to ensure that the conversation is not interrupted.

Applicants should anticipate the questions that interviewers might ask. Questions about strengths and weaknesses are common. Rehearsing these in advance will enable an applicant to discuss them confidently during an interview. Many websites help applicants prepare for interviews by providing sample interview questions and a variety of possible answers (including best and worst responses). First impressions are important. Arriving for the interview about 20 minutes early is advisable. Appearance, communication skills, and politeness are qualities that an employer will be observing. Prior to the interview, some organizations invite candidates to take part in a simulated test involving multiple simulated care situations. In these situations, employers observe how the candidates communicate with actor clients, how they manage difficult situations, and how they overcome ethical dilemmas. Even if applicants have impressive references, they must be prepared for these types of interviews.

An interview is a two-way street: it presents an opportunity for an employer to learn about a prospective employee, and it also allows an applicant to learn about the organization and the specific position. It is a good idea to decide in advance the information one hopes to obtain about a position and to come to the interview with prepared questions. Potential questions to ask employers might focus on how the employer supports transition of new graduates and the employer's commitment to professional development of staff. Applicants should also ask questions that help them learn more about the employment situation (e.g., nurse-to-client ratio, nursing workload, team structure, and the number of full- and part-time nurses in the practice setting). If the applicant has come from another city or province, they might want to ask whether the organization provides assistance with relocation, securing work for a spouse, or finding schooling or childcare for their children.

Even when an applicant is unsuccessful in securing a position, these interviews should be viewed as a learning experience. It is also important to learn to handle rejection well by reflecting on the interview questions and thinking about better answers that one could have provided to the interviewers; carrying out a postinterview analysis of what went right and what went wrong can also be helpful. To get through what may seem like a long and frustrating experience, applicants need to stay positive and focus on the main objective of their job search—finding an exciting and rewarding position that will lead to future career opportunities.

Mentoring

An essential element in career development is mentoring, which is an elusive experience that many people never find. A good mentor–mentee relationship is a rare occurrence and is probably the one factor that ensures successful transition into the workplace (Shellenbarger & Robb, 2016). Mentorship allows for a close relationship in which the new employee can ask any question and discuss any topic without censure. The mentor, often an experienced and expert nurse, facilitates the mentee's entry into the system by explaining the expectations of the role and the intricacies of the culture. As a role model, the mentor models successful behaviours for the role to which the novice aspires (Shellenbarger & Robb, 2016). Many talented people have built successful careers without the benefit of a mentor. However, most people will find that progress becomes significantly easier through the mentoring process.

Mentoring is an intangible relationship that cannot be orchestrated, but rather must happen spontaneously. This expectation increases the difficulty of promoting mentoring within an organization, since mentorship may not be subject to management strategies such as delegation or assignment. Nevertheless, organizations must use the mentoring relationship to promote staff development and an organizational culture that fosters the expectation that senior staff will mentor junior ones. Organizational leaders often ask senior staff in the organization to oversee the progress of junior members and to advise them about appropriate ways to succeed in the system. Junior members can seek out several senior people who can advise them about different aspects of the job. This gives the junior person a variety of alternatives to use in planning career advancement.

RESEARCH FOCUS
Mentorship and Transition to Practice

A descriptive qualitative study involving seven Canadian provinces explored 42 new graduate nurses' and 28 nurse leaders' perspectives on transition to practice (Regan, Wong, Laschinger et al., 2017). The researchers discovered that positive transition to practice is facilitated by support offered through formal orientation, appropriate mentors, and a constructive workplace culture that fosters learning and feedback. Barriers to transition to practice included inconsistent mentors and unrealistic workloads due to staffing shortage, uncivil or intimidating senior nurses, and short orientation—for example, "4 or 5 orientation shifts" versus "21 buddied shifts" (p. 249). The researchers called for increased organizational support for transition to practice and resources that foster professional development among existing and new graduate nurses.

Source: Regan, S., Wong, C., Laschinger, H. K., et al. (2017). Starting out: Qualitative perspectives of new graduate nurses and nurse leaders on transition to practice. *Journal of Nursing Management, 25,* 246–255. https://doi.org/10.1111/jonm.12456.

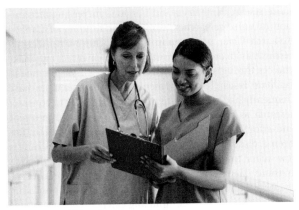

(istock.com/Wavebreakmedia)

Whichever career a nurse aspires to—be it clinical practice, research, management, education, or another field—mentorship is one key to success. An organization that can capture this ideal and make it work will be well on the way to creating a positive and supportive workplace.

 APPLYING CONTENT KNOWLEDGE

What does "mentoring" mean to you? Identify a significant mentor(s) in your life. How did this mentor assist you in developing your career?

BUILDING A RESEARCH CAREER: PATHWAY TO SUCCESS

A career in research can be an exciting prospect. Imagine being at the centre of a team that generates new ideas, tests better ways of doing things, and develops knowledge—being a nurse researcher is one of the most rewarding ways to spend one's life as a nurse. Nurse researchers today work in highly interdisciplinary teams that collaboratively address issues related to nursing and health. For example, an interdisciplinary team consisting of nurses, psychologists, physicians, anthropologists, social workers, exercise physiologists, and dietitians might collaborate to design a project aimed at promoting independence among community-dwelling older adults. As with any other plan to advance one's nursing career, choosing a research career requires postgraduate education. Such preparation is even more crucial than it is for other career paths in nursing, since the role of the researcher requires the acquisition of a new set of skills in addition to those required to be a nurse.

Currently, there are many opportunities available to nurses wishing to become researchers. These opportunities will likely increase in the near future as evinced by an increasing number of schools of nursing that are becoming more research intensive, and Canada's increasing recognition of nurse researchers through the funding of Canada Research Chair positions in nursing. Those who identify research as an area of interest early in their career can make choices throughout their education and initial practice to facilitate research development. In the past, nurses have frequently had to wait until mid-career or later to consider research as an option. Because of the time commitment and effort needed to become a researcher, this delay has been a disadvantage, leaving new researchers with only a few years to contribute after completing their research training. Hence, some schools of nursing are encouraging baccalaureate nursing students to consider becoming researchers earlier in their nursing careers. The purpose of this strategy is to ensure that the next generation of nurse

researchers has longer and more sustained and impactful research careers (Nehls & Rice, 2014).

 RESEARCH FOCUS

Early Entry into Doctoral Programs in Nursing

Based on their literature analysis on early entry into doctoral programs in nursing, Nehls and Rice (2014) reiterated that the mean age of graduates from doctoral programs in nursing is in the mid-40s, while the mean age of graduates from all other doctoral programs is in the early 30s. This is because the mean age of assistant professors in nursing is in the 50s, which is about 20 years older than the mean age of assistant professors in other fields of study. As a result, doctoral-prepared nurses have less time in which to contribute significantly to the discipline of nursing. While some schools of nursing have developed baccalaureate-to-doctorate entry, this strategy has some issues. Nehls and Rice (2014) interviewed 24 doctoral students who entered their PhD programs with a baccalaureate degree. The researchers discovered that decisions for early entry into a PhD program included involvement in research activities at the undergraduate level, encouragement from faculty members to consider higher education at the PhD level, and positive experiences with a research-intensive undergraduate course. Nehls and Rice (2014) also found that early-entry students are faced with the challenge of becoming nurses and doctoral students simultaneously; feel they do not have sufficient clinical experience to be able to teach nursing after completing their doctorate; and sometimes drop out of the doctoral program to gain practice experience. Most students that took part in Nehls and Rice's (2014) study emphasized the need for assurance of financial support before undertaking doctoral studies.

Source: Nehls, N., & Rice, E. (2014). Early entry to a doctoral degree in nursing program: Analysis of student experiences. *Journal of Nursing Education, 53*(4), 223–228. https://doi.org/10.3928/01484834-20140327-01.

Opportunities for Students

Undergraduate and graduate nursing programs provide many opportunities to gain an idea of what it would be like to work in research. Students who think they might be interested should test their interest and aptitude by taking advantage of these opportunities. In all university schools of nursing and in many college programs, there are faculty members who undertake research. These faculty members frequently receive grants to offset the cost of research and can hire students as research assistants. Experience as a research assistant may involve all aspects of the research process, from assisting with the creation of grant proposals, to data collection, entry, and analysis, to writing articles to report the results. Some schools encourage students to select a research project instead of a clinical or management experience to meet course requirements. In other cases, students may be assigned to a faculty research program specifically to gain hands-on experience as part of a nursing research course.

Most provinces offer opportunities for summer studentships in research, for which both undergraduate and graduate students may apply, with a faculty or community supervisor. These are funded in various ways by agencies such as the British Columbia Patient Safety and Quality Council, by health authorities or provincial ministries of health, or by universities themselves. The purpose of summer studentships is to introduce outstanding undergraduate or graduate students to career opportunities in research by giving them an educational experience in an active research program, often as part of a multidisciplinary team.

As part of their involvement in research, students typically collect data from research participants by conducting interviews or collecting physiological (e.g., blood pressure, weight, or frailty level) or subjective information through questionnaires or measurement tools. Other students may carry out literature reviews (e.g., concept analyses, scoping or systematic reviews) on an assigned topic and develop a paper or presentation from this work. Still others learn to enter and clean data, run statistical tests on the computer, and master a variety of software programs used in research, such as the Statistical Package for the Social Sciences (SPSS) or NVivo (qualitative data analysis software). These experiences help students to clarify whether a career in research appeals to them. Studentships also assist nursing schools with identifying excellent students who have the potential for advancement in research. Schools of nursing then actively recruit these students for graduate school.

In the past, most nursing graduate schools did not welcome students who had recently completed an undergraduate program, believing that students needed several years of experience to prepare for graduate work. This view is now considered outdated. Forward-thinking graduate programs recruit at least some of their students directly from undergraduate programs as part of their mission to build research capacity in the next generation of researchers. Federal granting agencies in Canada also promote these goals by requesting researchers to provide opportunities for undergraduate and graduate students to become part of the research team at different levels (e.g., research assistant, study coordinator, postdoctoral fellow). All these

efforts aim to prepare nurse researchers of the future. With a baccalaureate degree in nursing and some research experience, it is possible to find a position in nursing research at the level of research assistant or associate, project coordinator, or data collector. However, a more central role in the research team requires further preparation.

RESEARCH FOCUS

The Researching Older Adults' Repositioning (ROAR) study aimed to explore community-dwelling older adults' views on the restructuring of primary and community care services (Hulko, Mirza, & Seeley, 2020). This regional study was funded by an Interior Health Evidence-Informed Practice Grant and involved one small city and nine surrounding rural communities. With the goal of building research capacity among students, the ROAR team involved four undergraduate students who played an active role in recruitment, data collection, and analysis. The students recruited participants by identifying and connecting with community organizations and groups to send information about the study, organizing trips to various community sites, and providing information to potential participants. Students then took part in observing, co-leading, and eventually leading supervised interviews and focus groups with older adults. As the sample included First Nation Elders and Sikh older adults, students learned about cross-cultural considerations in research, including culturally safe ways to engage with Elders. One student was involved in data transcription and organization processes, while another assisted with data analysis using NVivo (e.g., coding and searching data). The ROAR team then acquired two subsequent knowledge translation grants (C² and Reach) from the Michael Smith Foundation for Health Research, which included undergraduate students as co-applicants. One student took part in a writing weekend to learn about the interpretation and dissemination phase of research and scoping reviews in particular. One student even accompanied the ROAR team to the annual conference of the Canadian Association on Gerontology.

Building a Track Record in Research

Research is a competitive business. All researchers find themselves in competition for scarce funding throughout their careers. Nurses who aspire to become researchers must begin as early as possible to build a record of accomplishment that will help them succeed. Success in research requires creativity, intelligence, and commitment. Students can demonstrate that they possess these characteristics through key indicators such as grades, research experience, publications, grants, awards, recommendations, and research plans. Graduate programs, granting agencies, award and scholarship committees, universities, and private foundations all use these indicators to award entry to graduate school, funding, academic positions, and scholarships. The criteria are weighted differently, depending on the circumstances. For instance, publication might be considered desirable for a novice researcher but will be required for more senior applicants.

In most competitions for funding, be it for a research grant, a scholarship, or salary support, the key indicators of success provide the basis for ranking candidates. In some cases, additional criteria might be considered, such as oral presentations or interviews that offer applicants scope for personal expression. It is not enough just to have a brilliant idea; a prospective research candidate must also be able to inspire decision makers with the assurance of success. Since success in the past is the most dependable indicator of future success, this criterion will always count heavily with decision makers. For most aspiring researchers, the first opportunity to accumulate some indicators of success (other than grades) is in an undergraduate program where students are encouraged to gain research experience and present or publish their work. Faculty in undergraduate programs should be alert to finding students with research potential. They should identify them early and make sure the students are aware of enrichment opportunities that will help them succeed. Since research contributes to the development of nursing as a discipline, it is the responsibility of all nurses to prioritize the development of research capacity in nursing.

When making decisions regarding experiences and opportunities that arise during graduate school, students should always keep the key indicators of success in mind and set their priorities accordingly. Every student should expect to publish papers written to meet course requirements and should apply for awards and scholarships whenever possible, not only for financial need. Every research activity undertaken should have the potential to provide an opportunity to disseminate findings through writing for publication. These are important goals that faculty supervisors and students should plan together, thus maximizing the graduate school experience to enhance the likelihood of future success.

Choosing a Graduate Program

Every province in Canada now has graduate programs in nursing. A complete listing can be obtained from the Canadian Association of Schools of Nursing. Nurses who aspire to pursue an advanced practice career in clinical practice should choose a program with a strong clinical

base and faculty members who are actively involved in clinical practice research. Many universities now offer NP programs at the master's level. However, post-RN and post-graduate educational levels also exist. In the future, there may be opportunities to enroll in other types of doctoral programs in nursing, such as a Doctor of Nursing (DN), which is a clinically based doctoral program. However, such programs may be difficult to support alongside PhD programs, since Canada has a small number of doctoral-prepared nursing faculty.

APPLYING CONTENT KNOWLEDGE

While existing nursing doctoral programs in Canada offer the PhD, the University of Toronto plans to launch Canada's first DN program in the fall of 2021. The program will prepare nurse leaders for health care, policy, and teaching roles. How do you see a DN-prepared nurse's role in the Canadian health care system? Which program would you choose if you wanted to pursue doctoral education? Provide a rationale for your answer.

Nurses who are considering a research career should choose one of the universities in Canada that has a doctoral program, since a PhD is the minimum requirement for a research career. Most graduate programs require students to complete a master's degree first, but some allow direct entry into a doctoral program. Information about these programs, including course requirements, residency, and funding opportunities, can be found on these universities' websites. Some of the factors to look for in a graduate program (master's or doctoral) include:

- Track records of key graduate faculty;
- Success rate of graduate students;
- Match between research underway in the school or clinical practice of faculty and the student's area of interest;
- Library and computer resources available to students;
- Opportunities for "apprenticeship" in a research-intensive environment and/or an outstanding clinical practice setting; and
- Availability of funding for graduate students.

Good clinical settings that support the development of excellence in practice can be found in conjunction with many of the graduate programs across Canada. University-associated health centres can often provide excellent clinical experience for graduate students in a variety of clinical specialties. Nurses interested in advanced practice should seek out facilities where opportunities are provided for community-based and/or acute care experiences. Settings where nurses can function as members of interdisciplinary teams provide good experience for students. For example, the University of Ottawa has the Centre for Research on Health and Nursing, a collaborative project between the university and the Canadian Nurses Association, where decision makers, knowledge users, and researchers collaborate with health care scientists at the university to improve patient care and outcomes.

Not every university lists nursing research centres on their websites, but this does not mean there are no research centres on campus involving nursing researchers. One example is the Collaboratory for Educational Research and Development, a centre for excellence in nursing education research at Thompson Rivers University. While there are several nursing-based research centres, most universities also house interdisciplinary research centres built around different research areas, such as perinatal research, gerontology, or nursing work–life balance. These centres bring together researchers from several disciplines who work together to address issues arising from the research area. Research centres often have career scientists at the hub who provide leadership to the interdisciplinary teams. Team members often include academic researchers, clinicians, clinical researchers, and students from a number of disciplines. The Trent Centre for Aging and Society (at Trent University) is one such centre; it houses two Canada Research Chairs and consists of staff, community members, as well as faculty and students from at least 10 different departments (e.g., geography, philosophy, sociology, nursing, English literature, etc.).

Some research centres cross specialties. For example, the University of Manitoba lists tens of research centres, institutes, facilities, and groups. Nursing researchers are involved in the Centre on Aging, the Manitoba Centre for Health Policy, and the Institute of Cardiovascular Sciences, which is a hospital-associated research hub. Other research centres operate in partnership with the community, the government, the health care system, or all of them combined. An example of this is the Centre for Excellence in Indigenous Health at the University of British Columbia, which is linked with Indigenous communities, the First Nations Health Authority, educational partners, nonprofit groups, and the government. There are also methodology based research centres such as the International Institute for Qualitative Methodology at the University of Alberta and the National Collaborating Centre for Methods and Tools at McMaster University.

Research centres can be the best environment for students to learn about research. Graduate students will experience a rich environment replete with colleagues from both nursing and other disciplines, resources (intellectual and fiscal), support from a variety of mentors, and the opportunity to develop their own interests and skills while contributing substantively to the research program of the centre. The interdisciplinary nature of the health research environment prepares students for the world at large, as the Canadian Institutes of Health Research (CIHR) are established on an interdisciplinary model. A graduate student who wants to pursue a research career may decide on a graduate school that houses a research centre in their area of interest.

If possible, prospective students should visit the campus of the potential graduate school and engage in meaningful conversations with key people; these might include students, research faculty, clinical specialists, and graduate program administrators. For students wishing to develop a clinical specialty area, there should be faculty practicing in that area who can supervise graduate students. For doctoral students, one or more potential supervisors must be available in the student's area of research interest. Applicants should take the time to outline a tentative area of research interest prior to visiting the school. This outline gives a focus to the ensuing conversations and enables a prospective student and the faculty member to assess whether a good match is likely. The outline will no doubt change as the student becomes more familiar with the chosen field and becomes aware of other opportunities. If students are unable to visit in person, they may collect information from websites or through email or phone conversations with research faculty, graduate students, and administrators.

Financing Graduate Education

In spite of the shift toward encouraging nurses to enter graduate school at an early age, most are at least 5 years beyond the baccalaureate degree before they begin. Many nurses received their basic education in diploma programs and therefore have reentered the educational system as postdiploma students in a baccalaureate program. Most of these students did not consider research or advanced practice as an option prior to reentering the system. Postdiploma students frequently continue their education to advance their current job within the health care system. Left with student loans to repay, mortgages, and children, nurses may not see a viable way to become full-time graduate students. The result is that most nurses enter graduate education as part-time students. This presents a difficult issue for the development of research capacity, when the best research training occurs in the context of an apprenticeship model.

Most universities maintain recruitment funds to attract the very best graduate students. A proactive strategy for student recruitment is crucial for any faculty desiring to be competitive. Once outstanding students are recruited, the next step is to provide them with funding to continue, preferably from a federal source. One of the indicators of excellence in a graduate program is the number and proportion of students who hold awards from granting agencies outside the university. This is an important question to ask when applying to a graduate school. The issue for schools of nursing revolves around helping applicants sort out the factors related to funding so they can make good choices. There is no doubt that future career scientists need to be full-time students for at least part of their graduate programs in order to qualify for funding opportunities that will increase their chances of success after graduation. As well, full-time study allows students to be immersed in research long enough to get a good grounding in the operation of a research program.

Today, there are unprecedented sources of funding available from federal granting agencies in Canada to support graduate education in nursing. To qualify, however, an applicant must be a full-time student working with a supervisor whose research excellence is recognized. Some of the awards available to students are substantial; together with allowable extra teaching or research funding that can be arranged by faculty, these awards can provide students with a decent salary, enabling most to commit to full-time study. The key issue is to identify students with potential for success, link them with supervisors who will help them secure funding, and arrange for them to receive any "top-up" funding that will ensure their success. Such sources of funding all provide students with an alternative to maintaining a position outside the university, which often takes priority over educational goals.

Other sources of funding for graduate students can be found within the university, in faculty research grants and from teaching and research assistantship funds. Teaching assistantships are available in several faculties, and graduate students commonly teach undergraduates in most university departments. This is a career-developing experience as well as a useful source of income. Research assistantships are also part of most university budgets, but these may be limited in number; they are designed to be a learning experience whereby students are assigned to assist faculty members with their research. Funded research projects are yet another source of funding and require the student to carry out part of the research, often data collection, under the supervision of a project director.

Getting the Most Out of Graduate Education

Graduate programs aim to provide advanced knowledge in the discipline and increase skills in practice and research. These programs often focus on the development of leaders, be they advanced practitioners, educators, policymakers, managers, or researchers. In a practice discipline like nursing, undergraduate programs prepare graduates for beginning practice by providing them with the necessary knowledge and skills. Graduate programs focus not only on building the knowledge base beyond the beginning level, but also on providing the skills for advanced practice and for knowledge development through research and theory building.

In Canada, master's programs have evolved to the point where they focus primarily on advanced practice, with some attention to leadership and management. These programs require students to specialize in an area of practice rather than attempt to increase skills and knowledge in all areas of nursing. Canadian doctoral programs provide the opportunity to focus even more specifically on an area for research and knowledge development. Skills developed in doctoral programs relate mainly to research and theory building.

Graduate programs in the United States of America are much more course-based than their Canadian counterparts. Master's programs are typically one to two years in length and require both course work and advanced practice. Courses tend to be in the clinical specialty area, theory, and research, and are often designed to meet requirements for specialty certification from the professional association. American doctoral programs also have extensive course requirements in such areas as philosophy, theory, clinical specialization, research, and cognate areas related to the research.

Canadian programs also offer specialization at the master's level and opportunities for advanced practice. However, they tend to have fewer practice hours and fewer specialty courses than the American programs and are not coordinated with requirements for specialty certification to any great extent. Since there are only a handful of specialty certification programs in Canada, most master's programs have not incorporated completion of a clinical specialty certification as part of the program. Doctoral programs in Canada tend to be more flexible than American programs, as they focus more on the student's specific research needs. Canadian graduate programs primarily follow the apprenticeship model.

Once into a graduate program, students with goals for research development will find many opportunities to develop particular skills and areas of knowledge. Most important, however, is finding appropriate mentorship within the faculty. Mentorship is a critical element of the apprenticeship model, as students learn by working alongside faculty members in research and practice. As students become acquainted with the resources available in the faculty, they will meet a number of individuals who can provide mentorship for different purposes (e.g., how to carry out specific statistical analyses, how to engage Indigenous communities in research, how to carry out systematic reviews).

The first year of any postgraduate program should provide students with opportunities to investigate all potential resources. Social functions for faculty and students are a good place for networking, as are research presentations, information sessions, lunch-and-learns, conferences, and faculty meetings. Important also are opportunities to communicate with other students, particularly those who are farther along in the program. This is one area in which the full-time student has a definite advantage over the part-time student, who may be on campus just to attend classes. There are sources of information available to all students through the faculty's website, newsletter, bulletin boards, or social media page (e.g., Facebook, Twitter, Instagram). These are important ways to track what is happening that might provide opportunities to develop.

Opportunities for development are particularly rich within research centres, since graduate students in the centre share a common area of interest and work closely with the research faculty. Students in a research centre have access to any faculty or staff within the centre. This access makes networking easier than it is for students in the larger faculty. Advanced practice students may not have this same opportunity to interact in a smaller group with experts in their field of interest. However, they can always apply for part-time research assistant positions within a research centre to gain exposure to new research projects, researchers, and other resources that might be of interest to them. Students might even get the opportunity to present or co-present their work at a conference. Attending and/or presenting at conferences also provides additional networking opportunities.

Postdoctoral Studies

The idea of a postdoctoral fellowship following completion of a PhD program is still new for nurses. Historically, the doctoral degree was considered sufficient preparation for a research career. It is still considered so in some disciplines, particularly in the humanities, but other disciplines such as science and medicine have used the postdoctoral fellowship as an essential piece of research training for decades. Graduate students play a valuable role in the professor's research. They take on a piece of the research as their own thesis project while working alongside the professor and others to carry out the work of the entire research program. Postdoctoral students typically seek out external opportunities to work with other regional, national, or international scholars for a period of 1 to 3 years as a way to continue their development and set up an independent program of research. Universities and industry recruit and employ postdoctoral fellows to fill academic and research positions. Often there is keen competition among postdoctoral fellows for the best jobs, but there is also keen competition among employers for the best postdoctoral opportunities.

There has long been a shortage of doctoral-prepared nurses to fill jobs in education and research. Nursing schools often recruit doctoral students for clinical or management positions while they are still PhD candidates (i.e., before they have completed their doctorates). Many faculty members are hired with master's degrees and are then persuaded by their deans to go on to complete a PhD. Often, these faculty members continue to work full or part-time throughout the duration of their PhD programs. Such nurses are likely to be older than graduate students in other disciplines and often have family and other commitments that make it difficult for them to leave the workforce for a period of several years to complete a PhD and postdoctoral fellowship. Their career trajectory is very different from that of their colleagues in other disciplines. However, the scene is shifting in nursing, as more and more younger nurses pursue doctoral education earlier in their careers. This change has come about thanks to the opportunities created by schools of nursing that allow baccalaureate nursing graduates to apply to a master's program or fast-track into a PhD program without having to complete a master's degree first. This option is most appealing to those interested in pursuing research careers.

Across North America, since the 1960s, the majority of graduates of doctoral programs have assumed academic positions without the benefit of postdoctoral fellowships. Many of these graduates were not successful in launching research programs following their PhD training. Since the main purpose of doctoral education is to train researchers, this has been a waste of talent. Numerous explanations have been offered for this problem. Some of these include heavy teaching loads in nursing programs; the scarcity of role models; unrealistic expectations for productivity in research, teaching, clinical practice, and community service; and the lack of good mentoring available to new academics. Some universities' efforts to recruit doctoral-prepared nurses into nonresearch, teaching-stream positions have also contributed to this trend.

A postdoctoral fellowship provides protection from competing priorities, particularly in teaching and clinical practice, because obligations in these areas are either greatly reduced or absent altogether. A fellowship gives the new graduate time to focus on research prior to assuming all the responsibilities of a full-time academic. Today, the expectation for faculty members at research-intensive universities is that they will complete a postdoctoral fellowship in a recognized research institution prior to taking up a research-focused university appointment. The intent of this strategy is to hire professors who possess advanced research training and have had the time to launch their program of research and develop research networks. So when these researchers are hired, they already have a strong portfolio of grants and publications, which will act as the foundation for securing further grants to establish their research programs.

In Canada, the shift to postdoctoral fellowships as the expectation for PhD graduates has taken place since doctoral programs began in the 1990s. The first graduates of the new Canadian programs in the early 1990s succeeded in obtaining funding for postdoctoral fellowships, and the movement began with them. Several of these early graduates have gone on to become career scientists with salary awards from federal sources. They, in turn, have developed successful research programs and are now supervising graduate students and postdoctoral fellows.

What is the expected outcome of a successful postdoctoral fellowship for the individual researcher? It varies somewhat depending on the goals of the researcher, but there are a few common outcomes that should be attained. These include:

- Publications: Each postdoctoral fellow should expect to publish two to three articles per year while holding a postdoctoral fellowship. At least one of these articles should come from the PhD thesis. Others will relate to work done during the postdoctoral fellowship. For instance, the research unit in which a postdoctoral fellow is conducting research will provide opportunities for the fellow to obtain experience in writing articles for publication from data already in place within the unit. Several team members may become coauthors on these articles.
- Grants: A major goal for a postdoctoral fellow involves obtaining research grant funds to support the early development of a research program.
- Skill development: A postdoctoral fellowship is the time for continued development in research techniques and skills. Instrument development and refinement, new analytical techniques, and discussion and debate of methodologies, whether quantitative or qualitative, are examples of the possibilities.
- Network of colleagues: A postdoctoral fellow should expand their network of colleagues beyond that already developed during the doctoral program. This can be done in a variety of ways, including attending conferences, visiting other research centres, participating in online discussions with experts in the field, and receiving and providing feedback on research and publications.

Career Scientists

The next phase in a research career after a postdoctoral fellowship is obtaining a beginning-level position as a career scientist. In Canada, this is a grant-supported position wherein all or part of an individual's salary is provided by the granting agency to the employer (university or other research institution) to ensure that the incumbent can spend the majority of time in direct research activities. Due to a shortage in nursing faculty across the country, many institutions hire nurses without postdoctoral preparation into research positions. These nurses, who have limited research training, are at a disadvantage when competing with postdoctoral-prepared nurses for research funding. They may also have difficulty thriving as career scientists, especially if they have a large teaching workload in addition to their research obligations. To become more competitive, these individuals must often seek research mentors or support from their universities through seed funding so they have a better chance of being awarded provincial and federal grants.

CASE STUDY

In the last 5 years, the School of Nursing at Thompson Rivers University has hired several doctoral-prepared nurses into professorial positions. Many have successfully secured national tri-agency grants (CIHR, Social Sciences and Humanities Research Council of Canada), while others have been awarded provincial grants. In order to enhance faculty members' competitiveness at the national level, the university held a competition in 2019 and awarded five Health Research Cluster Grants to research teams consisting of university-based researchers and practice partners from the Royal Inland Hospital and/or Interior Health (regional health authority). These renewable grants (worth $24,000 per year) also included support for three undergraduate students per health cluster (i.e., research capacity building for a total of 15 undergraduate students). Projects being undertaken include oncology emergencies, Indigenous health, care transitions of older adults, wound innovations, and role transition of newly graduated RNs.

Career scientists are eligible for many sources of funding that include ministries of health and health research foundations such as the Alberta Foundation for Medical Research or the Michael Smith Foundation for Health Research in British Columbia. These provincial awards are intended to equip researchers to compete for national awards. A career award from the CIHR provides salary funding for 5 years at a time, renewable with proof of adequate productivity. Career scientists are reviewed on a regular basis and must meet the terms of their awards for funding to continue. One prestigious award for exceptional emerging researchers is that of the Canada Research Chair Tier II, which universities award to early-career scientists in a particular field of study.

Career scientist awards are progressive in nature, with expectations of productivity and excellence increasing at each level. Scientists are judged on the quality of their research; their grants, publications, and presentations; awards and recognition; and the accomplishments of their students and associates. This is a demanding career. Research scientists are hard-working, dedicated individuals living competitive lives for whom risk taking is an everyday activity. However, a research career is also rewarding and has many positive attributes, not the least of which is the opportunity to make discoveries that improve the human condition and add to the knowledge base of the nursing profession.

SUMMARY OF LEARNING OBJECTIVES

- In their positions, advanced practice nurses (e.g., CNSs and NPs) use advanced clinical competencies and an expert knowledge base to influence or make complex decisions related to diagnoses and treatments.
- To be employable, students must develop their professional identities as nurses; be adaptable and self-efficacious; use social networks; and exhibit cognitive, clinical, and professional capabilities along with humanistic characteristics.
- A résumé or CV must be clear and accompanied by a reference letter. While social media provides unique opportunities to share CVs, given the relational nature of nursing, personal social networks are still an ideal way to seek employment.
- During an interview, applicants should ask questions about transition (e.g., mentorship), supports for professional development, and the employment situation.
- Some schools of nursing encourage baccalaureate nursing students to consider becoming researchers earlier in their nursing careers to support longer and more sustained and impactful research careers. However, early-entry PhD students often face challenges related to simultaneously becoming nurses and doctoral students.
- Students build their track records through grades, research experience, publications, grants, awards, recommendations, and research plans. These indicators enable nurses to attend graduate schools and secure funding, get hired into academic positions, and win scholarships.

- Due to a shortage in doctoral-prepared nursing faculty, Canada has been able to sustain only PhD programs in nursing. However, it is possible that schools of nursing will introduce other types of doctoral programs (e.g., a clinically based doctoral program).
- University-associated research centres provide excellent interdisciplinary practice and research experiences to graduate students. Such centres often have career scientists who provide leadership to the research teams associated with the centre.
- While most universities maintain recruitment funds to attract outstanding students, it is important to support these students through recognized supervisors and federal funding sources. This will allow students to commit to full-time study without having to maintain employment outside the university.
- The nursing faculty shortage has often led nursing schools to recruit doctoral students to fill jobs in education and research. However, research-intensive schools recruit candidates with postdoctoral preparation so that these individuals can be more successful in establishing and maintaining funded programs of research.
- Postdoctoral fellowships provide doctoral graduates with time to focus on research and build research careers. Researchers without postdoctoral training often seek research mentors or seed funding from their universities or regional organizations so they can become more competitive for provincial and national grants.

CRITICAL THINKING QUESTIONS

1. Describe the difference between NPs and CNSs.
2. What issues should students consider to become employable upon graduation?
3. How can nursing students and new graduates market themselves for possible employment opportunities?
4. What types of activities are important in building a record of research accomplishments?
5. What should prospective graduate students consider when choosing a graduate program?
6. What factors influence the decision to consider early entry into a doctoral program and what difficulties do early-entry doctoral students face?

REFERENCES

Bandura, A. (1995). Exercise of personal and collective efficacy in changing societies. In A. Bandura (Ed.), *Self-efficacy in changing societies* (pp. 1–45). Cambridge, UK: Cambridge University Press.

Canadian Nurses Association. (2019). *Advanced practice nursing: A Pan-Canadian framework*. Ottawa, ON: Author. Retrieved from http://www.cna-aiic.ca/-/media/cna/page-content/pdf-en/apn-a-pan-canadian-framework.pdf.

Casey, K., Fink, R., Jaynes, C., et al. (2011). Readiness for practice: The senior practicum experience. *Journal of Nursing Education, 50*(11), 646–652. https://doi.org/10.3928/01484834-20110817-03.

Fugate, M., Kinicki, A. J., & Ashforth, B. E. (2004). Employability: A psycho-social construct, its dimensions, and applications. *Journal of Vocational Behavior, 65*, 14–38.

Haroun, L. (2016). *Career development for health professionals: Success in school and on the job* (4th ed.). St. Louis, MO: Elsevier.

Hulko, W., Mirza, N., & Seeley, L. (2020). Older adults' views on the repositioning of primary and community care. *Canadian Journal on Aging*. https://doi.org/10.1017/S0714980819000540.

Mirza, N., Manankil-Rankin, L., Prentice, D., et al. (2019). Practice readiness of new nursing graduates: A concept analysis. *Nurse Education in Practice, 37*, 68–74. https://doi.org/10.1016/j.nepr.2019.04.009.

Nehls, N., & Rice, E. (2014). Early entry to a doctoral degree in nursing program: Analysis of student experiences. *Journal of Nursing Education, 53*(4), 223–228.

Pillai, A. A. (2014). *Ready, set, practice: A study of generational differences and their impact on senior baccalaureate nursing student perceived readiness to practice* (Publication No. 3666545) [Doctoral dissertation, Capella University]. ProQuest Dissertations Publishing.

Shellenbarger, T., & Robb, M. (2016). Effective mentoring in the clinical setting. *American Journal of Nursing, 116*(4), 64–68. https://doi.org/10.1097/01.NAJ.0000482149.37081.61.

Staples, E., Ray, S. L., & Hannon, R. A. (2016). *Canadian perspectives on advanced practice nursing*. Toronto, ON: Canadian Scholars' Press.

Staples, E., & Ray, S. L. (2016). A historical overview of advanced practice nursing in Canada. In E. Staples, S. L. Ray, & R. Hannon (Eds.), *Canadian perspectives on advanced practice nursing* (pp. 1–2). Toronto, ON: Canadian Scholars' Press.

Taylor, L. (2016). *How to develop your healthcare career: A guide to employability and professional development*. West Sussex, UK: John Wiley & Sons.

Truth and Reconciliation Commission of Canada. (2015). *Truth and Reconciliation Commission of Canada: Calls to Action*. Winnipeg, MB: Author. Retrieved from http://trc.ca/assets/pdf/Calls_to_Action_English2.pdf.

Zimmerman, B. J. (2002). Becoming a self-regulated learner: An overview. *Theory Into Practice, 41*(2), 64–70. https://doi.org/10.1207/s15430421tip4102_2.

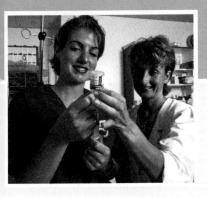

Monitoring Standards in Nursing Education

Cynthia Baker

e http://evolve.elsevier.com/Canada/Ross-Kerr/nursing

LEARNING OBJECTIVES

After reading this chapter, you will be able to:
- Describe the development of standards to monitor the quality of nursing education in Canada.
- Discuss the nature and role of quality assurance in higher education.
- Describe the accreditation and approval of nursing education programs in Canada.
- Examine the impact of quality assurance on nursing education in Canada.

OUTLINE

KEY TERMS

accreditation
approval
criteria
educational standards

institutional review
quality assurance

PERSONAL PERSPECTIVES

Standards for nursing education in Canada were initially created by nursing leaders to address the lack of evidence-informed education at hospital training schools. Introduced in 1874 by Dr. Mack at the St. Catharines General Hospital, the hospital training school was the dominant model for nursing education in Canada until the 1970s. Hospital training schools incorporated an apprenticeship approach to learning, which resulted in quality issues stemming from the use of student nurses for delivering most of the hospital's nursing services. Although the significant inadequacies of hospital-based training were well documented in the national Weir Report published in 1932, little changed. Nursing leaders in the first half of the twentieth century, however, were deeply concerned and advocated for separating the education of nurses from service.

In 1919, when hospital training schools still dominated nursing education, The University of British Columbia introduced the first baccalaureate program for nurses in Canada. In the following two decades, baccalaureate programs increased slowly but steadily across the country. In 1942, the heads of the university schools of nursing in Canada met in Montreal and created the Provisional Council of University Schools and Departments of Nursing, which later became the Canadian Association of Schools of Nursing. Key objectives adopted at this meeting were to promote additional baccalaureate programs for nurses and to develop national standards for nursing education. In 1957, the organization published *Desirable Standards for Nursing Education in Canada*. This document was the precursor of the national accreditation program for the baccalaureate programs of nursing launched in 1987. The goal of accrediting nursing education programs was, and continues to be, to foster high-quality nursing education in Canada in the interest of helping Canadians be healthy.

HISTORY OF THE DEVELOPMENT OF STANDARDS FOR NURSING EDUCATION

Standards for schools of nursing in Canada emerged over nearly half a century ago as a deliberate mechanism introduced by nursing leaders to improve nursing education nationally. The historical context of standard development for nursing education will be outlined in this chapter to provide a background on **quality assurance** mechanisms that emerged in nursing education.

Hospital Training Schools

Nursing education programs in Canada were originally developed in hospital schools of nursing primarily as a way to staff the hospitals. In 1874, Dr. Mack at St. Catharines General Hospital in Ontario established the first of these programs in the country and brought two of Florence Nightingale's instructors from England to help set it up (Pringle, Green, & Johnson, 2004). Although Florence Nightingale promoted independent schools of nursing that did not have any administrative or educational links to a hospital, the Mack Training School for Nurses led to an explosion of such hospital-based training programs across Canada. While Dr. Mack's purpose was to increase the educational preparation of nurses, hospital schools rapidly became the standard means of staffing hospitals, regardless of their size. The only registered nurses in the hospitals were the head nurses, supervisors, and the director of nursing. Nursing students received instruction from a few nurses, who taught courses like anatomy, physiology, and nursing arts (basic procedures) in the classroom, and from physicians, who taught courses about diseases and medical or surgical treatments. Clinical supervision of students was provided by head nurses and supervisors.

Hospital training schools in Canada continued to proliferate in the 1940s and early 1950s, despite the Weir Report's recommendations in 1932 that called for major reforms of nursing education and for nursing to be administered separately from the hospitals. Dr. Helen Mussallem, who was to become the executive director of the Canadian Nurses Association in 1963, began publishing research in 1957 that demonstrated significant issues with hospital-based nursing education in Canada. This work culminated in her groundbreaking study, commissioned by the landmark Royal Commission on Health Services (Mussallem, 1965). Chaired by Justice Emmett Hall, the commission itself resulted in the establishment of Canada's universal health care system (Hall, 1964) and also affected nursing education. Based on her research findings, Mussallem (1965) strongly recommended a shift from hospital training, and the Hall Commission identified an urgent need to restructure nursing education. The commission concluded that in light of the education in all other professions, the apprenticeship-type education system in nursing required examination. They therefore called for a complete separation of nursing education from nursing services. In the decades following the Royal Commission Report, jurisdictions across Canada moved nursing education from hospital training schools to universities and colleges.

Nursing leaders, such as Isabel Adams Hampton Robb and Mary Adelaide Nutting in the United States, recognized the need to monitor standards of education, and professional nursing associations in both the United States and Canada advocated for nurses to assume a monitoring role. Their goal was to devise a system involving **approval** for new nursing programs, the creation of standards for existing programs, and regular inspection to ensure that standards continued to be met.

University Education for Nurses

Despite the rapid growth and dominance of hospital training schools noted earlier, The University of British Columbia launched the first baccalaureate program in nursing in Canada in 1919, and five university certificate programs were initiated in 1920 (Kirkwood & Bouchard, 1992). During this period, nursing leaders saw university-based education of nurses as an opportunity for the profession to set standards to gain greater control over the quality of nursing education. As a result, university programs in nursing increased slowly but steadily across Canada between 1920 and 1949 (Kirkwood & Bouchard, 1992).

Nursing Education Standards

The creation of university schools of nursing in the first half of the nineteenth century led to the development of standards to monitor and improve the quality of nursing education. In September 1941, 14 university nursing educators representing eight universities met with executives of the Canadian Nurses Association at McGill University to discuss wartime needs but also "to seize the present opportunity to bring about some long-desired developments" (Kirkwood & Bouchard, 1992, p. 5). A second meeting of nursing educators representing 11 universities followed in June 1942, during which the Provisional Council of University Schools and Departments of Nursing was formed. This organization became the Canadian Association of University Schools of Nursing (CAUSN), and in 2002, the Canadian Association of Schools of Nursing (CASN).

At their inaugural meeting in June 1942, the small band of nursing educators who launched the association specified the following four objectives for their organization:

- Determine desirable standards for university schools of nursing to meet;
- Improve standards of existing schools;
- Support the development of new university programs of nursing; and
- Strengthen international relationships between university schools of nursing.

Ten years later, the association adopted its statutes and regulations, which identified the creation of standards for university schools of nursing as a key mandate of the organization. As a result, in 1957, the association published a precursor to a national **accreditation** program in a booklet titled *Desirable Standards for Canadian Schools*

of Nursing. These standards addressed the educational preparation of faculty, resources, classroom infrastructure, and teaching.

Hospital schools of nursing, which dominated nursing education in Canada for almost a century, no longer exist in any of the provinces. The phasing out of these programs began in the 1970s, when the governments of New Brunswick, Ontario, Quebec, and Saskatchewan closed their hospital schools. The remaining provinces with hospital schools phased them out during the 1980s and early 1990s. Initially, nursing education moved either to 4-year baccalaureate programs at universities or 2-year diploma programs at educational institutions offering higher education, such as community colleges. None of the territories had hospital schools, but there were college diploma programs in both the Northwest Territories and Nunavut. In 2004, these two territories joined forces to form the Registered Nurses Association of the Northwest Territories and Nunavut.

Immediately following the release of the Hall Commission Report, new baccalaureate programs of nursing were created in universities across the country. By 1988, all provinces except for Prince Edward Island, which offered only one diploma program, had developed one or more university programs. On November 9, 1988, the provincial government of Prince Edward Island announced a decision to phase out their diploma nursing education for the 4-year baccalaureate degree program, a move that was supported by the professional nursing association, nurses' unions, employers and educators alike ("Baccalaureate Education," 1989, p. 10). With the official opening of the baccalaureate degree in September 1992, Prince Edward Island became the first province in Canada to achieve the goal of a baccalaureate degree as the minimum preparation for entry into nursing. This represented the initial step in a move to the baccalaureate degree as entry to practice in all jurisdictions of Canada, except for Quebec.

The goal following the release of the commission's report was for about 25% of nurses to earn their baccalaureate degrees in preparation for administrative, supervisory, and instructor positions and for 75% of nurses to earn diplomas in preparation for bedside nursing (Mussallem, 1965). By the end of the 1970s, however, the entry-level education that nurses needed had become a major topic of debate among nursing organizations, regulators, educators, governments, and community colleges. With the increasing complexity of nursing care and the expansion of nursing roles, provincial and national nursing associations adopted positions in support of the baccalaureate degree as the entry-to-practice requirement. Jurisdictions across the country then began to adopt the baccalaureate as the entry-to-practice requirement for registered nurses. By 2000, this goal had been achieved across the country, with the exception of Quebec. However, to address an acute shortage of nurses, the Saskatchewan government reopened diploma seats briefly, as did the governments of Alberta and Manitoba.

An important factor facilitating the move to the baccalaureate as entry-to-practice requirement in several provinces was the establishment of collaborative baccalaureate programs of nursing offered jointly through partnerships between community colleges and universities. In 1985, for example, the University of Alberta and Red Deer College began planning a collaborative 4-year baccalaureate program that was later extended to include other schools in the province (Wood, 2011). In British Columbia, the University of Victoria, in partnership with the colleges offering nursing diploma programs, developed a joint collaborative degree program. Collaborations continued to grow throughout the Western provinces.

Similar changes unfolded in Central, Eastern, and Northern Canada. In Newfoundland, in the early 1990s, all college schools were collaborating with Memorial University, and Dalhousie began partnerships with two institutions that had offered diploma programs in 1995. The College of Nurses of Ontario adopted the degree as the entry requirement in 1998, with 2005 set as the effective date, and this decision was endorsed by the provincial cabinet in 2000. All 22 colleges in Ontario began developing collaborative programs in partnership with universities to meet the 2005 requirement. Colleges in the territories also established partnerships with degree institutions in the South. Aurora College, for example, in the Northwest Territories is in partnership with the University of Victoria. In New Brunswick, no provincial collaborations were established, as the diploma schools of nursing were closed in 1989, although the University of New Brunswick developed a collaborative partnership with Humber College in Ontario. The diploma schools in New Brunswick, however, were incorporated into the two universities in the province. Similarly, as already noted, Prince Edward Island phased out its sole diploma program entirely and replaced it with a 4-year university degree program.

QUALITY ASSURANCE IN HIGHER EDUCATION

Standards are at the heart of programs that assess and monitor the quality of higher education. What quality represents, however, is relative, and definitions of the concept are diverse. Harvey and Green (1993) grouped definitions of quality into five categories. In some definitions, quality means exceptional, connoting something special. In others,

quality is conceptualized as value for money, implying high standards at a low cost. A number of definitions of quality identify it as perfection, in which a set of specifications are met perfectly. For others, quality represents transformation. Finally, quality is also understood as fitness of purpose. Evaluations of higher education typically reflect a fitness of purpose understanding of quality, which is judged based on the extent to which a given purpose is met (Liu, 2016). Standards are developed to reflect the particular purpose specified. They may, however, range from minimal expectations to ideal depending on the objectives of the evaluation.

Standards for evaluating programs of higher education initially focused on inputs to education such as libraries, qualifications of faculty, and admission requirements. In the 1980s and 1990s, there was a move in the United States to review what students were learning and the outcomes of education programs as well as the structure and processes of these programs (Phillips, 2019). Thus, there has been a greater incorporation of outcomes in **educational standards** internationally. A study within social work, for example, examined self-efficacy as a student outcome within education programs (Holden, Barker, Rosenberg, & Onghena, 2007). Within nursing, entry-to-practice competencies are often an outcome of education programs that are assessed in a quality assurance review (College and Association of Registered Nurses of Alberta, 2008).

Although quality assurance in higher education is a relatively recent phenomenon, it has burgeoned in the last two decades in Canada and internationally. Currently, Canadian nursing education programs may be assessed and monitored through several such systems. These include internal **institutional reviews**, external evaluations conducted by regional or provincial/territorial governments, accreditation reviews by the national CASN accreditation program, and reviews by provincial/territorial regulatory bodies through approval processes.

INSTITUTIONAL REVIEWS, ACCREDITATION, AND APPROVAL

Internal and government reviews of education are concerned with assuring the academic quality of departments, schools, and faculties of higher education. As universities are autonomous in academic matters, they determine their own quality assurance standards and procedures and couple their review with an external assessment based on the relevant provincial quality assurance mechanisms. **Accreditation** of nursing programs fosters continuous quality improvement as well as quality assurance. It is a national and voluntary process used by many health and other professions to monitor and enhance the quality of professional education. It is also used to monitor and enhance the quality of service agencies, such as hospitals, long-term care facilities, and home care organizations. Provincial approval processes for nursing education are a regulatory and legislative mechanism to support the public protection mandate of health professional regulation. In contrast with accreditation, program approval is a legislated and regulatory process that is unique to nursing, conducted in provinces and territories in Canada and in state jurisdictions in the United States. In the next section, each of these quality assurance mechanisms will be examined in greater detail and situated in a broader context.

Institutional and External Reviews

Higher education in Canada falls under provincial and territorial jurisdiction, and universities receive the authority to grant degrees from provincial legislation, although a few universities still retain charters. The university itself determines the standards and processes for conducting an institutional review of departments and faculties, and the province sets the quality assurance mechanism of the accompanying external review. There is, however, national support for a Canadian Degree Qualifications Framework and thus a shared understanding of quality in higher education across the country. Thus, Canadian universities develop and maintain periodic internal quality assurance policies and procedures, developed within the framework of external reviews required by provincial or regional authorities, that reflect the national Canadian Degree Qualifications Framework.

The internal quality assurance policies and procedures of the university focus on its academic programs. Typically, these policies and procedures include an assessment of the program's curriculum and the satisfaction of its students and involve a self-evaluation and a review by peers. As these periodic reviews apply to all programs offered by the university, baccalaureate, master's, and doctoral programs in nursing must undergo such assessments.

Guidelines of Good Practice in Accreditation

Accreditation of schools and education programs is a national external quality review process to systematically assess academic institutions and academic programs against a predetermined set of standards or **criteria**. It is recognized and promoted internationally as a key mechanism to advance the quality of health professional education. The landmark *Lancet* study by Frenk, Chen, Bhutta et al., (2010), for example, identified accreditation as a key process for transforming health professional education in order to strengthen health care systems. Similarly, the World Health Organization's (WHO) international guidelines for transforming and scaling up health professional education

state that national accreditation programs of health professional education and training should be introduced where they do not exist, and strengthened where they do (World Health Organization, 2013, p. 14).

In some countries, accreditation of health professional education is undertaken by a government ministry or agency. In Canada, as in the United States, accreditation is "outside of the government structure and is focused on professionally driven standards carried out in nongovernmental associations" (Phillips, 2019, p. 2). The *Guidelines for Good Practice* of the Association of Accrediting Agencies of Canada (2015) specify that an accreditation agency must incorporate the principles of both quality assurance and continuous quality improvement into their program. To achieve the latter, the criteria or standards and procedures should consider the school's internal mechanisms for addressing unmet expectations, as well as provide effective follow-up on the outcomes of the external review (International Network for Quality Assurance Agencies in Higher Education [INQAAHE], 2016).

Both national and international guidelines emphasize that an accreditation review process must be transparent, fair, and objective and respect confidentiality. The process must also include a self-assessment and an on-site peer review conducted by reviewers who both meet the qualifications defined by the agency and have completed a reviewer training program (INQAAHE, 2016). Moreover, best practice guidelines specify that accreditation decision making must be an independent process carried out by a panel of appropriately qualified decision makers who assess and measure institutions and education programs objectively in relation to predetermined expectations (INQAAHE, 2016).

Accreditation is not only a systematic evaluation process, but also a time-defined status that notifies the public that an institution or program has met accepted national standards of quality (Phillips, 2019, p. 1). Accreditation therefore promotes accountability of education programs to consumers and stakeholders. For example, the accreditation of a given education program provides assurance to prospective students that the program they are applying for has met national standards. Similarly, the public is assured that the school produces health professionals who have received the educational preparation they need for professional practice.

As accreditation standards represent the quality expectations for an educational institution its curriculum, and student outcomes, the standards must incorporate the perspectives of educators, educational institutions, regulators, practitioners, and employers in the professional field (Phillips, 2019). The creation and revision of accreditation standards, therefore, must be informed by an ongoing dialogue among educators, assessors, professional associations, and regulatory bodies (Phillips, 2019). The *Guidelines of Good Practice* developed by the INQAAHE (2016) explicitly specify that the standards or criteria must have been subject to reasonable consultation with stakeholders and must also be revised at regular intervals to ensure relevance.

Accreditation of Nursing Education

In 1972, the CASN was designated the national accrediting agency for baccalaureate programs of nursing. It was not until 1987, however, that the first baccalaureate program of nursing was accredited at the faculty of nursing at the Université de Montréal (Kirkwood & Bouchard, 1992). The work of developing the standards for the program was carried out by a highly engaged committee living in different provinces at a time when there was no email, Dropbox, teleconferencing, or funding for travel and very few existing accreditation programs in Canada. By 1994, however, the program was well established, and 12 baccalaureate programs of nursing had been accredited (McBride, 1994). In 2002, the number had increased to 30. Although initially most of the programs seeking accreditation were in Ontario, Quebec, and Nova Scotia, there was a steady increase in accredited programs across the country. As of 2019, 105 baccalaureate programs of nursing located in every province of Canada as well as the Northwest Territories were accredited. Accredited programs are posted on the CASN accreditation website and receive a certificate. Schools also receive a seal that they may post on their website indicating that a given program is accredited.

In addition to the accreditation of baccalaureate programs of nursing, the CASN has recently developed an accreditation program for bridging programs aimed at internationally educated nurses (IENs) as part of a project sponsored and funded by Health Canada. The purpose of creating this program was to address inconsistencies in IEN bridging programs and to promote national standards. As a result, a number of bridging programs are now accredited. The CASN is also launching a national accreditation program for master's and post-master's nurse practitioner programs and, in collaboration with the Canadian Association of Practical Nurse Educators (CAPNE), an accreditation program for practical nurses. It does not currently, however, offer accreditation of master's or doctoral programs.

⚇ APPLYING CONTENT KNOWLEDGE

Do you think accreditation should be offered for master's and doctoral programs? Why or why not?

Evolution of the Accreditation Program

CASN accreditation of baccalaureate programs was introduced for two main reasons: (1) to support and improve standards of baccalaureate and graduate nursing programs in CASN member schools and (2) to recognize programs that have been reviewed and met specific standards (Canadian Association of Schools of Nursing [CASN], 1989, p. 1). A major objective guiding the initial development of the accreditation program was to identify criteria that would ensure an education program was preparing practitioners who could deal effectively not only with existing problems but also with future health problems (French, 1982, p. 2). The vision guiding the initiative was to promote nursing education that was responsive to societal needs with criteria that would support curricular development and change (French, 1982). To this end, Dr. Moyra Allen at McGill University developed the initial criterion-based framework for the accreditation program. Three guiding criteria were selected: (1) relevance, which referred to the trends in society that have an impact on the health needs of the community; (2) accountability, defined as the extent to which the program teaches students that the primary responsibility in nursing is to the patient; and (3) relatedness, the extent to which parts of the program support and build on other parts, thereby promoting the achievement of goals. A fourth criterion, uniqueness, was subsequently adopted. Uniqueness was defined as "the extent to which a program capitalizes on the resources within its particular setting" (Canadian Association of University Schools of Nursing, 1978, p. 3).

In 2002, with the advent of collaborative programs and the move to the baccalaureate degree as the entry-to-practice requirement in most Canadian jurisdictions, a national accreditation task force was struck to conduct an extensive review of the accreditation program. This resulted in the adoption of a major change in 2005. The new framework was organized around two sets of standards, one concerned with the educational unit and the other with the education program. The educational unit incorporates the administrative structures, processes, and resources supporting a nursing education program as well as the internal and external environment in which it is delivered (CASN, 2015). In the case of collaborative programs, each institution offering the program is considered to be an educational unit and is assessed against the standards. The education program standards incorporate the curriculum and program framework, program evaluation and program outcomes (CASN, 2015).

The basic philosophy underpinning the initial development of the accreditation program continued to guide it and the four criteria developed by Dr. Allen provide the quality dimension of the accreditation standards. Thus, respect for the uniqueness of education programs remains a key quality expectation, as does the accountability of graduates, the interconnectedness of the program and the program structure, as well as the current relevance of the program and its administrative structure.

In terms of relevance, the Truth and Reconciliation Commission of Canada (2015) specifically addresses entry-level nursing education, calling for an urgent and major response from schools across the country. As a result, the CASN Baccalaureate Accreditation Program has threaded expectations for nursing education based on the report, particularly in standards related to the curriculum and to teaching and learning. These standards address Call to Action 24, for example, which states that all nursing students must learn about Indigenous health issues and Indigenous teachings and practice. In addition, in order to engage in relationships that are authentic, reciprocal, and meaningful, Dr. Lisa Bourque Bearskin (2016), representing the Aboriginal Nurses Association of Canada (which has since become the Canadian Indigenous Nurses Association), emphasized that nursing graduates need knowledge and skills in intercultural competency, human rights, and anti-racism, all of which are incorporated in the accreditation standards.

Many schools of nursing in Canada offer more than one baccalaureate program. For example, schools of nursing may offer a 4-year program, a program for practical nurses to become baccalaureate-prepared nurses, and a shorter advanced standing baccalaureate program for students who have already completed a degree in another discipline. For the purpose of an accreditation review, a nursing education program is defined as "a course of study that has a single and unique university degree conferred on the student by a single degree-granting institution, a single curriculum framework, and a single sequence of defined courses with single course descriptions and specified options that are designed to meet a single and specified set of program outcomes" (CASN, 2015, p. 7). If an institution or a collaboration undergoing an accreditation review offers more than one baccalaureate program meeting this definition, each one is assessed against the education program standards and receives a separate accreditation decision (CASN, 2015).

The standards of both the educational unit and education program are broad statements of expectations that are followed by descriptors—which provide more detail to further delineate them—and then key elements—which are the observable and measurable qualitative or quantitative indicators of the standard. In addition, an interpretation of each key element identifies the types of evidence that would demonstrate that the key element is being met. The extent to which the key elements of a given standard are

being met determines whether the standard is judged to be met, partially met, or unmet (CASN, 2015).

Because many baccalaureate programs were being offered collaboratively by universities and colleges, it was decided that a separate accreditation decision should be made for the educational unit standards and for the education program standards. In the case of collaboratively delivered programs, each education unit is reviewed and receives its own accreditation decision; the collaborative program, however, is assessed against the education program standards and receives a single accreditation decision that applies to the program in all educational units involved in delivering this program (CASN, 2015).

Reviews and revisions of the baccalaureate accreditation program were carried out on an ad hoc basis between 1987 and 2009. In 2012, however, a policy was adopted that the Advisory Committee on Accreditation Policy—a standing committee of the CASN with representation from education, regulation, employers, and other health professions—must conduct a major review involving national stakeholder consultation every 7 years to ensure the relevance of the program and propose updates if needed. Proposed changes of the accreditation standards resulting from such a review are adopted by the CASN Council at the annual general meeting of the association.

The nurse practitioner and the practical nurse accreditation programs are based on the same framework of standards as the baccalaureate program. However, the interpretation and evidence requirements may differ. For example, schools must demonstrate that the entry-to-practice competencies specified by the school's jurisdictional regulatory body are integrated into the curriculum. But the competencies for each nursing group may differ. For instance, the standards for IEN bridging programs are specific to bridging programs. The standards are based on an extensive literature review; an extensive national consultation among multiple stakeholders to determine the quality expectations for this particular type of nursing education program; and a national stakeholder evaluation of the standards.

Decision Making

The CASN Accreditation Bureau (CAB) is the decision-making body for the CASN accreditation program. While it must function within the regulations and in compliance with the policies of the Association, CAB operates at arm's length from the CASN Board of Directors, and from the CASN Council to ensure the independence of accreditation decisions. No member of the Board of Directors nor of Council may be a member of the accreditation bureau. Moreover, there is a formal, independent appeal process, and the governance bodies of the CASN may not interfere in any way with an accreditation decision made by CAB.

The accreditation bureau is a standing committee of the CASN Council and consists of 10 members. Five are selected through formal processes from the following constituencies: regulation, service agencies, faculty of other health professions, students, and the community at large; another five are chosen from among nursing faculty elected by member schools at Council. One elected faculty member is officially designated bilingual, but there is a requirement that at least five members of CAB be sufficiently bilingual to read and review comprehensive reports written in French. All members of CAB act and vote as individuals and not as representatives of a given group.

Monitoring the Quality of Collaborative Programs

As noted, the major revisions of the CASN accreditation program adopted in 2005 were in part a response to the unique challenges of monitoring the quality of collaborative nursing education programs. The collaborative programs themselves identified issues with maintaining the quality of their education programs. These often stemmed from the differing cultures, priorities, goals, and aspirations of the colleges and universities that entered into collaboration. In 2004, Molzahn and Purkis identified challenges based on their experience in a collaboration in British Columbia. These challenges stemmed from major differences in the cultures of universities and colleges: universities are traditionally committed to promoting scholarship and research, while colleges focus strongly on providing access to opportunity. These differences could lead to challenges with coming to an agreement on academic policy, such as admission criteria and standards for progressing through the program.

Orchard (2004) stressed the importance of national standards to foster high-quality programs across the country to meet current and future health care needs, regardless of whether the educational delivery model was a collaborative program or a standalone university model. Strategies recommended to enhance collaborations included clear legal agreements between the institutions to address mutual expectations in advance. Another issue identified as critical was the need for collaborative partners to reach agreement on evaluation and review processes to monitor and demonstrate quality (Molzahn & Purkis, 2004).

Relationships Among Accreditation Agencies

In 1994, the CASN was among the founding members of the Association of Accreditation Agencies in Canada (AAAC), and the association continues to participate as a member of this organization. AAAC currently has a membership of 27 national accrediting bodies of professional education. The AAAC determines the guidelines for good practice in accreditation in Canada and also provides its members with an online reviewer training program. All CASN reviewers complete this general program as well as a supplementary training provided by the CASN that is specific to the CASN accreditation review process and program.

In 2008, a mutual recognition agreement was established between the CASN accreditation program and the Commission on Collegiate Nursing Education (CCNE), an autonomous accreditation agency in the United States. The accreditation program is reviewed and renewed on a regular basis, most recently in 2016. The CCNE program was created by the American Association of Colleges of Nursing (AACN), although it operates independently of the AACN. This mutual recognition is helpful to graduates of accredited programs in Canada or the United States applying to master's or doctoral programs in the other country.

Accreditation Costs

When the CASN accreditation program was being developed, a concern for its founders was how it should be financed. In 1977, the CASN submitted a proposal to the W.K. Kellogg Foundation for possible funding; however, support was not obtained. The foundation was approached again in 1979, but by 1980, there were strong indications that support would not be forthcoming. Consequently, the CASN proceeded with plans to implement the program, and a special fee that was assessed to all university nursing programs was kept in reserve to support accreditation. When the CASN first implemented the accreditation program in 1987, each school was charged an additional fee based on an estimate of the amount of involvement of the association with the nursing program. It was soon recognized that a more structured and systematic funding approach was needed, so the CASN Council decided that the program should be implemented on a cost-recovery basis. To do so, the CASN's annual membership fees includes a fee to support the accreditation program. In addition, the CASN also established a fee schedule for schools that undergo accreditation reviews. These fees have not been increased since 2006. In addition, a school or a collaboration undergoing an accreditation review pays the costs of travel and lodging for the review team (CASN, 2008).

Besides the cost of the accreditation review, the process can also be time consuming for schools, which is a cost in itself. Completing a self-study report, organizing the reviewers' site visit, and hosting a review team represent additional demands on staff, faculty, and administrators. This process has been monitored since the accreditation program was first developed. Although the plan was to create an accreditation program that could be implemented with minimal effort, cost, and time, an early evaluation of the program reported that the schools found the self-study process to be very time consuming, "even though it increased awareness and stimulated discussion about the programme among faculty and students" (Thomas, Arseneault, Bouchard et al., 1992, p. 41). Thomas and Arseneault (1992) concurred that the self-study is time consuming and increases faculty workload, but noted that schools also found the process rewarding because it fosters self-development and quality improvement.

Schools continue to report that preparing for an accreditation review is time consuming, although less so than in the past, and also that they find the process to be valuable. In the last decade, efforts to streamline and reduce the demands on schools have included a paperless program with documents transmitted electronically through secure portals, electronic templates with guidelines to facilitate documentation of the self-study, and an accreditation 101 course for schools to assist them with preparing for an accreditation review.

Approval of Nursing Education

In Canada, constitutional responsibility for education, the delivery of health care, and the regulation of health professions rests with the individual provinces and territories. Consequently, policies and mechanisms for monitoring standards in nursing education may be defined by each province. This responsibility is delineated in legislation that regulates the profession. In all provinces except Quebec, responsibility for monitoring standards in nursing education has been assumed by the provincial/territorial regulatory body. Approval is, therefore, a mandatory process carried out by provincial/territorial regulatory nursing bodies as part of their public protection mandate. The focus of approval is often on ensuring that entry-to-practice competencies are met and that patient safety is ensured, but there has been considerable diversity from one jurisdiction to another. Moreover, frameworks and approaches to approval have changed over time.

The approval mechanism was designed to ensure compliance with the minimum standards required to adequately prepare students to enter practice. What constitutes both minimal standards and adequate preparation, however, has been controversial. In the days when almost all nursing students were hired in the hospitals where they had been trained, few questions were asked about the adequacy of their preparation or minimal standards. Hospital training emphasized mastery of tasks, procedures, and the ability to perform these in a given hospital setting at the time. As the profession of nursing became more complex, it was clear to most educators that more in-depth learning was needed. The requirement for comprehensive patient assessments, patient monitoring, clinical reasoning, communication, collaboration, teamwork, patient advocacy, and patient safety were critical aspects of the new registered nurse student's education and contextual to the various places where

a nurse might work, so a variety of exposure was required. Nurses did not remain in the hospitals where they trained for as long, and thus the seamless transition from student to registered nurse among hospital-trained nurses was less and less achievable. Although there has been general acknowledgement that new graduates are not expert practitioners, what should be expected of them has been subject to considerable research and debate. Transition-to-practice theory (Duchscher, 2018) has been used extensively to guide acute-care residency programs in the United States. Developed through a series of studies of new graduates employed in Canadian hospitals, the theory is based on evidence that 12 months is approximately the length of time that a new graduate needs to integrate the professional role of a registered nurse and become a competent member of the interprofessional team.

In the last decade, three approaches have been used in the approval of nursing education programs in Canada. In one, the regulatory body develops approval standards, conducts the review of the nursing programs in its jurisdiction, determines whether or not the programs are approved, and monitors this process. In the second, there is a blended or integrated approach with the CASN accreditation program for baccalaureate programs of nursing. In this approach, the CASN accreditation process and standards are used for the approval program, but the approval decision is made by the regulatory body independently of the accreditation decision, and this decision reflects the regulatory mandate. In the third approach, the CASN accreditation program and the CASN accreditation decision provide the process, standards, and approval decision for the regulatory body.

In recent years, baccalaureate programs of nursing have tended to follow the second integrated approach, in which accreditation and approval are carried out jointly using the CASN accreditation program, but with the regulatory body making the approval decision. In 2005, the College of Registered Nurses of Nova Scotia was the first to develop and implement this joint accreditation–approval process. The memorandum of understanding is reviewed and revised on a regular basis, with the most recent being signed in 2016. The Association of Registered Nurses of Newfoundland and Labrador adopted a similar blended process in 2008, in which the CASN accreditation program is used as the basis for approval, but with provisions to evaluate additional requirements consistent with the regulatory mandate. More recently, a memorandum of understanding for an integrated approach was agreed on by the CASN and the Saskatchewan Registered Nurses Association in 2015, the College of Registered Nurses of Manitoba in 2018, and the College and Association of Registered Nurses of Alberta in 2019. An integrated approach will be piloted in New Brunswick as the result of an agreement signed in 2019.

In contrast to these other regulatory bodies, the College of Nurses of Ontario (CNO)—which fulfills the registration and discipline functions for the three regulated nursing groups in Ontario—changed accreditation models in January 2019. The CNO moved from a model in which the CASN accreditation program and accreditation decision served as the approval program for baccalaureate education in Ontario to an independent approval program for the three regulated nursing groups (registered practical nurses, registered nurses, and nurse practitioners) in their jurisdiction. In 2000, when the baccalaureate degree became the entry-to-practice requirement for registered nurses, the CNO voted to designate the CASN accreditation program to supplant program approval in Ontario, and a memorandum of understanding was signed with the CASN in 2001. With the growth of education programs for both registered practical nurses and nurse practitioners in Ontario, the CNO initiated approval programs for each of these, which then led to the development of an approval framework that would be applicable to the nursing education programs for each of the three regulated nursing groups. The program structure, processes, and outcomes provide the organizing framework for the approval program standards (College of Nurses of Ontario, 2019).

The College of Nurses of British Columbia also implements an approval program for baccalaureate programs of nursing in the province that is independent of CASN accreditation. However, to reduce duplication of effort, a joint committee mapped the standards of the accreditation program with the standards of the approval program so that a recently accredited program is not evaluated on the overlapping standards. This policy was enacted in 2013.

The approval process, when conducted independently of a CASN accreditation review, typically involves the submission of a self-study report, documentary evidence related to specified approval standards, or both. This step of the process is followed by an on-site visit or interviews by teleconference conducted by persons designated by the regulatory body. Reviewer findings are reported to the regulatory body, and final approval decisions are made by the council of the college or association.

IMPACT OF QUALITY ASSURANCE ON NURSING EDUCATION

Nursing education standards delineate and clarify quality expectations for education programs; the evaluation of nursing education programs against these standards fosters quality improvement. The impact of standards in several areas of the CASN accreditation program provide examples of such quality improvement.

An important question raised in the past concerned the effect of accreditation on research productivity. The process of accreditation in itself was not found to promote research without the inclusion of standards related to research productivity. Since the adoption of the 2005 accreditation program, CASN accreditation standards have explicitly emphasized faculty scholarship as well as institutional support for faculty scholarship (CASN, 2015). As a result, over the last 10 years there has been a steady growth in research activities and in the dissemination of research findings among programs undergoing an accreditation review. This growth has been especially evident among college partners of collaborative programs and among non-research-intensive universities, where scholarship is not typically supported or fostered by the institution.

Accreditation standards related to interprofessional education (IPE) have promoted the introduction of IPE in curricula, not only in nursing but also in six other health professions in Canada. In 2008, Health Canada funded phase one of an initiative to promote the integration of IPE in health professional education. This initiative brought together eight accreditation organizations for six professions: medicine, nursing, pharmacy, physical therapy, occupational therapy, and social work. Guiding principles were developed by the accrediting bodies for the integration of interprofessional education into accreditation programs. In phase two, explicit guidelines for developing accreditation interprofessional education standards were created, and each of the accreditation organizations, including nursing, adapted and integrated these into their respective programs (Interprofessional Education Collaborative, 2019). As a result, a pan-Canadian approach developed through interprofessional collaborations is being used to foster IPE in programs of nursing. Although IPE has increased significantly in nursing education, there has been no evaluation of the impact of this approach on the collaborative practice of graduates of these programs.

> **APPLYING CONTENT KNOWLEDGE**
>
> Have you been part of an accreditation process in your nursing education? What do you think the process would be like? Challenges and benefits?

Although the monitoring and assessment of nursing education programs in Canada by external bodies has enhanced the programs' quality, as noted earlier, the demands of providing reports and producing the required evidence has increased the workload of faculty, staff, and administrators in Canadian schools of nursing. However, these schools are not alone in their experience. While quality assurance of higher education is recent, it has grown substantially around the world, as has the need for individual programs to undergo multiple reviews (Council for Higher Education Accreditation, 2016). As a result, institutions of higher education in a number of countries have called for less time-consuming processes to ensure and enhance quality. Greater collaboration among quality assurance programs is being proposed to reduce some of the demand, and this approach has been promoted in the assessment and monitoring of nursing education in Canada. In addition, the international quality principles put forward by the Council for Higher Education Accreditation (2016) suggest that in the future there will be a move to more streamlined external reviews and less in-depth retesting of standards that were well met in the previous review. In light of these international principles, the CASN accreditation program is currently piloting processes to streamline accreditation by simplifying evidence requirements and removing unnecessary demands on schools while maintaining the rigour and quality of the accreditation review (Baker, 2019).

CONCLUSION

Canadian nurses and nursing bodies have long upheld a commitment to promoting high-quality nursing education through the creation of standards, the assessment of schools of nursing against these standards, and the evaluation of nursing education programs as part of quality improvement and quality assurance measures. Although the accreditation process imposes financial and time demands on nursing schools, evaluations of the accreditation process indicate that it is valued for the quality enhancement it produces and for the public recognition it brings. As part of their

mandate to protect the public, regulatory bodies in Canada are similarly committed to ensuring that nursing education programs comply with regulatory standards. Although evaluation of the quality of nursing education originally targeted entry programs for registered nurses, education standards of other regulated nursing groups are now being monitored by accreditation and approval mechanisms.

> ### APPLYING CONTENT KNOWLEDGE
>
> 1. Why are standards for nursing education programs important for nursing students?
> 2. How could the process of accreditation and institutional program review be streamlined without abandoning the goal of quality?
> 3. What role should nursing students play when the nursing program they are enrolled in is under review?

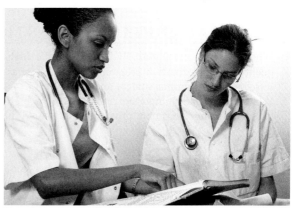

(istockphoto.com/Simone van den Berg)

SUMMARY OF LEARNING OBJECTIVES

- The development of standards for nursing education arose from the desire of nursing leaders to address quality issues with hospital training schools for nursing.
- The introduction of standards for nursing education in 1957 was associated with advocacy by the leadership of the profession for nursing education to be provided by educational institutions separately from nursing service.
- The concept of quality is relative, and quality assurance has multiple definitions. In the evaluation of programs of higher education, quality is often understood to refer to fitness of purpose.
- Standards and criteria are developed to monitor quality. They articulate predetermined expectations about quality. Programs, services, and institutions are assessed against these expectations.

- Nursing education programs in Canada are monitored for quality through a number of mechanisms, including institutional reviews, accreditation, and approval.
- Accreditation is a national process used around the world to monitor the quality of professional education and other services such as health care institutions. It is recognized internationally as a key mechanism to improve the quality of health professional education in a given country.
- National guidelines for good practices in accreditation are published by the Association of Accreditation Agencies of Canada and internationally by the International Network for Quality Assurance Agencies in Higher Education.
- The Canadian Association of Schools of Nursing (CASN), which became the accrediting body for

baccalaureate degree programs of nursing in 1972, first implemented the program in 1987. As of 2019, there are 105 accredited baccalaureate degree programs of nursing in Canada.

- The CASN recently launched an accreditation program for bridging programs for internationally educated nurses. The CASN is also piloting an accreditation program for nurse practitioner programs and practical nurse programs.
- Approval of nursing education programs is carried out by provincial/territorial nursing regulatory bodies in support of their public protection mandate, based on legislation in their jurisdiction.
- Three approval approaches have been used in Canada in the last decade. (1) An independent approach—the regulatory body independently develops approval standards and conducts a review of programs in its

jurisdiction. (2) A blended or integrated approach with CASN accreditation—the CASN standards and process are used but the regulatory body is engaged in the process. The process may include additional standards, and the regulatory body makes an approval decision that is independent of the accreditation decision. (3) The CASN accreditation program—the CASN accreditation decision provides the process, standards, and approval decision for the regulatory body.

- Assessment of education programs against predetermined quality expectations is a mechanism that fosters quality improvement.
- Over the last decade, the effects of accreditation standards related to scholarship and interprofessional education demonstrate the impact that monitoring standards can have in promoting continuing quality improvement.

CRITICAL THINKING QUESTIONS

1. What are the most important indicators of a high-quality nursing education program that should be assessed to ensure optimal student outcomes?
2. What are the most important indicators of a high-quality nursing education program that should be

assessed to ensure optimal outcomes for employers of new graduates?
3. How does an accreditation review benefit nursing students both present and future?

REFERENCES

Association of Accrediting Agencies of Canada. (2015). *Guidelines for good practice.* Retrieved from http://www.otapta.ca/pdfs/Home/Guidelines%20for%20Good%20Practice%20-%20Final%20March%202015.pdf.

Baccalaureate education comes to PEI. (1989). *The Canadian Nurse, 85*(3), 10. Retrieved from https://www.canadian-nurse.com/.

Baker, C. (2019). *Executive Director's report to Council.* Retrieved from https://www.casn.ca/2019/11/executive-director-annual-report/.

Bourque Bearskin, R. L. (2016, March 1). Through the lens of truth and reconciliation: Next steps. *Canadian Nurse.* Retrieved from https://www.canadian-nurse.com/en/articles/issues/2016/march-2016/through-the-lens-of-truth-and-reconciliation-next-steps.

Canadian Association of Schools of Nursing. (1989, September). *CASN Newsletter.* Ottawa, ON: Author.

Canadian Association of Schools of Nursing. (2008). *Accreditation.* Ottawa, ON: Author. Retrieved from https://www.casn.ca/accreditation/casn-and-accreditation/.

Canadian Association of Schools of Nursing. (2015). *CASN accreditation program manual.* Ottawa, ON: Author. Retrieved from www.casn.ca.

Canadian Association of University Schools of Nursing. (1978). *Development of a method to promote growth and change in university schools of nursing and nursing in general.* Ottawa, ON: Author.

College and Association of Registered Nurses of Alberta. (2008). (KEEP) *Continuing Competence Program.* Retrieved from http://www.nurses.ab/CARNA.

College of Nurses of Ontario. (2019). *Nursing education program approval.* Retrieved from http://www.cno.org/en/become-a-nurse/nursing-education-program-approval/.

Council for Higher Education Accreditation. (2016). *International quality principles: Toward a shared understanding of quality.* Retrieved from https://www.chea.org/sites/default/files/pdf/Principles_Papers_Complete_web.pdf.

Duchscher, J. B. (2018). Stages of transition and transition shock. *Nurses Professional Development, 34*(4), 228–232. https://doi.org/10.1097/NND.0000000000000461.

French, S. (1982). Design for accreditation of educational programs in nursing. In M. S. Henderson (Ed.), *Recent advances in nursing No. 4: Nursing education* (pp. 81–102). London, UK: Churchill Livingstone.

Frenk, J., Chen, L., Bhutta, Z. A., et al. (2010). Health professional education for a new century: Transforming education to strengthen health systems in an interdependent world. *The Lancet, 376*, 1923–1958. https://doi.org/10.1016/S0140-6736(10)61854-5.

Holden, G., Barker, K., Rosenberg, G., & Onghena, P. (2007). Assessing progress toward accreditation raised objectives: Evidence regarding the use of self-efficacy as an outcome in the advanced research concentration curriculum. *Research on Social Work Practice, 17*(4), 456–465.

International Network for Quality Assurance Agencies of Higher Education. (2016). *Guidelines of good practice.* Retrieved from www.inqaahe.org/guidelines-good-practice.

Interprofessional Education Collaborative. (2019). *Vision and mission.* Retrieved from https://www.ipecollaborative.org.

Kirkwood, R., & Bouchard, J. (1992). *"Take counsel with one another": A beginning history of the Canadian Association of University Schools of Nursing, 1942–1992.* Ottawa, ON: Canadian Association of University Schools of Nursing.

Hall, E. (1964). *Royal commission on health services.* Ottawa, ON: Government of Canada.

Harvey, L., & Green, D. (1993). Define quality. *Assessment and Evaluation in Higher Education, 18*(1), 9–34.

Liu, S. (2016). Quality assurance and institutional transformation (pp. 15-46). In *Higher education quality assessment and university change: A theoretical approach.* Singapore: Springer. https://doi.org/10.1007/978-981-10-0789-7_2.

McBride, W. (1994, Summer). Executive director's message. *CASN Newsletter,* 2–3.

Molzahn, A. E., & Purkis, M. E. (2004). Collaborative nursing education programs: Challenges and issues. *Canadian Journal of Nursing Leadership, 17*(4), 41–55.

Mussallem, H. (1965). *Nursing education in Canada.* Ottawa, ON: Royal Commission on Health Services.

Orchard, C. (2004). Commentary: The case for national standards. *Canadian Journal of Nursing Leadership, 17*(4), 54–55. https://doi.org/10.12927/cjnl.2004.20313.

Phillips, S. (2019). *Accreditation: Realities, challenges, and opportunities.* Retrieved from https://www.ncbi.nih.gov/books/NBK435959.

Pringle, D., Green, L., & Johnson, S. (2004). *Nursing education in Canada: Historical review and current capacity.* Ottawa, ON: Nursing Sector Study Corporation. Retrieved from https://www.mycna.ca/~/media/nurseone/page-content/pdf-en/nursing_education_canada_e.pdf.

Thomas, B., & Arseneault, A. (1992). Organizing your school for accreditation. *Canadian Journal of Nursing Research, 24*(2), 58–59. Retrieved from https://cjnr.archive.mcgill.ca/article/view/1153.

Thomas, B., Arseneault, A., Bouchard, J., et al. (1992). Accreditation of university nursing programmes in Canada. *Canadian Journal of Nursing Research, 24*(2), 33–48.

Truth and Reconciliation Commission of Canada. (2015). *Truth and Reconciliation Commission of Canada: Calls to action.* Retrieved from http://trc.ca/assets/pdf/Calls_to_Action_English2.pdf.

Wood, M. (2011). *Survey of nursing education in Canada.* Toronto, ON: University of Toronto Press.

World Health Organization. (2013). *Transforming and scaling up health professionals' education and training.* Retrieved from https://www.who.int/hrh/resources/transf_scaling_hpet/en/?.

PART V

Canadian and International Nursing

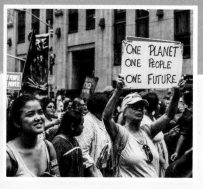

25

Global Nursing: Emerging Issues and Events Locally and Beyond

Barbara Astle

e http://evolve.elsevier.com/Canada/Ross-Kerr/nursing

LEARNING OBJECTIVES

After reading this chapter, you will be able to:
- Describe the impact of key health-related issues on health systems and health status globally.
- Discuss the impact of recent global nursing events on the evolution of the nursing profession.
- Identify and discuss the major national health issues affecting the nursing profession in Canada.
- Discuss the contribution of national nursing initiatives led by Canadians.

OUTLINE

KEY TERMS

Anthropocene epoch
antimicrobial resistance
antimicrobial stewardship
climate change
COVID-19
Ebola
H1N1

health equity
immigration
migration
noncommunicable diseases
novel coronavirus
opioid misuse
pandemic

planetary health
refugee
SARS
superbugs
Sustainable Development Goals
vaping

PERSONAL PERSPECTIVES

Climate Change—What is Nursing's Role?

As a student nurse, I learned about **planetary health** as it relates to **climate change** in my global health course. During the summer, working in Northern British Columbia as an employed student nurse, I started to understand how climate change affected me as a nurse and the health of the community. The location where I was working was experiencing forest fires so severe and uncontrollable that they impacted the air quality index. Consequently, I noticed an increase in the number of children and older persons with respiratory symptoms being admitted to our rural hospital. At the nursing station, we were discussing how changes in the environment, brought on by the fires, directly influenced the health of the community at large. I asked the question, How do you think this relates to climate change? This led to an in-depth conversation about the importance of understanding the effects of climate change and its impact on human health and the health of our planet. Also, what can Canadian nurses do to influence climate change at a local level that will have an impact globally?

INTRODUCTION

This chapter focuses on the key local and global issues, events, and various initiatives where the nursing profession in Canada has played a key role in facilitating further understanding locally, nationally, and globally in the twenty-first century. It is critical that nurses, in their role of promoting social justice and the achievement of **health equity** as a primary goal, understand the implications for nursing practice within diverse populations in Canada and also appreciate the responsibilities and potential contributions that Canadian nurses make globally. Health equity refers to the "absence of systematic disparities in health (and its key social determinants) that are systematically associated with social advantage/disadvantage" (Braveman & Gruskin, 2003, p. 256).

GLOBAL IMPACT OF KEY HEALTH-RELATED ISSUES ON THE HEALTH SYSTEM

Pandemics

Awareness of the need to plan for, and expect, global and national pandemics has always been a concern in global health. In the past few decades, the world has witnessed a number of pandemics that have made us realize more than ever that we are only a "plane ride away" from being affected (Lees, 2015; Skolnik, 2021). A **pandemic** is defined as the worldwide spread of a new disease (World Health Organization [WHO], 2010a). Nurses are often the first health care providers to encounter someone with possible symptoms of an infectious disease. In order to effectively care for their clients, nurses need to be informed of presenting symptoms; local, national, and global protocols; and global travel advisories and restrictions.

SARS

Canada has experienced several infectious disease outbreaks that have led to system-wide reforms with global health implications. In the past few decades, Canada has witnessed the emergence of diseases that have had a distinct impact on the Canadian population, revealing how quickly an outbreak can spread globally. In 2003, **SARS** (severe acute respiratory syndrome) was first seen in Canada in individuals returning from Hong Kong, with Toronto being the region most severely affected. SARS is caused by a type of virus known as a coronavirus. This virus belong to the same family of viruses that causes mild to moderate upper respiratory illnesses like the common cold (Canada. com Health, 2019).

Initially, there was speculation that the virus causing SARS may have crossed from wildlife to humans; however, it now seems that it developed from one or more animal viruses into a new strain (Canada.com Health, 2019). At the time, in 2003, Canada was not prepared to deal with the severity of a pandemic locally, provincially, or nationally (Low, 2004). The Public Health Agency of Canada (PHAC) quickly realized the inefficiencies in the Canadian health care system and took major steps following the resolution of this emergency to critically assess and analyze the international surveillance system (Government of Canada, 2004). As a result, there were many lessons learned in Canada from the SARS outbreak that improved public communications strategies, improved coordination among various levels of government, enhanced surveillance mechanisms, and increased experts in human resources in order to be prepared for such global emergencies in the future (Government of Canada, 2004).

H1N1

In 2009, the WHO declared a global pandemic of the **H1N1** virus. H1N1 originated from animal influenza viruses (WHO, 2010b) that appeared to be unrelated to seasonal human H1N1 viruses. This pandemic was a new strain of the influenza virus and began with a rash of cases in Mexico. It then spread quickly to other countries around the globe, including Canada. On June 11, 2009, the threat to global health was determined to be significant, and the WHO raised the level of alert to phase 6 (Table 25.1), the highest level that it can declare. Phase 6 implies that community-level outbreaks have taken place in at least one other country in a different WHO region from the original outbreak. Throughout the summer, the WHO and national health agencies continued to carefully monitor this quickly evolving global health situation.

A second outbreak of H1N1 began in September 2009. Mass immunization campaigns were implemented in all provinces and territories in Canada. This outbreak tapered off by January 2010. A total of 428 deaths occurred in Canada, with over 8,000 people admitted to hospital—1,500 of these people ended up in intensive care units owing to respiratory complications. Globally, there were approximately 14,300 deaths. The role of PHAC in coordinating information and connecting with its provincial counterparts was evident during this pandemic. Some of the key issues that were highlighted during this pandemic included vaccine production, availability, and procurement; organization and roll-out of mass public health campaigns; communication and coordination at all levels of government; and ethical issues relating to vaccine distribution and prioritizing.

Ebola

Between 2014 and 2016, West Africa faced the "largest and most complex Ebola outbreak since the virus was first discovered in 1976" (WHO, 2014). In Canada, PHAC was placed on alert as to how such a highly contagious virus could possibly be transmitted to humans here and in other parts of the world. **Ebola** is a viral disease caused by Ebola filovirus, a highly infectious and rapidly fatal disease with a high mortality rate (WHO, 2014). The WHO worked quickly to develop key components of a public health response to control Ebola (WHO, 2014).

No cases have been recorded in Canada; however, human outbreaks of Ebola continue to emerge in Africa, particularly in the Democratic Republic of the Congo, with

TABLE 25.1	World Health Organization Pandemic Phases
Phase	**Explanation**
1	No animal influenza virus circulating among animals has been reported to cause infection in humans.
2	An animal influenza virus circulating in domesticated or wild animals is known to have caused infection in humans and is therefore considered a specific potential pandemic threat.
3	An animal or human–animal influenza reassortant virus has caused sporadic cases or small clusters of disease in people, but has not resulted in human-to-human transmission sufficient to sustain community-level outbreaks.
4	Human-to-human transmission of an animal or human–animal influenza reassortant virus able to sustain community-level outbreaks has been verified.
5	The same identified virus has caused sustained community-level outbreaks in two or more countries in one WHO region.
6	In addition to the criteria defined in phase 5, the same virus has caused sustained community-level outbreaks in at least one other country in another WHO region.
Post-peak period	Levels of pandemic influenza in most countries with adequate surveillance have dropped below peak levels.
Possible new wave	Level of pandemic influenza activity in most countries with adequate surveillance rising again.
Post-pandemic period	Levels of influenza activity have returend to the levels seen for seasonal influenza in most countries with adequate surveillance.

Source: World Health Organization. (2009). The WHO pandemic phases. In *Pandemic influence preparedness and response: A WHO guidance document* (p. 11). Retrieved from https://apps.who.int/iris/bitstream/handle/10665/44123/9789241547680_eng.pdf.

the eleventh and most recent outbreak occurring on June 1, 2020 (Government of Canada, 2020b; WHO, 2020e). In Canada, PHAC works on a global, national, and provincial/territorial level with the WHO to track Ebola outbreaks (Government of Canada, 2020b). There is a well-established protocol to follow if a confirmed case of Ebola in Canada were ever to emerge. This protocol involves notifying the Pan American Health Organization (PAHO) and the WHO as part of the International Health Regulations. These regulations were revised in 2005 and are coordinated by the WHO, with its primary aim "to keep the world informed about public health risks and events" (Centers for Disease Control and Prevention, 2019, para. 5).

COVID-19

On March 11, 2020, the Director-General of the WHO declared **COVID-19** a pandemic (WHO, 2020a). The formal name of the **novel coronavirus** that causes COVID-19 was designated by the International Committee on Taxonomy of Viruses on February 11, 2020 as SARS-CoV-2 (severe acute respiratory syndrome coronavirus 2) (WHO, 2020b). Because of the previous association of the acronym with the 2003 SARS pandemic in Canada, that same day the WHO also announced that the disease would be referred to as COVID-19 to prevent confusion (WHO, 2020b). This is the first pandemic caused by a coronavirus (WHO, 2020b).

The speed with which COVID-19 spread globally is a lesson in how an unknown outbreak can rapidly overwhelm the world. The novel coronavirus that causes COVID-19 is believed to have originated in Wuhan, China (WHO, 2020a). The first case was reported in someone who had visited a wet market in early December 2019. Early reports indicated that the virus was transmitted from a bat to the person, although this theory has not been decisively proven (Lai, Shih, Ko et al., 2020; Maron, 2020). By the end of December 2019, several people had presented to hospitals in Wuhan with a pneumonia-like illness (Huang, Wang, Li et al., 2020). On January 1, 2020, the Chinese government reported a cluster of the illness, and the WHO moved to help China address the outbreak through in-country support. On January 7, the first positive identification of novel coronavirus was made (Chen, Zhou, Xuan et al., 2020). The first case of the illness outside of China was reported in Taiwan on January 13 (WHO, 2020a). China instituted a city-wide lockdown of Wuhan on January 23 (Lau, Khosrawipour, Kocbach et al., 2020). By the end of February 2020, 2 months after the notification of the new illnesses, the virus had spread to several more countries. By March 11, a total of 114 countries had reported 118,000 cases of COVID-19 and 4,291 deaths, prompting the declaration of a pandemic by the WHO (WHO, 2020a). With the declaration of the pandemic, several countries quickly moved to contain the virus and mitigate its spread. However, despite these efforts, the virus continued to spread. In Canada, the first case of COVID-19 was reported on January 27, 2020, and the first death occurred on March 9 (Government of Canada, 2020a). Canada restricted travel on March 16 and negotiated a temporary closure of the Canada–US border on March 26, the first time the border has been closed since Confederation (Government of Canada, 2020a). By March 31, a total of 7,708 cases and 90 deaths had been reported (Government of Canada, 2020a). Several provinces declared states of emergency, and international flights were first curtailed then cancelled altogether. Social distancing (later called physical distancing) was implemented, and all schools and nonessential businesses were closed. People were instructed to stay home and not to go to work unless they provided an essential service, leading to huge economic uncertainty. Globally, as of August 6, 2020, 7 months after the first cases were reported in China, the world has seen more than 18.5 million confirmed cases and over 700,000 deaths attributed to COVID-19 (WHO, 2020d). Early in the pandemic, on March 3, 2020, the Director-General of the WHO reported a global death rate of 3.4%; by comparison, seasonal flu generally kills far fewer than 1% of those infected (WHO, 2020c). However, the accuracy of reporting on the impact of COVID-19 during the pandemic was acknowledged as an issue due to lack of access to testing and challenges with reporting cause of death. A postpandemic reflection and in-depth review of the world's response is required to fully understand the impacts of this particular global pandemic.

The major pandemics in the past 25 years, including SARS, H1N1, and the still-unfolding COVID-19 pandemic, have revealed how quickly a disease can threaten global health. Since 2003–2004, there has been increasing awareness and acknowledgement that all countries have a role to play in being responsible to strengthen health care systems and to identify and control the spread of public health threats and disease outbreaks (Centers for Disease Control and Prevention, 2019). Since the early part of this century, many scientists have been warning that the world was overdue for a pandemic of a magnitude similar to that of the influenza outbreak of 1918–1920. The introduction of International Health Regulations has been a major step in changing the way public health threats and disease outbreaks are detected and reported worldwide.

However, despite advances in International Health Regulations, any lessons learned from the SARS, H1N1, and Ebola pandemics earlier in this century and the current COVID-19 pandemic will again radically change health care, society, and global pandemic readiness for years to come. It is uncertain where, when, or how the final pages of the COVID-19 pandemic story will be written, as the situation continued to unfold at the time of publication.

Immigration and Migration Trends Changing Ethnocultural Diversity Worldwide

During the twenty-first century, global **immigration** and **migration** have steadily increased. There are many reasons that people relocate within a country (migration) or move to another country (immigration). Internally displaced people within their own country may move because of environmental disasters, such as forest fires, floods, drought or hurricanes. The movement of people or internally displaced people to another country may also be due to conflict, violence, or persecution (United Nations High Commissioner of Refugees Canada, 2019). People may move because of civil unrest, such as that in Syria or Venezuela, or persecution for their ethnicity, such as the Rohingya people in Myanmar, who do not have citizenship in that country and thus are considered noncitizens (Blakemore, 2019). Other reasons include gender discrimination (Amnesty International, 2019) and economic factors, such as migrant workers from Central America who travel to the United States or Canada for a better livelihood. Someone who is forced to leave their country of origin for fear of being persecuted is known as a **refugee**.

As a result of these global immigration and migration trends, the ethnocultural diversity of countries worldwide is changing, including in Canada. According to the 2016 Canadian Census, nearly 1 in 5 people in Canada were born outside of the country (Statistics Canada, 2017). Canada ranks second to Australia as the country with the largest proportion of foreign-born citizens. Since the 2001 Census, Canada's largest groups of immigrants have remained essentially unchanged—the Middle East and Asia are the primary source countries of immigrants. This increasing diversity brings the global issues much closer to home and affects our health care system.

HIV/AIDS

HIV/AIDS continues to be a significant global concern, particularly in sub-Saharan Africa, where nearly 1 in every 25 adults is living with HIV (Government of Canada, 2017). Progress in eradicating this health concern is occurring as the incidence of HIV/AIDS is declining. For example, between 2000 and 2015, there was a 45% decrease in HIV infections. From 2015 until 2017, 1.1 million people died from AIDS-related causes globally, in contrast to 2 million in 2000 alone. Moreover, between 2000 and 2015, there was a 45% decrease in new infections. In 2016, fewer people were dying of AIDS-associated illnesses, and 17.3 million people living with HIV had access to antiretroviral therapy (Government of Canada, 2017). The reasons for this progress are effective public awareness campaigns and prevention programs; improved access to health services through strengthened health systems; and scaled-up access to new medications and treatments. Canada has actively participated in the global response to HIV/AIDs, acknowledging the importance for universal access to HIV treatment, prevention measures, and care and support (Government of Canada, 2017).

Global Tobacco Control

May 21, 2003 was a historic day for global public health. At the 56th World Health Assembly, the WHO's 192 member states unanimously adopted the world's first public health treaty, the WHO Framework Convention on Tobacco Control. Negotiated under the auspices of the WHO, this new treaty was the first legal instrument designed to reduce tobacco-related deaths and disease worldwide. The treaty required countries to impose restrictions on tobacco advertising, sponsorship, and promotion; establish new packaging and labelling of tobacco products; establish clean indoor air controls; and strengthen legislation to clamp down on tobacco smuggling (WHO, 2003).

The WHO Framework Convention on Tobacco Control is now 25 years old. Since 2003, tobacco control efforts have experienced both progress and setbacks. Globally, tobacco use disproportionately affects low- and middle-income countries (WHO, 2019a), and in Canada it remains the leading cause of premature death and disease. It is estimated that over 4 million Canadians use tobacco, which is around 17% of the population. On the positive side, Canada has developed a Tobacco Strategy that seeks to reduce tobacco use to less than 5% by 2035 (WHO, 2019a). The Tobacco Strategy consists of is a 5-year commitment to help Canadians who smoke to (1) quit or reduce the harms of their addiction to nicotine and (2) protect the health of nonsmokers and young people from the dangers of tobacco use (Government of Canada, 2019b).

On November 9, 2019, the Canadian government adopted new regulations to give tobacco products and packages a standardized and plain appearance (Government of Canada, 2019c, 2020c). The underlying premise of such a move was to reduce the appeal of tobacco products to protect all Canadians, especially adolescent and younger adults, from being induced to use them and the possibility of developing an addiction. Globally, at least 13 other countries have approved similar actions (Government of Canada, 2019c). (Refer to the "Key Health Issues in Canada" section to learn about other related health issues, such e-cigarettes and vaping, currently impacting the nursing profession.)

Global Influences on Health and Safety

The World Trade Center attacks on September 11, 2001, and subsequent terrorist attacks in Sri Lanka and New Zealand in 2019 have continued to change the way we view international and domestic safety and security. Air travel continues to pose a security issue, with ongoing restrictions on travel to and from certain countries. These changes have all been the product of increased vigilance within the global security community. It is now standard for all those working in a health profession to stay apprised of global issues, changing regulations, and new health concerns. Nurses should also keep current about the safety and security conditions of the places they might travel for their own health and safety. For example, the Government of Canada (2019d) maintains a website that provides current travel advice and advisories.

Planetary Health and Climate Change

As we continue to witness disruptions in our climate and ecosystems during the **Anthropocene epoch**, it is clear that humans are having a significant impact on the planet, which is ultimately affecting the health of our population globally (Horton & Lo, 2015). In response to these global environmental changes, there is an emerging movement to addressing another dimension of global health called **planetary health.** Planetary health recognizes that human health and well-being must be understood as part of the health of the ecosystems we depend on and not as something separate. The Rockefeller Foundation–*Lancet* Commission defined planetary health as

> *the achievement of the highest attainable standard of health, well-being, and equity worldwide through judicious attention to the human systems—political, economic, and social—that shape the future of humanity and the Earth's natural systems that define the safe environmental limits within which humanity can flourish. Put simply, planetary health is the health of human civilisation and the state of the natural systems on which it depends… The concept of planetary health is based on the understanding that human health and human civilisation depend on flourishing natural systems and the wise stewardship of those natural systems.* (Whitmee, Haines, Beyrer et al., 2015, p. 1974)

With this upsurge of interest in planetary health, the Planetary Health Alliance developed a set of 12 cross-cutting principles as a curriculum development guide for educators (as cited in Stone, Myers, & Golden, 2018). These principles for planetary health education are important alongside understanding how Indigenous peoples in Canada have been protecting the Earth for the well-being of the community through Indigenous sovereignty (Manuel & Derrickson, 2017). As a result, nurse educators should employ the principles of planetary health and Indigenous sovereignty in global health curricula, nursing practice, research, and leadership.

Alongside these changes in our ecosystems, far more attention is now being given to changes in our climate, which have consequences for the well-being, health, and livelihood of the Canadian population (Bush & Lemmen, 2019; Intergovernmental Panel on Climate Change, 2014). The biggest threat to human health and survival in the twenty-first century is climate change (Watts, Amann, Ayeb-Karlsson et al., 2017; Whitmee, Haines, & Beyrer

et al., 2015). Recently, *Canada's Changing Climate Report* (CCCR), commissioned by Environment and Climate Change Canada, documented changes across Canada in temperature, permafrost, snow, and freshwater in addition to Canada's three oceans (Bush & Lemmen, 2019). For example, the CCCR found that Canada's annual average temperature has warmed by 1.7°C since 1948 (Bush & Lemmen, 2019). The CCCR was the first report to assess "how Canada's climate has changed, why, and what changes are projected for the future" (Bush & Lemmen, 2019, p. 428).

In Canada, climate change has dominated the agendas of governments officials and health care providers (Bush & Lemmen, 2019; Canadian Nurses Association [CNA] & Canadian Medical Association, 2009; Canadian Public Health Association, 2019) as well as professional nursing associations (CNA, 2017a; Kalogirou, Morin, & Martin, 2019; Nurses and Nurse Practitioners of British Columbia, 2019; Registered Nurses' Association of Ontario [RNAO], 2019a). The Canadian Association of Nurses for the Environment (2020) has provided eco-literacy information on climate change, and the International Council of Nurses (ICN, 2018) has acknowledged the need global for awareness and responsibility for the effects of climate change. In their position statement, the CNA (2017) emphasized that nurses "have a role in supporting adaptation and mitigation with respect to climate change through nursing practice, research, administration, education and policy" (para. 1). As well, on a provincial level, the Nurses and Nurse Practitioners of British Columbia (2019) has articulated how important it is that nurses speak to the health of our environment, a sentiment echoed by the RNAO (2018).

The Paris Agreement was adopted by all 195 participating member states and the European Union on December 12, 2015, at the United Nations Framework Convention on Climate Change with the intention of addressing the mitigation, adaptation, and finance of greenhouse gas emissions. The long-term temperature goal of the Paris Agreement is to keep the global average temperature to well below 2°C above preindustrial levels, and to limit the temperature increase even further to 1.5°C, with the intention of reducing the effects and risks of climate change. As of 2020, 189 Parties have ratified of the 197 Parties to the Convention (United Nations Climate Change, 2020). In addition, the WHO remains committed to supporting the Paris Agreement, as well as supporting the building of climate-resilient health systems and monitoring national progress in protecting the health of the population from climate change (WHO, 2019b).

Moving from UN Millennium Development Goals to UN Sustainable Development Goals

In 2000, the United Nations (UN) member states agreed on eight Millennium Development Goals (MDGs) to address key global health and development issues (United Nations, 2015) with a target date of 2015 to meet these goals. While many countries met the target dates for the MDGs, gaps remained between and within countries, particularly in structurally vulnerable states. To build on the MDGs, the UN General Assembly in September 2015 adopted 17 **Sustainable Development Goals** (SDGs), listed in Box 25.1 (see also Chapter 1, Figure 1.2). Not only are the SDGs distinct to each country, but they also promote human prosperity as well as protecting the planet.

A national framework has been developed globally to attain these goals, and Canada continues to be active in the global push to achieve these goals. It is important that nurses recognize their role in attaining the SDGs. The ICN (2017) has stated that "nurses, as the primary providers of healthcare to all communities in all settings, are key to the achievement of the SDGs" (p. 3).

Noncommunicable Diseases

Noncommunicable diseases, also called chronic diseases, continue to be a major contributor to premature death in Canada and around the world, but they especially affect low- and middle-income countries (WHO, 2018). The WHO estimates that noncommunicable diseases cause the deaths of 41 million people globally each year, which corresponds to 71% of all deaths worldwide. The primary noncommunicable diseases are cardiovascular diseases (stroke and heart attacks), cancers, chronic respiratory diseases, and diabetes. In Canada, chronic diseases affect 44% of adults over 20 years of age, with hypertension and osteoarthritis ranking as the two most prevalent chronic conditions (Government of Canada, 2019f).

 APPLYING CONTENT KNOWLEDGE

1. Discuss the impact that the emergence of the Ebola crisis has had on the Canadian health system response locally, nationally, and globally.
2. What factors have influenced the attainment of the SDGs?

GLOBAL NURSING LEADERSHIP IMPACT ON THE NURSING PROFESSION

World Health Organization

Nursing and Midwifery

In 2002, the WHO recommended a collaborative action framework to support in-country efforts to enhance the capacity of nursing and midwifery services to contribute to national health goals. The *Strategic Directions for Nursing*

BOX 25.1 The 17 Sustainable Development Goals Adopted by the UN General Assembly

1. End poverty in all its forms everywhere.
2. End hunger, achieve food security and improved nutrition, and promote sustainable agriculture.
3. Ensure healthy lives and promote well-being for all at all ages.
4. Ensure inclusive and equitable quality education and promote lifelong learning opportunities for all.
5. Achieve gender equality and empower all women and girls.
6. Ensure availability and sustainable management of water and sanitation for all.
7. Ensure access to affordable, reliable, sustainable, and modern energy for all.
8. Promote sustained, inclusive, and sustainable economic growth, full and productive employment, and decent work for all.
9. Build resilient infrastructure, promote inclusive and sustainable industrialization, and foster innovation.
10. Reduce inequality within and among countries.
11. Make cities and human settlements inclusive, safe, resilient, and sustainable.
12. Ensure sustainable consumption and production patterns.
13. Take urgent action to combat climate change and its impacts.
14. Conserve and sustainably use the oceans, seas, and marine resources for sustainable development.
15. Protect, restore, and promote sustainable use of terrestrial ecosystems, sustainably manage forests, combat desertification, halt and reverse land degradation, and halt biodiversity loss.
16. Promote peaceful and inclusive societies for sustainable development, provide access to justice for all, and build effective, accountable, and inclusive institutions at all levels.
17. Strengthen the means of implementation and revitalize the global partnership for sustainable development.

Source: United Nations. (n.d.). *About the Sustainable Development Goals.* Retrieved from https://www.un.org/sustainabledevelopment/sustainable-development-goals/.

---

and Midwifery Services report recommended the following five key result areas for a concentration of effort between 2002 and 2008 (WHO, 2002):

1. Health planning, advocacy, and political commitment;
2. Management of health personnel for nursing and midwifery services;

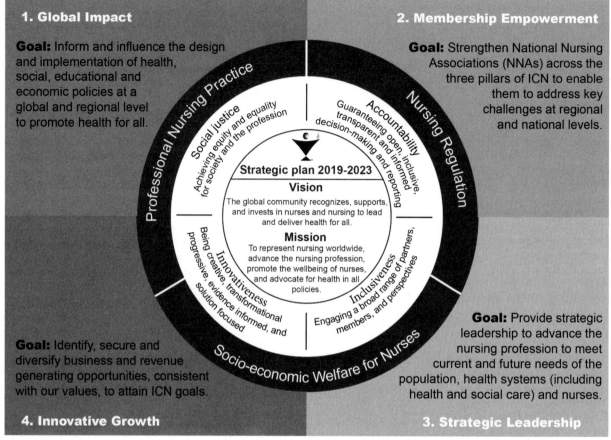

1. Global Impact

Goal: Inform and influence the design and implementation of health, social, educational and economic policies at a global and regional level to promote health for all.

2. Membership Empowerment

Goal: Strengthen National Nursing Associations (NNAs) across the three pillars of ICN to enable them to address key challenges at regional and national levels.

Goal: Identify, secure and diversify business and revenue generating opportunities, consistent with our values, to attain ICN goals.

Goal: Provide strategic leadership to advance the nursing profession to meet current and future needs of the population, health systems (including health and social care) and nurses.

4. Innovative Growth

3. Strategic Leadership

Professional Nursing Practice · Nursing Regulation · Socio-economic Welfare for Nurses

Social justice · Achieving equity and equality for society and the profession

Accountability · Guaranteeing open, inclusive, transparent and informed decision-making and reporting

Innovativeness · Being creative, transformational progressive, evidence informed, and solution focused

Inclusiveness · Engaging a broad range of partners, members, and perspectives

Strategic plan 2019-2023

Vision
The global community recognizes, supports, and invests in nurses and nursing to lead and deliver health for all.

Mission
To represent nursing worldwide, advance the nursing profession, promote the wellbeing of nurses, and advocate for health in all policies.

Fig. 25.1 *International Council of Nurses Strategic Plan, 2019–2023.* (**Source:** International Council of Nurses)

3. Practice and health system improvement;
4. Education of health personnel for nursing and midwifery services; and
5. Stewardship and governance. (pp. 10–11)

A recent update, in 2016, consisted of a collaborative initiative between the ICN and the WHO to launch the Global Strategic Directions for Strengthening Nursing and Midwifery 2016–2020 (WHO, 2016a). These new strategic directions aim to ensure that the nursing and midwifery workforce "contributes to Universal Health Coverage and the Sustainable Development Agenda by ensuring equitable access to skilled and motivated nursing and midwifery workforces within performing and responsive health systems" (WHO, 2016b, para. 2). The four key themes of the strategic directions are shown in Figure 25.1. Dr. Frances Hughes, the ICN's Chief Executive Officer, emphasized that because nursing and midwifery are the largest health personnel group in many countries, investment in this initiative was paramount.

New Director-General and Refocus on SDGs

In 2017, Dr. Tedros Adhanom Ghebreyesus was appointed as WHO Director-General, succeeding Dr. Margaret Chan, who had been in the position since 2007 (WHO, 2017a). His vision is a global commitment to sustainable development that will be achieved through the SDGs. His vision addresses the economic, social, and political determinants of health, which will lead to improved quality of life globally: "We need a WHO—fit for the 21st century—that belongs to all, equally. We need a WHO that is efficiently managed, adequately resourced and results driven, with a strong focus on transparency, accountability and value for money" (WHO, 2019c, para. 1).

International Council of Nurses

The ICN is a federation of more than 130 national nurses' associations representing more than 20 million nurses globally. Founded in 1899, the ICN is the world's first and

TABLE 25.2 Four Key Thematic Areas of the Global Strategic Directions for Nursing and Midwifery 2016–2020	
Theme 1	Ensuring an educated, competent, and motivated nursing and midwifery workforce within effective and responsive health systems at all levels and in different settings
Theme 2	Optimizing policy development, effective leadership, management, and governance
Theme 3	Working together to maximize the capacities and potentials of nurses and midwives through intraprofessional and interprofessional collaborative partnerships, education, and continuing professional development
Theme 4	Mobilizing political will to invest in building effective evidence-based nursing and midwifery workforce development

Source: World Health Organization. (2016). *Global strategic directions for strengthening nursing and midwifery 2016–2020.* Retrieved from https://www.who.int/hrh/nursing_midwifery/global-strategic-midwifery2016-2020.pdf.

widest-reaching international organization for health care providers. The organization is operated by nurses and leads nurses internationally, working to ensure quality nursing care for all, sound health policies globally, the advancement of nursing knowledge, and the presence worldwide of a respected nursing profession and a competent and satisfied nursing workforce (ICN, 2019a). In Canada, the CNA is the official member of the ICN. The mission of the ICN is to:

- Represent nursing worldwide;
- Advance the nursing profession;
- Promote the well-being of nurses; and
- Advocate for health in all policies. (ICN, 2019b, para. 1)

The vision of the ICN is that "the global community recognizes, supports and invests in nurses and nursing to lead and deliver health for all" (ICN, 2019b, para. 2). In the ICN's strategic plan for 2019–2023, four areas of focus are identified (Table 25.2).

ICN Strategic Priorities

The ICN identified 10 strategic priorities to integrate and align nursing with global health priorities (Table 25.3). For the period 2017 to 2020, the ICN named distinctive health topic priorities for global advancement and focus. The intention behind these priorities was to influence the WHO and other high-level decision-making bodies so that nurses could participate in policy setting, decision making, and implementation of national and international strategies and policies (ICN, 2019c).

Projects: Leadership for Change

The ICN also has a long history of implementing projects that are supported by external funding and technical assistance from various sectors and organizations. The focus of these projects are to:

- Extend capacity to deliver initiatives addressing the SDGs;

- Provide global platforms for the ICN to synergize with other organizations to deliver access to specialize knowledge and research on key nursing and health topics; and
- Support programmatic activity on today's critically important global issues. (ICN, 2019d, para. 1)

The ICN developed one such project in 1995, the Leadership for Change (LFC) program. With this program, the ICN set out to help nurses gain the leadership skills needed to implement organizational change in order to improve nursing practice and achieve better health outcomes. An important element of this program is to work closely with the national nurses' associations to act upon the specific needs of the countries in which the programs are being implemented. To date, the LFC programs have been implemented in more than 40 countries (ICN, 2019d). Other projects include the Girl Child Education Fund; Global Nursing Leadership Institute; Lesotho

TABLE 25.3 Strategic Priorities of the International Council of Nurses	
Priority	**Health Topics**
1	Universal health coverage
2	Noncommunicable diseases
3	Primary health care
4	Human resources for health
5	Person-centered care
6	Patient safety
7	Antimicrobial resistance
8	Mental health
9	Immunization
10	Sustainable Development Goals

Source: International Council of Nurses. (2019). *ICN strategic priorities.* Retrieved from https://www.icn.ch/nursing-policy/icn-strategic-priorities.

Organizational Development Project; Nursing Policy Leadership Programme; Tuberculosis/Multidrug-resistant TB/MDR-TB project; and eHealth & International Classification for Nursing Practice (ICN, 2019d).

International Center for Human Resources in Nursing

The International Center for Human Resources in Nursing was established in 2006 by the ICN and the Florence Nightingale International Foundation. The centre is dedicated to strengthening the nursing workforce globally through the development, ongoing monitoring, and dissemination of comprehensive information, standards, and tools on nursing human resources policy, management, research, and practice. The centre's mission is to improve the quality of patient care through advancing nursing and health care services, and staff have produced valuable global research on health human resources in nursing (International Center for Human Resources in Nursing, 2015).

WHO Chief Nursing Officer

Over the past decade, the global nursing community has called for greater leadership and representation at the WHO. This call was met in 2017 when Director-General Dr. Tedros Adhanom Ghebreyesus named Elizabeth Iro—a nurse and midwife and most recently the secretary of health of the Cook Islands—to the newly created position of Chief Nursing Officer (McSpedon, 2018). This appointment was a significant milestone, marking Director-General Ghebreyesus' promise to ensure that nurses are included as part of the senior leadership team, both at the policy-making tables and in the community (McSpedon, 2018). Dr. Ghebreyesus emphasized that nurses are critical to achieving universal health coverage and the SDGs. This WHO mandate aligns with the goals of the ICN and the International Confederation of Midwives.

Nursing Now 2020 Campaign

The ICN's most recent initiative was the launching of the Nursing Now campaign in 2017. Its aim was to raise the status and profile of nurses globally and to "empower nurse to take their place at the heart of tackling 21st century health challenges" (Nursing Now, 2019a, para 2). The campaign, a program of the Burdett Trust, consisted of a 3-year collaboration between the ICN and the WHO that coincided in 2020 with the International Year of the Nurse and Midwife as well as the two-hundredth anniversary of the birth of Florence Nightingale and two flagship reports. On April 7, 2020, World Health Day, the WHO released the *State of the World's Nursing Report 2020*. This report, the first of its kind, is a landmark resource for the nursing profession that provides evidence to support a stronger justification for governments to invest in nursing (Nursing NOW, 2019b; WHO, 2020f). The other flagship report, on the state of the world's midwifery (its third edition), will be launched in 2021 (International Confederation of Midwives, 2019).

Commonwealth Nurses Federation

The Commonwealth Nurses Federation (CNF) is a working group founded in 1973 under the umbrella of the Commonwealth Ministers of Health. As a federation of national nursing and midwifery associations from Commonwealth countries, the group is involved in promoting high standards of professional practice. The specific objectives of the CNF are to:
- Influence health policy;
- Develop nursing networks;
- Improve nursing standards and competence; and
- Strengthen nursing leadership throughout the Commonwealth. (Commonwealth Nurses Federation, 2019)

Lillian Carter Center for Global Health and Social Responsibility

The Lillian Carter Center for Global Health and Social Responsibility (formerly the Lillian Carter Center for International Nursing) has as its mission the improvement of the health of vulnerable people worldwide through nursing education, research, practice, and policy. The Center focuses on enhancing the impact of nursing globally through targeted international academic exchanges; partnerships fostering scholarship; the creation of a forum for exploration of issues relating to the global supply, demand, distribution, and quality of the nursing workforce worldwide; and increasing access to relevant training and education (Emory University, 2019).

Focus on Health Human Resources Globally

Health human resources are an urgent issue for health care systems globally. The ICN has made human resources for health a strategic priority, stating that "the world cannot help to achieve the Sustainable Development Goals, Universal Health Coverage and other health goals without looking at the Human Resources for Health" (ICN, 2019c). The ICN bases their current efforts toward health human resources on the document that resulted from the Fourth Global Forum on Human Resources for Health in Dublin in 2017, which was founded on the 2030 Agenda for Sustainable Development. This landmark event was co-organized by Ireland's Department of Health, Department of Foreign Affairs and Trade, the Health Service Executive of Ireland, the Global Health Workforce Network, Trinity College Dublin, and the WHO. The forum culminated in the Dublin declaration, an affirmation of the global call for many initiatives, such as the importance for all "relevant stakeholders to strengthen their collaboration to expand and transform investments in the health and social workforce, with particular emphasis on empowering women and advancing youth employment" (Fourth Global Forum on Human Resources for Health, 2017, p. 7).

👤 APPLYING CONTENT KNOWLEDGE

1. How does the WHO Chief Nursing Officer's global leadership position align within the ICN's Health for All policy?
2. What role do nurses in Canada play in promoting universal health coverage and the WHO's Sustainable Development Goals?

KEY HEALTH ISSUES IN CANADA

Health care systems in Canada have been increasingly contending with serious emerging health issues, some of which are based upon changes in health practices and others influenced by federal government policies. The most pressing health issues of the past decade (2010–2019) included the increased use of e-cigarettes, also known as **vaping**; the legalization of cannabis; **opioid misuse**, which has developed into a crisis; **antimicrobial resistance;** and **medical assistance in dying** (MAID). Each of these issues is highlighted below.

Vaping

In Canada, there has been a recent upsurge in the number of people opting to replace tobacco smoking with vaping, or electronic cigarettes (e-cigarettes), particularly among youth (Health Canada, 2019). Vaping is defined as the "act of inhaling and exhaling an aerosol produced by a vaping product such as an e-cigarette" (Health Canada, 2019, para. 10) Vaping does not burn the way cigarette smoking does; instead, it heats a liquid into a vapour, which subsequently turns into an aerosol. The substances contained in the vapour can be flavourings and/or nicotine.

Public health experts in Canada had originally envisioned e-cigarettes as a stop-smoking aid for adults. However, in September 2019, Health Canada issued an advisory, warning Canadians of the potential risk of pulmonary illness associated with vaping products. This warning stemmed from the recently reported cases in the United States of severe pulmonary illness and numerous deaths associated with the use of vaping products. While the sources of the illnesses reported are unknown, the US Centers for Disease Control and Prevention purport that

the cause of the illnesses is likely chemical exposure. The Government of Canada continues monitoring available health surveillance systems and data sources in Canada for signs of severe pulmonary illness that could be related to vaping (Health Canada, 2019, para. 6).

Nurses need to be aware that vaping does have health risks and that its short- and long-term effects currently remain unknown (RNAO, 2019b). As part of taking a patient's health history, nurses and other health care providers should ask whether patients have used or still use drugs from any source, whether legal or illegal. In addition, when caring for a patient who exhibits respiratory symptoms of unknown origin, nurses should ask about the use of vaping products, such as e-cigarettes, liquids, and refill pods and/or cartridges. In addition, Dr. Doris Grinspun (2019), the Chief Executive Officer of the RNAO, has emphasized that the research conducted by the RNAO "found insufficient evidence that e-cigarettes are an effective smoking cessation tool." Grinspun has advocated that nurses need to protect Canadians from the harmful substances in vaping products by calling on our governments to act. The RNAO (2019b) has also suggested that nursing join with the Canadian Cancer Society in advocating for an increase in the legal age to purchase vaping products from 18 to 21 years.

Cannabis Legalization

In October 2018, the Canadian government legalized recreational cannabis with the proclamation of the *Cannabis Act* (Balneaves, 2019, para. 2). This move follows in the footsteps of many US states and the country of Uruguay. The new legislation allows Canadians to legally access recreational cannabis and controls how it is distributed, produced, and sold in Canada. The primary intention of this legislation was to protect the public from harms posed by interactions with the justice system and the illegal cannabis market. Before legalization, when Canadians had a health condition that required cannabis, they could, with support from a nurse practitioner or physician, register at a licensed producer and have a 30 day supply of cannabis shipped to their home. With legalization, patients can now purchase cannabis for therapeutic purposes directly from websites and stores without needing to provide medical documentation or register with a licensed producer.

While accessing medical cannabis has become easier, it has also led some patients to purchase cannabis without first consulting a health care provider, resulting in medical conditions whereby cannabis is contraindicated and thus causes unfavourable drug interactions. For example, medications like clobazam and warfarin are known to cause interactions with certain cannabinoids. Cannabidiol can also adversely affect the immune systems of patients with compromised immunity. Those who use large amounts of cannabis and also have a family history of psychotic illness such as schizophrenia are at higher risk of experiencing the untoward psychological effects of cannabis (Di Forti, Quattrone, Freeman et al., 2019). Lastly, many patients are now trying to determine—on their own—the correct choice of cannabis, formulation, and dose for their specific medical condition (Balneaves, 2019, para. 8).

In terms of the role of nurses and other health care providers, the health professions are acknowledging the importance of providing appropriate care for patients using cannabis. In turn, more educational initiatives are being dedicated to improving health care providers' knowledge of medical and recreational cannabis. For instance, since 2017, the CNA has been working on the creation of a national nursing framework on the legalization of cannabis with a grant from Health Canada's Substance Use and Addictions Program; in addition, the CAN has led the development of online modules, annual interactive thinktank sessions, supplementary resources, and knowledge translation products to increase nurses' knowledge, understanding, and awareness of cannabis (CNA, 2019a). In addition, other resources are available to assist health care providers with understanding the new cannabis legal system through the Government of Canada (2019g). This increased understanding of the current evidence will assist nurses and other health care providers with ensuring that clients obtain accurate information, in an equitable and appropriate manner, about the potential risks and benefits of using medical cannabis (Balneaves, 2019, para. 13).

Opioid Misuse/Crisis

Like many other countries, Canada is currently facing the urgent challenge of reducing the harm associated with the misuse of opioids (Government of Canada, 2019h; Taha, Maloney-Hall, & Buxton, 2019). More than 15,393 people have lost their lives as a result of apparent opioid-related deaths since January 2016, leading to a public health emergency in Canada (Government of Canada, 2019i).

Taha, Maloney-Hall, and Buxton (2019) conducted a review of the peer-reviewed and grey literature from 2013 to 2019 to examine current responses to the opioid crisis, lessons learned, and the knowledge gap that still remains to be addressed according to the Canadian Drugs and Substance Strategy. They concluded that there is no clear "one-size-fits-all" response to this crisis and that it is important to acknowledge the "uniqueness" of individual communities, sex and gender issues, Indigenous peoples, youth and correctional populations, as well as the larger impact of opioid misuse on society and families. This situation is evolving as the health care community continues to

---

BOX 25.2   Recommended Actions for Nurses to Address the Opioid Crisis in Canada

1. Optimize assessment skills related to substance use and misuse.
2. Educate individual clients, families, and the public regarding substance use and misuse.
3. Optimize pain management skills.
4. Support palliative and end-of-life clients' and families' use of opioids to control pain.
5. Encourage best practices in harm reduction strategies.
6. Refer to community resources.
7. Respond to overdose.
8. Adopt a trauma-informed approach.
9. Destigmatize addiction.
10. Collaborate interprofessionally and intersectorally to address the crisis.

Source: Canadian Association of Schools of Nursing. (2017). *Nurses' role in combating the opioid crisis in Canada.* Ottawa, ON: Author. Retrieved from https://www.casn.ca/wp-content/uploads/2017/09/Nurses-Role-in-Combating-the-Opioid-CrisisFINAL-EN-1.pdf.

---

learn about new interventions and services, and evaluates how the overall system responds.

Nursing organizations in Canada have acknowledged that the increasing misuse of and addiction to prescription and illicit opioids is a growing public health crisis, including the Canadian Association of Schools of Nursing (CASN, 2017) and the CNA (2019b), the national and global professional voice of Canadian nursing. In 2017, the CASN hosted regional workshops for registered nurses (RNs) and nurse practitioners (NPs) to better understand this growing epidemic and to examine the perspectives on ethical, legal, and harm reduction strategies. This series of meetings resulted in 10 recommended actions, which are listed in Box 25.2.

The federal government committed to investing $10.7 million in projects for treatment and harm reduction and research initiatives (CNA, 2019b). They also "approved injectable hydromorphone for use as a treatment for adults with severe opioid use disorder and added diacetylmorphine to the federal government's list of drugs for an urgent public health need" (CNA, 2019b, para. 1). These medications improve and stabilize the health of people using opioids. The CNA publicly stated its supported of the federal government's actions to address the opioid crisis (CNA, 2019b). The CNA has taken the position that the opioid crisis has had such devastating effects on individuals, families, and communities in Canada that a comprehensive approach is needed. Such an approach encompasses strategies for prevention and improved access to treatment, including harm reduction.

Antimicrobial Resistance

There is growing concern worldwide that infections like tuberculosis or pneumonia, which were previously treatable with a standard course of antimicrobials (e.g., antifungal agents or antibiotics), are becoming increasingly resistant to those drugs (CNA, 2019c, para. 1). Antimicrobial resistance arises "when microorganisms such as bacteria, viruses, fungi and parasites change in ways that render the medications used to cure the infections ineffective," due to the misuse or overuse of antimicrobials (WHO, 2017b, para. 2). **Superbugs,** defined as microorganisms that are resistant to many antimicrobials, pose a major public health threat both locally and globally (WHO, 2017b, para. 2). These infections have the potential to spread to others, resulting in more deaths, and are becoming an economic burden on the health care system (Council of Canadian Academies, 2019).

The CNA (2019c) has strongly advocated for delineating the critical role nurses must play in the fight against antimicrobial resistance. The role of nurses includes:

(1) Assessing and monitoring signs and symptoms of infections and side effects of antimicrobials;

(2) Prescribing and de-prescribing judiciously antimicrobials by authorized nurse prescribers and NPs, who can be stewards;

(3) Acting as stewards for microbiology and laboratory testing;

(4) Educating patients and the public about when it is appropriate to use antimicrobials and responding to any other patient concerns; and

(5) Implementing infection prevention and control practices. (CNA, 2019, para. 2)

Antimicrobial stewardship is the cautious use of antimicrobials to improve infection cure rates, decrease unnecessary exposure to them, minimize the emergence of antibiotic resistance, reduce adverse drug reactions, and lower health care costs (American Nurses Association & Centers for Disease Control and Prevention, 2017). In addition, Ashcroft (2019) stated that nurses can assume a personal role in antimicrobial stewardship by acting as role models. For example, nurses can make conscious decisions to choose antibiotic-free food, avoid antimicrobial cleaning products, and not administer antibiotics for illnesses that are most likely viral.

Medical Assistance in Dying

MAID has been legal in Canada since 2016, following the royal assent of Bill C-114. The CNA was instrumental in shaping the federal policy, bringing together a taskforce of members from provincial, territorial, and federal governments, nursing associations, and regulatory bodies to provide their expertise on the development of the National

---

BOX 25.3   Purpose of the National Nursing Framework on Medical Assistance in Dying in Canada

Medical assistance in dying (MAID) has been legal in Canada since 2016. Nurse practitioners, physicians, pharmacists, and "persons aiding practitioners" (including nurses) are permitted to help those who have explicitly requested MAID. This framework was developed with several purposes in mind:

- To raise awareness among nurses of the change in the federal law, which now permits MAID in certain circumstances and within regulatory direction.
- To guide nurses in reflecting on ethical issues that may occur as they care for persons considering MAID in various practice settings.
- To reinforce sound ethical nursing practice.
- To outline the role of nurses (i.e., NPs as compared to registered nurses, licensed practical nurses and registered psychiatric nurses) in MAID and to support nurses in their practice as they work with persons considering and receiving MAID and their families and interprofessional health-care teams (in alignment with regulatory direction in relevant jurisdictions).
- To raise the visibility of the profession's contribution to end-of-life care decision making and care that includes MAID.
- To be a resource that supports nurse regulators, clinical nurse leaders, administrators/employers and interprofessional health-care teams to develop policies, guidelines, processes and services which use the knowledge and skills of nurses appropriately to provide or aid in MAID.
- To be a nursing resource for entry to practice and continuing education on MAID.

Source: Canadian Nurses Association. (2017b). *National Nursing Framework on Medical Assistance in Dying in Canada* (p. 4). Retrieved from https://www.cna-aiic.ca/-/media/cna/page-content/pdf-en/cna-national-nursing-framework-on-maid.pdf. © Canadian Nurses Association. Reprinted with permission. Further reproduction prohibited.

Nursing Framework on Medical Assistance in Dying in Canada (CNA, 2017b). The purpose of the framework is outlined in Box 25.3. This seminal document was intended to be a supplement to specific employer and regulatory standards, policies, guidelines, and practices in various Canadian jurisdictions. It is important that nurses be aware that they must consult with their individual employer and regulatory bodies for specific direction. In addition, this framework is a guide for RNs, registered psychiatric nurses, licensed/registered practical nurses, and NPs. Chapter 13 discusses the MAID legislation and its legal impact on nursing.

MAJOR NURSING INITIATIVES IN CANADA

Health Human Resources

In Canada, one of the greatest ongoing challenges in health care is maintaining a sufficient and stable supply of health care providers. A CNA report estimates that Canada will be short almost 60,000 full-time equivalent RNs by 2022 if new policies are not implemented to curb such a situation (CNA, 2014). The CNA has been a leader in developing research plans and policies to address Canada's RN shortage. The CNA's solutions are based on a planning model that aligns with provincial, territorial, and federal policies calling for a population health needs–based approach to health human resources planning. These solutions include:

- Increasing RN productivity;
- Reducing RN annual absenteeism;
- Increasing enrollment;
- Improving the retention of practicing RNs;
- Reducing attrition rates in RN entry-to-practice practice programs; and
- Reducing international in-migration. (CNA, 2014, p. 3)
  Please see Chapter 17 for more discussion on health human resources and nursing.

Canadian Nurses Association

The CNA is a federation of 13 jurisdictions across Canada representing more than 135,000 nurses in provincial and territorial nursing associations and colleges; licensed/registered practical nurses; registered psychiatric nurses; independent RNs from Ontario and Quebec; retired nurses; the Canadian Nursing Students' Association; and the Canadian Network of Nursing Specialties. As the national and global professional voice of Canadian nurses, the CNA's mission is advancing the practice of nursing and the profession to improve health outcomes in a publicly funded, not-for-profit health system. The CNA carries out its mission by unifying the voices of nurses; strengthening nursing leadership; promoting nursing excellence and a vibrant profession; advocating for health policy and quality health systems; and serving the public interest (CNA, 2019d). The goals of the CNA are to:

- Promote and enhance the role of nurses to strengthen nursing and the Canadian health system;
- Shape and advocate for health public policy provincially/territorially, nationally, and internationally;
- Advance nursing leadership for nursing and for health; and
- Broadly engage nurses in advancing nursing and health. (CNA, 2019d, para. 3)

RNAO Nursing Best Practice Guidelines Program

In 1999, the RNAO, in partnership with the Ontario Ministry of Health and Long-Term Care, launched the Nursing Best Practice Guidelines (BPG) Program (RNAO, 2019c). Today, the BPG Program is an Ontario flagship of excellence that is nationally and globally known for its leading role in BPG development, implementation science and practice, and clinical and health work context evaluation. This program has enabled health systems and organizations to focus on clinical and patient care excellence while employing the most recent research to inform practice and optimize outcomes. The BPG Program has been influential in advancing government priorities as well as outcomes for organizations, patients, providers, and health systems. There are currently 50 published guidelines, a toolkit, and an educator's resource to support implementation. A number of these publications are available in French and other languages. Several countries, including Spain, Italy, and Chile, have adopted the BPGs or are in the process of becoming Best Practice Spotlight Organizations (RNAO, 2019d). Some examples of recent guidelines include adopting eHealth solutions, implementation strategies, and assessment and interventions for perinatal depression (RNAO, 2019e).

WHO Collaborating Centres

The WHO Collaborating Centres are institutions such as research institutes, parts of universities, or academies that are designated by the Director-General to carry out activities in support of the organization's programmes. There are 800 WHO Collaborating Centres in over 80 member states working with the WHO in areas such as nursing, mental health, nutrition, communicable diseases, occupational health, and health technologies (WHO, 2019d). In nursing, there are 42 PAHO/WHO Collaborating Centres specifically focused on nursing and midwifery (McMaster, 2019b).

In Canada, there is one PAHO/WHO Collaborating Centre in Nursing, at the McMaster University School of Nursing. This PAHO/WHO Collaborating Centre focuses on primary health care and health human resources and was re-designated as a centre in 2015. In addition, this centre has provided data to support two key reports, the *State of the World's Nursing Report* and the *State of the World's Midwifery*. This centre also works collaboratively with institutions in the Global Network of WHO Collaborating Centres for Nursing and Midwifery and faculty internally across various disciplines (McMaster University, 2019).

International Research Collaborations at Canadian Universities

Many Canadian universities and faculties of nursing are active in global research projects (Canadian Coalition for Global Health Research, 2019). In addition, nursing students and faculty members have numerous opportunities to become involved in global health placements and other initiatives both at home and internationally (Canadian Society for International Health, 2019).

Nursing Now 2020 Campaign in Canada

Nursing Now Canada was launched at an event co-hosted by the CNA and the ICN on June 2, 2019, in Vancouver, British Columbia, as part of the 3-year Nursing Now 2020 campaign to raise the profile of nursing globally (CNA, 2019e). In attendance were Barbara Stillwell, Nursing Now's Executive Director; Claire Betker, CNA President; Robin Buckland, Chief Nursing Officer of Indigenous Services Canada; and Marilee Nowgesic, Chief Executive Officer of the Canadian Indigenous Nurses Association (CINA). To be accepted as a national group, Nursing Now Canada required the support of a federal government chief nursing officer—which it received from Indigenous Services Canada—and the CNA as the national professional nursing association. This multi-stakeholder collaboration led to Canada being successful in its application, with an important element being the partnership with CINA.

Nursing Now Canada is based on an action plan with three pillars:
1. Nursing leadership pillar: To establish a comprehensive Canadian hub of leadership development;
2. Chief nursing officer pillar: To establish federal, provincial, and territorial chief nursing officers in positions of leadership (i.e., reporting to their respective deputy and assistant deputy ministers of health); and
3. Indigenous pillar: To support and enable the current and future nursing and midwifery workforce to provide culturally safe care across Canada. (CNA, 2019e)

APPLYING CONTENT KNOWLEDGE

1. How can the CNA successfully promote policies to combat the nursing shortage in Canada?
2. In the Nursing Now 2020 campaign, the main object was to raise the profile of nursing globally. As a nurse or nursing student, what do you think you can do to raise the profile of nursing locally, provincially, nationally, and globally?

CONCLUSION

The Canadian nursing community continues to play a prominent role in local, national, and global contexts through its support of the global health and nursing agenda. The role of Canadian nursing is evident from its active participation and engagement in global organizations such as the ICN and WHO; other national nursing organizations such as the CNA; and institutions representing civil society, nongovernmental organizations, academia, and interprofessional health care organizations.

SUMMARY OF LEARNING OBJECTIVES

- Global health issues that impact nurses throughout the world include pandemics (such as SARS, HIV/AIDS, H1N1, Ebola); immigration and migration trends; tobacco control; and events that threaten global health and safety, including terrorism and climate change.
- The Sustainable Development Goals were developed in 2015 by the WHO as a means to ensure that the goals not met by the Millennial Development Goals remained foremost on the agendas of WHO member states. The goals focus not only on prosperity but also on environmental safety and climate integrity.

- Global nursing leadership that influences the nursing profession includes work by the WHO, which has set the strategic direction for nursing and midwifery through a collaboration with the ICN. In 2017, the WHO instituted the new position of Chief Nursing Officer. The ICN made human resources for health a strategic priority. Other leadership comes from the Commonwealth Nurses Federation and the Lillian Carter Center for Global Health and Social Responsibility.
- Major health issues in Canada include medical assistance in dying, vaping, antimicrobial resistance, cannabis

legalization, and the opioid misuse crisis. Nurses work front and centre in promoting health public policy in these areas.

- National initiatives in place to address national and international health issues include health human resources planning; the work of the CNA; the Best Practice Guidelines Program, developed and maintained by the RNAO and operationalized in several countries; membership in WHO Collaborating Centres; international research collaborations within Canada to respond to existing issues; and participation in the Nursing Now 2020 initiative. The Canadian focus of the Nursing Now 2020 campaign consisted of three pillars: a nursing leadership pillar, a chief nursing officer pillar, and an Indigenous pillar.

CRITICAL THINKING QUESTIONS

1. Discuss the impact that changing global demographics and migration patterns are having on global health.
2. The WHO has appointed a Chief Nursing Officer to provide leadership globally. Why is this leadership position critical to global nursing?
3. What can Canadian nurses do to influence climate change policy locally and globally?

REFERENCES

American Nurses Association & Centers for Disease Control and Prevention. (2017). *Redefining the antibiotic stewardship team: Recommendations from the American Nurses Association/Centers for Disease Control and Prevention Workgroup on the Role of Registered Nurses in Hospital Antibiotic Stewardship Practices.* Retrieved from https://www.cdc.gov/antibiotic-use/healthcare/pdfs/ANA-CDC-whitepaper.pdf.

Amnesty International. (2019). *Who we are.* Retrieved from https://www.amnesty.org/en/who-we-are/.

Ashcroft, M. (2019, November 18). Nurses are critical in effective antimicrobial stewardship. *Canadian Nurse.* Retrieved from https://canadian-nurse.com/en/articles/issues/2019/november-2019/nurses-are-critical-in-effective-antimicrobial-stewardship.

Balneaves, L. (2019, July 8). Medical cannabis in Canada since legalization. *Canadian Nurse.* Retrieved from https://www.canadian-nurse.com/en/articles/issues/2019/july-2019/medical-cannabis-in-canada-since-legalization.

Blakemore, E. (2019, February 8). Who are the Rohingya people? *National Geographic.* Retrieved from https://www.nationalgeographic.com/culture/people/reference/rohingya-people/.

Braveman, P., & Gruskin, S. (2003). Defining equity in health. *Journal of Epidemiology in Community Health, 57*(4), 254–258. https://doi.org/10.1136/jech.57.4.254.

Bush, E., & Lemmen, D. S.(Eds). (2019). *Canada's changing climate report.* Ottawa, ON: Government of Canada. Retrieved from https://changingclimate.ca/site/assets/uploads/sites/2/2020/06/CCCR_FULLREPORT-EN-FINAL.pdf.

Canadian Association of Nurses for the Environment. (2020). *Advocacy and issues.* Retrieved from https://cnhe-iise.ca/issues.html.

Canadian Association of Schools of Nursing. (2017). *Nurses' role in combating the opioid crisis in Canada.* Retrieved from https://www.casn.ca/wp-content/uploads/2017/09/Nurses-Role-in-Combating-the-Opioid-CrisisFINAL-EN-1.pdf.

Canadian Coalition for Global Health Researchers. (2019). *About us.* Retrieved from https://www.ccghr.ca/about/.

Canada.com Health. (2019). *SARS (severe acute respiratory syndrome).* Retrieved from https://bodyandhealth.canada.com/channel/infection/sars/sars-severe-acute-respiratory-syndrome.

Canadian Nurses Association. (2014). *Tested solutions for eliminating Canada's registered nurse shortage.* Retrieved from https://cna-aiic.ca/-/media/cna/page-content/pdf-en/rn_highlights_e.pdf.

Canadian Nurses Association. (2017a). *Climate change and health position statement.* Retrieved from https://www.cna-aiic.ca/~/media/cna/page-content/pdf-en/climate-change-and-health-position-statement.pdf.

Canadian Nurses Association. (2017b). *National nursing framework on medical assistance in dying in Canada.* Ottawa, ON: Author. Retrieved from https://www.cna-aiic.ca/-/media/cna/page-content/pdf-en/cna-national-nursing-framework-on-maid.pdf.

Canadian Nurses Association. (2019a). *Canadian Nurses Association approved for Health Grant to lead development of national nursing framework on the legalization of cannabis.* Retrieved from https://www.cna-aiic.ca/en/news-room/news-releases/2019/canadian-nurses-association-approved-for-health-canada-grant-to-lead-development-national-nursing-framework-on-the-legalization-of-cannabis.

Canadian Nurses Association. (2019b). *Canadian Nurses Association supports steps taken by the federal government in addressing the opioid crisis.* Retrieved from https://www.cna-aiic.ca/en/news-room/news-releases/2019/canadian-nurses-association-supports-steps-taken-by-the-federal-government-in-addressing-the-opioid-crisis.

Canadian Nurses Association. (2019c). *Antimicrobial resistance (AMR).* Retrieved from https://www.cna-aiic.ca/en/policy-advocacy/antimicrobial-resistance-amr.

Canadian Nurses Association. (2019d). *About us*. Retrieved from https://www.cna-aiic.ca/en/about-us.

Canadian Nurses Association. (2019e). *Canada joins the global Nursing Now campaign*. Retrieved from https://www.cna-aiic.ca/en/news-room/news-releases/2019/canada-joins-the-global-nursing-now-campaign.

Canadian Nurses Association & Canadian Medical Association. (2009). *Joint position statement: Environmentally responsible activity in the health-care sector*. Retrieved from https://www.cna-aiic.ca/-/media/cna/page-content/pdf-en/jps99_environmental_e.pdf.

Canadian Public Health Association. (2019). *Climate change and human health*. Retrieved from https://www.cpha.ca/climate-change-and-human-health.

Canadian Society for International Health. (2019). *International projects*. Retrieved from http://www.csih.org/en/programs/international-projects.

Centers for Disease Control and Prevention. (2019). *International Health Regulations (IHR)*. Retrieved from https://www.cdc.gov/globalhealth/healthprotection/ghs/ihr/.

Chen, N., Zhou, M., Xuan, D., et al. (2020). Epidemiological and clinical characteristic of 99 cases of 2019 novel coronavirus pneumonia in Wuhan, China: A descriptive study. *The Lancet, 395*, 507–513. https://doi.org/10.1011/s0140-6736(20)30211-7.

Commonwealth Nurses Federation. (2019). *About*. Retrieved from https://www.commonwealthnurses.org/About.html.

Council of Canadian Academies. (2019). *When antibiotics fail: The expert panel on the potential socio-economic impacts of antimicrobial resistance in Canada*. Retrieved from https://cca-reports.ca/wp-content/uploads/2018/10/When-Antibiotics-Fail-1.pdf.

Di Forti, M., Quattrone, D., Freeman, T. P., et al. (2019, May). The contribution of cannabis use to variation in the incidence of psychotic disorder across Europe (EU-GEI): A multicentre case-control study. *The Lancet, 6*(5), 427–436. https://doi.org/10.1016/S2215-0366(19)30048-3.

Emory University. (2019). *Lillian Carter Centre for Global Health and Social Responsibility*. Retrieved from http://www.nursing.emory.edu/centers-and-initiatives/lillian-carter-center/index.html.

Fourth Global Forum on Human Resources for Health. (2017, November 13–17). *Dublin Declaration on Human Resources for Health: Building the Health Workforce of the Future*. Royal Dublin Society, Dublin, Ireland. Retrieved from https://www.icn.ch/sites/default/files/inline-files/Dublin_Declaration-on-HumanResources-for-Health.pdf.

Government of Canada. (2004). *Chapter 1: Learning from SARS: Renewal of public health in Canada—Introduction* [Archived]. Retrieved from https://www.canada.ca/en/public-health/services/reports-publications/learning-sars-renewal-public-health-canada/chapter-1-introduction.html#learning.

Government of Canada. (2017). *HIV/AIDS in developing countries*. Retrieved from https://www.international.gc.ca/world-monde/issues_development-enjeux_developpement/global_health-sante_mondiale/hiv_aids-vih_sida.aspx.

Government of Canada. (2019b). *Canada's tobacco strategy*. Retrieved from https://www.canada.ca/en/health-canada/services/publications/healthy-living/canada-tobacco-strategy.html.

Government of Canada. (2019c). *The government of Canada implements commitment to plain packaging for tobacco products*. Retrieved from https://www.canada.ca/en/health-canada/news/2019/05/the-government-of-canada-implements-commitment-to-plain-packaging-for-tobacco-products.html.

Government of Canada. (2019d). *Travel advice and advisories*. Retrieved from https://travel.gc.ca/travelling/advisories.

Government of Canada. (2019f). *Prevalence of chronic diseases among Canadian adults*. Retrieved from https://www.canada.ca/en/public-health/services/chronic-diseases/prevalence-canadian-adults-infographic-2019.html.

Government of Canada. (2019g). *Talk about cannabis: Cannabis in Canada: Get the facts*. Retrieved from https://www.canada.ca/en/health-canada/services/drugs-medication/cannabis/resources.html.

Government of Canada. (2019h). *Opioid-related harms and deaths in Canada*. Retrieved from https://www.canada.ca/en/health-canada/services/substance-use/problematic-prescription-drug-use/opioids/data-surveillance-research/harms-deaths.html.

Government of Canada. (2019i). *National report: Apparent opioid-related deaths in Canada*. Retrieved from https://health-infobase.canada.ca/datalab/national-surveillance-opioid-mortality.html.

Government of Canada. (2020a). *Coronavirus disease (COVID-19) outbreak update*. Retrieved from https://www.canada.ca/en/public-health/services/diseases/2019-novel-coronavirus-infection.html

Government of Canada. (2020b). *Update on the outbreak of Ebola virus disease in the Democratic Republic of the Congo*. Retrieved from https://www.canada.ca/en/public-health/services/diseases/ebola.html.

Government of Canada. (2020c). *Tobacco Products Regulations: Plain and Standardized Appearance*. Retrieved from https://www.canada.ca/en/health-canada/services/health-concerns/tobacco/legislation/federal-regulations/products-regulations-plain-standardized-appearance.html.

Grinspun, D. (2019, September 30). Grinspun: Clamp down on the sale and promotion of vaping product. *Ottawa Citizen*. Retrieved from https://ottawacitizen.com/opinion/columnists/grinspun-clamp-down-on-the-sale-and-promotion-of-vaping-products.

Health Canada. (2019). *Information update—Health Canada warns of potential risk of pulmonary illness associated with vaping product*. Retrieved from https://healthycanadians.gc.ca/recall-alert-rappel-avis/hc-sc/2019/70919a-eng.php.

Horton, R., & Lo, S. (2015). Planetary health: A new science for exceptional action. *Lancet, 386*, 1921–1922. https://doi.org/10.1016/S0140-6736(15)61038-8.

Huang, C., Wang, Y., Li, X., et al. (2020). Clinical features of patients infected with 2019 novel coronavirus in Wuhan, China. *The Lancet, 395*, 497–506. https://doi.org/10.1016/S0140-6736(20)30183-5.

Intergovernmental Panel on Climate Change. (2014). *Climate change 2014: Summary for policymakers*. Retrieved from https://www.ipcc.ch/.

International Center for Human Resources in Nursing. (2015). *Introduction to the International Center for Human Resources in Nursing.* Retrieved from https://ifna.site/international-center-for-human-resources-in-nursing/.

International Confederation of Midwives. (2019). *The state of the world's midwifery 2021: Concept note.* Retrieved from https://www.internationalmidwives.org/assets/files/general-files/2020/06/sowmy2021-concept-note_2020.pdf.

International Council of Nurses. (2017). *Nurses: A voice to lead: Achieving the SDGs.* Retrieved from https://www.icnvoicetolead.com/sdgs/nurses-role/.

International Council of Nurses. (2018). *Nurses, climate change and health: Position statement.* Retrieved from https://www.icn.ch/sites/default/files/inline-files/ICN%20PS%20Nurses%252c%20climate%20change%20and%20health%20FINAL%20.pdf.

International Council of Nurses. (2019a). *Who we are.* Retrieved from https://www.icn.ch/who-we-are.

International Council of Nurses. (2019b). *ICN mission, vision and strategic plan.* Retrieved from https://www.icn.ch/who-we-are/icn-mission-vision-and-strategic-plan.

International Council of Nurses. (2019c). *ICN strategic priorities.* Retrieved from https://www.icn.ch/nursing-policy/icn-strategic-priorities.

International Council of Nurses. (2019d). *Leadership for change (LFC).* Retrieved from https://www.icn.ch/what-we-do/projects/leadership-change-lfc.

Kalogirou, M. R., Morin, J., & Martin, W. (2019). Climate change—A nursing concern. *Alberta RN, 75*(1), 32–33.

Lai, C.-C., Shih, Z.-P., Ko, W.-C., et al. (2020). Severe acute respiratory syndrome coronavirus 2 (SARS-CoV-2) and coronavirus disease-2019 (COVID-19): The epidemic and the challenges. *International Journal of Antimicrobial Agents, 55*(3), 1–9. https://doi.org/10.1016/j.ijantimicag.2020.105924.

Lau, H., Khosrawipour, V., Kocbach, P., et al. (2020). The positive impact of lockdown in Wuhan on containing the COVID-19 outbreak in China. *Journal of Travel Medicine, 27*(2). https://doi.org/10.1093/jtm/taaa037.

Lees, W. D. (2015). Faith in the face of fear. *Trinity Western Magazine*(26), 24–27. Retrieved from https://www.twu.ca/trinity-western-magazine-26.

Low, D. E. (2004). *SARS: Lessons from Toronto. In Learning from SARS: Preparing for the next disease outbreak: Workshop Summary.* Washington, D.C.: The National Academies Press. pp. 63-70.

Maron, D.F. (2020, April). "Wet markets" likely launched the coronavirus. Here's what you need to know. *National Geographic.* Retrieved from https://www.nationalgeographic.com/animals/2020/04/coronavirus-linked-to-chinese-wet-markets/.

Manuel, R., & Derrickson, R. (2017). *The reconciliation manifesto: Recovering the land and rebuilding the economy.* Toronto, ON: James Lorimer & Company.

McMaster University. (2019). *International partnerships.* Retrieved from https://nursing.mcmaster.ca/community/international-partnerships/paho-who-collaborating-centre.

McSpedon, C. (2018). The World Health Organization's Chief Nursing Officer. *American Journal of Nursing, 118*(9), 69–70. https://doi.org/10.1097/01.NAJ.0000544986.95312.c6.

Nurses and Nurse Practitioners of British Columbia. (2019). *Engaging BC nurses with climate change issues.* Retrieved from https://www.nnpbc.com/pdfs/policy-and-advocacy/position-statements/PS-NNPBC-Climate-Change-Issues.pdf.

Nursing Now. (2019a). *Nursing Now campaign.* Retrieved from https://www.nursingnow.org/.

Nursing Now. (2019b). *State of the world's nursing report: Webinar invitation from WHO, ICN and Nursing Now.* Retrieved from https://www.nursingnow.org/state-of-the-worlds-nursing-report-webinar-invitation-from-who-icn-and-nursing-now/.

Registered Nurses' Association of Ontario. (2018, November 15). *Urge the Ontario government to protect health by developing a strong climate change plan.* Retrieved from https://rnao.ca/policy/action-alerts/climate_change_plan.

Registered Nurses' Association of Ontario. (2019a). *Fighting climate change: Sign the pledge.* Retrieved from https://rnao.ca/news/fighting-climate-change-sign-pledge.

Registered Nurses' Association of Ontario. (2019b). *RNAO calls for end to the selling and promotion of vaping products.* Retrieved from https://rnao.ca/news/rnao-calls-end-selling-and-promotion-vaping-products.

Registered Nurses' Association of Ontario. (2019c). *RNAO Nursing Best Practice Guidelines.* Retrieved from https://rnao.ca/sites/rnao-ca/files/2019_ENGLISH_PANELS.pdf.

Registered Nurses' Association of Ontario. (2019d). *RNAO Best Practice Spotlight Organizations* (BPSO). Retrieved from https://rnao.ca/bpg/bpso.

Registered Nurses' Association of Ontario. (2019e). *Guidelines.* Retrieved from https://rnao.ca/bpg/guidelines.

Skolnik, R. (2021). *Global health 101* (4th ed.). Burlington, MA: Jones & Bartlett Learning.

Statistics Canada. (2017). *Focus on geography series, 2016 census.* Retrieved from https://www12.statcan.gc.ca/census-recensement/2016/as-sa/fogs-spg/Index-eng.cfm.

Stone, S. B., Myers, S. S., & Golden, C. D. (2018). Cross-cutting principles for planetary health education. *The Lancet, 2,* 92–193. https://doi.org/10.1016/S2542-5196(18)30022-6.

Taha, S., Maloney-Hall, B., & Buxton, J. (2019). Lessons learned from the opioid crisis across the pillars of the Canadian drugs and substances strategy. *Substance Abuse, Treatment, Prevention, and Policy, 14,* 32. https://doi.org/10.1186/s13011-019-0220-7.

United Nations. (2015). *The Millennium Development Goals report 2015.* Retrieved from https://www.un.org/millenniumgoals/2015_MDG_Report/pdf/MDG%202015%20rev%20(July%201).pdf.

United Nations Climate Change. (2020). *Paris Agreement—Status of ratification.* Retrieved from https://unfccc.int/process/the-paris-agreement/status-of-ratification.

United Nations High Commissioner of Refugees Canada. (2019). *What is UNHCR?* Retrieved from https://www.unhcr.ca/what-we-do/about-unhcr/.

Watts, N., Amann, M., Ayeb-Karlsson, S., et al. (2017). The Lancet countdown on health and climate change: From years of inaction to global transformation for public health. *The Lancet, 391*(10120), 581–630. https://doi.org/10.1016/S0140-6736(17)32464-9.

Whitmee, S., Haines, A., Beyrer, C., et al. (2015). Safeguarding human health in the Anthropocene epoch: Report of The Rockefeller Foundation–*Lancet* Commission on planetary health. *Lancet, 386*, 1973–2028. https://doi.org/10.1016/S0140-6736(15)60901-1.

World Health Organization. (2002). *Nursing midwifery services: Strategic directions 2002–2008.* Geneva, Switzerland: Author.

World Health Organization. (2003). *An international treaty for tobacco control.* Retrieved from http://www.who.int/features/2003/08/en/index.html.

World Health Organization. (2010a). *What is a pandemic?* Retrieved from https://www.who.int/csr/disease/swineflu/frequently_asked_questions/pandemic/en/.

World Health Organization. (2010b). *What is the pandemic (H1N1) 2009 virus?* Retrieved from https://www.who.int/csr/disease/swineflu/frequently_asked_questions/about_disease/en/.

World Health Organization. (2014). *Geographic distribution of Ebola virus disease outbreaks in humans and animals.* Retrieved from https://www.who.int/csr/disease/ebola/global_ebolaoutbreakrisk_20140818-1.png.

World Health Organization. (2016a). *Global strategic directions for strengthening nursing and midwifery 2016–2020.* Retrieved from https://www.who.int/hrh/nursing_midwifery/global-strategic-midwifery2016-2020.pdf.

World Health Organization. (2016b) *Government Chief Nursing and Midwifery Officers discuss strategies on the future of nursing and midwifery workforce.* Retrieved from https://www.who.int/hrh/news/2016/discuss_strategies/en/.

World Health Organization. (2017a). *Dr. Tedros takes office as WHO Director-General.* Retrieved from https://www.who.int/news-room/detail/01-07-2017-dr-tedros-takes-office-as-who-director-general.

World Health Organization. (2017b). *What is antimicrobial resistance?* Retrieved from https://www.who.int/features/qa/75/en/.

World Health Organization. (2018, June 1). *Noncommunicable diseases.* Retrieved from https://www.who.int/news-room/fact-sheets/detail/noncommunicable-diseases.

World Health Organization. (2019a). *WHO report on the global tobacco epidemic, 2019: Offer help to quit tobacco use.* Retrieved from https://apps.who.int/iris/bitstream/handle/10665/326043/9789241516204-eng.pdf.

World Health Organization. (2019b). *Climate change.* Retrieved from https://www.who.int/health-topics/climate-change#tab=overview.

World Health Organization. (2019c). *"Together for a healthier world": Dr. Tedros Adhanom Ghebreyesus' vision.* Retrieved from https://www.who.int/dg.

World Health Organization. (2019d). *Collaborating centres.* Retrieved from https://www.who.int/about/who-we-are/structure/collaborating-centres.

World Health Organization. (2020a). *Timeline of WHO's response to COVID-19.* Retrieved from https://www.who.int/news-room/detail/29-06-2020-covidtimeline.

World Health Organization. (2020b). *Naming the coronavirus disease (COVID-19) and the virus that causes it.* Retrieved from https://www.who.int/emergencies/diseases/novel-coronavirus-2019/technical-guidance/naming-the-coronavirus-disease-(covid-2019)-and-the-virus-that-causes-it.

World Health Organization. (2020c). *WHO Director-General's opening remarks at the media briefing on COVID-19—3 March 2020.* Retrieved from https://www.who.int/dg/speeches/detail/who-director-general-s-opening-remarks-at-the-media-briefing-on-covid-19---3-march-2020.

World Health Organization. (2020d). *Coronavirus (COVID-19) Dashboard.* Retrieved from https://covid19.who.int/.

World Health Organization. (2020e). *New Ebola outbreak detected in northwest Democratic Republic of the Congo; WHO surge team supporting the response.* Retrieved from https://www.who.int/news-room/detail/01-06-2020-new-ebola-outbreak-detected-in-northwest-democratic-republic-of-the-congo-who-surge-team-supporting-the-response.

World Health Organization. (2020f). *State of the world's nursing report 2020.* Retrieved from https://www.who.int/publications/i/item/9789240003279.

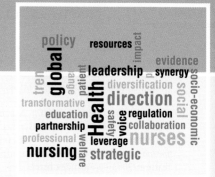

Internationalization in Canadian Nursing

Ndolo Njie-Mokonya

ⓔ http://evolve.elsevier.com/Canada/Ross-Kerr/nursing

LEARNING OBJECTIVES

After reading this chapter, you will be able to:
- Understand internationalization of nursing in Canada within the context of health human resources outcomes and globalization.
- Describe strategies and activities whereby Canadian nursing practice has become internationalized.
- Identify nursing practice and education challenges confronting internationally recruited nurses in Canada.
- Describe internationally recruited nurses' contributions to nursing in Canada.

- Describe the ethical implications of international nurse recruitment.
- Understand nursing's role in integrating internationally educated nurses to the care team.
- Understand international nurse recruitment within the context of a health human resources framework.
- Understand current research exploring internationalization of nurses in Canada.

OUTLINE

KEY TERMS

credential evaluation
globalization
international recruitment
internationally educated nurses
licensure
migration

nurse migration
nursing regulatory bodies
nursing shortage
patient experience
patient safety
transition

PERSONAL PERSPECTIVES

My interest in researching the experience of internationally educated nurses in the Canadian health care system comes from my personal experience as an immigrant student in Canada within a Bachelor of Science in Nursing program. Having completed more than 15 years of nursing practice and clinical practicum instruction in the Canadian health care system, I have had the opportunity to observe firsthand the difficulties experienced by nursing students from immigrant communities during their clinical practicums. As a nursing student who completed her elementary education in a West African nation, I knew that my educational background differed from that of my nursing school peers. For example, I encountered one such difference when I wrote my first exam in the nursing program. The exam consisted of only multiple-choice questions, but I had been used to a long-answer exam style. This disadvantage, coupled with the fact that I am a visible minority, rather fortified my will to succeed. I knew that the only way to successfully complete the nursing program and become a nurse in Canada was to adapt to the ways of learning and nursing as taught within the academic program here. Therefore, my interest in this topic was derived from the experiences and challenges I faced in practice settings in Canada, particularly as an immigrant student nurse in a university program. Furthermore, as a current graduate student, I became increasingly aware of how knowledge creation strengthens our understanding of concepts and theory. This belief has served as an impetus for me to examine this under-researched area of nursing practice. It is for these reasons that making explicit the knowledge of internationally educated nurses from their own perspectives is of utmost importance.

INTRODUCTION

This chapter addresses how nursing transcends national and international boundaries and examines the development of nursing in other countries. The effects of internationalization in Canadian nursing will be explored within the context of international nurse recruitment and **migration. Nurse migration** for the purposes of employment dates back many decades. International nurse recruitment by Western countries, including Canada, has occurred as a result of economic **globalization** and a predicted nurse shortage in the workforce. A synopsis of why nurse recruiters continue to recruit internationally to sustain local nursing positions in their various countries will be described, followed by a discussion of ethical implications related to international nurse recruitment. Then, a synopsis of research and published work that describes the impact of international nurse recruitment for **internationally educated nurses** (IENs), nursing practice, and education will be presented. Understanding the value of IENs and the factors that influence their recruitment are likely to inform policies and legislation that support their integration and increase awareness of the socioeconomic and political factors that influence the nursing profession itself.

GLOBAL NURSE MIGRATION

Predicted global nurse shortages have led developed countries like Canada, the United States, the United Kingdom, and Australia to undertake and establish international nurse recruitment practices (Edge & Hoffman, 2013). For instance, the American Association of Colleges of Nursing has predicted that the registered nurse (RN) workforce will grow from 2.9 million in 2016 to 3.4 million in 2026. They are projecting a need for 203,700 new RNs every year until 2026 to address the **nursing shortage** resulting from baby boomer retirements and increasing health care demands (American Association of Colleges of Nursing, 2019). In the United Kingdom, the National Health Service has predicted a shortage of 40,000 nurses (Geissler, 2019). Similarly, the Australian government has predicted a shortage of 85,000 nurses by 2025 (Health Workforce Australia, 2014). In Canada, despite 1.4% growth in the number of regulated nurses entering the workforce between 2017 and 2018, this represents a decrease from the annual supply rate of 2.2% in 2014 (Canadian Institute for Health Information [CIHI], 2019). A nurse shortage of about 60,000 full-time RN positions is still predicted by 2022, particularly in the care of seniors and in community work settings (Canadian Nurses Association, 2019).

Other factors that have contributed to increasing nurse shortages in developed countries are an aging nursing population, reduced hours worked by nurses, a decrease in the allotment of full-time university nursing positions, increased co-morbid conditions, and the use of technology and increasing health care service needs; as a result, governments have been forced to fill these vacancies through **international recruitment** (Buchan, 2006; Konno, 2006; Squires, Ojemeni, & Jones, 2016). In Canada, 8.5% of the regulated nurse workforce is made up of IENs, an increase from 7.8% over the last 5 years (CIHI, 2019). This increase translates to 36,189 IENs. Within the context of forecasting and health systems planning, the predicted nursing shortage partly contributes to increased mobilization among these skilled workers and global migration due to nurse recruitment.

The aging population in Canada is another major contributor to the growing demand for health care services and the added pressure placed on health human resources to meet this demand. Consequently, the government has predicted a greater need for nurses in the workforce, which has implications both for nurses who supply such services and for the population requiring nursing services. For example, according to recent Statistics Canada population predictions, seniors will make up one-quarter of the Canadian population by 2036 (Statistic Canada, 2019). These predictions imply that the nursing workforce itself is rapidly aging as well. Hence, nurses at any stage of their careers—be it the early, mid-, or late phase—are likely to influence the supply of nurses. From 2014 to 2018, nurses under the age of 40 increased from 38.9% to 43.6% of the RN workforce; nurses from ages 40 to 59 decreased from 49% to 45.2%; and nurses over 60 years of age decreased slightly from 12% to 11.2% (CIHI, 2019).

Figure 26.1 shows the trend for the nursing workforce by age group from 2014 to 2018. The figure shows that most nurses currently within the workforce are between the ages of 40 and 59. For nurses under 40 years of age, it is unknown what proportion accounts for the millennials and postmillennial age groups. Expected nurse shortages in the next few decades due to an aging workforce, according to Canadian regulated nurse supply predictions, is highly foreseeable if trends remain unchanged. This will continue to reinforce the practice of international nurse recruitment in Canada to address these predicted nurse shortages.

Likewise, the increasingly aging population in Canada is likely to contribute to the rising demands for nursing services. As patients live longer with two or more comorbidities and an increasing need for health services, it will translate into longer stays in hospital and an increased demand for care within the home and in the community (CIHI, 2019; Squires, Ojemeni, & Jones, 2016). In addition, as health service delivery shifts from predominantly hospital-based to more community-based models, home care and primary care—including outpatient treatment centres, home care services, and long-term care (CIHI, 2017)—are creating increasing demands for nurses within community and primary care practice settings. The cumulative

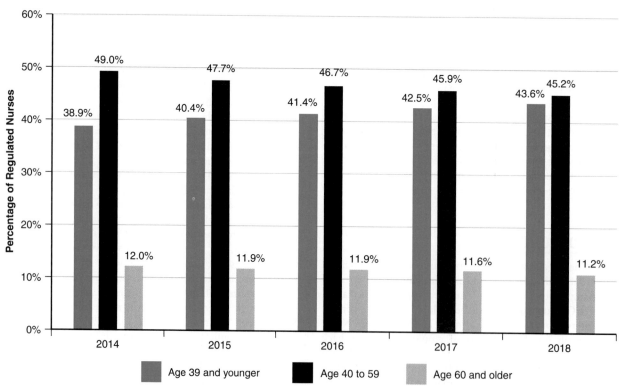

Fig. 26.1 Registered nurse workforce in Canada by age group, 2014–2018. (**Source:** Canadian Institute for Health Information. (2019). *Nursing in Canada, 2018: A lens on supply and workforce.* Ottawa, ON: Author.)

effect of these trends is an increasing demand for nursing services. The CIHI (2017) has reported that "these trends challenge health system planners and decision-makers as they balance changes in service delivery while continuing to provide a level of service and care that considers access, quality and appropriateness alongside the cost of delivering care" (p. 22). The next two sections consider the socioeconomic and political factors that sustain international nurse recruitment as well as the discourses surrounding the ethical effects of international nurse recruitment.

ACTIVITIES THAT FOSTER THE MOBILIZATION OF NURSES

International Policies and Migration Laws

Several international policies and agreements between developed and underdeveloped nations have fostered the mobilization of skilled workers, including nurses, in the global market. In 2008, the Canadian government, through its immigration policies, implemented programs that facilitated the migration of skilled workers within certain professional classes and levels of education to meet employment demands and to strengthen the economy in the long term (Citizenship and Immigration Canada, 2009). Two such programs were the Canadian Experience Class program in 2008 and the Foreign Credential Recognition program in 2009 (Human Resources and Skills Development Canada [HRSDC], 2009). For instance, the Foreign Credential Recognition program facilitated the recognition of skilled workers' credentials to support their integration into their respective professional occupations (HRSDC, 2009).

Another mechanism promoting credential recognition within Canada uses the labour mobility provisions of the Canadian Free Trade Agreement (Internal Trade Secretariat, n.d.). The labour mobility provisions target "barriers specific to national workforce migration within regulated professions" (Nelson, Verma, Hall et al., 2011, p. 2) to promote national professional credential recognition between provinces and the establishment of "occupational competency as the ideal assessment criteria of professionals" (Nelson, Verma, Hall et al., 2011, p. 2). In addition, once the credentials of internationally recruited health care providers (including nurses) are recognized in one province, they are accepted throughout Canada.

Although migration laws attempt to accurately describe the immigration status of IENs, nurse migration remains complex, as most IENs enter Canada through the immigration points system as spousal dependents or under the Live-in Caregiver Program (Blythe and Baumann, 2009; Nelson, Verma, Hall et al., 2011). In response to the federal economic plan, nomination programs were developed within the provinces to further attract IENs. Despite the skilled worker laws and agreements promoting nurse recruitment, the mobility of nurses and their credential transferability have given rise to ethical implications pertaining to the portability of their nursing skills and an ability for "professional associations and regulators to manage the challenges of skill recognition and workplace integration" (Nelson, Verma, Hall et al., 2011, p. 5). Therefore, the ethical implications of the transferability of nursing skills as a result of international recruitment merits further consideration.

Ethical Implications of International Nurse Recruitment

There are documented concerns surrounding the ethical and social injustices of international recruitment and nurse migration, particularly for nurses who migrate from underdeveloped countries (Canadian Nurses Association, 2017; International Council of Nurses [ICN], 2019; Li, Nie, & Li, 2014; Nelson, Verma, Hall et al., 2011; Shaffer, Bakhshi, & Alvarez, 2019; Squires, 2008). Nurses are included on the list of preferred skilled workers permitted to immigrate to Canada as a way to sustain international economic cooperation (Shaffer, Bakhshi, & Alvarez, 2019; Nelson, Verma, Hall et al., 2011). This international cooperation is partly attributed to the frequent global demand for nurses to fill workforce vacancies as well as the perceived portability of nursing knowledge and skills to meet these demands (Sherwood & Shaffer, 2014; Squires, 2008; Zolot, 2019). Sherwood and Shaffer (2014) explored the ethical implications that underlie this assumption by situating international nurse recruitment within the context of providing quality and safe care. With **patient safety** being foundational to quality and ethical care, the authors argued that the transferability of IEN nursing knowledge requires more than merely gaining employment in the host country, stating that "nurses from different countries may have differing philosophical views of nursing and beliefs about human rights and social justice that influence ethical safe practice" (Sherwood & Shaffer, 2014, p. 49).

The role of nurses, their scopes of practice, their nursing education, and the health care systems within which they work vary among nations (Njie-Mokonya, 2014; Baumann, Blythe, Kolotylo, & Underwood, 2004). Ensuring consistency in role and competency when making recruitment decision is vital to enhance safe patient care in the host countries especially since nurses are a key part of the health care system; in fact, they are the largest group of regulated health professional within the health care system (RNAO, 2016).

Furthermore, within the context of patient safety and the appropriateness of skill transferability, the competency of IENs and their role inconsistencies must be considered during their integration and **credential evaluation** programs (Sherwood & Shaffer, 2014). In addition, IENs must be evaluated to ensure that they fully grasp the health care systems into which they have been recruited (Njie-Mokonya, 2014). For example, Njie-Mokonya (2014) used the following quote from a study participant to illustrate the importance of ensuring that IENs understand new models and systems of health care delivery:

> *Institutions who hire IENs need to make emphasis on interdisciplinary and available community services . . . if I didn't go to the bridging program here in Canada, I wouldn't have understood how Canadian system works, e.g., what's free and not free; health coverage, community services etc. particularly for psychiatric patients who need to go back into the community.* (p. 81)

A second quote from another participant in the same study (Njie-Mokonya, 2014) exemplifies how IENs need time to adapt to new work environments:

> *They use acronyms here and you wonder what they are talking about, despite the need to write things out for someone new—it is a different language [referring to professional abbreviations]. If you don't know what it means during the induction session, with time you eventually figure it out. When you ask, you look like you don't know. They use abbreviations like ADL, CCAC, and ALC. They use it every day, even with orientation presentations, in fact throughout the presentation.* (p. 90)

Within the discourse of skill transfer and patient safety and advocacy, simply recruiting a person who holds a nurse title from oversees is inadequate. As nurse migration and international recruitment continues owing to workforce demands, IENs will continue to secure employment globally (Tulenko, 2012). Given that health care systems are increasingly complex and vary among nations, it remains to be seen whether educational and professional practice standards can be instituted internationally (Baumann, Blythe, Kolotylo, & Underwood, 2004; Nelson, Verma, Hall et al., 2011).

Nurses can be identified among preferred skilled workers recruited to occupy vacant job positions internationally. However, socioeconomic and ethical challenges exist when nurses are recruited from underdeveloped to developed countries, depleting the poorer nations of their own qualified health care workers. The "brain gain, drain waste" phenomenon is said to occur when health care workers migrate to Western nations and then are seemingly not used to their full capacity owing to the legislative and licensing requirements that must be met (Bourgeault, Neiterman, Lebrun

RESEARCH FOCUS

Does International Nurse Recruitment Promote Patient Safety?

Employment trends suggest that recruiting IENs who hold the title of "registered nurse" can both address staffing needs and ultimately ensure that the standards of patient care are met. While some IENs are recruited directly into health care organizations, others gain employment through health recruiting agencies that assist in staffing these health care organizations. Is the recruitment of health care providers holding a registered nurse title adequate for meeting patient care needs? Sherwood and Shaffer (2014) examined the role of IENs in providing quality and safe care in the workforce. The authors found that, owing to differences in educational preparation, professional standards and scopes of practice, and differing nursing philosophies, IEN practice competencies presented concerns with patient safety. The authors suggested that the quality of support IENs receive during their **transition** into new work environments can determine their ability to adapt to the environment and positively contribute to providing quality and safe care to patients.

Source: Sherwood, G. D., & Shaffer, F. A. (2014). The role of internationally educated nurses in a quality, safe workforce. *Nursing Outlook, 62*(1), 46–52. https://doi.org/10.1016/j.outlook.2013.11.001.

et al., 2010). An intersection of pull–push variables facilitate these movements. For example, nurses may migrate out of their home countries in pursuit of the *pull* factor from industrialized countries, such as the prospects of better career opportunities and professional growth (Jose, 2010; Li, Nie, & Lie, 2014; Sherwood & Shaffer, 2014) as well as reunion with family (Blythe & Baumann, 2009; Squires, 2008). These *pull* factors are facilitated by *push* conditions in the health care and economic systems of the source countries, which causes nurses to leave for better employment conditions and wages overseas. Sherwood and Shaffer (2014) have cited push conditions like "low wages, limited job and professional growth opportunities, lack of resources in the work environment" (p. 47) in addition to gender discriminatory against women (Nichols, Davis & Richardson, 2010) and a disadvantaged health care system structure (Kingma, 2007).

Even though the ICN (2008) supports the migration rights of individual nurses who are in pursuit of career advancement, the Council stands against depleting poorer countries of their valuable health workers and the recruitment of nurses into poor work conditions in the West.

Ethical concerns arise when nurses are recruited from low-income and underdeveloped countries that are dealing with their own struggling health care systems. Inattention to the detrimental effects of recruitment within poor countries is likely to increase nurses' desire to leave their countries because of poor work conditions and to seek better work and career progression opportunities abroad (Li, Nie, & Li, 2014). Both the recruiting and source countries need to remain aware of the ethical implications of international nurse recruitment from the perspective of social responsibility. Migration policies and programs must be balanced with the individual and professional responsibility to give back to society, especially in underdeveloped countries. Global inattention to this dilemma will cause nurses from less developed countries to continue leaving for better employment prospects, leaving the source countries in worse condition (Li, Nie, & Li, 2014).

 APPLYING CONTENT KNOWLEDGE

Identify and discuss the social responsibility factors that should be considered by nursing associations, nurse leaders, and nurse recruiters before they engage in international recruitment in order to minimize the negative effects in source countries.

EXPERIENCES OF INTERNATIONALLY EDUCATED NURSES IN DESTINATION COUNTRIES

Practice Challenges

IENs experience practice and educational challenges upon arrival in their destination countries. Some of the challenges that IENs experience before obtaining their regulated nurse license include credential evaluation (Allan & Westwood, 2016); low licensure exam pass rates (Covell, Neiterman, & Bourgeault, 2016; Hall, Stevens, & Meleis, 2015); and access to bridging programs where "gaps in their training or education is matched to those of local graduates" (Neiterman, Bourgeault, Peters et al., 2018). Even after successfully obtaining their RN **licensure**, IENs experience challenges such as understanding medical and professional terminology (Lum, Bradley & Valeo, 2015; Njie-Mokonya, 2014; O'Neil, 2011); being unaware of professional standards and the extent of a nurse's scope of practice (Jose, 2011; Blythe & Baumann, 2009; Sherwood & Shaffer, 2014; Njie-Mokonya, 2014); having weak communication skills and lack of proficiency in the English language (Yi & Jezewski, 2000); and facing cultural and nonverbal communication obstacles that can create confusion in social interactions (Bola, Driggers, Dunlap, & Ebersole, 2003; Tregunno, Peters, Campbell, & Gordon, 2009; Yi & Jezewski, 2000).

A study by Bola, Driggers, Dunlap, & Ebersole (2003) illustrates how differences in the interpretation of cultural norms between an IEN and their locally trained counterparts can influence how nonverbal cues such as eye contact are interpreted. The authors demonstrated this difference by conceptualizing cultures as being either high context or low context. High-context cultures attach greater meaning to nonverbal communication cues such as eye contact, while low-context cultures attach less meaning to nonverbal cues and more meaning to words. Given the verbal and nonverbal communication challenges faced by IENs, it can be expected that communication extends beyond an IEN's capacity to speak English with their patients and colleagues. They must also be familiar with the organizational hierarchy, the health care system, and culture of Canadian society in order to function efficiently as a health care provider (Njie-Mokonya, 2014).

While skilled worker immigration policies support skill transferability, IENs often migrate without a full understanding of nursing practices, standards, and educational preparation before trying to obtain licensure in their new country. One study has suggested that the majority of IENs in Canada arrive with immigrant visas (Baumann, Blythe, Rhéaume, & McIntosh, 2006) and that other IENs are issued work visas under the Live-In Caregiver Program (Bourgeault, Neiterman, Lebrun et al., 2010; Blythe & Baumann, 2009). With limited Canadian work experience and low initial licensure pass rates (Salami & Nelson, 2014; Kolawole, 2009), IENs may instead seek alternate employment to familiarize themselves with Canadian culture and the health care system in their new province or territory (Njie-Mokonya, 2014) as well as to improve their communication skills (Covell, Neiterman, & Bourgeault, 2016). In Njie-Mokonya's (2014) study, one IEN described her approach to gaining familiarity with the Canadian health care system and how it facilitated her integration experience after obtaining her RN licensure:

> I worked as a nanny and as a care aid with a community agency, so I already had some integration into the Canadian culture. I had a feel of how nursing worked in Canada . . . by the time I started working as an RN I have had some exposure to the health care system. (p. 80)

IENs seem to have better transition experiences as nurses when they have gained previous work experience as live-in nannies or as unregulated care providers in Canada, when they have past experience migrating to another country first, and when they have previously worked in similar specialties (e.g., in an operating room) (Njie-Mokonya, 2014).

National and international studies have documented IENs' experiences of marginalization, racism, and cultural shock after securing employment in their host countries. Research studies and reports on the experiences of IENs in Canada and overseas have suggested that they often feel discriminated against at work (Dico-Bloom, 2004; Kingma, 2008; Neiterman & Bourgeault, 2015; Njie-Mokonya, 2014; Tregunno, Peters, Campbell, & Gordon, 2009; Turrittin, Hagey, Guruge et al., 2002) and experience communication barriers caused by strong accents (Njie-Mokonya, 2014). Furthermore, their experiences of discrimination appear to be universally consistent.

In Njie-Mokonya's (2014) study, IENs reported experiencing incivility from nurses, physicians, and patients and their families. One IEN narrated her experience with a physician, describing it as discriminatory: "Sometimes they [referring to surgeons] are mean to me . . . they will ask, 'Are you Canadian?' I think the hospitals should hire Canadians first. I need to learn to speak up more" (p. 74). Another IEN from a different hospital reported similar experiences of nurse–physician impoliteness, stating, "Some surgeons or anesthetists if they don't like you, they treat you badly . . . they don't talk to you, so this hinders communication" [referring to communication about patient care] (p. 74). Similarly, another IEN described her experience of working on a ward where she did not feel accepted: "I don't feel part of the team, I received poor report[s] from the staff, and I have less time to spend with patients and families. I did not receive help from other nurses" (p. 74). Yet another IEN felt that her accent posed an issue of trust both to patients and to her nursing colleagues:

> Patients don't feel trust right away because of accent . . . they're more suspicious; they ask about your training . . . they're afraid, but after doing your job well, they trust you. With my nursing colleagues, they didn't trust initially because of my accent. They verify with other nurses about my abilities and knowledge to provide care. (Njie-Mokonya, 2014, p. 97)

The documented challenges that IENs face once employed have been attributed to differences in scope of practice (McGillis Hall, Jones, Lalonde et al., 2015), educational preparation (Blythe & Baumann, 2009), and professional language comprehension (Njie-Mokonya, 2014). Neiterman and Bourgeault's (2015) study has suggested similar unwelcoming experiences, with more IENs than other internationally trained health care providers experiencing racism. Marginalizing experiences negatively influence IENs' integration into their workplaces and often lead to feelings of isolation and frustration. Integration

programs that lack comprehensive support structures for IENs as they transition into Canadian work settings are likely to leave them with substandard attitudes towards their colleagues and workplaces (O'Brien-Pallas & Wang, 2006).

Furthermore, the ability of IENs to seamlessly engage in professional communication is often hindered due to their accents. Accents pose a hindrance because the relational nature and professional work life of nurses consists of constant communication with patients, families, other nurses, and interprofessional team members involved in patient care. IENs who spoke English as a second language encountered barriers in both written (e.g., proper spelling) and expressive (e.g., spoken fluency in English or French) communication with other health care team members or with patients (Njie-Mokonya, 2014). In addition, Njie-Mokonya (2014) found that the issue of language comprehension was bidirectional. In other words, some IENs experienced challenges understanding their patients' accents, particularly those of French-speaking patients or their families, and vice versa, where the patients, families, or Canadian-trained nurse colleagues had difficulties understanding the IENs when they spoke because of their accent.

In the same study by Njie-Mokonya (2014), IENs described the challenges they had with communication, particularly during telephone conversations while giving or receiving orders or during transfer of accountability to or from other teams involved with patient care. As one IEN who worked in the operating room stated:

> I was anxious about being understood . . . or getting verbal report or messages for surgeons from the floor nurse. I never did floor nursing, so I do not know the order of ward routine. It is difficult to interrupt surgeon during their surgical procedures, so I take the message. Still learning, not comfortable with phone call situations, I don't want to put patients in danger. (Njie-Mokonya, 2014, p. 96)

Others discovered that the complexity of professional language was more challenging than daily English, which was shocking to some and caused them anxiety. As one participant noted:

> Some IENs are less confident, they feel like they didn't practice English language enough, I think we are just overwhelmed with all the information . . . not really nursing information, but not being fluent in English or French triggers nervousness . . . About language, language has to be absorbed; professional language is different in that it is not taught in school; you have to work to attain a comfort level. (Njie-Mokonya, 2014, p. 96).

In addition to enrolling in bridging programs, IENs will seek alternative employment as a strategy to adapt to the

Canadian culture, obtain different patient care experiences, and improve language proficiency (Njie-Mokonya, 2014; Neiterman, Bourgeault, & Covell, 2017). For instance, in a study by Neiterman, Bourgeault, and Covell (2017) examining bridging programs targeted at IENs, they identified challenges developing content to match the diverse needs of these IENs. The need to learn the nuances of professional language and culture may explain why IENs seek other employment outside of nursing to develop competence in communicating with nurses and other health care providers.

 APPLYING CONTENT KNOWLEDGE

Given the benefit of bridging programs, present an argument for the need to offer mandatory socialization programs just before, or immediately following, the hiring of IENs into the Canadian workforce.

Since Njie-Mokonya's work in 2014, other Canadian authors (Lum, Bradley & Valeo, 2015; Lum, Dowedoff & Englander, 2016) have published work that examines IEN competence in oral communication. Their findings suggest similar experiences of unfamiliarity with professional language and how it varies with day-to-day communication in English. Lum and her colleagues have stated that "having a general knowledge of an official language, such as English or French in Canada, does not necessarily mean that a new immigrant will be familiar with, and can apply language skills appropriately, within the practice context" (Lum, Dowedoff & Englander, 2016, p. 345). While IENs arrive in a country with hopes of integrating into the nursing work life and environment, little do they know how much time will be needed to fully integrate into the professional health care culture of that country. Yet, they do not see the need for added communication training (Lum, Dowedoff, & Englander, 2016) either with bridging training or alternative employment in order to attain a level of professional communication competence. Likewise, bridging programs are a key means to improving professional language and communication skills when creating support programs for IENs to facilitate their integration.

Marginalization appears to be more prevalent in social professions, such as nursing, where professional distinction and hierarchy are present (Hall, Stevens & Meleis, 1994). For example, depending on the work environment, a nursing team could consist of an RN, a registered practical nurse, a nurse manager, and an advanced practice nurse, all of whom could come from various ethnic backgrounds. Hall, Stevens, and Meleis (1994) describes marginalization as "the process through which persons are peripheralized

on the basis of their identities, associations, experiences, and environments" (p. 25). From this definition, one could describe IENs as being different from other nurses based on their racial or ethnic background as well as their past nursing experiences. In addition, within the nursing profession, distinctions are further enhanced in terms of qualifications and positions that create and sustain distinct boundaries (Hall, Stevens, & Meleis, 1994). An IEN who sounds and looks different from other nurses and is working in a new position in a new environment and new country could fit into the above-described peripheralized criteria. Even though discriminatory experiences are not unique to IENs, an understanding of marginalizing tendencies, particularly given the social nature of the nursing profession, can facilitate the creation of appropriate support policies and educational programs for the integration of IENs as well as raising awareness among their Canadian-trained colleagues.

RESEARCH FOCUS

Internationally Educated Nurse Occupation Trends in Destination Countries

The supposed portability of IEN competencies and skills has been identified as one reason for their recruitment. But is it true that the "once a nurse, always a nurse" attitude suggest that a nurse trained in a specialty (e.g., maternity nurse) can work in that specialty anywhere? IENs as well as their employers have reported barriers to matching their competencies with the educational and credential evaluation requirements in their destination countries. A study by Salami, Meherali, and Covell (2018) explored the occupational mobility of 14 baccalaureate-prepared IENs after they arrived in Canada. The authors found that these IENs followed the employment path of becoming licensed practical nurses while pursuing their credential evaluation. For these IENs, it was the easier employment option. These findings suggest that IENs do experience barriers to gaining employment as RNs. The IENs also experience deskilling and dissatisfaction with their employment experience in their new country.

Source: Salami, B., Meherali, S., & Covell, C. L. (2018). Downward occupational mobility of baccalaureate-prepared, internationally educated nurses to licensed practical nurses. *International Nursing Review, 65,* 173–181.

Educational Challenges

When nurses are recruited internationally to fill positions in host countries, they must possess the required professional preparation that is equivalent to the educational preparation and clinical competencies required of nurses in the host countries, requiring IENs to augment their education and clinical skills. This gap is due to inconsistencies in nursing educational preparation (Blythe & Baumann, 2009) and scope of practice in the source countries (McGillis Hall, Jones, Lalonde et al., 2015; Sherwood and Shaffer, 2014; Njie-Mokonya, 2014; Jose, 2011). In Canada, some IENs enroll in bridging educational programs to address gaps in their training or education (Neiterman, Bourgeault, & Covell, 2017, p. 23). And yet there is scarce nursing literature comprehensively examining the impact of educational bridging programs for IENs. Fortunately, there is growing interest in this subject, resulting in more published work by Canadian and international authors on the structure of bridging programs as well as the experiences of IENs who enroll in these bridging programs (Atack, Cruz, Maher, & Murphy, 2012; Canadian Association of Schools of Nursing, 2012; Lum, Dowedoff, & Englander, 2016; Neiterman, Bourgeault, & Covell, 2017; Xu & He, 2012).

Ontario is the destination of choice for nearly 40% of the skilled workers who migrate to Canada every year, with many health care providers among them (Government of Ontario, 2013). Since 2003, the Ontario government has invested over $240 million in bridging education programs (Government of Ontario, 2013). In Canada, unlike Australia or the United Kingdom, bridging programs receive public funding, since international health care providers immigrate into the country under the skilled worker program (Xu & He, 2012).

CASE STUDY

Common Initial Workplace Experiences Among Internationally Educated Nurses

Kate is a 35-year-old IEN. She has been a licensed RN in Ontario for a little over 6 months. She completed her university degree in nursing from the Philippines where she worked as an operating room nurse for 5 years before emigrating to Canada. Upon her arrival in Ontario, she enrolled in a bridging college program for IENs, completed her practicum hours as required by the College of Nurses of Ontario, and successfully secured employment with a local hospital, where she did her practicum as an operating room nursing student. Despite her past work experience as an operating room nurse in the Philippines, she has experienced challenges integrating with her team at work. She does not feel welcomed by them, and her knowledge as a nurse is questioned by the care team. As the charge nurse working with Kate, what factors would you consider exploring with her to ensure a positive work experience?

According to the Canadian Association of Schools of Nursing, there are approximately 35 bridging programs in Canada that IENs can attend (Canadian Association of Schools of Nursing, 2012). Indicators that are evaluated in order for IENs to successfully obtain their professional licenses are credentials, professional competencies, and language proficiency (Neiterman, Bourgeault, & Covell, 2017). Bridging programs are routinely recommended to internationally educated health care providers, including nurses, when any of the three assessed criteria do not match the levels of their colleagues who were trained in Canada. It has been a challenge to establish an appropriate format for the bridging programs that will match the individual needs of internationally trained health care providers (Bourgeault et al., 2010), since IENs come with varying educational backgrounds (Blythe & Baumann, 2009) and scopes of practice (McGillis-Hall et al., 2015). These factors may contribute to variations in the program structure despite provincial financial investments in the bridging programs.

RESEARCH FOCUS

Transition Program Analysis for Internationally Educated Nurses: Lessons to Be Learned

Transition programs in Canada and overseas that offer complementary courses to IENs to match their competencies and education and that perform credential evaluation vary in structure, content, and program length. These inconsistencies have been attributed to the varying experiences that IENs bring to their destination countries, such as differences in educational preparation, scope of practice, working language proficiency, and cultural differences. In view of a growing trend to manage IEN transition programs nationally as well as systematically to best support workforce challenges, can lessons be learned from international practices? A review by Xu and He (2012) evaluated IEN transition programs in Canada, the United States, the United Kingdom, and Australia—the four highest-recruiting nations for IENs. The authors found differences such as when the transition programs were required or implemented (i.e., prelicensure versus postlicensure). Looking at the similarities and differences to both approaches as well as the pros and cons, the authors' findings suggest a move towards nationally supervised standardized programs that are transparent and equitable as well as including rigorous competency assessments that meet practice standards.

Source: Xu, Y., & He, F. (2012). Transition programs for internationally educated nurses: What can the United States learn from the United Kingdom, Australia, and Canada? *Nursing Economics, 30*(4), 215–239.

Neiterman et al., (2017) identified four challenges with the bridging programs. The challenges were developing a curriculum that addresses diverse participant needs, identifying optimal format for program delivery, obtaining clinical placements for participants, and financial sustainability for programs within community colleges and institutions (Neiterman, Bourgeault, & Covell, 2017, p. 26). Despite these challenges, IENs contribute positively to **patient experience** (Njie-Mokonya, 2016). In addition, IENs in the Neiterman et al. study reported that attending the bridging programs was beneficial to them, as they were able to form valuable networks and gain Canadian experience. IENs have also reported increased awareness of the Canadian health care system and available programs pertaining to patient care, especially patient discharge and community support programs (Njie-Mokonya, 2014).

CONTRIBUTION OF INTERNATIONALLY EDUCATED NURSES TO NURSING IN CANADA

The ongoing recruitment of IENs in Canada reflects the growing diversity of Canada's population. As previously discussed, this growing diversity has led to increasing disparities in the delivery of health care services, particularly among patients from different ethnic backgrounds (Njie-Mokonya, 2016). The multilingual capabilities of IENs uniquely positions them to enhance the patient experience and thus strengthens the health care service teams they are a part of. The ICN (2013) supports health care service teams made up of diverse health care providers to promote the provision of culturally appropriate care to all patients. When IENs are part of nursing teams, they are likely to share insights about other cultures with their Canadian-trained nurse colleagues and could provide language translation services to both the care team and family members. Such positive patient experience is a valuable factor in supporting quality health care service as well as in assisting patients from different ethnic backgrounds. When IENs and patients share the same ethnic background, it positively impacts patient experience. Njie-Mokonya (2016) concluded that

> Their [IENs'] fluency in other languages resulted in better patient and family experiences with the health care system; explaining procedures and the plan of care to patients and families in their mother tongue, rather than English, helped alleviate anxiety about their hospital stay. (p. 10)

A culturally diverse nursing team adds value to hospital care and is likely to improve the quality of care received by patients from diverse ethnic backgrounds.

INTERNATIONAL NURSE RECRUITMENT WITHIN THE HEALTH HUMAN RESOURCES FRAMEWORK

Nurses and nursing students in Canada need to be aware of the effects of globalization, especially the societal changes that have increased the health care needs of the population (e.g., aging, diversity) and thus created a demand for international nurse recruitment. How these socioeconomic factors intersect with the social responsibility that accompanies international nurse recruitment can be discussed within a health human resources framework. This discussion will be guided by O'Brien-Pallas, Murphy, & Birch's (2007) conceptual framework for health system and health human resources planning.

The health system and health human resources planning framework consists of three main constructs within a broader socioeconomic, political, geographical, and technological health system context. According to O'Brien-Pallas, Murphy, and Birch (2007), these three constructs are as follows:

1. *Population health needs* describes the changes of the population and its health care needs over time. For instance, both age distribution and the health needs of the population fluctuate over time depending on the age group, people's level of education, and the nature of the community (i.e., urban, rural, or remote);

2. *System design* includes planning and forecasting and describes nursing supply and health care service delivery. System design also evaluates service production capacity by the levels of services needed and available nurses and non-nurses required (e.g., allied health and service technicians) to deliver such services; and

3. *Resource deployment and utilization* describes nurse retention and the different health service delivery outcomes (i.e., health, provider, and system outcomes). (p. 9)

Discussing international nurse recruitment within the context of resource deployment and utilization construct allows practices and anticipated outcomes to be examined in order to support the integration of IENs following their recruitment into the Canadian health care system. Resource deployment and utilization also involves professional incentives, such as suitable work hours and flexibility, workload, and job satisfaction; personal factors, such as financial need and family support systems; and nurses' intentions of leaving the profession as well as the impact on who continues to nurse and on nurse leaders and recruiters (O'Brien-Pallas, Murphy, & Birch, 2007).

Projected nurse shortages influence the decision to recruit internationally, with recruitment facilitated by international trade agreements and migration laws to leverage forecasted economic agendas. Within the resource deployment and utilization portion of the health system and health human resources planning framework, better work conditions are used to recruit IENs under both national and provincial programs as a means to mitigate nurse shortages and improve nursing service and provider outcomes within the health care system.

The effective deployment and utilization of IENs is important for efficient system delivery outcomes within IENs' respective provincial destinations. Nonetheless, the challenges IENs face with integration; undergoing the necessary credential and competency evaluation in order to successfully pass their licensure exams; and the transition from novice to experienced nurse within the workplace can impact and delay the goals of ensuring adequate health human resources in response to meeting provider and system service outcomes. Njie-Mokonya (2014) reported that IENs indicated needing an average of 2 years to feel fully integrated and recognized as RNs in Canada. This suggests that, despite successfully obtaining their licenses as RNs, the support systems within the workplace are still necessary to facilitate their transition within the health care system. However, examining international nurse recruitment and its impact on the health system and provider outcomes remains to be explored. The health system and health human resources planning framework are yet to be "tested on other provider groups so that the impact of substituting different providers can be evaluated" (O'Brien-Pallas, Murphy, & Birch, 2007, p. 13).

The current trend of recruiting IENs to address projected nurse shortages in Canada and internationally is likely to continue. Consequently, efforts should continue to be directed at increasing professional education, retaining existing nurses within the workforce, and evaluating provincial credential and licensing practices to facilitate the international recruitment and migration of skilled workers. Advancing increased social responsibility within the nursing profession can begin with nursing educational schools, whereby cultural values and mutual respect are discussed openly. The challenges that IENs face in their destination countries and the cost implications of integrating into both a new country and new place of work can be discussed in a broader context because many Canadian-trained nurses travel to other destinations to practice nursing. A full collaboration by professional associations, **nursing regulatory bodies**, nurse advocates, and political and educational stakeholders is vital for effective and comprehensive results that will support nurse recruitment from other countries.

Nurse shortages are a common concern globally, and the need for nursing services internationally is on the rise. As the Canadian population ages, people are living longer while also facing comorbidity and complex health conditions. Technological innovations and models of care beyond the traditional hospital environment are increasingly being supported within community settings. Statistics show that IENs often migrate to Canada using spousal visas without revealing their nursing status until they arrive in Canada. As a result, the government does not have an accurate estimate of how many IENs enter the country each year.

Canada can learn several important lessons from the experiences of other countries that recruit many IENs, including Australia and the United Kingdom. First, IENs that go through transition programs in Canada should be identified and an evaluation of the supports they require during their transition should be understood. Second, it may be misleading to recruit IENs based solely on their RN title and assumed transferability of skills and competencies. There are many workplace difficulties face by IENs in terms of adapting to Canadian scope of practice, culture, and professional language. Adopting posthire upgrade programs (rather than bridging programs), as is the case in the United Kingdom (Xu & He, 2012), is likely to lead to better outcomes for IENs. The posthire upgrade programs combine both theoretical and practical knowledge for IENs and tailor their upgrade education to their areas of practice and employment. A known challenge facing bridging programs in Canada is the ability to streamline them, since a single type of program content and structure may not fit the needs of all IENs who make Canada their destination. The mismatches in program content and structure are due to variances in scopes of practice, educational preparation, and the extent of patient and team engagement in their countries of origin. An upgrade program is likely to leverage and raise IENs' knowledge and competencies to that of their Canadian nurse colleagues in a time-effective, workplace-oriented way, giving IENs an opportunity to determine their areas of improvement. The impact of IEN recruitment on health systems has yet to be comprehensively evaluated. Additional research and collaborative work will offer more conclusive decisions about the impact of internationalization within Canadian nursing.

APPLYING CONTENT KNOWLEDGE

1. How can IENs' knowledge and experience be leveraged and maximized in the workplace?
2. What are some factors that employers should consider and what kind of changes can they implement after hiring IENs to support their transition in the workplace?

SUMMARY OF LEARNING OBJECTIVES

- Given the increasing diversity of the Canadian population, IENs make a valuable addition to nursing service teams.
- There are lessons to be learned from other countries on how best to implement, structure, and regulate IEN transition programs.
- IENs come with varying scopes of practice, varying degrees of patient and family interaction, and varying educational preparation, leading to unpleasant workplace experiences among IENs.
- IENs experience higher levels of marginalization in the workplace compared with their nurse colleagues and other internationally educated health care providers.
- Ethical dilemmas associated with international nurse recruitment and push–pull factors that facilitate nurse migration calls for nurse leaders to demonstrate a higher level of social responsibility.

CRITICAL THINKING QUESTIONS

1. What are some of the advantages and disadvantages of recruiting nurses from overseas?
2. What are some social responsibility actions and political considerations to be taken by nurse leaders, political groups, and professional nursing associations to positively influence international nurse recruitment?
3. How can Canadian-trained nurses and nurse administrators facilitate and support IEN transition in the workplace?
4. What are two advantages and two disadvantages of bridging versus upgrade programs for IENs?

REFERENCES

Allan, H. T., & Westwood, S. (2016). English language skills requirements for internationally educated nurses working in the care industry: Barriers to UK registration or institutionalized discrimination? *International Journal of Nursing Studies, 54,* 1–4.

American Association of Colleges of Nurses. (2019). *Fact sheet: Nursing shortage.* Retrieved from https://www.aacnnursing.org/News-Information/Fact-Sheets/Nursing-Shortage.

Atack, L., Cruz, E. V., Maher, J., & Murphy, S. (2012). Internationally educated nurses' experiences with an integrated bridge program. *Journal of Continuing Education in Nursing, 43*(8), 370–378.

Baumann, A., Blythe, J., Rhéaume, A., & McIntosh, K. (2006). *Internationally educated nurses in Ontario: Maximizing the brain gain.* Hamilton, ON: McMaster University.

Baumann, A., Blythe, J., Kolotylo, C., & Underwood, J. (2004). *Building the future: An integrated strategy for nursing human resources in Canada: The international nursing labour market.* Ottawa, ON: Nursing Sector Study Corporation. Retrieved from https://cna-aiic.ca/~/media/cna/page-content/pdf-fr/international_nursing_labour_market_e.pdf.

Blythe, J., & Baumann, A. (2009). Internationally educated nurses: Profiling workforce diversity. *International Nursing Review, 56,* 191–197.

Bola, T. V., Driggers, K., Dunlap, C., & Ebersole, M. (2003). Foreign-educated nurses: Strangers in a strange land? *Nursing Management, 34*(7), 39–42.

Bourgeault, I. L., Neiterman, E., Lebrun, J., et al. (2010). *Brain gain, drain waste: The experiences of internationally educated health professionals in Canada.* Ottawa, ON: University of Ottawa.

Buchan, J. (2006). The impact of global nursing migration on health services delivery. *Policy, Politics, & Nursing Practice Supplement, 7*(3), 16S–25S.

Canadian Association of Schools of Nursing. (2012). *Towards a pan-Canadian planning framework for health human resources: A final report on the Pan-Canadian Framework for Guiding Principles and Essential Components for IEN Bridging Programs.* Ottawa, ON: Author. Retrieved from https://casn.ca/wp-content/uploads/2014/12/FinalReportPanCanadianFrameworkFinalVersion.pdf.

Canadian Institute for Health Information. (2017). *Regulated nurses, 2016: Report.* Ottawa, ON: Author. Retrieved from https://www.cihi.ca/sites/default/files/document/regulated-nurses-2018-report-en-web.pdf.

Canadian Institute for Health Information. (2019). *Nursing in Canada, 2018: A lens on supply and workforce.* Ottawa, ON: Author. Retrieved from https://www.cihi.ca/sites/default/files/document/regulated-nurses-2018-report-en-web.pdf.

Canadian Nurses Association. (2017). *International trade and labour mobility: Position statement.* Ottawa, ON: Author. Retrieved from http://www.cna-aiic.ca.

Canadian Nurses Association. (2019). *Health human resources report.* Ottawa, ON: Author. Retrieved from https://www.cna-aiic.ca/en/nursing-practice/the-practice-of-nursing/health-human-resources.

Citizenship and Immigration Canada. (2009). *Facts and figures—Immigration overview: Permanent and temporary residents, 2008.* Retrieved from https://qspace.library.queensu.ca/bitstream/handle/1974/8469/2008_CIC_Facts%20and%20Figures%20-%20Immigration%20Overview%20-%20Permanent%20and%20Temporary%20Residents.pdf?sequence=12&isAllowed=y.

Covell, C. L., Neiterman, E., & Bourgeault, I. L. (2016). Scoping review about the professional integration of internationally educated health professionals. *Human Resources for Health, 14*(38). https://doi.org/10.1186/s12960-016-0135-6.

Dico-Bloom, B. (2004). The racial and gendered experiences of immigrant nurses from Kerala, India. *Journal of Transcultural Nursing, 15*(1), 26–33.

Edge, J. E., & Hoffman, S. J. (2013). Empirical impact evaluation of the WHO Global Code of Practice in the international recruitment of health personnel in Australia, Canada, UK and USA. *Globalization and Health, 9*, 60. https://doi.org/10.1186/1744-8603-9-60.

Geissler, H. (2019, May 20). NHS hospital crisis: Britain needs twice as many student nurses. Express. Retrieved from https://www.express.co.uk/news/uk/1129647/nurse-shortage-nhs-rcn-40-000-shortage-act-now.

Government of Ontario. (2013). *Helping skilled immigrants in Ontario succeed.* Retrieved from https://news.ontario.ca/mci/en/2013/11/helping-skilled-immigrants-in-ontario-succeed.html.

Hall, J., Stevens, P., & Meleis, A. (1994). Marginalization: A guiding concept for valuing diversity in nursing knowledge development. *Advances in Nursing Science, 16*(4), 23–41.

Health Workforce Australia. (2014). *Australia's Future Health Workforce – Nurses detailed report.* Retrieved from https://www1.health.gov.au/internet/main/publishing.nsf/Content/34AA7E6FDB8C16AACA257D9500112F25/$File/AFHW%20-%20Nurses%20detailed%20report.pdf.

Human Resources and Skills Development Canada. (2009). *A pan-Canadian framework for the assessment and recognition of foreign qualifications.* Ottawa, ON: Author. Retrieved from https://www.canada.ca/en/employment-social-development/programs/foreign-credential-recognition/funding-framework.html.

Internal Trade Secretariat. (n.d.). *Labour mobility.* Ottawa, ON: Author. Retrieved from https://www.cfta-alec.ca/labour-mobility/.

International Council of Nurses. (2008). *Position statement: Ethical nurse recruitment.* Geneva, Switzerland: Author.

International Council of Nurses. (2013). *Position statement: Scope of nursing practice.* Geneva, Switzerland: Author.

International Council of Nurses. (2019). *International Council of Nurses 2019 international workforce forum.* Geneva, Switzerland: Author.

Jose, M. M. (2011). Lived experiences of internationally educated nurses in hospitals in the United States of America. *International Nursing Review, 58*, 123–129.

Kingma, M. (2007). Nurses on the move: A global overview. *Health Services Research, 42*(3 Pt. II), 1281–1298.

Kingma, M. (2008). Nurse on the move: Diversity and the work environment. *Contemporary Nurse, 28*(1–2), 198–206.

Kolawole, B. (2009). Ontario's internationally educated nurses and waste in human capital. *International Nursing Review, 56*, 184–190.

Konno, R. (2006). Support for overseas qualified nurses in adjusting to Australian nursing practice: A systematic review. *International Journal of Evidenced-Based Healthcare, 4*(2), 83–100.

Li, H., Nie, W., & Li, J. (2014). The benefits and caveats of international nurse migration. *International Journal of Nursing Sciences, 1*(2014), 314–317.

Lum, L., Bradley, P., & Valeo, A. (2015). Challenges in oral communication for internationally educated nurses. *Journal of Transcultural Nursing, 26*(1), 83–91.

Lum, L., Dowedoff, P., & Englander, K. (2016). Internationally educated nurses' reflections on nursing communication in Canada. *International Nursing Review, 63*, 344–351.

McGillis Hall, L., Jones, C., Lalonde, M., et al. (2015). Not very welcoming: A survey of internationally educated nurses employed in Canada. *GSTF Journal of Nursing and Health Care, 2*(2), 60–65.

Neiterman, E., & Bourgeault, I. L. (2015). The shield of professional status: Comparing internationally educated nurses' and international medical graduates' experiences of discrimination. *Health, 19*(6), 615–634. https://doi.org/10.1177/1363459314567788.

Neiterman, E., Bourgeault, I. L., & Covell, C. L. (2017). What do we know and not know about the professional integration of international medical graduates (IMGs) in Canada? *Healthcare Policy, 12*(4), 18–32. https://doi.org/10.12927/hcpol.2017.25101.

Neiterman, E., Bourgeault, I., Peters, J., et al. (2018). Best practices in bridging education: Multiple case study evaluation of postsecondary bridging programs for internationally educated health professionals. *Journal of Allied Health, 47*(1), e23–e28.

Nelson, S., Verma, S., Hall, L., et al. (2011). The shifting landscape of immigration policy in Canada: Implications for health human resources. *Heath Care Policy, 7*(2), 60–67.

Nichols, B., Davis, C. R., & Richardson, D. R. (2010). International models of nursing. In Institute of Medicine (Ed.), *The Future of nursing: Leading change, advancing health* (Appendix J, pp. 565–642). Washington, D.C.: National Academies Press.

Njie-Mokonya, N. (2016). Internationally educated nurses' and their contribution to the patient experience. *Online Journal of Issues in Nursing, 21*(1), 1–17. https://doi.org/10.3912/OJIN.Vol21No01Man05.

Njie-Mokonya, N. (2014). *Exploring the integration experiences of internationally educated nurses (IENs) within the Canadian health care system* [Master's thesis]. University of Ottawa.

O'Brien-Pallas, L., & Wang, S. (2006). Innovations in health care delivery: Responses to global nurse migration—A research example. *Policy, Politics, & Nursing Practice, 7*(3 Suppl.), 49S–57S. https://doi.org/10.1177/2F1527154406292854.

O'Brien-Pallas, L., Murphy, G., & Birch, S. (2007). *Health human resources modelling: Challenging the past, creating the future.* Ottawa, ON: Canadian Health Services Research Foundation.

O'Neill, F. (2011). From language classroom to clinical context. The role of language and culture in communication for nurses using English as a second language. *International Journal of Nursing Studies, 48*, 1120–1128. https://doi.org/10.1016/j.ijnurstu.2011.02.008.

Registered Nurses' Association of Ontario. (2016). *Mind the safety gap in health system transformation: Reclaiming the role of the RN*. Toronto, ON: Author. Retrieved from https://rnao.ca/mind-the-gap.

Salami, B., & Nelson, S. (2014). The downward occupational mobility of internationally educated nurses to domestic workers. *Nursing Inquiry*, *21*(2), 53–161. https://doi.org/10.1111/nin.12029.

Shaffer, F., Bakhshi, M., & Alvarez, T. (2019). The role of nurses in advancing the objectives of the global compacts for migration and on refugees. *Nursing Administration Quarterly*, *43*(1), 10–18. https://doi.org/10.1097/NAQ.0000000000000328.

Sherwood, G. D., & Shaffer, F. A. (2014). The role of internationally educated nurses in a quality, safe workforce. *Nursing Outlook*, *62*(1), 46–52. https://doi.org/10.1016/j.outlook.2013.11.001.

Squires, A. (2008). Ethical international recruitment: Many faces, one goal. *Journal of Nursing Management*, *39*(9), 16–21. https://doi.org/10.1097/01.NUMA.0000335253.23789.98.

Squires, A., Ojemeni, M., & Jones, S. (2016). Exploring longitudinal shifts in international nurse migration to the United States between 2003 and 2013 through a random effects panel data analysis. *Health Resources for Health*, *14*(1), 21.

Statistics Canada. (2019). *Population projections for Canada, provinces and territories: 2009 to 2036. Highlights*. Ottawa, ON: Author. Retrieved from https://www150.statcan.gc.ca/n1/pub/91-520-x/91-520-x2010001-eng.htm.

Tregunno, D., Peters, S., Campbell, H., & Gordon, S. (2009). International nurse migration: U-turn for safe workplace transition. *Nursing Inquiry*, *16*(3), 182–190.

Tulenko, K. (2012). *Insourced: How importing jobs impacts the healthcare crisis here and abroad*. Dartmouth, NH: Dartmouth College Press.

Turrittin, J., Hagey, R., Guruge, S., et al. (2002). The experiences of professional nurses who have migrated to Canada: Cosmopolitan citizenship or democratic racism? *International Journal of Nursing Studies*, *39*(6), 655–667.

Xu, Y., & He, F. (2012). Transition programs for internationally educated nurses: What can the United States learn from the United Kingdom, Australia, and Canada. *Nursing Economics*, *30*(4), 215–239.

Yi, M., & Jezewski, M. A. (2000). Korean nurses' adjustment to hospitals in the United States of America. *Journal of Advanced Nursing*, *32*(3), 721–729.

Zolot, J. (2019). International nurse migration: Nurses' dual role as migrants caring for other migrants. *American Journal of Nursing*, *119*(6), 16. https://doi.org/10.1097/01.NAJ.0000559791.78619.8b.

GLOSSARY

accessibility The availability of insured health services to any eligible Canadian within a reasonable time and distance. (Chs. 1, 11)

accreditation A national program that promotes excellence in the quality of nursing education and assists programs with identifying strengths and weaknesses. (Ch. 3)

accreditation An objective third-party assessment of an organization, service, institution, or program against standards of excellence to identify what is being done well and what needs improvement. (Ch. 24)

action Steps based on values, principles, and policies that will establish the context and resources for moving forward in diverse contexts. (Ch. 14)

active euthanasia An action designed to intentionally cause death (e.g., medically assisted dying). (Ch. 15)

advanced practice nursing Pertains to the two clinical roles in Canada for registered nurses: the clinical nurse specialist (CNS) and the nurse practitioner (NP). Both roles require extensive clinical experience and postgraduate education (usually at the master's level). The advanced education allows practitioners to provide both direct and indirect client care. Direct client care pertains to working with individuals, families, and communities to achieve health outcomes; indirect activities provide clinical expertise through care coordination and consultation with other health care providers. (Chs. 22, 23)

advocacy To bring voice and action on issues that determine the quality of care, ethics, health policy, and equity. (Ch. 18)

allyship The practice of people from dominant or privileged groups taking action to reject and dismantle the conditions of oppression. (Ch. 14)

alumnae Groups of individuals who have graduated from a program of study. (Ch. 20)

Anthropocene epoch The geological period that began 8,000 years ago whereby the collective activities of human beings have substantially altered Earth's surface, atmosphere, oceans, and systems of nutrient cycling. (Ch. 25)

antimicrobial resistance When microbes mutate and become resistant to the antimicrobials (e.g., antibiotics, antifungals) typically used to treat and eradicate them. This resistance is usually due to the overuse of antimicrobials, resulting in the ability of microbes to spread and infect others. The term given to these highly resistant microbes is "superbugs." (Ch. 25)

antimicrobial stewardship The idea that cautious use of antimicrobials is required to improve infection cure rates, decrease unnecessary exposure to antimicrobials, minimize the emergence of antibiotic resistance, reduce adverse drug reactions, and lower health care costs. (Ch. 25)

anti-oppressive practice Going beyond accepting and valuing diversity, anti-oppressive practice involves taking actions that seek to dismantle the forces and conditions that produce marginalization and colonization. These actions are strategic and occur within a framework of accountability. (Ch. 14)

apothecary Historically, a person who had some knowledge of medicinal plants and who could thus provide some basic care. Early pharmacists were often called apothecaries. (Ch. 2)

applied ethics Specific application of ethical ideas to particular situations in, for example, nursing or medicine. (Ch. 15)

appropriate technology Scientifically sound and socially acceptable methods, human and physical resources, funds, facilities, equipment, tools, and techniques. (Ch. 11)

approval Formal approval of a prelicensure educational program of nursing by the regulatory body in the program's jurisdiction. (Ch. 24)

artificial intelligence The intelligence or understanding generated by technology rather than humans. Artificial intelligence (AI) is an innovative approach that can be considered both a process and a tool. AI as a process refers to the use of sophisticated technology systems incorporating complex algorithms and programming that synthesize and analyze vast amounts of information, seeking patterns, matches, and answers to queries. AI is fundamentally grounded in machine learning. An example of an AI tool is Watson, the groundbreaking tool developed by IBM that is in use by health care organizations around the world to help answer a variety of clinical, productivity, and other questions. (Ch. 10)

associations Nonprofit professional organizations that advance the interests of a profession and its members through advocacy and professional development. Where permitted, professional associations may also include regulatory functions. (Ch. 3)

autonomy The ability and right of people to choose without interference from external influences. (Ch. 15)

awareness A consciousness and acknowledgement of privilege that includes taking responsibility for one's own ongoing learning. (Ch. 14)

bargaining agent A union certified by the labour board to negotiate collective agreements on behalf of a group of employees. (Ch. 19)

bargaining unit(s) A group that has bargaining rights within a union and is certified under each province's or territory's labour relations legislation. (Ch. 19)

beliefs What a person considers to be true. (Ch. 15)

beneficence Ethical principle of doing what is best for the patient and avoiding or preventing harm. (Ch. 15)

best practice guidelines A synthesis from research translated into evidence-informed guidelines for practice at the point of care. (Ch. 12)

bias   Showing prejudice or favour toward one person or group over another. (Ch. 14)

big data   The large, highly variable, and complex data sets that are arriving at an ever-higher speed or rate; commonly used software tools (traditional database tools) do not have the capability to efficiently manage and process these data. (Ch. 6)

borrowed theories   Theories that have been used to explain nursing's specific knowledge base but from a different philosophical context. Borrowed theories come from other applied sciences such as psychology, sociology, and anthropology. (Ch. 7)

Canadian Federation of Nurses Unions   A nonprofit lobbying federation of the majority of nurses' unions in Canada and the Canadian Nursing Students' Association, representing nearly 200,000 nurses and student nurses. (Ch. 19)

capacity   The legal capacity to make medical decisions; an individual's age and mental competence to understand the nature and ramifications of their own decision making. (Ch. 13)

certification   The recognition of certain educational standards, activities, or other requirements indicating that a practitioner has obtained more than the minimal entry-to-practice requirements. Often used to describe the qualifications of a nurse who has specialized, but not always. (Ch. 21)

change management   The processes, systems, structures, technologies, and values used by all members of an organization to enact any change that will happen, or is happening, in the organization. Change management involves operational, psychological, and cultural approaches. (Ch. 12)

cisgender   A person whose gender identity aligns with their sex assigned at birth. (Ch. 5)

cisnormativity   The commonplace assumption that all people are cisgender and that everyone accepts this as "the norm." The term is used to describe prejudice against trans people that is less overt and direct and more widespread and systemic in society, organizations, and institutions. This form of systemic prejudice may even be unintentional and unrecognized by the people or organizations responsible. (Ch. 5)

client   Various terms refer to the people with whom nurses work: patient, client, and consumer. Client implies collaboration, partnership, and a strengths focus and is consistent with anti-oppressive practice. (Ch. 14)

climate change   Long-term changes in local, regional, and global weather patterns that have major consequences for the health and well-being of all life on Earth. (Ch. 25)

clinical information systems   Technology solutions—either specific standalone solutions or a component system of a larger enterprise system—that support the planning, delivery, management, and evaluation of clinical care. (Ch. 10)

clinical intelligence   The understanding that arises from the analysis of information generated though clinical practice. (Ch. 10)

cloistered (noncloistered) order of nuns   Cloistered nuns are nuns who are part of a religious order that prohibits its members from leaving their convent, while noncloistered nuns are nuns who do not have to stay within the confines of the convent or cloister. The term cloister is often used to describe where cloistered nuns live. Historically, cloistered nuns were devoted to the care of the sick and lived within the walls of the hospital. The hospital and its attached land were usually surrounded by a high stone wall that protected the nuns' privacy. (Ch. 2)

code of ethics   A statement of moral contract or duty. A necessary and central mark of a profession that develops later, a code of ethics lays out the social contract between the profession and the public that it serves. (Ch. 3)

collective agreement   Also known as a contract, it is the document negotiated between the employer and union for a "collective" group of employees. (Ch. 19)

collective bargaining   Meetings that take place between an employer and a union to mutually negotiate, develop, or amend a collective agreement. (Ch. 19)

colonialism   A practice in which a colonial power sets up colonies or settlements elsewhere (in other countries or territories) for the political and economic benefit of the colonizing country. (Ch. 6)

colonization   The process of settling on the land and establishing control over the Indigenous people of an area. (Ch. 14)

competency, competencies   The state of possessing the skills and abilities to practise as a nurse; the skills and abilities, including professionalism, required to meet the requirements of practice. (Chs. 6, 9)

comprehensiveness   No eligible Canadian can be charged (in whole or in part) for any medically necessary insured benefit, including in-hospital care accessed through physicians, health providers, and government-sponsored dental services. (Chs. 1, 11)

conceptions of (the nature of) nursing   Knowledge in the discipline of nursing that is created from thinking about nursing in a different manner than in an evidence-informed base or scientific base. Contribute to how nursing is expressed by nurses and seek to explain what nurses know. (Ch. 7)

conceptual framework   The organization or matrix of concepts that provides a focus for investigation or analysis. (Ch. 6)

confidentiality   The requirement or promise to maintain the privacy of any information provided and to prevent the unauthorized release of the information. (Ch. 13)

consent   In the context of health care, it means agreeing to allow treatment. Valid consent must relate to the treatment, be informed, and be given voluntarily, and the patient must have the capacity to consent to the proposed treatment. (Ch. 13)

consequentialism   Ethical theory that what is right or wrong is determined by the outcomes or consequences of a person's actions. (Ch. 15)

continuous quality improvement   A management philosophy that focuses on a systematic way to increase quality, reduce waste, involve staff in improvement work, and meet customer expectations. (Ch. 12)

COVID-19   The name given to the novel coronavirus disease that was declared a pandemic by the WHO on March 11, 2020. It is not certain how the virus that causes it developed, but most of the early cases have been traced back to a wet market in Wuhan, China. (Ch. 25)

credential evaluation The process of appraising foreign qualifications. (Ch. 26)

credentialling The process of obtaining, verifying, and assessing the qualifications of a practitioner to provide care or services in or for a health care organization. Credentials are documented evidence of licensure, education, training, experience, or other qualifications. Some credentialling is voluntary and done after initial education, licensure, and registration of the individual. It can be professional or specialty specific. (Ch. 21)

criteria The required elements that define a particular principle or standard by which something may be judged or decided. (Ch. 24)

critical perspective A perspective based on a mode of inquiry that seeks to understand and challenge the status quo. It also seeks to understand and explain the role of power in relationships and how power influences the status quo. (Ch. 18)

Crusades A series of religious wars that occurred in the Middle Ages between the years 1096 and 1272. (Ch. 2)

cultural awareness A consciousness, acknowledgement, and commitment to learning about groups of people where there are common values and ways of thinking and acting. (Ch. 14)

cultural blindness A focus on "similarities" as a way to deny diversity and the inability to recognize the uniqueness of individual people or groups. (Ch. 14)

cultural competence The ongoing process of building awareness of one's own cultural identity and views on different cultures with the goal of bringing this awareness into action for sensitive and safe practice. (Ch. 14)

cultural humility An awareness of one's own limitations regarding what can actually be known about the "culture" of another person. Culture is a lived, dynamic experience, so one can only know what another chooses to share. It requires a need to be curious in relationships with others and a willingness to seek out information. Also known as being relational. (Ch. 6)

cultural knowledge Understanding some of the characteristics, history, values, beliefs, and behaviours of another group of people. (Ch. 14)

cultural pluralism When smaller groups of people within a larger society maintain their unique cultural identities, and their values and practices are accepted by the wider society. (Ch. 14)

cultural safety Gaining an understanding of others' health beliefs and practices so that health care actions work toward equity and avoid discrimination. An encompassing approach to bring sensitivity into action of the history and context of client/community beliefs, values, attitudes, and behaviours. (Ch. 14)

cultural sensitivity Being attuned to others' concerns and needs arising from historical contexts, held within the beliefs, values, attitudes, and behaviours of a group of people. (Ch. 14)

cultural skill The practice of communicating awareness, knowledge, understanding, and sensitivity; part of the ongoing process of cultural competency. (Ch. 14)

cultural understanding Development of knowledge about the values, beliefs, and actions of a group of people. (Ch. 14)

culture Expression of common values and ways of thinking and acting that differ from those of another group. (Ch. 14)

data science A broad field of study that combines expertise in a particular domain of knowledge with programming skills, mathematics, and statistics to enable the review, analysis, and extraction of valuable knowledge and insights from data. It is geared toward helping individuals and organizations make better decisions. (Ch. 6)

decentralized To move away from the centre. Health care that is decentralized moves the responsibility for decision making and administration of programs and services away from a central authority and closer to end users/patients/communities. (Ch. 1)

decolonization Practices concerned with dismantling the systematic oppression of Indigenous peoples, Indigenous culture, and the sites of oppression imposed by colonization. For example, the Truth

and Reconciliation Commission of Canada's Calls to Action are part of a decolonization strategy. (Chs. 6, 14)

deductive A type of scientific reasoning that begins with a general statement or hypothesis and examines the possibilities to reach a specific, logical conclusion. It moves from a broad idea to a specific conclusion. (Ch. 6)

deontology Ethical theories that hold the belief that certain acts are intrinsically right or wrong and are the product of reason. (Ch. 15)

devolved The result of delegating or shifting power for decision making from a higher to a lower level of government (e.g., from federal to provincial/territorial). (Ch. 1)

digital health An umbrella term that refers to the overall domain of health care facilitated by digital technologies. It encompasses such terms as eHealth, mHealth, and uHealth. Digital health is evolving rapidly in response to the fast pace of technological innovation. Examples include robotics, smart technology, virtualization of health services, and nanotechnology. (Ch. 10)

dignity Recognition of the worth of others and of their deserving of respect. (Ch. 15)

discipline A unique body of knowledge that is taught or researched at the university level. (Ch. 3)

diversity Variety and uniqueness in dimensions of experience and understating, here considered in term of race, immigrant or refugee status, access to health care, sexual diversity, ethnicity, gender, and disability. (Ch. 14)

Doctor of Nursing (DN) A more recent degree type that focuses on developing skills in translating research into practice, applying research knowledge in decision making, and developing and implementing clinical innovations to make an impact on the health care system, improving care delivery, and advancing nurse education and scholarship. (Chs. 22, 23)

Doctor of Philosophy (PhD) A PhD is the traditional doctorate, the highest university degree awarded to students following the completion of a comprehensive examination and dissertation with an oral defense. PhD graduates are expected to make significant contributions to their field of study through ongoing research and scholarship. (Ch. 22)

Doctorate of Nursing Practice (DNP) In the United States, the DNP is transitioning to be the entry-level point for advanced practice nurses, including nurse anesthetists. This degree is designed to enhance the leadership abilities of nurses who work in either a clinical setting or administration. (Ch. 22)

doctrine of double effect An ethical concept used as a justification for situations in which there are both good and bad effects; in health care, the focus is on the intention of the health care provider. (Ch. 15)

dominant discourses In health care, it includes the ideas we have about what health is and what determines health as well as the policies and practices produced by these ideas within the specific social, economic, and political context in which they are produced. For example, in the early 1990s, a population health and health promotion discourse emerged. (Ch. 6)

duty of care The reasonable degree of skill and knowledge and degree of care that is reasonably expected of a normal, prudent practitioner of the same experience in the same setting. Professional standards of practice offer clues of the expected duty of care. (Ch. 13)

duty of fair representation A legal term whereby a union is given the exclusive right to represent a group of employees. In return, the union must not act in an arbitrary or discriminatory manner and must represent the employees in good faith. (Ch. 19)

Ebola A highly infectious viral disease caused by the Ebola filovirus. It has an extremely high mortality rate. (Ch. 25)

educational standards A level of quality or attainment against which an educational institution or educational program is compared. (Ch. 24)

eHealth Health care services facilitated by the use of electronic technologies. eHealth was initially used to describe the adoption of technology to support and optimize health care delivery. However, the term eHealth has been subsequently

subsumed by the term digital health. (Ch. 10)

electronic health record A digital record that provides an integrated and comprehensive collection of a person's encounters with the health care system, including a patient's health history. (Ch. 13)

electronic medical record The digital or computer equivalent to the patient chart, these are computer-based patient records specific to a single clinical practice or setting such as a hospital, clinic, or doctor's office. These are sources of communication between various health care providers within a practice environment. (Ch. 13)

embodiment From relational ethics; body and mind are viewed as one and inseparable. (Ch. 15)

empiricism A philosophical school of thought that has contributed to epistemology. The philosophy that claims that knowledge stems entirely from sensory experiences. (Ch. 6)

employability The process individuals undertake to prepare themselves to fulfill the specifications of a job. (Ch. 23)

engagement From relational ethics; refers to the capacity to connect with others in a meaningful relationship. (Ch. 15)

entry to practice The minimum requirements set by a profession's regulators that a professional must meet in order to be allowed to apply for registration or licensure in a profession. In nursing, entry to practice in most provinces and territories is a baccalaureate degree from a recognized degree-granting institution, usually a university. (Ch. 21)

epistemology, epistemological The branch of philosophy concerned with the theory of knowledge and how we come to know about the world and the nature of evidence. Relating to the study of the nature, origin, and limits of human knowledge. (Chs. 5, 6, 7)

equality When everyone receives the same resources, treatment, services, and so on. Equality is about fairness but assumes that everyone has the same needs and therefore requires the same level and types of access. (Ch. 1)

equity When everyone receives the resources, treatments, services, and so

on that they require. Equity means that some people will receive more supports or services in order to narrow gaps or "differences" in health or health status. (Ch. 1)

equity-oriented health care Practices that promote equity. Equity is the ability of people to have access to equal opportunity—it is about justice and fairness; however, it is not the same as equality. Health equity means that there are no remediable or unfair differences between people that intrude on their ability to access health care. (Ch. 6)

ethical awareness In this context, recognition of the ethical implications of all nursing actions and the first step in moral action. (Ch. 15)

ethical dilemma Choice between two mutually exclusive courses of action, neither of which is preferable nor unilaterally acceptable. (Ch. 15)

ethics A branch of philosophy that involves the formalized study of right and wrong for the purpose of bringing about the "good" in society; concerned with what ought to be, not with what is. (Ch. 15)

ethnicity The state of belonging to a social group that shares common cultural patterns (e.g., beliefs, values, customs, behaviours, traditions). (Ch. 14)

ethnocentrism A type of cultural prejudice in which a dominant group subordinates the cultural values, beliefs, and behaviours of others, with the dominant group believing that theirs are the best, preferred, and most superior ways. (Ch. 14)

euthanasia Putting to death, by painless methods, a person who is terminally ill or severely disabled, either by omission of an act or commission. (Ch. 15)

everyday ethics Day-to-day ethical choices of nurses that involve the development of moral perspectives and decisions that are made in relationship with patients, families, colleagues, communities, and the environment at large. (Ch. 15)

exam blueprint For a certification exam, a plan describing what topics will be covered and how they will be tested. (Ch. 21)

feminist perspective A critical perspective with gender as the focus of inquiry and influence. (Ch. 18)

fidelity Keeping promises; foundational to trust. (Ch. 15)

fiduciary relationship A relationship of trust in which there is an obligation or duty to act in the best interests of the patient. (Ch. 15)

filtered research evidence A summary of the findings of primary research studies. (Ch. 9)

gamification The use of design principles that are commonly employed in the commercial technology–based gaming industry to engage consumers in tools and resources that support health in a less formal and more interactive manner. Gamification is often used in the development of health resources for youth to increase interest, engagement, accessibility, and social relevance. (Ch. 10)

gender bias Behaviour that shows favouritism toward one gender over others and includes both prejudicial attitudes and discrimination. (Ch. 5)

globalization Integration of local and national interests into the global market economy. When something becomes globalized, it has the ability to have an international or global effect or influence on other countries. (Ch. 26)

grand theories General concepts that pertain to the overall nature and goals of professional nursing. A grand theory is a synthesis of scholarly research, professional experience, and insights from theoretical pioneers. (Ch. 6)

gross domestic product Total value of goods and services produced in a country in a year. It reflects a country's economic strength and prosperity. (Chs. 1, 10)

H1N1 A pandemic originating from animal influenza viruses, unrelated to seasonal human H1N1 viruses. It resulted in 14,300 deaths worldwide in 2009. (Ch. 25)

Hall Commission Report Common name given to the *Report of the Commission on Health Services*, a commission led by Emmett Matthew Hall, a Supreme Court of Canada judge. The Hall Commission was established in 1961 and produced two reports that were published in 1964. (Ch. 20)

health equity The ability of all people to reach their full health potential through fair access to resources, opportunities, and support without being disadvantaged by any economic or socially determined circumstances. (Chs. 11, 25)

health promotion The process of enabling people to increase control over and improve their health and of developing environments and conditions that foster health. (Ch. 11)

heteronormativity A cultural or social framework, often implicit, wherein all human beings are considered heterosexual and this is "the norm." Heteronormativity not only enforces strict norms about sexuality but also reinforces strict gender roles within society. (Chs. 5, 6)

heuristic A simple mental shortcut that assists with problem solving and decision making. (Ch. 6)

homophobia A broad term referring to the irrational fear or hatred of, and discrimination against, people based on their sexual orientation. (Ch. 5)

human-factors research A field that focuses on applying what is known about human behaviour, abilities, limitations, and other characteristics to the design of systems, tasks and activities, environments, and equipment and technologies. With its emphasis on user- or person-centered design, it can help to ensure that health care is a good fit with the people, the tasks, and the environments involved and that the care provided is safe, effective, and efficient. As an example, ergonomics uses human-factors research to allow a person to successfully live and function in their home after a significant health challenge. (Ch. 6)

illness prevention Activities to avert ill health or injury (e.g., early detection to limit the consequences of disease), limit the effects of disease or injury, and prevent recurrence. (Ch. 11)

immigrant In Canada, a person who has chosen to live in the country, who has been accepted for entry by the Government of Canada, and who may apply for permanent residency. (Ch. 14)

immigration The act of moving permanently to a foreign country. (Ch. 25)

incidental instruction Teaching and learning that takes place at the time of a naturally occurring incident. (Ch. 20)

indigenization The recognition of the validity of Indigenous worldviews, knowledge, and perspectives; the opportunities for indigeneity to be expressed; and the incorporation of Indigenous ways of knowing and doing into institutions, agencies, and organizations. For example, in education, indigenization is more than simply inserting a course into a curriculum; it also involves ongoing dismantling of colonizing processes and practices (ongoing decolonization). (Ch. 6)

inductive hermeneutic An interpretive approach to the exploration of problems that arise when dealing with human actions and the products of such actions (for instance, human texts). (Ch. 6)

inflow The number of nurses who are entering the profession. (Ch. 17)

informed consent To meet the requirement of informed consent, a patient must be provided with information concerning the nature of the treatment and its gravity, the expected benefits of the treatment, the material risks and material side effects of the treatment, alternative courses of action, and the potential consequences of not having the treatment. (Ch. 13)

infrastructure support Elements within a research setting that are required to conduct the research. This includes systems and funding that support researchers to identify funding and partnership opportunities, prepare grant applications to successfully compete for funding, and manage the finances of grants. It also includes systems that ensure the ethical conduct of research within institutions. Also included is infrastructure such as computers, space to conduct research, space and equipment for graduate students and trainees associated with a particular research study, and specialized equipment or space (e.g., interview rooms with one-way mirrors, equipment to monitor physiological status). (Ch. 8)

institutional review One of the processes to assess and monitor nursing education in Canada. (Ch. 24)

interdisciplinary collaboration Individuals from different academic disciplines or fields—such as psychology, political science, and sociology—working together from their respective branches of knowledge on the same topic. (Chs. 11, 16)

interdisciplinary research Research conducted by a team of researchers from different disciplines that draws on and adapts the unique knowledge and approaches to research from each of the disciplines. (Ch. 8)

international recruitment The act of enlisting workers from other countries. (Ch. 26)

internationally educated nurses Registered nurses who have completed their original nursing education at a nursing program in a country other than Canada. (Ch. 26)

interpretive knowledge The subjective viewpoints or experiences that explain the facts (e.g., numbers) being examined. For example, if a researcher is seeking to understand the growing rates of anxiety and depression among postsecondary students, then the researcher could interview students in those settings to gain knowledge about their experiences and thus better inform the researcher's interpretation of these numbers. (Ch. 6)

interprofessional collaboration When health care (or social care) providers consistently work together interdependently to provide health care (or social care) services. To work together in this manner, care providers must understand their own and each others' roles and responsibilities while sharing accountability for outcomes. (Chs. 16, 18)

interprofessional education Commonly referred to as IPE. When health care and/ or social care providers, educators, or students come together to learn about, from, and with one another to improve collaboration and the quality of services provided. (Ch. 16)

interprofessional learning The learning that arises from interprofessional education, where students, providers, and educators interact to learn about each other while learning from and with each other. (Ch. 16)

intersectionality The ways in which a person's social and political identities combine to create unique modes of discrimination and privilege. An approach to viewing people's collective experience of oppression. (Ch. 14)

intersectoral collaboration The joint work of organizations in the public,

nonprofit, and private sectors to achieve changes that cannot effectively be realized through the actions of any single sector. (Ch. 11)

intraprofessional collaboration Collaboration that occurs within a single profession. Also known as uniprofessional. (Ch. 16)

justice Respecting the rights of others; making fair decisions. (Ch. 15)

knowledge mobilization The active process of moving knowledge from research into use in practice and policy. Methods include the engagement of knowledge users in the process of conducting research and creating new knowledge, synthesis of research findings, and other activities to encourage the use of research findings. (Ch. 8)

knowledge transfer The sharing of knowledge and research findings between people or organizations. Unlike the related concepts of knowledge translation and knowledge mobilization, knowledge transfer does not include the application and uptake of knowledge. (Ch. 8)

knowledge translation The active process of putting knowledge into use. This extends beyond the dissemination of research findings to methods that make the research findings applicable and ultimately used in practice to improve health and health services. Another term for this is knowledge mobilization. (Ch. 8)

labour relations legislation Federal, provincial, and territorial Acts that set out the laws regulating union–employer relationships. (Ch. 19)

lean quality management A continuous quality improvement approach built from the tools and approaches of the successful Toyota management system of continuous improvement. Lean is not an acronym. (Ch. 12)

LGBTQ2 A shortened acronym that incorporates both sexual orientation and gender identity. Represents lesbian, gay, bisexual, transgender, queer, and two-spirit people. The longer acronym, LGBTQQIP2SAA, is meant to refer to the entire spectrum of lesbian, gay, bisexual, trans, queer, questioning, intersex, pansexual, two-spirit, and asexual

communities and their allies. (Chs. 5, 11, 14)

liberalism A political doctrine whereby the protection and enhancement of the freedom of the individual is deemed the central problem of politics. (Ch. 6)

licensure The process by which an individual is granted permission to use a protected title (such as "registered nurse"). It is a mandatory requirement for being able to practice one's profession as specified by the legislation of the province or territory. In Canada, each province and territory determines the requirements for nurse licensure, which includes the ability for the public to access the registered nurse's information (full name, credentials, and other relevant details) in a public register maintained by the regulatory body. (Chs. 21, 26)

licensure examination The required examination that applicants must pass to become a nurse in Canada. Registered nurses must pass the NCLEX-RN exam. In the province of Quebec, registered nurse applicants write the Ordre des infirmières et infirmiers du Québec (the Quebec Professional Exam). Licensed (or registered) practical nurses in Canada must pass the Canadian Practical Nurse Registered Examination. Nurse practitioners (registered nurses with extended class) must pass one of three specialty exams —primary care, pediatric, or adult—after they have completed their specialty education. (Ch. 21)

linguistic interpretation Understanding based on language. (Ch. 14)

macro-level factors In the Health Canada Interprofessional Education for Collaborative Patient-Centred Practice Framework, macro-level factors refer to links at the system level that influence interprofessional education and collaborative practice, such as politics, socioeconomics, and culture. (Ch. 16)

mandatory licensure The legal requirement for a member of a profession, such as a nurse, to (1) obtain a license to practice before being allowed to use the protected title of the profession, (2) possess the requisite skills of the profession, and (3) be accountable for safe, ethical, and competent treatment of patients and clients for whom the licensee cares. All nurses who practice in

Canada must have mandatory licensure. (Ch. 21)

mandatory registration   Statutory requirement for practice within a jurisdiction. Registration with a regulatory body signifies that a nurse has satisfied all necessary entry-to-practice requirements. (Ch. 3)

marginalization   Directly or indirectly created inequalities in health and health care experienced by individuals or groups owing to complex social and political factors. (Ch. 5)

market economy   A system whereby the laws of supply and demand—not government—direct the production of goods and services. Supply includes natural resources, capital, and labour. Demand includes purchases by consumers, businesses, and the government. (Ch. 6)

meso-level factors   In the Health Canada Interprofessional Education for Collaborative Patient-Centred Practice Framework, meso-level factors refer to links at the organizational level that influence interprofessional education and collaborative practice, such as between teaching and the health organizations themselves. (Ch. 16)

meta-analysis   The use of statistical methods to synthesize or combine results across several studies. (Ch. 9)

metaparadigm   The central aspects of a discipline that function as a framework from which the more formal conceptual structures develop. In nursing, the concepts of the metaparadigm are nursing, health, environment, and person. (Ch. 6)

mHealth   The delivery of health care services through mobile technology such as smartphones and tablets. (Ch. 10)

micro-level factors   In the Health Canada Interprofessional Education for Collaborative Patient-Centred Practice Framework, micro-level factors refer to connections between students, educators, and health care providers that influence interprofessional education and collaborative practice. Micro-level factors in education relate to teaching, whereas micro-level factors in the practice setting refer to interactions. (Ch. 16)

microaggressions   Subtle, often automatic, and unconscious verbal and nonverbal slights, insults, and disparaging messages directed toward people in relation to their gender, age, disability, and cultural or racial group membership. (Ch. 14)

migration   The movement of people within or across jurisdictions. It includes national or international movement, which can be initiated by individual choice or due to other factors such as war and violence. (Chs. 25, 26)

moral distress   A "discomforting" experience that a nurse encounters when prevented from doing what they believe is right. (Ch. 15)

morality   Choices and behaviour that are in accordance with people's values and what they believe to be right or wrong, or good. Sometimes used interchangeably with ethics. (Ch. 15)

multiculturalism   The diverse ancestry of citizens and, in the Canadian context, policy that supports the ideals of equality and mutual respect among the population's ethnic and cultural groups. (Ch. 14)

multidisciplinary research   Research conducted by a team of researchers from different disciplines. Differences with respect to knowledge and how knowledge is generated in that discipline are maintained by researchers on the team, and the research benefits from the various perspectives. (Ch. 8)

multilateral agencies   Organizations formed by three or more countries (e.g., UNICEF). (Ch. 11)

mutuality   From relational ethics; a relationship in which neither the patient nor the nurse is harmed. (Ch. 15)

negligence   Failure to exercise the degree of care that a person of ordinary prudence, based on reasonable standard, would exercise under the same or similar circumstances. (Ch. 13)

neocolonial   Relating to or characterized by the use of economic, political, cultural, or other pressures to control or influence other countries. It is a process of indirect control rather than direct control (colonial). (Ch. 6)

neocolonialism   The continued exercise of indirect economic and political influence over a country or people in the absence of formal political control (i.e., colonial methods). (Ch. 6)

neoliberalism   A political ideology espousing freedom from or movement away from a welfare state to free markets and deregulation of financial markets, privatization, and individualism. (Chs. 6, 19)

New France   The areas of North America that were colonized by France. "New France" was first used to refer to the St. Lawrence Valley and parts of today's Atlantic provinces. It later included large parts of the current American Midwest and Louisiana. (Ch. 2)

Next Generation NCLEX   The updated version of the current NCLEX-RN blueprint to reflect decisions made by nurses and interactions between nurses and patients to meet patient outcomes. The new exam will become available in 2023. (Ch. 21)

newcomer   A person who arrives in a new country to settle there for a variety of reasons and with a variety of background experiences. (Ch. 14)

nonbinary   A person whose gender identity does not align with a binary understanding of gender such as man or woman. Nonbinary people may redefine gender or decline to define themselves as gendered altogether. (Chs. 5, 8)

noncoercion   From relational ethics; refers to creating an environment in which people are encouraged and free to make choices without force. (Ch. 15)

noncommunicable diseases   Another term for chronic diseases. The major noncommunicable diseases are cardiovascular diseases (stroke and heart attack), cancer, chronic respiratory diseases, and diabetes. (Ch. 25)

nonmaleficence   Ethical principle of doing no harm. (Ch. 15)

normal school   Historically, the name used to identify an educational institution for training teachers. (Ch. 20)

normative ethics   Concerned with the provision of a moral framework composed of values, principles, virtues, and ideals that establish what ought to be done. (Ch. 15)

novel coronavirus   The name given to a new coronavirus that had not been seen in humans before. The novel coronavirus that causes COVID-19 belongs to the same family of viruses that cause the common cold and seasonal influenza in humans. However, not all coronaviruses cause illness. (Ch. 25)

nuns Female members of religious orders. Nuns who were devoted to the care of the sick were often referred to as nursing sisters. (Ch. 2)

nurse migration Nurse movement within or across jurisdictions. (Ch. 26)

nurse practitioner Specialized registered nurses who practise at an advanced level within an extended class license and who meet additional education, experience, and exam requirements set by their provincial or territorial licensing body. Within this role, nurse practitioners order and interpret diagnostic tests and make diagnoses in order to prescribe medications and recommend treatments. (Ch. 22)

nursing body of knowledge Knowledge specific to nursing, created about nursing-specific activities, processes, and interventions. (Ch. 7)

nursing data science An emerging domain of study that focuses on managing what was formerly known as "big data." Data science, and more specifically nursing data science, draws on new approaches, methodologies, and tools to manage vast amounts of information generated in health care to inform nursing and health care practice. (Ch. 10)

nursing data standards The recommended or prescribed format and representation of nursing data to enable consistent capture, storage, management, comparison, and evaluation of nursing data to inform care. (Ch. 10)

nursing informatics The use of information and communication technologies (ICT) and digital tools to support the planning, delivery, evaluation, and management of nursing care. (Ch. 10)

nursing order A religious organization, sometimes called a religious nursing order, within which members live according to the rules set by the order and devote their lives to the care of the sick. For example, the Augustines and the Grey Nuns are nursing orders devoted to the care of the sick. Other types of religious orders have different areas of focus. For example, the Ursulines are a religious teaching order devoted to educating children. (Ch. 2)

nursing organizations Nursing organizations include unions, professional associations, and regulatory colleges that help direct the course of the nursing profession and its capacity to influence policy and politics. (Ch. 18)

nursing regulatory body Organizations within Canadian provinces and territories that determine registration and licensure criteria for registered nurses and confirm the eligibility of applicants or members to practise in their jurisdiction. (Ch. 26)

nursing-sensitive outcomes Outcomes that are within the control of a nurse. An example would be decubitus ulcer rates. (Ch. 12)

nursing shortage Situations whereby nurse demand supersedes its supply. (Ch. 26)

Nursing Sisters "Nursing Sisters" (with both initial letters capitalized) is the name used to refer to Canadian nurses who took care of soldiers during World War I, World War II, and the Korean War. After the Korean War, the term was replaced by "nurses." (Ch. 2)

nursing theories Explanations of phenomena, in either a scientific or naturalistic context, through the lens of professional nursing. Nursing theories were developed to help nurse educators and scholars try to articulate the essence of what nursing did and what it was. (Ch. 7)

occupation Habitual employment or what a person does for a living. (Ch. 3)

Organisation for Economic Co-operation and Development A 36-country international collaboration founded in 1961 to stimulate economic progress and world trade. (Ch. 17)

omics The integration of a number of disciplines, including genomics, proteomics, and metabolomics, to name a few. Key is the blending together of features of biological knowledge that reflect the complexity and diversity of living systems in context over time. (Ch. 6)

ontology The study of the nature of being. In nursing, ontology is the study of the experience of being a nurse. Several nursing scholars point to the importance of "knowing as being," where the epistemology (knowing) of nursing

is inextricably linked to the ontology (being) of nursing. Knowing is a way of being. (Chs. 6, 10)

opinion leader A person viewed by practitioners as trustworthy and likeable. Through their opinions they influence how others practise. (Ch. 9)

opioid misuse Misuse and addiction to prescription and/or illicit opioids. It has resulted in a public health crisis in Canada. (Ch. 25)

oppression The practice of one group or individual using power to maintain privilege and dominance over another. (Ch. 14)

outcomes standards or criteria Standards to help measure the outcomes of care delivered. (For example, did the wound heal?) Aggregate data on wound healing would allow clinicians to evaluate how they are doing and to continuously improve practice. (Ch. 12)

outflow The number of nurses who have left the profession. (Ch. 17)

palliative sedation The practice of lowering consciousness in those near death to relieve refractory symptoms. (Ch. 15)

pandemic The global spread of a new disease. (Ch. 25)

paradigm A distinct set of concepts or thought patterns, including theories, research methods, postulates, and standards, describing what constitutes legitimate contributions to a discipline. A *paradigm shift*, a concept identified by American physicist and philosopher Thomas Kuhn, is an important change that happens when the usual way of thinking about or doing something is replaced by a new and different way. (Ch. 6)

passive euthanasia Enabling death through omission or an intervention or withdrawal of an intervention; letting people die. (Ch. 15)

paternalism Deciding what is best for patients without their fully informed consent or full participation. (Ch. 15)

patient experience An individual patient's experiences with, and within, the health care system. (Ch. 26)

patient safety A field of practice that advocates for the reduction of errors among practitioners within the health care system. (Chs. 12, 26)

patient–family engagement A proactive organizational approach to involving patients and families in the design and planning of health care. (Ch. 12)

permissive licensure Allows those practitioners who do not have licensure to practice in the profession. Nurses must meet specified standards but are not required to gain licensure through examination or testing. Practitioners cannot use the protected title (e.g., "nurse") but can perform the skills of the profession. No longer exists in Canada. (Ch. 21)

personalized medicine The application of innovative technological advances in gene sequencing and molecular data that enables the customized adaptation of care (disease prevention and treatment) to each individual. Examples of personalized medicine include the treatment of cancer and other life-threatening diseases. (Ch. 10)

philosophical thinking A method of thinking reflectively in a systematic way about the human condition or parts thereof. It encompasses questions about the meaning of nursing, what nursing does (epistemology) or ought to do (ethics), and why nursing exists (metaphysics). (Ch. 7)

planetary health Interactions between humans and the planet that impact health and well-being worldwide. (Ch. 25)

policy A statement about what ought to be done. (Ch. 9)

policy influence To influence the direction taken by governments, organizations, and senior decision makers. (Ch. 18)

politics A process of influence whereby the decisions and actions of people in a position of power impact another group of people with less power. (Ch. 18)

population health The health of a population as measured by health status indicators and as influenced by interrelated conditions and factors across the lifespan. (Ch. 11)

portability The principle that health service benefits remain in effect for eligible Canadians who are in transit or relocating between provinces and/or territories. (Chs. 1, 11)

portals Designated locations on a website where centralized access to specific services, such as access to secure or private information and resources, may be made available. In health care, portals are often used to allow patients to access resources such as patient education, preoperative and postoperative checklists, and diagnostic test preparation. Patients may also be directed to a secure login location where they can access personal health records, test results, or other private health information. (Ch. 10)

positive professional image The state wherein the professional discipline is proudly marketed by its members, acknowledged by the public, and recognized by other health care disciplines as powerful, influential, of critical importance to the health care system, and worthy of respect. (Ch. 4)

power The capacity to influence others based on position, values, and resources. (Ch. 18)

practice readiness The state of possessing and adequately exhibiting cognitive, professional, and clinical capabilities to meet the entry-level competencies for which an individual is educated. (Ch. 23)

practice-based evidence The insight generated through examination of trends in the practice of nursing and delivery of care to clients rather than relying on traditional research-based evidence. Practice-based evidence is recognized as having both validity and relevance in terms of supporting decisions about health care and nursing practice. (Ch. 10)

praxis process The coming together of theory and practice; it is a blend of critical reflection and action within a theory and research-driven practice. (Ch. 6)

precision health care Expert medical and nursing services in the area of wellness, screening, and education; it is about treatment as well as the prediction and prevention of disease. (Ch. 6)

prejudice A negative attitude about a person or group without factual data. (Ch. 14)

privacy The right of an individual to control how, when, and with whom their personal information is shared. (Ch. 13)

privilege A right or advantage granted to only one individual or group that provides unearned advantage over other people based on being born in a certain group. White privilege is institutionalized preferential treatment of white people, potentially to the detriment of people of colour. From the perspective of Western medical knowledge and training, medicine privileges Western ideas about knowledge over Indigenous ideas. (Ch. 14)

private-duty nurses Historically, private-duty nurses were nurses who provided services to clients in their homes. When taking care of patients, they often took care of the entire needs of the household, especially if the patient was the mother. (Ch. 20)

privatization The shift to private-sector ownership of health care facilities and services (e.g., hospitals, MRI clinics) within the traditionally publicly operated Canadian health care system. (Ch. 1)

process standards or criteria The manner in which work gets accomplished or the internal processes that are in place to achieve work. (Ch. 12)

profession A paid occupation that involves specialized training and formal qualification. Characteristics include a definition of the profession, self-regulation, service to others, applied knowledge that must be learned through formal education, and a code of ethics. (Ch. 3)

professional brand image Where members speak of their discipline and market themselves using language that consistently reflects power, purpose, collaborative influence, evidence-informed competencies, knowledge building, advocacy, and activism for health policy change. (Ch. 4)

professional image How the public and other health care disciplines see, recognize, imagine, or understand nursing, individual nurses, and the discipline as a whole. Professional image is a perception upon which the public builds opinions, beliefs, and attitudes about what nurses are and what they do. Image evokes impressions, builds reputations, and constitutes a marketable brand that reflects worth, value, and symbolic meanings granted to nurses by others. (Ch. 4)

professional image enactment The observable professional behaviour that brings professional image to life; professional image is dependent upon consistent and committed performance of nursing practice competencies during all interactions. (Ch. 4)

professional image marketing Whereby members actively engage in broadly disseminating a professional nursing image in order to strategically transform public and disciplinary understanding of the nursing role, leveraging this image for greater policy influence. (Ch. 4)

professional responsibility language The language included in collective agreements between unions and employers that provides for nurses to have a formal procedure to address staffing, policies, and practice in their work environments. It is a forum for nurses to bring forward their concerns when they are assigned work that is inconsistent with proper patient care. (Ch. 19)

professional self-identity The attributes, qualities, characteristics, roles, ways of being, and functions that combine to build the self-concept that individual nurses and the discipline as a whole believe to represent the essence of what it means to be a nurse. (Ch. 4)

program approval Outcome of a review of the curricula and program of study in a nursing school whereby a regulatory college or association is assured that graduates will be able to meet the entry-to-practice competencies necessary for safe practice. Required for graduates to write licensing examinations. (Ch. 3)

public administration Health services administered by a nonprofit public administrative system (Chs. 1, 11)

public image of nursing A viewpoint held by members of the public that is overly simplified, influenced by stereotypical images, emphasizes the interrelational domains of nursing, and reflects limited awareness of the empirical, evidence-informed domains of nursing practice. (Ch. 4)

public participation Individual and community involvement in the planning and operation of their health care and the health of their communities. (Ch. 11)

quality assurance A process of assessment to ensure that an organization or program is providing the best possible service and/or product(s).

Involves a focus that checks for errors and compliance with standards through audit-type procedures. (Chs. 12, 24)

quality improvement Actions used to improve the outcomes at the recipient level (e.g., in health care, the patient is the recipient) by improving processes to increase the value of services, improving responsiveness of the system, and enhancing overall outcomes of care for the patient. (Ch. 12)

race A social classification based on an imagined hierarchy of human value that relies on phenotypes, skin colour, and other expressions of group membership. (Ch. 14)

racializing The categorization of people by race, which leads to bias, discrimination, and limited opportunities for diversity. (Ch. 14)

racially visible Observable diversity by way of colour. (Ch. 14)

racism A form of prejudice in which members of one cultural group perceive themselves to be superior to another cultural group. (Ch. 14)

Rand formula A law stipulating that union dues are mandatory. This prevents individuals from opting out of paying dues while having the benefits of collective bargaining, such as wages, health care benefits, and working conditions. (Ch. 19)

reductionist Refers to an analysis or description of a complex phenomenon in terms of its simplest or fundamental constituents. (Ch. 6)

refugee A person forced to leave their home country because of a fear of persecution or war. (Chs. 1, 14, 25)

registered nurses Self-regulated health care providers who work autonomously and in collaboration with others, enabling individuals, families, groups, communities, and populations to attain their optimal level of health. (Ch. 1)

registration The result of meeting the required elements of a profession to ensure safe, competent, and ethical practice. For example, in Canada, each province and territory sets registration requirements for nurses, but they tend to require most of the following: proficiency in English or French, evidence of a clear criminal record, evidence of passing the licensure examination, proof of Canadian

citizenship, completion of an acceptable program at an educational institution, and recent example of safe practice (usually gained in the educational process). (Ch. 21)

regulated nurses In Canada, refers to all registered nurses (including nurse practitioners), licensed or registered practical nurses, and registered psychiatric nurses. (Ch. 17)

regulatory colleges Nonprofit organizations with statutory obligations to protect and serve the public through maintenance of a registry of members, establishment of continuing education and practice recency requirements, management of member misconduct, and approval and monitoring of curricula and nursing programs. (Ch. 3)

relational practice Practices and activities based on the foundational context of relationships and contextual realities. (Ch. 14)

Research Chair An award of financial support to a researcher's research program that, in addition to the researcher's grant funding, supports research and training of graduate students and postdoctoral fellows. The financial support provides the researcher with time away from teaching, allowing them to devote their time to doing research and training graduate students. The Research Chair may be financed by a government funding program (e.g., the Canada Research Chairs program), sponsorship from a private-sector company, or an individual donor. Some universities also have internal funding to create Research Chairs. (Ch. 8)

research dissemination Sharing or spreading research findings to other researchers and potential knowledge users. (Ch. 8)

research synopses A brief summary of the methods and findings of one study. May include a critique or appraisal of the research methods. (Ch. 9)

robotics The domain of study and the development of using automated or remotely controlled devices (rather than humans) to perform specific tasks. Examples in health care include robotic surgery, where a surgeon may be geographically distant from the location where the actual surgery is performed and using robots to perform routine tasks such as retrieving supplies or assisting in patient transfers. (Ch. 10)

royal commission   A systematic inquiry sponsored by the federal government or a provincial government. Royal commissions are normally established to examine a topic in depth and thus provide evidence for governmental policymaking or action. (Ch. 20)

SARS   SARS, or sudden acute respiratory syndrome, is a viral disease caused by a coronavirus. SARS first appeared in China in November 2002 and within a few months had spread worldwide. There has been no known transmission of SARS anywhere in the world since 2004. (Ch. 25)

scientific theories   Theories that describe, explain, or predict phenomena using specific observation, measurement, and evaluation methodologies. Theories seek to explain the natural world using generally agreed upon protocols and methods that provide data that can either be verified or replicated using one of the three aforementioned methodologies. (Ch. 7)

scope of practice   Specific actions, procedures, or processes that can be performed by a health care provider specific to their education level, practice type, and competency. Usually identified in a regulation specific to a health profession. (Chs. 13, 21)

self-efficacy   One's belief in their ability to respond appropriately to a situation. (Ch. 23)

self-regulated learning   An active, self-directive process in which learners set goals and plan, monitor, and reflect on their progress toward achieving their goals. (Ch. 23)

settler colonialism   Colonialism that functions through the replacement of Indigenous populations with an invasive settler society that over time develops a distinctive identity and sovereignty. (Ch. 6)

sexual orientation   How people think of themselves and identify in terms of their sexual attraction to other people. (Ch. 14)

smart devices   Devices connected to networks that enable the user to remotely perform a wide variety of tasks. Examples include smartphones or tablets where users can communicate with others,

manage their banking needs, obtain remote health care services, and more. Other examples include smart watches that monitor health and generate alerts in the event of a health event; smart glasses that provide additional information and feedback to the wearer and to networked locations, as desired; and smart home devices that enable the performance of many tasks (turning lights on or off, activating home alarm, controlling thermostat, controlling oven or stove, etc.). (Ch. 10)

social construction   A term used to reflect how individuals, through their interactions with one another, construct an understanding and knowledge of the world to form the basis of reality (i.e., "truth"). (Ch. 5)

social determinants of health   The social and economic factors that impact the conditions in which people are born, grow, work, live, and age. (Ch. 11)

social justice   The practice of fair and equitable relations between people and society (in particular, the distribution of wealth, opportunities, and privileges). (Chs. 11, 14, 15)

social safety net   Publicly funded services (such as welfare, health care, and unemployment insurance) that enhance socioeconomics, security, and equality in society, often targeting people who are low income, vulnerable, and older. (Ch. 1)

specialization   An area of concentration that focuses on a particular area of clinical nursing practice, and whose foci are related to the age (gerontological nursing), issue (infection control), a disease (cancer), or practice specialty (maternity nursing). Nurses who specialize take advanced education and/ or certification to become experts in their specialized field. (Ch. 21)

spiritual   Relates to the human spirit or soul as opposed to physicality. Spirituality is a desire to find deeper meaning, direction, and truth, believed by some to be inherent in all people. Some people hold the belief that spirituality is one dimension of the self that is integrated with other aspects of the self and that these dimensions are inextricably linked to one another; the physical, emotional, spiritual, and mental aspects of self. (Ch. 6)

skill mix   The combination of all formal caregivers participating in nursing care for an individual patient or client. (Ch. 17)

standardized data   The accurate, consistent, and comparable data that are generated when data standards are applied and which enable effective analysis of nursing and health care. (Ch. 10)

stereotyping   The application of generalizations to a person based on their belonging to a group without exploring their individual values, beliefs, and behaviours. (Ch. 14)

structural violence   The systematic ways in which social structures harm or otherwise disadvantage individuals. It is often subtle and invisible; usually there is no one specific person who can (or will) be held responsible, and therefore it can be difficult to address. (Ch. 6)

structural and systemic factors   The policies, processes, and practices embedded within health and social systems that challenge the ability of people to achieve health and social equity. (Ch. 6)

structural standards or criteria   The relationships that exist between the available human and material resources within a healthcare setting. Examples include the philosophy of the institution, the structure of an organization and staffing patterns. (Ch. 12)

superbugs   Microorganisms that have become resistant to antimicrobials and no longer respond to standard antimicrobial treatments. Resistance develops as a result of the overuse or misuse of antimicrobials. (Ch. 25)

sustainability   The ability of a system to meet the needs of current and future generations. (Ch. 1)

Sustainable Development Goals   Seventeen development goals adopted by all UN member states in 2015 with the goal of ending poverty, protecting the planet, and improving the lives and prospects of everyone by 2030. (Ch. 25)

systematic review   A summary of all available high-quality research about a particular practice issue, including a critique of the research methods used in the publications being reviewed. (Ch. 9)

tacit knowledge   The knowledge we possess that is generated from personal experience and context. It is the most difficult to write down, articulate, and present in a tangible form. (Ch. 6)

telehealth The use of technology to provide services to remote and isolated clients. In Canada, telehealth is delivered extensively through videoconferencing platforms that link health care providers to clients in the North. Services include teleophthalmology, telepsychiatry, teledermatology, telecardiology, and more. (Ch. 10)

tenure track A period of time or pathway to promotion and tenure for newly hired professors at Canadian universities. A professor who achieves tenure gains permanent employment at the university. Tenure protects a professor who might engage in controversial research from being fired without cause. (Ch. 22)

theorizing The way in which we engage with each other as knowers and the way in which we approach our work with individuals, families, and communities. (Ch. 6)

therapeutic lying The deliberate deception of patients for reasons considered to be in their best interests. (Ch. 15)

tort A wrongful act by which an individual has been harmed. Persons so injured can legally claim monetary damages as a remedy. (Ch. 13)

total quality management An earlier version of continuous quality improvement (CQI) that focused on an organizational approach to creating a culture of CQI. (Ch. 12)

trans (transgender) An umbrella term that describes people with diverse gender identities and gender expressions that do not conform to stereotypical ideas about what it means to be a girl/woman or boy/man in society. It includes but is not limited to people who identify as transgender, transsexual, cross-dressers, or gender nonconforming (gender variant or genderqueer). (Chs. 5, 14)

transdisciplinary research Research conducted by teams of researchers from two or more disciplines. Typically, team members come from the health sciences, social sciences, humanities, and natural sciences. Boundaries between disciplines

with respect to knowledge and how knowledge is generated are transcended, and new ways of generating knowledge and solving problems are created. (Ch. 8)

transition A process that consists of movement from one state or condition to another. (Ch. 26)

translational gap or relevance gap The gap that exists between the theories used in nursing practice and the perceived relevance or importance of the knowledge created by these theories. (Ch. 7)

uHealth The ubiquitous nature of technology in regard to supporting health care. As technology has been largely adopted by the world, its widespread availability among populations has enabled more innovative use of technology (even basic or more primitive forms) to support the delivery of health services. (Ch. 10)

unions Organizations that negotiate working conditions, such as pay and hours of work, and advocate for appropriate staffing and other factors that impact the work life of their members. (Ch. 3)

universal health care The provision of a core set of health services to all citizens of a country regardless of ability to pay. (Ch. 1)

universality The principle that all eligible Canadian residents are entitled to receive the same health benefits without discrimination. (Chs. 1, 11)

upstream A focus on improving fundamental social and economic structures through policies and other measures to decrease the barriers to achieving full health potential. (Ch. 11)

vacancy rates A calculation of the number of job positions that are unfilled for a particular profession. (Ch. 17)

values Beliefs and ideals that individuals, groups, and societies consider important or core. (Ch. 15)

vaping Inhaling and exhaling an aerosol made from a mixture of specific products, including flavourings and/ or nicotine, and delivered through an e-cigarette. (Ch. 25)

veracity The principle of telling the truth. (Ch. 15)

virtualization The provision of health care services using technology that links providers and clients/consumers. Examples include telehealth or online encounters with a physician or nurse. Future innovations will include holographic virtual care to help optimize accessibility and efficiency. (Ch. 10)

virtue ethics Ethical theory that focuses on the moral character of the person rather than moral actions. (Ch. 15)

visible minority Another term for people of colour; that is, people who are neither Indigenous nor white. (Ch. 14)

vocation Sometimes defined as a calling, it is a profession characterized by strong ideals such as service to others, search for perfection, deference to authority, caring for others, and self-sacrifice. A view of nursing that has been especially enduring and that was supported by apprenticeship models of nursing education. (Ch. 3)

Weir Report Name often given to the *Report on Nursing Education* written by G.W. Weir in 1932. (Ch. 20)

welfare state A system whereby the government (the state or a well-established network of social institutions) plays a key role in the protection and promotion of the economic and social well-being of its citizens. It is based on the principles of equality of opportunity, equitable distribution of wealth, and public responsibility for those unable to provide for themselves. For example, in the welfare state, education and health services are provided at no or low cost to all citizens. (Ch. 6)

white supremacy A historically based, institutionally perpetuated system of exploitation and oppression of continents, nations, and people of colour by white people and nations of the European continent for the purpose of maintaining and defending a system of wealth, power, and privilege. (Ch. 14)

worldview A view of the world used for living in the world. It is a comprehensive model or framework of ideas, values, and attitudes about the world, oneself, and life in the world. (Ch. 6)

PHOTO CREDITS

The following photo credits are for the images at the start of each chapter.

Chapter 1
© CanStock Photo Inc./corund

Chapter 2
Archives de la Ville de Montréal. BM99-1_02P04

Chapter 3
istock.com/monkeybusinessimages

Chapter 4
istock.com/SDI Productions

Chapter 5
Marcia Porter, Memorial University Faculty of Nursing

Chapter 6
istock.com/Halfpoint

Chapter 7
istock.com/peepo

Chapter 8
istock.com/Oliver Le Moal

Chapter 9
iStock.com/FatCamera

Chapter 10
iStock.com/metamorworks

Chapter 11
iStock.com/SDI Productions

Chapter 12
iStock.com/fstop123

Chapter 13
iStock.com/Don Bayley

Chapter 14
iStock.com/HamidEbrahimi

Chapter 15
iStockphoto.com/monkeybusinessimages

Chapter 16
iStock.com/Goodboy Picture Company

Chapter 17
iStock.com/JohnnyGreig

Chapter 18
The University of Victoria

Chapter 19
© Canadian Federation of Nurses Unions

Chapter 20
UTARMS, University of Toronto Faculty of Nursing, A1988-0005/10003

Chapter 21
Courtesy of Tammie R. McParland

Chapter 22
Courtesy of Dr. Laurie Freeman

Chapter 23
iStock.com/sturti

Chapter 24
University of New Brunswick/Joy Cummings

Chapter 25
iStock.com/andyparker72

INDEX

Page numbers followed by *f* indicate figures; *t*, tables; *b*, boxes.